Clinical Paediatric Nephrology

Clinical Paediatric Nephrology

Second edition

Edited by

R. J. Postlethwaite FRCP
Consultant Paediatric Nephrologist
Royal Manchester Children's Hospital, Pendlebury, Manchester

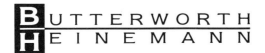

Butterworth-Heinemann Ltd
Linacre House, Jordan Hill, Oxford OX2 8DP

 A member of the Reed Elsevier plc group

OXFORD LONDON BOSTON
MUNICH NEW DELHI SINGAPORE SYDNEY
TOKYO TORONTO WELLINGTON

First published 1986
Second edition 1994

British Library Cataloguing in Publication Data
Clinical Paediatric Nephrology. – 2Rev.ed
  I. Postlethwaite, R. J.
  618.9261

ISBN 0 7506 1347 5

Library of Congress Cataloguing in Publication Data
Clinical paediatric nephrology / edited by R. J. Postlethwaite. – 2nd ed.
  p. cm.
  Includes bibliographical references and index.
  ISBN 0 7506 1347 5
  1. Paediatric nephrology. I. Postlethwaite, R. J.
  [DNLM: 1. Kidney Diseases—in infancy & childhood. WS 320 C6412 1944]
  RJ476.K5C563 1994
  618.92′61—dc20
  DNLM/DLC   93–44212
  for Library of Congress   CIP

Typeset by Datix International Limited, Bungay, Suffolk
Printed and bound in Great Britain by Bath Press Ltd, Avon

Contents

Contributors

Arbus, G.S. MD FRCPC
Assistant Professor of Pediatrics
University of Toronto;
Staff Physician
Hospital for Sick Children
Toronto
Ontario
Canada

Beattie, T.J. MB CHB FRCP(Glasg)
Consultant Paediatrician and Nephrologist
Royal Hospital for Sick Children
Yorkill
Glasgow;
Hon. Clinical Senior Lecturer
University of Glasgow
Glasgow, UK

Brodehl, J. MD
Professor of Paediatrics
Kinderklinik
Medizinische Hochschule Hannover
Hannover
Germany

Chambers, T.L. FRCP
Consultant Physician
Paediatric Department
Southmead General Hospital
Westbury-on-Trym
Bristol, UK

Chevalier, R.L. MD
Professor, Director of Research and Vice-Chair
Department of Pediatrics
University of Virginia
Charlottesville
Virginia, USA

Dickson, A.P. MB ChB FRCS(Ed)
Consultant Paediatric Urologist/Surgeon
University of Manchester School of Medicine
Booth Hall Children's Hospital
Blackley
Manchester, UK

Dillon, M.J. MB FRCP DCH
Consultant Physician and Nephrologist
Institute of Child Health
University of London
London, UK

Farine, M. MD FRCPC
Staff Nephrologist
Division of Nephrology;
Assistant Professor of Pediatrics
The Hospital for Sick Children
University of Toronto
Toronto
Ontario
Canada

Fish, A.J. MD
Professor of Pediatric Nephrology
University of Minnesota
Minneapolis, Minnesota, USA

Gordon, I. MB BCh FRCR
Consultant Radiologist
Department of Paediatric Radiology
The Hospital for Sick Children
Great Ormond Street;
Senior Lecturer in Diagnostic Radiology
Institute of Child Health
London, UK

Gough, D.C.S. FRCS FRCS(E) FRACS DCH
Consultant Paediatric Urologist
Salford Health Authority
Royal Manchester Children's Hospital
Pendlebury
Manchester, UK

Grupe, W.E. MD
Professor and Vice-President for Medical
    Education
Project Hope
Health Education Science Center
Virginia, USA

Guignard, J.-P. MD
Professor of Paediatrics;
Director of Paediatric Nephrology
Centre Hopitalier Universitaire Vaudois
Lausanne
Switzerland

Haycock, G.B. MB BChir, FRCP DCH
Rothschild Professor of Paediatrics and
    Honorary Consultant Paediatric
    Nephrologist
United Medical and Dental Schools of Guy's
    and St Thomas' Hospitals
Guy's Hospital
London, UK

Jodal, U. MD
Consultant Paediatric Nephrologist
Department of Paediatrics
Göteborg University
East Hospital
Göteborg
Sweden

Kalia, A. MD
Associate Professor
Division of Pediatric Nephrology
Department of Pediatrics
University of Texas Medical Branch
Galveston
Texas, USA

Lendon, M. PhD FRCPath
Senior Lecturer in Paediatric Pathology;
Honorary Consultant
Department of Pathology
Royal Manchester Children's Hospital and
    Department of Pathological Sciences
University of Manchester
Manchester, UK

Lewis, M.A. MRCP
Consultant Paediatric Nephrologist
Royal Manchester Children's Hospital
Pendlebury
Manchester, UK

Meadow, S.R. MA FRCP DCH
Professor of Paediatrics and Child Health
St James's University Hospital
Leeds, UK

Moss, G. MRCP
Consultant Paediatrician
Sheffield Childrens' Hospital
Western Bank
Sheffield, UK

Mughal, Z. MB ChB MRCS MRCP DCH
Consultant Paediatrician;
Honorary Senior Lecturer in Child Health
Department of Paediatrics
St Mary's Hospital
Manchester, UK

Mundy, A.R. MS FRCS MRCP
Professor of Urology
Guy's Hospital
London, UK

Postlethwaite, R.J. FRCP
Consultant Paediatric Nephrologist
Royal Manchester Children's Hospital
Pendlebury
Manchester, UK

Price, D.A.
Senior Lecturer in Child Health;
Honorary Consultant in Paediatric
 Endocrinology
Royal Manchester Children's Hospital
Pendlebury
Manchester, UK

Rigden, S.P.A. FRCP
Consultant Paediatric Nephrologist
Guy's Hospital
London, UK

Robson, A.M. MD FRCP
Medical Director
Children's Hospital
New Orleans
Louisiana, USA

Savage, J.M.
Consultant Paediatric Nephrologist
The Queen's University of Belfast
Institute of Clinical Sciences
Belfast, UK

Schärer, K.
Professor of Paediatrics;
Head
Division of Paediatric Nephrology
Department of Paediatrics
University of Heidelberg
University Children's Hospital
Heidelberg
Germany

Smellie, J.M. MA DM FRCP DCH
Senior Lecturer in Paediatrics
University College Hospital
London;
Honorary Consultant Paediatrician
University College Hospital
The Hospital for Sick Children
Great Ormond Street and Guy's Hospital
London, UK

Super, M.
Consultant Clinical Geneticist
Royal Manchester Children's Hospital
Pendlebury
Manchester, UK

Taylor, C.M. MB FRCP DCH
Consultant Paediatrician and Nephrologist
Department of Nephrology
The Children's Hospital
Ladywood Middleway
Ladywood
Birmingham, UK

Travis, L. B. MD FAAP CDE
William W. Glauser Distinguished Professor of
 Pediatrics and Director of Pediatric
 Nephrology
Department of Pediatrics
The University of Texas Medical Branch at
 Galveston
Galveston
Texas, USA

Trompeter, R.S. MB FRCP
Consultant Paediatric Nephrologist
Department of Paediatric Nephrology
The Hospital for Sick Children
Great Ormond Street
London, UK

van Gool, J.D.
Pediatric Renal Centre
University Children's Hospital
Utrecht
The Netherlands

Vehaskari, V.M. MD
Professor of Pediatrics
Director of Pediatric Nephrology
Louisiana State University
Medical Center
New Orleans
Louisiana, USA

White, R.H.R. MA MD FRCP DCH
Senior Research Fellow
Department of Nephrology
The Children's Hospital
Birmingham;
Emeritus Professor of Paediatric Nephrology
University of Birmingham, UK

Wraith, J.E. MB ChB FRCP
Consultant Paediatrician
Willink Biochemical Genetics Unit
Royal Manchester Children's Hospital
Pendlebury
Manchester, UK

Preface

This textbook remains more modest in ambition than classical encyclopaedic textbooks. It aims to provide a non-specialized paediatrician with up-to-date information about common paediatric nephrological problems. The need for such a text has been confirmed by the success of the first edition. The focus remains clinical with the emphasis on clinical presentation, differential diagnosis, evaluation and treatment. Pathogenesis and pathology are less extensively discussed but there is enough detail to allow understanding of the clinical management.

The medical aspects of paediatric urology such as wetting, urinary tract infection, obstructive and non-obstructive urological abnormalities and calculi are much commoner than almost any paediatric nephrology problem such as glomerulonephritis. With the advent of antenatal detection of urological problems this is even more true. This was the justification for including some paediatric urology topics in the first edition and this coverage has been increased in the second edition.

Hopefully armed with this text the non-specialist paediatrician will be able to approach any common paediatric nephrological or urological problem with confidence and know when to ask for specialist help.

1

Haematuria

S.R. Meadow

Blood in the urine is a common manifestation of urinary tract disorder. Macroscopic haematuria refers to urine in which blood is visible as either a red or brownish colour. Microscopic haematuria refers to urine in which ordinary visual inspection is normal but blood is detected either by microscopy or chemical tests. The advent of more sensitive chemical tests has led to more children with microscopic haematuria being discovered.

Definition

Normally very few red cells are excreted in the urine. They are believed to pass into the urine via the glomerulus, their pliable form allowing them to be squeezed through capillary basement membranes. The normal red cell excretion rate increases with age and is greater after exercise.

The definition of abnormal haematuria is somewhat arbitrary and will depend upon the methods used for its detection. Surveys of microscopic haematuria in children suggest that it is unwise to pay much attention to a 'trace' reading on the dipstix. Similarly a child who merely has a reading of 'small' (1 +) on one occasion and has normal samples thereafter is unlikely to have a significant problem or to benefit from investigation. Readings greater than a trace, or more than 5 red cells per mm^3 which persist for more than four days should be regarded as abnormal.[1]

Tests for haematuria

Appearance

The urine has a pink to red colour when fresh but develops a hazy smoke or brown-coloured tinge on standing. The brown colour comes from the methaem derivative of the oxidized haem pigment. A very small quantity of blood can discolour urine, e.g. 0.5 ml of blood in 500 ml of urine is visible. Blood also causes urine to be hazy or obviously cloudy. Usually the blood is present in the same concentration in all specimens of urine collected at about the same time, but for localized lesions, for instance in the urethra, there is value in the 'three glass test' in which examination of an initial specimen of urine, a mid-stream specimen of urine and a terminal specimen of urine may disclose that blood is only present in, for instance, the initial specimen. Other causes of red urine are common and the more important of these are shown in Table 1.1.

Chemical tests

Most tests depend on the peroxidase-like activity of haemoglobin, as shown below:

$$\text{H}_2\text{O}_2 + \text{Chromogen} \xrightarrow{\text{Haemoglobin peroxidase activity}} \text{Oxidized chromogen (highly coloured)} + \text{H}_2\text{O}$$

Orthotolidine is commonly used as the chro-

Table 1.1   Other causes of red urine

Foods, particularly beetroot and berries (anthocyanins) and confectionery containing vegetable dyes

Drugs, e.g. Pyridium (phenazopyridine), phenindione, phenothiazines, rifampicin, desferrioxamine, phenolphthalein* and anthraquinone laxatives (e.g. Dorbanex: danthron).

Haemoglobinuria

Myoglobinuria

Urates, which in high concentration may produce a pinkish tinge

*Reddish colour only in alkaline urine.

mogen. The most convenient tests to use are the 'dipstix' tests which incorporate chemically impregnated paper sections on a plastic strip.[2] These dipstix, e.g. those marketed by Ames Co. and by Boehringer, are easy to use but it is important to follow the instructions closely. The stick should be dipped briefly in the urine, excess fluid tapped off and strict attention paid to the time interval printed on the container before comparing the resultant colour with the colour chart – for blood it is usually 40 s. Delayed reading produces false positive reactions. Theoretically, since the test depends on free haemoglobin, it should react more vigorously if the red cells have haemolysed but in practice this is not important because when there is significant haematuria some of the red cells will always have lysed and there will be sufficient free haemoglobin to cause a positive test.

The chemical test will be positive for haemoglobinuria, for instance following intravascular haemolysis, in the absence of haematuria. It also reacts positively to myoglobin in the urine, for instance after rhabdomyolysis. The test is less sensitive in urines with high specific gravity and in urine containing large amounts of reducing agent such as ascorbic acid. Conversely some oxidizing agents, e.g. hypochlorite and microbial peroxidases associated with urinary tract infection, may cause false positive results. The dipstix chemical tests for blood are *very* sensitive. Some may feel that they are too sensitive. As mentioned earlier, it is unwise to pay much attention to the 'trace' reading on the dipstix. A child who merely has a reading of 'small' or '1 + ' on one occasion and has subsequent normal specimens is unlikely to benefit from investigation. It should be remembered that normal people excrete some red cells in

their urine and that, after exertion or other stress, the excretion rate may rise; depending on the concentration and chemical constitution of the urine, the test may become positive. However, persistent readings greater than trace are abnormal.

Microscopy

Abundant red cells are easy to identify by microscopy; the characteristic biconcave disc appearance of many of the cells, their lack of granularity and the fact that they are slightly smaller than white blood cells makes identification simple (Figure 1.1). However, when red cells are scanty, identification is extremely difficult because the red cells become misshapen in the urine and it is impossible to differentiate them from other unidentified small objects. To overcome this problem the urine may be centrifuged:[3] 10 ml urine is centrifuged for 5 min at $750 \times g$, 9.5 ml of supernatant is removed and the deposit resuspended in the remaining 0.5 ml urine. Red cells should be easily identified if they are present, but quantitation 'per high power field' has many problems. Even with careful attention to technique and using counting chambers to enumerate the cells, problems remain. One technician in one laboratory using a standard technique can produce reproducible results, but different technicians using different microscopes in different laboratories produce tremendous variation. It is estimated that the variability factor is greater than 80 times, which means that there can be no universally accepted standards for red cells per mm^3 in centrifuged urine. Standardization is possible for the examination of well-mixed but uncentrifuged urine examined in a counting chamber; there should not be more than 5 red cells per mm^3. What this amounts to in practice is that, if one is certain of seeing a few red cells in the 0.9 mm^3 of a Fuchs–Rosenthal counting chamber, then there is an excess of red cells. In practice there will also be a positive reaction on the dipstix test. If the dipstix test is negative, it is highly unlikely that the objects being seen on microscopy are red cells!

Red cells haemolyse fast in standing urine, particularly when the urine is of low specific gravity or with an alkaline pH. Therefore, these conditions are more likely to be associated with false negatives on microscopy, though the chemical test should still be positive.

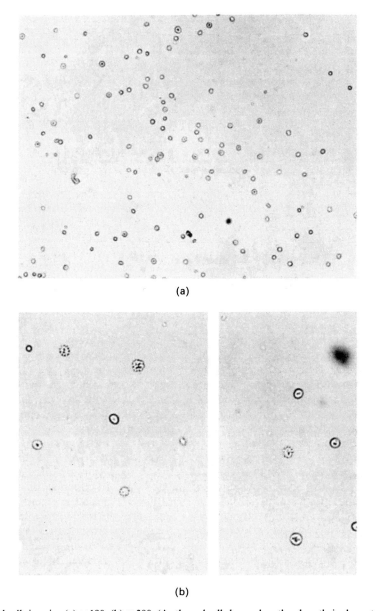

(a)

(b)

Figure 1.1 Red blood cells in urine (a) × 190, (b) × 300. (As the red cells haemolyse they lose their characteristic biconcave disc appearance and develop a crinkled edge and variable shape)

Red cells from the lower urinary tract maintain their form and their colour better than those that are distorted in their passage through the glomeruli. With experience one can distinguish between red cells originating from the kidneys and those from the lower urinary tract.[4] A phase contrast microscope allows this differentiation more easily,[5] but using a simple microscope much the same effect can be obtained by racking the condenser very low and examining the cells in different lighting conditions to display their shape better. Red cells from the glomerulus show great variation in shape, size and haemoglobin content. Those from the lower urinary tract resemble a sample to which a fresh drop of blood has been added from a pricked finger: the cells tend to be of uniform shape and size and have a definite red/pink colour.

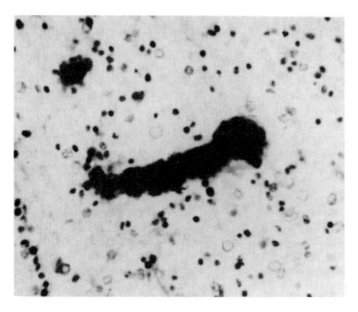

Figure 1.2 A red cell/granular cast (× 300). Many misshapen disintegrating red cells can also be seen

These differences allow urine with moderate (or greater) amounts of haematuria to be analysed in automated haematological analysers to define the morphological appearance of the red cell and differentiate between glomerular and non-glomerular origin. Such auto-analysis has the advantage of not requiring an experienced skilled technician.[6–8]

It is important to search carefully for casts when trying to localize the origin of haematuria. Casts originate in the renal tubules and have a matrix composed of Tamm–Horsfall mucoprotein. Hyaline casts are associated with proteinuria, and a few such casts may be found in concentrated early morning samples from healthy people. Cellular casts may contain epithelial or blood cells. White blood cells (WBC) casts indicate a renal origin of leucocytes and are indicative of pyelonephritis or other inflammatory diseases. Red blood cell (RBC) casts are always pathological and usually indicate glomerular bleeding. Epithelial casts are formed by desquamated cells from the epithelial lining of the tubule. Epithelial cell casts are often present with RBC or WBC casts. Red cell casts as they disintegrate take up a granular appearance (Figure 1.2). Thus red cell/granular casts in the urine mean that the blood has originated from the kidneys. Often the casts are seen best peripherally near the edge of the coverslip. The identification of casts is of such importance in

localizing haematuria that, if casts are not seen on an uncentrifuged specimen, then a centrifuged deposit should be examined for casts. Casts may get broken up by centrifugation, but their characteristic tube-like appearance should still be visible. In general, the greater the concentration of casts the more severe the renal disorder.

Measurement of red cell excretion rate by a timed collection of urine (Addis count)[9] has gone out of fashion in most countries because of the errors associated with the method, which include problems with an accurately timed collection of urine, variable methods of centrifugation and resuspending the cellular deposit, difficulties in identifying red cells by microscopy, and haemolysis and disintegration of red cells in the lengthy collection of urine. It is more usual to rely on a combination of chemical tests and microscopy of a fresh random sample of urine, preferably a morning sample.

Clinical presentations

For the family, macroscopic haematuria is an alarming occurrence which usually leads the parents to seek medical help fast, irrespective of whether the child has other symptoms. This presentation will be most common for doctors, though with the increasing sensitivity and use of dipstix tests as a routine test, an increasing number of children are coincidentally found to have microscopic haematuria while being examined for another reason. These two different clinical presentations will be considered separately, though there is clearly an overlap in the causes since their only difference is the degree of haematuria. Moreover, some vigilant relatives will notice a very small degree of urine discoloration which for another family would only come to light as a result of tests being performed on the urine.

Macroscopic haematuria

If the child has haematuria at the time of the consultation, assessment is fairly straightforward. However, when it is merely a story of red urine with no adequate chemical or microscopic test of the urine previously done, and the urine test at the time of the consultation is normal, assessment is more problematic. Assuming that the child seems normal and is healthy on examination, then it may be best to instruct the parent how to use a dipstix test and to send them away with the test plus instructions to either check the urine regularly or at the time that it is next discoloured in order to verify haematuria.

Causes

The causes of haematuria are shown in Table 1.2. The following points should be remembered when taking the medical history, examining the child and considering further investigation.

Table 1.2 The main causes of haematuria

Infection
  Including tuberculosis, schistosomiasis and adenovirus

Trauma

Glomerulonephritis

Hypercalciuria ± calculus

Congenital abnormality
  Including cysts, hydronephrosis and diverticula

Vascular
  Including arteritis and infarction

Tumour

Bleeding disorder

Chemical cystitis, e.g. cyclophosphamide

Exercise induced

Factitious

More than 50% of children presenting with gross haematuria have a readily apparent cause.[10]

A third of urinary tract infections are said to be associated with haematuria, though usually this is microscopic rather than overt macroscopic haematuria. However, some children with bacterial urine infections present with macroscopic haematuria, and urinary infection is the commonest cause of macroscopic haematuria, accounting for 49% of cases of macroscopic haematuria in children.[10] As with all urine infections, other symptoms and signs may be negligible. It is conventional to diagnose urinary tract infection only if more than 10^5 organisms per ml (i.e. 10^8/litre) are cultured, but it is becoming increasingly recognized that lesser growth of an organism may cause trouble for some children.

Viruses are not often considered to be a cause of urine infection, but an important cause of haematuria is acute haemorrhagic cystitis particularly associated with adenovirus type 11 and type 21 which causes a short self-limiting disease characterized by gross haematuria and symptoms of bladder inflammation. Usually the macroscopic haematuria has gone by the fifth day, though microscopic haematuria may persist for 2 or 3 days more.[11] Tuberculosis is a most rare cause of haematuria in Western countries, though it should still be considered in someone with prolonged ill health or tuberculosis elsewhere. Schistosomiasis (bilharziasis) is an important cause of haematuria in Middle Eastern countries and in tropical Africa, the ova causing a granulomatous inflammatory reaction of the bladder and the lower urinary tract.

Trauma sufficient to cause haematuria will usually be associated with an obvious history of a damaging event and also with bruising or other signs of external injury.

Glomerulonephritis is an easy diagnosis when associated with other symptoms and signs of an acute nephritic syndrome, but a vast number of subclinical cases of glomerulonephritis present merely with haematuria.

Calculi are uncommon in children but they may present with haematuria alone, i.e. no colic. Conversely, the occurrence of pain at the time of haematuria does not necessarily mean the presence of a renal stone because profuse bleeding can cause colic from the clots of blood passing down the ureter and some of the other causes of haematuria are themselves associated with pain.

Idiopathic hypercalciuria (without) stone formation may cause haematuria.[12,13] For those with symptoms, the commonest presentation is isolated haematuria which may be gross or microscopic; calcium stones are much less common. Measurements of urinary calcium excretion is mandatory.[14,15]

The finding of an anatomical abnormality on X-ray examination does not necessarily mean that this is the cause of the bleeding. It is debatable how often hydronephrosis or bladder diverticula cause bleeding in the absence of infection. However, it is certain that they sometimes do.

Vascular causes are rare and usually the cause is apparent from the rest of the history: thus the striking picture of renal vascular thromboses in a neonate or of arteritis associated with a multisystem disorder.

Urinary tract tumours are uncommon. A third of children with a nephroblastoma (Wilms' tumour) have microscopic haematuria, but macroscopic haematuria is rare. It must be exceedingly uncommon for a tumour to be diagnosed as a result of a child presenting with haematuria.

Children with bleeding disorders, such as haemophilia or thrombocytopenia, may develop gross haematuria and commonly have microscopic haematuria. In many countries sickle cell haemoglobinopathy is a more important cause of haematuria and spontaneous haematuria, usually from the left kidney, is a well-recognized association of sickle cell trait; it is thought to result from infarction of the renal collecting systems.[16,17]

Some of the chemicals causing haematuria are listed in Table 1.3. Some cause the haematuria by affecting coagulation, others by direct renal damage and others by irritation of the bladder. The cytotoxic drug cyclophosphamide is particularly notorious for causing a chemical cystitis which may progress to severely inflamed and ulcerated bladder mucosa. This is more likely if the child is not passing much urine because of low fluid intake.

There is still some argument about the cause of exercise-induced haematuria. Although earlier reports suggested that the bladder was the source of the haematuria, it seems more likely that the source is glomerular. It is a transient haematuria coming on immediately after severe exercise and has disappeared within 48 h. It is as if the normal increase in red cell excretion associated with exercise has been excessive and therefore haematuria is seen.

Factitious haematuria is most commonly the result of the child or the parent (usually the mother) adding blood to the urine sample after it has been passed, though occasionally haematuria is the result of instruments being inserted into the urethra.[18] Such haematuria will usually have a lower urinary tract appearance unless, as sometimes happens, the mother herself has genuine renal haematuria and substitutes her own urine specimens for that of the child. Forensic laboratories will be able to determine the type of blood, human or animal meat, and distinguish between blood originating from the child or the parent.[19] If there is doubt that the urine sample has originated from the child a loading dose of vitamin C may be given which causes the child's urine to react positively to the vitamin C detector dipstix, so confirming that at least some of the child's urine is in the sample under investigation.[20]

Table 1.3   Drugs and chemicals which may cause haematuria

Anticoagulants

Antibacterials
  Ampicillin
  Kanamycin
  Methicillin
  Penicillin
  Polymyxin
  Sulphonamides

Other drugs
  Aspirin
  Amitriptyline
  Benzotropine mesylate
  Chlorpromazine
  Colchicine
  Cyclophosphamide
  Indomethacin
  Phenylbutazone
  Trifluoperazine

Solvents
  Carbon tetrachloride
  Phenol
  Turpentine

Metals
  Copper sulphate
  Lead
  Gold
  Phosphorus

NB. Many other drugs, poisons and ingested substances may occasionally cause haematuria. Thus, whenever haematuria is being investigated and the child may have ingested a drug or poison, that substance should be checked carefully in a pharmacopoeia for the possibility of causing haematuria.

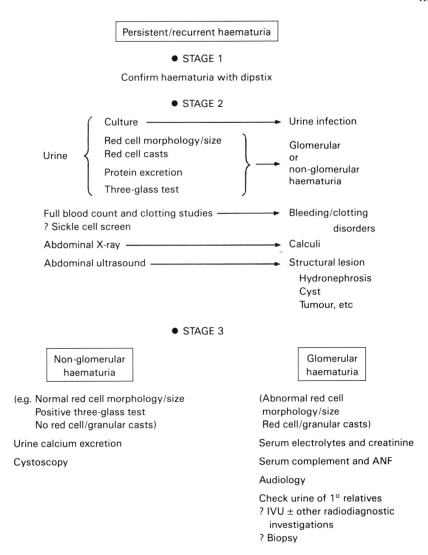

Figure 1.3 A scheme for the investigation of haematuria that has persisted or recurred for over 1 month

Other features of particular importance in the history are: lower urinary tract symptoms of dysuria and frequency are likely to be associated with bladder or urethral inflammation, whereas upper abdominal or loin pain is more likely to be associated with glomerulonephritis or a vascular or structural abnormality of the kidney. Preceding or accompanying upper respiratory tract infection makes glomerulonephritis more likely. Family history of renal disorder (cystic disease, Alport's syndrome and other less serious forms of familial nephritis) tends to run true to type and to be of similar severity. The ethnic background and travels of the family are relevant to implicating sickle-cell disease, chronic tuberculosis and schistosomiasis.

Evaluation

Macroscopic haematuria is such an alarming occurrence for the parents that prompt investigation (stages 1 and 2 in Figure 1.3) is likely to be indicated. The urgency is less with microscopic haematuria and it is usual to document its presence over at least 1 month before embarking on further evaluation. Bearing in mind the probable causes of haematuria, a systemic approach to history, examination and further investigation is possible. A relevant history will be taken.

A thorough physical examination is also important and, in particular, it is imperative to check the blood pressure and examine the abdomen and genitalia carefully. Usually no abnormalities are found, but the presence of hypertension or oedema at the time of haematuria might suggest an acute nephritic syndrome. The presence of anaemia would be a worrying feature suggesting more chronic disease.

The presence of haematuria is verified first by dipstix testing; and the three-glass test is performed. The type (origin) of haematuria is identified by either microscopy or automated blood analyser. If no casts are seen, then the urine should be centrifuged to see if casts are present in the centrifuged deposit. Of the other routine urine tests, that for proteinuria is the most relevant. There can be appreciable haematuria in dipstix testing and on microscopy without a positive reading of the Albustix test for protein. In general, the finding of proteinuria, particularly if persistent, points towards a renal origin for the proteinuria and a less favourable prognosis than for the child who merely has haematuria without any proteinuria.

Further investigation

Careful and skilled examination of the urine must precede any further investigation and must be considered together with the history and findings on physical examination.

For most children it will be appropriate to culture the urine for infection and to arrange for imaging of the kidney. But even those may be inappropriate when the history and examination have pointed clearly to an alternative firm diagnosis, e.g. acute post-infectious glomerulonephritis. Full blood count, clotting studies and, where appropriate, sickle cell screening tests should be performed. Abdominal X-ray will exclude radio-opaque calculi. The form of any further radiodiagnostic investigation will depend to some extent on local facilities and expertise. Ultrasound is likely to be the first choice, though an intravenous urogram or other imaging technique may be needed for the child with persisting glomerular haematuria.

Tests for the diagnosis of acute nephritic syndrome and other forms of glomerulonephritis are described elsewhere (see Chapter 17). Tests of renal function in a well child with haematuria are likely to be normal and it is unlikely that anything more complicated than a serum creatinine level will be required in the first instance.

At this stage of assessment and investigation a probable diagnosis will have been established for most children with macroscropic haematuria and for a minority of those with microscopic haematuria. In children with non-glomerular haematuria, urine calcium excretion or, if normal, cystoscopy will identify a cause in most (stage 3, Figure 1.3). It is worth stressing that cystoscopy is indicated only for this very small group of patients. The practice of early cystoscopy for children with haematuria is to be deprecated; it is unlikely to identify a cause for the bleeding and subjects the child to unnecessary investigation and anaesthetic.

A case can be made out for extensive investigation including renal biopsy and arteriography but the experience is that, though such investigations may eventually display an abnormality, this abnormality is either not of great importance or not amenable to treatment, so that intensive investigation of the well child with haematuria is of little benefit to the child. If no cause is found, it is more sensible to discuss the problem with the anxious parents of the child, and to be optimistic since much haematuria is relatively transient. It is best to impress on them the rarity of renal failure and the fact that the child is healthy and has kidneys which work well and then to follow-up the child during the next few months with the parents testing the urine occasionally and a record being kept of the occurrence of any haematuria. If the haematuria persists either macroscopically or microscopically for at least a year, then it is probably worth investigating further as outlined below.

Recurrent haematuria

Usually the term is applied to children who have intermittent *macroscopic* haematuria, but many will have persisting or recurrent *microscopic* haematuria in between. Presumably there is another group of children who have recurrent microscopic haematuria unknown to their parents or doctors. Most of the causes of haematuria listed in Table 1.2 may cause recurrent haematuria but for the child presenting with recurrent haematuria most of the listed causes will be excluded either quickly or in the course of more detailed assessment and investigation. There is left a considerable number of children who have what is loosely called 'recurrent haematuria of childhood' or 'benign haematuria'[21] Boys are affected more often than girls and onset before the age of 2 is unusual. Many present with overt haematuria at the time of, or in the day or two following, an upper respiratory tract infection. For a few, haematuria also seems to be associated with increased physical activity. Most merely present with bright red urine which persists for two to five days. Approximately one-third have associated symptoms. Both loin pain and central abdominal pain are common and occasionally there may be vague arthralgia of the medium-sized joints and non-specific skin rashes. For many of the children, the urine is normal in between the bouts of haematuria, but a considerable proportion have persisting microscopic haematuria between the attacks of macroscopic haematuria. Most of them do not have persistent proteinuria.

In taking the history carefully, assessment of the family is important not only to detect severe forms of familial nephritis, such as Alport's syndrome, but because some forms of relatively benign haematuria have a familial tendency. It is worth checking the urine of all first-degree relatives of the patient.

It is usual for physical examination including measurement of the blood pressure, examination of the eyes and a check on the hearing, to be normal. Moreover, on routine testing, most children will not have proteinuria; the minority who do have proteinuria should have that assessed quantitatively as outlined elsewhere. It is of great importance to establish the origin of the blood – it is usually glomerular (stage 3, Figure 1.3). However if red cell morphology and the absence of casts suggest non-glomerular bleeding, urosurgical help may be appropriate.

It is likely that the child with recurrent haematuria will have had several samples of urine cultured, and intravenous urogram and measurement of the blood urea/creatinine and electrolytes fairly early on. Similarly a full blood count and coagulation tests will have been normal. Subsequently serum C3 and C4 complement will have been found normal and antinuclear factor negative. Even though the child may be well and leading a normal life, the occurrence of periodic haematuria is worrying for the family and for the physician.

Opinions differ about the need for renal biopsy. The relative indications vary from worrying clinical associations to the need to answer specific questions from the family about an older child's choice of career. Relative indications for biopsy include:

- Associated proteinuria or raised serum creatinine persisting for more than 1 month.
- Family history of glomerulonephritis.
- Persistence of recurrent haematuria for more than 1 year.
- Social/educational reasons.

When renal biopsy is thought appropriate it must be done in an experienced specialist unit with full facilities for expert processing and interpretation of the histology. It is mandatory to have the specimen studied by light microscopy, immunofluorescence and by electron microscopy.

In children who have had recurrent haematuria for at least a year, a variety of patterns may be recognized on the renal biopsy:

- In some the changes will be of a recognized glomerulonephritis, e.g. membranoproliferative glomerulonephritis, and the prognosis will reflect the prognosis of the specific diagnosis.
- Approximately 20% will show Berger's disease; these will have variable but usually mild changes on light microscopy, the main finding being marked mesangial deposits of IgA with IgG and C3 complement on immunofluorescence (see below). The group with this histology are particularly prone to have their bouts of haematuria immediately following a respiratory infection.
- Approximately 20% will have minimal or no abnormalities on light microscopy and immunofluorescence with a variety of changes in the glomerular basement membrane (see below).
- In some children there will be minimal changes on light microscopy with negligible changes on immunofluorescence and electron microscopy. There is every reason to expect a good prognosis for this group.

At the stage at which biopsy is being considered, it is probably worth ensuring that the child has a formal audiogram in addition to any simple clinical hearing tests, as deafness is a pointer to Alport's syndrome and also deserves early specialist help in its own right.

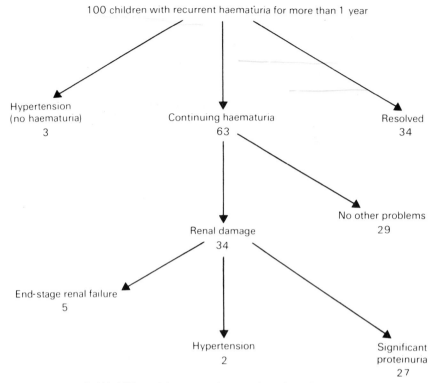

Figure 1.4 Long-term outcome in 100 children with recurrent haematuria (After Miller *et al.*[22])

It will be realized that though biopsy may yield considerable prognostic help and may enable one to advise the child and family more sensibly about future education, training and job selection, there are few implications for direct treatment since most of the renal disorders are not amenable to specific treatment yet. It is for this reason that decisions about the appropriateness and timing of biopsy will always take account of conflicting pressures from the family and referring doctor in deciding what is in the best interest of the child. Follow-up of children with recurrent haematuria reveals a significant incidence of complications in the form of hypertension, proteinuria and, rarely, renal insufficiency 7–10 years later; therefore it is probably wisest to arrange for the child to have a health check including measurement of the blood pressure and a check on the urine at least once a year throughout their childhood and then perhaps explain to the child at that stage that they must arrange for their own health checks thereafter. It is difficult to do this without causing needless alarm. Another difficult task is to make it clear to the family that a

normal life and normal activity should be followed even when bouts of haematuria follow physical activity.

It should be explained to the parents that although the activity causes the haematuria to show, it is not causing more damage to the kidneys or to the child – just as running causes a child with one leg slightly shorter than the other to display a limp which is not apparent when the child is merely walking, so haematuria becomes apparent on exercise without causing harm. But, however tolerant the family and skilful the physician, the physician usually ends up wishing that blood was not red and that no-one was aware of the intermittent bouts of haematuria.

The flow chart (Figure 1.4) shows the outcome 7–10 years after initial presentation of 100 consecutive children who had intermittent haematuria for at least 1 year and were referred to the Paediatric Nephrology Centres at Manchester and Leeds.[22] The conclusion from that study was that recurrent haematuria is not always 'benign' and that a less favourable prognosis is more likely if there is persisting micro-

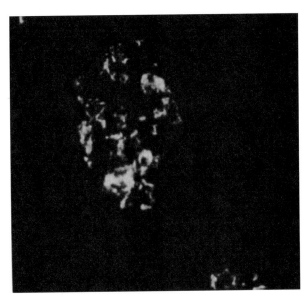

Figure 1.5 Mesangial deposits of IgA. Direct immunofluorescence with fluorescein isothiocyanate-labelled anti-IgA, × 300

scopic haematuria in between the attacks, proteinuria at onset or subsequently and, as might be expected, when the biopsy shows more marked changes.

Berger's disease (*mesangial IgA nephritis*)

Although this is a histological diagnosis, it is of particular relevance to the consideration of haematuria because of its relatively high incidence in patients of all ages who present with recurrent haematuria.[23,24]

The diagnosis is applied when the predominant finding on immunofluorescence of the renal biopsy is of granular deposits of IgA in the mesangium of the glomerulus. Commonly these deposits are also associated with IgG and C3 complement (Figure 1.5). Light microscopy tends to show mild mesangial proliferation with considerable focal variation, and electron microscopy shows mesangial hypercellularity with discrete finely granular electron-dense deposits within the mesangium.[25]

Clinical features
It is nearly twice as common in boys. Familial occurrence is rare but does occur occasionally. The mode range of onset is 5–10 years; occurrence below the age of 3 is rare. Commonly the condition presents with haematuria at the time

of, or closely following, an upper respiratory tract infection. There may be transient features of an acute nephritic syndrome but serum complement levels remain normal.[26]

It is quite common for children with Berger's disease to have abdominal pain at the time of the macroscopic haematuria; sometimes this is of a severity that leads to a laparotomy. Rarely there is also arthralgia. Some children have no symptoms apart from red urine.

Although the initial illness is usually short, microscopic haematuria may persist for many years interspersed with bouts of macroscopic haematuria at the time of upper respiratory tract infections. Other children have intermittent macroscopic haematuria with completely normal urine in between the bouts. Most bouts of haematuria are symptomless.

Since identification of mesangial IgA nephritis only became possible with the advent of immunofluorescence, there is a lack of very long-term follow-up studies of children with the condition. In the medium term, it seems that most children do not have progressive disease and that only a small minority progress to renal insufficiency within the first 10 years. However, if at onset there is a crescentic nephritis, the outcome is worse with one-third progressing to end-stage renal failure within two years. It is possible that the prognosis varies at different ages and may be worse in older children.[27,28] The study of 18-year-old army recruits in Singapore who had proteinuria or microscopic haematuria revealed a high incidence of mesangial IgA nephritis and follow-up showed that 8% developed end-stage renal failure within 3 years and a further 7% developed hypertension.

The similarity between the epidemiology, the clinical features and the clinical course led to the suggestion that Berger's disease might be considered as an example of Henoch–Schoenlein syndrome without the rash.[29] Certainly the histological features are identical and immunologically for both conditions serum IgA may be elevated, IgA-bearing lymphocytes increased and immune complexes containing IgA detected. From the clinical point of view a child with IgA nephritis should be followed up in much the same way as a child who has had Henoch–Schoenlein nephritis. The main difference seems to be that recurrent macroscopic haematuria is more common with Berger's disease than with Henoch–Schoenlein nephritis.

Basement membrane nephropathy

In the majority of children with recurrent haematuria and normal light microscopy and immunofluorescence it is possible to demonstrate changes in the glomerular basement membrane (GBM) on electron microscopy.[30] These changes fall into three group:

Group 1 – basement membrane nephropathy (lamellation type)
This is characterized by irregular and marked thickening of GBM accompanied by severe structural distortion. These changes are indistinguishable from the changes seen in Alport's syndrome.

Group 2 – basement membrane nephropathy (extensive attenuation type)
This is characterized by diffuse attenuation of GBM, and is a common finding in children with *mild* microscopic haematuria.[31]

Group 3 – idiopathic haematuria with minimal basement membrane alteration
This is characterized by slight variation in GBM thickness.

Extensive long-term experience, over 12 years,

for groups 2 and 3 is not yet available but preliminary data from several sources suggests a favourable prognosis in that renal impairment has not been reported in the early years of follow-up. This contrasts with the more serious prognosis for group 1 (see Chapter 23).

History and urine testing of family members may confirm a family problem in all three groups. In some, progression of renal disease and at least one affected subject with neural hearing loss suggest a diagnosis of Alport's syndrome. In other families, hearing loss and progressive renal failure are absent in the affected patients and their family members.[30] (Familial nephritis is reviewed fully in Chapter 23.) The outlook for patients with GBM changes without other affected family members is not known.

Microscopic haematuria

Increased use of multiple test dipstix for routine examination of urine together with the increased sensitivity of the haemastix portion of that test has led to many more children with microscopic haematuria coming to light. Often the child is undergoing a routine health check before a surgical procedure, at his school medical examination or during a clinic consultation. At other times the microscopic haematuria is uncovered during an acute admission for another problem and because the multitest dipstix includes a blood test as one of six or eight other tests on that strip.

As mentioned at the beginning of this chapter, it is normal to excrete some red cells each day and at times of stress rather more blood is excreted. Therefore, in the same way that proteinuria may appear transiently at the time of illness, fever, trauma or extreme exertion, so may microscopic haematuria.

The prevalence of microscopic haematuria in children is quite high. One of the largest screening surveys was done in Helsinki using the Ames haemastix test.[1] Performing this test at weekly intervals on a large number of children who were at school and believed to be well, revealed that 3.4% had a positive test on at least one occasion; 0.9% had two or more positive tests. In a smaller survey conducted some years earlier on 2100 Birmingham schoolchildren, it was found by the authors that 0.4% had microscopic haematuria persisting for more than 1 month. With the modern haemastix and their increased sensitivity, it is likely that be-tween 0.5 and 1% of children at school have microscopic haematuria persisting for at least 1 month. The causes of this haematuria are un-likely to be different from the causes considered in Table 1.2, but the severity of the cause will be less in many cases.[32] Thus some of the children will be recovering from extremely mild nephri-tis, others will have incurred minor trauma, etc.

Therefore, when assessing the child who has been found on casual examination to have mi-croscopic haematuria, the approach is just as for assessing any other form of haematuria. However, the degree of that microscopic haema-turia is relevant and there is no doubt that if there are abundant cells, and in particular any cast, on microscopy of the urine, then a more significant lesion is likely.[1,33]

A second important feature is the duration of the microscopic haematuria. If it is merely a temporary phenomenon which is present for a week or two and then goes, it is unlikely to be of importance and it is unlikely that the child will profit from extensive investigation if the rest of the history and physical examination are normal. If the microscopic haematuria persists for more than a month, some degree of further investigation is important along the lines men-tioned earlier when trying to detect a cause of macroscopic haematuria. The question is how far should that investigation be pursued. Our own experience of investigating, perhaps over-investigating, schoolchildren found to have mi-croscopic haematuria caused a lot of anxiety and investigation for the children with little apparent benefit. Therefore, it is reasonable to approach the problem of persisting or recurrent microscopic haematuria in much the same way as the problem of recurrent macroscopic haema-turia is approached and, in general, it is not necessary to consider renal biopsy until the microscopic haematuria has been present for at least 1 year.

The third important factor is the presence of proteinuria. As with microscopic haematuria, the larger surveys of microscopic haematuria show that the children who have associated proteinuria are more likely to have a poor prognosis.[34-36] The findings on renal biopsy when studied by light microscopy, immunofluo-rescence and electron microscopy help to iden-tify the small subgroup more likely to have marked renal disease leading to future renal impairment.

Conclusions

Throughout this chapter various different causes of haematuria have been considered, but it must be stressed that for the apparently well child who has macroscopic or microscopic hae-maturia and an unexceptional previous history, by far the most likely cause is glomerulonephri-tis. Glomerulonephritis is likely to be present in about 1% of children and, though it may not cause much illness in childhood, it is much less certain how benign it will be in later life. The Singapore study of nearly 70 000 army recruits found a 1.5% incidence of microscopic haematu-ria: over 90% of these had a renal biopsy which showed glomerulonephritis and during rela-tively brief follow-up of up to 5 years, 8 had developed renal failure. Acknowledging the dif-ferences in the epidemiology of renal disease that may exist between different races in differ-ent parts of the world, it is nevertheless wise to acknowledge that *persisting* haematuria, whether it be macroscopic or microscopic, is a reason for regular, though not necessarily fre-quent, follow-up health checks, since hyperten-sion and renal failure are worth detecting and treating early; such follow-up is all the more important if the haematuria is consistently large (rather than merely 1 + on dipstix testing) and if it is associated with proteinuria.

References

1. Vehaskari V.M., Rapola J., Koskimies O., Savilahti E., Vilska J. and Hallman N. Microscopic haematuria in schoolchildren: epidemiology and clinicopathologic evaluation. *J. Pediatr.* 1979, **95**, 676–684
2. Free A. and Free H. *Urinalysis in Clinical Laboratory Practice.* Cleveland, CRC Press, 1976
3. Schumann G.B. *Urine Sediment Examination.* Balti-more, Williams & Wilkins, 1980
4. Birch D.F. and Fairley K.F. Haematuria: glomerular or non-glomerular? *Lancet* 1979, **ii**, 845–846
5. Fassett R.G., Horgan B.A. and Mathew T.H. Detection of glomerular bleeding by phase-contrast microscopy. *Lancet* 1982, **i**, 1432–1434
6. Schichiri M., Oowada A., Nishio Y., Tomita K. and Shiigai T. Use of anutoanalyser to examine urinary red cell morphology in the diagnosis of glomerular haematu-ria. *Lancet* 1986, **ii**, 781–782
7. Gibbs D.D. and Lynn K.L. Red cell volume distribution curves in the diagnosis of glomerular and non-glomeru-lar haematuria. *Clin. Nephrol.* 1990, **33**, 143–147
8. De Caestecker M.P. and Ballardie F.W. Unexplained haematuria. *Br. Med. J.* 1990, **301**, 1171–1172

9. Addis T. The number of formed elements in the urinary sediment of normal individuals. *J. Clin. Invest.* 1926, **2**, 409–415

10. Ingelfinger J.R., Davis A.E. and Grupe W.E. Frequency and aetiology of gross haematuria in a general paediatric setting. *Pediatrics* 1977, **59**, 557–561

11. Mufson M.A., Belshe R.B., Horrigan T.J. and Zollar L.M. Causes of acute hemorrhagic cystitis in children. *Am. J. Dis. Child.* 1973, **126**, 605–609

12. Roy S., Stapleton F.B., Noe H.M. and Jerkins G. Haematuria preceding renal calculus formation in children with hypercalciuria. *J. Pediatr.* 1981, **99**, 712–715

13. Kalia A., Travis L.B. and Brouhard B.M. The association of idiopathic hypercalciuria and asymptomatic gross haematuria in children. *J. Pediatr.* 1981, **99**, 716–719

14. Stapleton F.B., Noe H.N., Roy S. and Jerkins G. Hypercalciuria in children with urolithiasis. *Am. J. Dis. Child.* 1982, **136**, 675–678

15. Kruse E., Kracht U. and Kruse U. Reference values for urinary calcium excretion and screening for hypercalciuria in children and adolescents. *Eur. J. Pediatr.* 1984, **143**, 25–31

16. Atkinson D.W. Sickling and haematuria. *Blood* 1969 **34**, 736–740

17. Liebman N.C. Renal papillary necrosis and sickle cell disease. *J. Urol.* 1969, **102**, 294–295

18. Meadow S.R. *Factitious Illness – The Hinterland of Child Abuse – Recent Advances in Paediatrics* No. 7. London, Churchill Livingstone, 1984

19. Meadow R. Management of Munchausen syndrome by proxy. *Arch. Dis. Child.* 1985, **60**, 385–393

20. Nading J.H. and Dival-Arnould B. Factitious diabetes mellitus confirmed by ascorbic acid. *Arch. Dis. Child.* 1984, **59**, 166–179

21. Ayoub E.M. and Vernier R.L. Benign recurrent hematuria. *Am. J. Dis. Child.* 1965, **109**, 217–223

22. Miller P. F. W., Speirs N. I., Aparicio S.R. *et al.* Long term prognosis of recurrent haematuria. *Arch. Dis. Child.* 1985 **60**, 420–425

23. Berger J. IgA deposits in renal disease. *Transplant Proc.* 1969, **1**, 939–944

24. Clarkson A.R., Woodroffe A.J., Bannister K.M. *et al.* The syndrome of IgA nephropathy. *Clin. Nephrol.* 1984, **21**, 7–14

25. Levy M., Gonzales S., Broyer M. and Habib R. Berger's disease in children. *Int. J. Paed. Nephrol.* 1982, **3**, 129–130

26. Southwest Paediatric Nephrology Study Group. A multi-centre study of IgA nephropathy in children. *Kidney Int.* 1982, **22**, 643–652

27. Waldherr R., Rambausek H., Michalk D. *et al.* Mesangial IgA nephritis – contrasting features in paediatric and adult patients. *Int. J. Paed. Nephrol.* 1982, **3**, 146

28. Emancipator S.N., Gazzo G.R. and Lamm M. IgA nephropathy: perspectives on pathogenesis and classification. *Clin. Nephrol.* 1985, **24**, 161–179

29. Meadow S.R. and Scott D.C. Berger disease – Henoch–Schoenlein syndrome without the rash. *J. Pediatr.* 1985, **106**, 27–32

30. Yum M. and Bergstein J.M. Basement membrane nephropathy: a new classification for Alport's syndrome and asymptomatic haematuria based on ultrastructural findings. *Human Pathol.* 1983, **14**, 996–1003

31. Lang S., Stevenson B. and Risdon R.A. Thin basement membrane nephropathy as a cause of recurrent haematuria in childhood. *Histopathology* 1990, **16**, 331–337

32. Dodge W.F., West E.F., Smith E.H. and Bunce H. III. Proteinuria and hematuria in school children: epidemiology and early natural history. *J. Pediatr.* 1976. **88**, 327

33. West C.D. Asymptomatic hematuria and proteinuria in children: causes and appropriate diagnostic studies. *J. Pediatr.* 1976, **89**, 173–182

34. Hisano S. and Ueda K. Asymptomatic haematuria and proteinuria: renal pathology and clinical outcome in 54 children. *Pediatr. Nephrol.* 1989, **3**, 229–234

35. Turi S., Visy M., Vissy A., Jaszai V., Czirbesz Z., Haszon I., Szelid Zs. and Ferkis I. Longterm follow-up of patients with persistent/recurrent isolated haematuria: a Hungarian multicentre study. *Pediatr. Nephrol.* 1989, **3**, 235–239

36. Vehaskari M.V. Asymptomatic hematuria – a cause for concern? *Pediatr. Nephrol.* 1989, **3**, 240–241

2

Proteinuria

A.M. Robson, V.M. Vehaskari

The association between renal disease and proteinuria was described by Richard Bright more than 150 years ago. This chapter briefly reviews current knowledge, relates it to the clinical aspects of proteinuria and outlines the appropriate management of the child found to have protein in the urine.

Renal handling of proteins

Filtration of protein

Plasma proteins cross the normal glomerular barrier, albeit in low concentrations. The ability of these proteins to enter the glomerular filtrate is related primarily to protein molecular size and charge.[1] Glomerular permselectivity based on molecular size results from the characteristics of the glomerular basement membrane which provides the mechanical barrier to filtration. The larger plasma proteins, such as globulins, are virtually excluded from the normal glomerular filtrate. Smaller proteins like albumin are filtered in low concentrations. Micropuncture studies in experimental animals indicate that the albumin concentration in the glomerular filtrate of mammalian kidneys may be as high as 2 mg/dl. If this figure can be extrapolated to the human kidney, then as much as 3.5 g of albumin are filtered each day by the kidneys of a healthy adult. Smaller proteins such as the peptide hormones, insulin or growth hormone, or derivatives of immunoproteins such as β_2-microglobulin can penetrate the

glomerular barrier with relative ease. They have a sieving coefficient in excess of 0.5, which means that their concentrations in the glomerular filtrate are at least 50% of those in the plasma.

Molecular charge also plays an important role in determining glomerular permeability to macromolecules. Negatively charged molecules are less able to penetrate the glomerulus than are neutral molecules of identical size: positively charged molecules have enhanced clearances.[2] This charge selectivity is due to glomerular polyanions which consist of the sialoproteins that line the surfaces of both the glomerular endothelial and epithelial cells, and glycosaminoglycans present in the glomerular basement membrane.[3] These fixed negative charge sites are believed to provide an electrical barrier which minimizes the transglomerular passage of relatively large molecules such as albumin, that carry a strongly negative charge at the physiological pH of 7.4.

Other factors which influence the ability of proteins to enter the glomerular filtrate include deformability of molecular shape and alterations in glomerular haemodynamics.[3] A decreased glomerular capillary blood flow increases albumin penetration of the glomerular barrier and entry of albumin into the urinary space. These effects are functional, not pathological, since restoration of blood flow promptly reverses the leaky state of the glomerular capillary wall.[4] The plasma concentration of a protein also affects the level of proteinuria. There is a straight-line relationship between the plasma concentration of a protein and the amount of that protein which appears in the urine.[5] This applies even to albumin. An increase in plasma albumin concentration to above normal levels will result in albuminuria even in persons with normal kidneys.

Tubular reabsorption

Almost all of the smaller proteins that are filtered through the glomeruli are reabsorbed by the proximal convoluted tubules.[1] As a consequence, normal urine contains negligible quantities of the peptide hormones or immunoglobulin fragments even though they are readily filtered. These proteins are reabsorbed by a process of endocytosis which operates at well below maximum rates in health. Indeed, metabolism by the kidney represents an important regulatory process for many of these proteins.

The proximal convoluted tubules also reabsorb most of the larger plasma proteins that are filtered. This mechanism is separate from that used to reabsorb the smaller proteins, and it remains uncertain whether albumin and globulins compete for the same transport sites or have separate reabsorptive mechanisms. Reabsorption of the larger proteins, too, is accomplished by a process of endocytosis followed by partial digestion of the protein in endocytic vacuoles. The catabolic products are returned to the circulation. This transport system operates at, or close to, its maximum rate in health. None of these filtered plasma proteins can be returned intact into the body protein pool.

Protein secretion

Forty per cent of normal urinary protein is of tissue rather than plasma origin. It is composed of a heterogeneous group of numerous proteins, many of which are glycoproteins. Some of these are derived from cells lining the urinary tract and have the potential of being important diagnostic indicators;[6] others are from non-renal tissues such as the accessory sex glands. The major protein in this group is uromucoid or Tamm–Horsfall protein which is excreted in amounts of 30–60 mg/day in the adult. This large glycoprotein is a major constituent of urinary casts. Histochemical studies suggest that it is added to the urine, primarily in the thick ascending limb of the loop of Henle, but it may be added at more distal sites too.

Protein in urine

Under normal conditions, approximately 60% of protein in normal urine is derived from plasma protein. This results from a balance between the amount of these proteins filtered and the amount reabsorbed.[1] Albumin predominates and constitutes about 40% of the total urinary protein with another 15% migrating on electrophoresis as α_1- or α_2-globulins. Numerous other proteins have been identified and include a variety of immunoproteins, peptides, enzymes, hormones and partially degraded plasma proteins. The proportions of the different proteins in urine can vary. For example, after severe exercise proteinuria may increase several-fold. This is due to increased albuminuria, so that after exercise albumin may represent as much as 80% of total urinary protein compared to the more normal value of 40%.

Measurement of proteinuria

Screening techniques

Dipstick methods

The development of the dipstick represents a major advance which has simplified the testing of urines for protein and has increased the frequency with which such tests are performed. The dipstick is impregnated with tetrabromophenol blue, buffered to pH 3.5. At a constant pH, the binding of protein to this reagent results in the development of a blue colour in proportion to the amount of protein present. The dipstick is yellow when the urine is protein free. With increasing concentrations of protein, the colour of the dipstick changes through yellow-green, to green, to a green-blue. Thus an approximate estimate of protein concentration can be obtained over a wide range of protein concentrations from as low as 10–15 mg/dl to more than 1000 mg/dl.[7]

The method has certain limitations (Table 2.1). Albumin demonstrates better binding characteristics to the dye than do other proteins, so that dipstick results correlate better with the level of albuminuria than with total proteinuria. Indeed, a negative dipstick test for protein does not exclude the presence in the urine of low concentrations of globulins, haemoglobin, Bence-Jones protein or mucoproteins. There is a considerable observer error in interpreting the

Table 2.1 Causes for misleading screening tests for proteinuria

False positive results	*False negative results*
Dipstick method	
Highly concentrated urine	Very dilute urine
Alkaline urine (pH > 8)	Acid urine (pH 4.5)
Gross haematuria, pyuria, bacteriuria	Non-albumin proteinuria
Dipstick left in urine too long	
Contamination and drugs	
Quaternary ammonium compounds such as antiseptics, chlorhexidine or benzalkonium	
Phenazopyridine	
Protein precipitation methods	
Highly concentrated urine	
Gross haematuria, pyuria, bacteriuria	
Drugs	
Radiographic contrast media	
Metabolites of tolbutamide and sulphonamides	
High levels of penicillin analogues or cephalosporins	

colour of the dipstick. In addition, the result of the dipstick test must be interpreted in relation to both the concentration and the pH of the urine. If a diuresis is induced to obtain a urine sample, the urinary protein concentration may be reduced to a level below the sensitivity of the dipstick (10–15 mg/dl) even in patients spilling up to 1.0 g of protein per day. Misinterpretation of such a false negative result can be avoided if any negative dipstick result for protein is viewed with caution in urines with a specific gravity of below 1.002. Conversely, under conditions of oliguria, with a urine specific gravity in excess of 1.025, a healthy person may register trace protein on the dipstick. Since the dipstick method for protein is pH dependent, a very acid urine (pH 4.5) can cause a false negative test and a very alkaline urine (pH > 8.0), a false positive result.

False positive tests for protein may also occur in the presence of gross haematuria, pyuria and bacteriuria; as a result of contamination of the urine with antiseptics such as chlorhexidine or benzalkonium which are the agents most frequently used for skin cleansing when obtaining a clean catch urine sample; any quaternary ammonium compound, such as a detergent, especially if present in high concentration; and a limited number of drugs, such as phenazopyridine. If the dipstick is kept in the urine too long, the buffer may be leached out and a false positive test may result. Finally, the concentration of urinary salts modifies the quantitative accuracy of the dipstick.

Despite these limitations the dipstick pro-

vides an excellent screening test for the presence of proteinuria.

Turbidometric methods

These methods are based on the principle that proteins are insoluble at an acid pH and are used either for screening purposes or for quantitating proteinuria. A variety of precipitating agents may be used including sulphosalicylic acid, trichloroacetic acid or sodium sulphate. For many years, patients used acetic acid (vinegar) to check urines for protein at home. These methods are simple and cheap but are less convenient than dipsticks for home use. Radiographic contrast media, the metabolites of tolbutamide and sulphonamides, high levels of cephalosporins or penicillin analogues and gross haematuria can result in false positive tests. Despite such disadvantages, the turbidometric methods are frequently used to confirm the dipstick result in routine screening.

Quantification of proteinuria

Laboratory methods

Measurement of the rate of protein loss in the urine is important in determining whether the patient requires a more extensive evaluation. Numerous methods are available to quantitate proteinuria.[8] Each has advantages and disadvantages. In addition, results will vary depending on the method used. The clinician must be aware of this when comparing data from different laboratories.

Turbidometric assays are reliable when the urine contains a relatively high protein concentration. Their simplicity, convenience and cost-effectiveness have made them attractive for the hospital laboratory. However, they have a relative lack of sensitivity and poor linearity of results over a wide range of concentrations and tend to give lower results for protein than those obtained by other methods. This has been attributed to an inhibitor in the urine. More recently a microturbidometric method has been developed. It uses benzethonium chloride as a precipitating agent and is more accurate. Unfortunately it is more complex and frequently requires multiple dilutions of the urine, making it less suitable for routine use. The Folin–Lowry and biuret methods have also proved to be reliable, especially when modified to avoid errors due to the presence in the urine of peptides or amino acids. There is an increasing trend, however, towards the dye-binding methods that involve one of a variety of dyes. These tend to have disadvantages similar to those described for dipsticks and may also interact with drugs such as gentamicin, kanamycin or miconazole to overestimate the level of proteinuria.

The typical laboratory method in widespread use today utilizes a turbidometric method modified for use in a clinical analyser. Benzethonium chloride is used to precipitate urinary protein in an alkaline medium. The resulting decrease in light transmission is measured in absorbance at 540 nm and the protein concentration in the sample is calculated by means of a standard curve or a mathematical function. The system is accurate and requires samples of less than 500 μl.

Normal values for proteinuria

It has been traditional when evaluating the proteinuric subject to measure the amount of protein excreted in a timed urine sample. Although it is well accepted that normal human urine contains small amounts of protein, it is difficult to define a precise upper limit for such proteinuria. Values are affected both by the conditions under which the urine was collected and by the laboratory method used to measure urinary protein concentration. For example, the level of albuminuria in normal children varies by age and sex; the variations in results that result from the method used to measure the

protein have already been discussed above. Furthermore there are differences in albumin excretion in urines collected during the day compared to those obtained at night.[9] It is not practical to develop 'normal' values which take into consideration each of these variables. Our guideline is that if the urine is collected with the patient at rest and afebrile, urinary protein excretion should not exceed 60 mg/m² body surface area per day. This value agrees well with the normal protein excretion rates in adults of up to 100 mg per day and applies to all age ranges except the first months of life when normal proteinuria typically is increased to as high as 240 mg m^{-2} day^{-1}.[10] Some reference sources suggest that normal values for urinary protein excretion may be as high as 150 mg m^{-2} day^{-1}. This higher value allows for some of the practical difficulties associated with urine collection which may not be obtained under ideal conditions. For example, during the period of collection the patient may not have been supine and may have had periods of vigorous exercise which would increase protein excretion markedly. We believe that the use of this more liberal value has potential for error and recommend that if urine protein excretion is to be quantitated the urine should be collected with the patient at rest when the lower 'normal' value applies.

For practical reasons, we obtain accurately timed overnight urine collections of approximately 12 h duration. The protein excretion rate is then extrapolated to a 24 h value by using the appropriate correction factor. For example, if the urine collection was obtained over an 11.5 h period, the urine protein excretion rate would be multiplied by 24/11.5 to obtain a 24 h value.

We do not think that there is any practical advantage in expressing urinary protein excretion per hour or per unit of body weight as advocated by some.

Urinary protein creatinine ratios

Obtaining accurate 12 or 24 h urine collections can be inconvenient and difficult to accomplish. In addition, quantitating urinary protein loss does not compensate for the effects that alterations in glomerular filtration rate (GFR) may have on the level of proteinuria. For example, a decrease in GFR due to progression of a renal disease may result in a decrease in proteinuria secondary to a decrease in the amount of protein filtered. Sometimes this can be so dramatic that it results in amelioration of the nephrotic syndrome. It may be misinterpreted as improvement rather than progression of the disease if changes in GFR are not monitored. In the past, attempts were made to prevent such errors by factoring urine protein excretion by GFR measured simultaneously. This is not practical for routine clinical use.

More recently, the use of single voided urine samples has been evaluated as an estimate of quantitative proteinuria.[11,12] For this purpose the concentration of both protein and creatinine are measured in the urine sample and protein levels are expressed per unit of urine creatinine (U_p/U_{cr} ratio). This technique has the advantages of not requiring timed urine samples and of not having to be corrected for body size. It assumes that creatinine excretion is directly related to body mass and is relatively constant throughout the day.[13]

Many studies have found that the amount of protein excreted in a 24 h urine correlates extremely well with the protein to creatinine ratio measured in random urine samples. It remains debated, however, whether random samples obtained during normal daytime activities or early morning samples are superior. The U_p/U_{cr} ratio is higher in samples produced when subjects are in an upright, as opposed to a recumbent, position.[14] Studies that included subjects with normal renal function as well as those with renal failure have shown that U_p/U_{cr} ratios from daytime samples correlated better with 24 h urine protein excretion values than did values from early morning samples.[14] In contrast, early morning samples had the better correlation when data was evaluated from normal subjects and from those with renal disease that was associated with normal glomerular filtration rates.[15]

Despite these differences, normal values for U_p/U_{cr} ratio obtained by different authors have agreed quite well. For example, one extensive investigation found that a protein to creatinine index [(mg protein × 10)/(mmol creatinine)] below 125 in a random urine sample excluded abnormal proteinuria. This is equivalent to the excretion of 110 μg protein/mg creatinine which is considered the upper range of normal in other studies. Both of these values correlate well with normal results published by others and with a normal urine protein excretion of less than 60 mg m^{-2} day^{-1}. If the laboratory

reports U_p/U_{cr} ratios as mg protein per mg creatinine, values less than 0.1 are normal, 0.1 to 1.0 represent mild proteinuria, 1.0 to 10 moderate proteinuria and those in excess of 10 heavy proteinuria.

We have observed misleading elevated U_p/U_{cr} ratios in some subjects with orthostatic proteinuria. Thus we believe the technique is of more value when monitoring the progress of proteinuria than in the initial evaluation of proteinuria. Our preference is to obtain both a 12 h protein excretion value and a U_p/U_{cr} ratio in the investigation of proteinuria and then to monitor serial values only for the U_p/U_{cr} ratio with urine samples being obtained under similar conditions at each follow-up visit.

Qualitative aspects of proteinuria

Measurements of individual proteins

Urinary protein can be characterized by electrophoresis, and accurate measurement of urinary levels of individual proteins, such as albumin, can be accomplished by radioimmuno- or immunochemical assay. Such measurements remain more of a research than a clinical tool but may have some clinical usefulness. For example, measurements of micro-albuminuria have been shown to be of value in predicting nephropathy in insulin-dependent diabetic subjects[16] and that these subjects demonstrate microheterogeneity of this albumin.[17] In addition, the measurement of urinary concentrations of small molecular weight proteins such as β_2-microglobulin may provide information of great clinical importance. Measurements of low-molecular-weight proteins in the urine appear to be a most sensitive indicator of even mild damage to the proximal tubule and can identify injury induced by nephrotoxic drugs such as the aminoglycoside antibiotics.[18] Commercial kits are available which facilitate measurement of urinary levels of β_2-microglobulin either by radioimmunoassay or by an enzymatic method. Normal urine should contain less than 0.37 mg/litre of this protein. Higher values indicate the presence of tubular injury or disease.

Sodium dodecyl sulphate gradient polyacrylamide gel electrophoresis (SDS PAGE) separates urinary proteins according to their molecular mass. The technique had been limited primarily to research applications until several methodological advances were made and a system suitable for commercial use was developed (PhastSystem-Pharmacia, Uppsala, Sweden). This permitted separation of proteins from 1 μl of unconcentrated urine in 2 h. Preliminary studies have shown that urines from patients in relapse from steroid-responsive nephrotic syndrome are characterized by bands of albumin and transferase. In contrast, samples from steroid-resistant nephrotic syndrome contain two additional bands of haptoglobin and IgG. Patterns of tubular proteinuria were found in children with proximal renal tubular abnormalities, whereas mixed patterns of glomerular and tubular proteinuria strongly suggested renal insufficiency.[19]

Protein selectivity indices

In health, the fractional clearances of many proteins are related in a linear fashion to the logarithm of the protein's molecular weight. Diseases such as glomerulonephritis which cause severe histological damage in the glomeruli are more likely to result in the urinary loss of larger plasma proteins such as globulins than are diseases such as minimal change nephrotic syndrome (MCNS), in which glomerular injury is not apparent. This is the theory behind measurement of protein selectivity. For these measurements, the clearances of a variety of proteins, typically albumin, transferrin, IgG and α_2-macroglobulin, are measured and their rates of loss or clearances are compared by one of several mathematical methods to derive a selectivity index.

Measurements of protein selectivity will separate *groups* of patients with different causes for their nephrotic syndrome. Patients with glomerulonephritis tend to have *non-selective* proteinuria with relatively high clearances of globulins and other large proteins; those with MCNS have *selective* proteinuria composed primarily of albumin. Unfortunately, there is considerable overlap in results, so that one cannot draw too firm conclusions from measurements of selectivity. For example, some patients with biopsy-proven glomerulonephritis have been shown to have a selective pattern of proteinuria.

Selectivity has also been used to predict a nephrotic patient's responsiveness to steroids. Selective proteinuria in children with nephrotic syndrome is associated with a high rate of response to steroid therapy. Unfortunately, this use of selectivity is not infallible either, so that

patients with congenital nephrotic syndrome of the Finnish type have selective proteinuria but are non-responsive to steroids.

There are many reasons for the problems associated with interpreting the results of protein selectivity. The renal clearances of only selected proteins are related to the protein's molecular size. In addition, the accurate measurement of many of the individual protein concentrations can be difficult. However, even the use of the latest immunonephelometric method for protein measurements does not resolve the problems.[20] In summary, it is apparent that many known, unknown and uncontrollable factors influence the filtration of proteins in the clinical setting and that measurements of selectivity cannot be used as a substitute for renal biopsy in any individual patient.

Prevalence of proteinuria

Studies of large populations of children have recorded that proteinuria may occur in anywhere from under 1% to more than 10% of these subjects. There are many reasons for such a variation. It is readily apparent that proteinuria is intermittent in the majority of children. For example, proteinuria was documented to occur in at least one sample in 10.7% of children evaluated in one study in which four urine samples were tested from each of 8954 schoolchildren aged between 8 and 15 years. However, only 0.1% of the population had all four urine samples positive for protein.[21]

Some of the factors which influence the reported prevalence of proteinuria include the subject's age and sex as well as the protein concentration required by the definition for proteinuria. These points are well illustrated in Figure 2.1, which shows that proteinuria was more common in girls and in older children. Whereas 56 out of 1000 12-year-old schoolgirls were found to have 10 mg/dl of protein in two out of three urine samples, only 2 per 1000 of these same subjects had protein levels of 100 mg/dl or more in all three of the samples.[22]

The School Health Law, passed in Japan in 1974, mandated urine screening of elementary and junior high school students for the detection of renal disease. It has generated a wealth of valuable data. In a study of 560 000 children in Tokyo, the prevalence of proteinuria was 0.08% in elementary schoolchildren and 0.37%

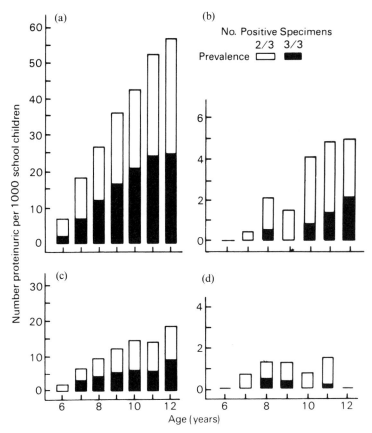

Figure 2.1 Prevalence of proteinuria in school-aged children showing the influence of age, sex, level of proteinuria and frequency at which proteinuria was documented (a) and (b) in girls; (c) and (d) in boys. With proteinuria of (a), (c) 10 mg/dl and (b), (d) 100 mg/dl (From the data of Dodge *et al.*[22])

in those attending junior high school.[23] Another study[24] involving 92 934 children found the prevalence of proteinuria to be 0.03% and that of haematoproteinuria 0.06%. Rates were somewhat lower in a second screening, but different criteria were used. These values are lower than the earlier published data from the USA, in which the prevalence of proteinuria was 0.942% in girls and 0.33% in boys.[22]

Mild glomerular changes of IgA nephropathy have been described in about one-third of children[25] and young adults[26] who have isolated proteinuria and who undergo a renal biopsy. Membranoproliferative glomerulonephritis (MPGN) has also been documented in about 12% of such children.[25] In general, the pathological abnormalities that were identified tended to be mild (as did the course of the MPGN), with proliferative changes being more frequent with increasing degrees of proteinuria. Changes

of MPGN have also been documented in another study of children with proteinuria as the sole urinary abnormality, although hypocomplementaemia was documented in these children, too.[24]

Intermittent proteinuria

By definition, intermittent proteinuria indicates that protein is detectable in only some of the urine samples from the proteinuric subject. This form of proteinuria may be related to posture (orthostatic proteinuria); alternatively, the proteinuria may occur at random when the proteinuria is referred to as being non-postural, intermittent proteinuria. Both postural or non-postural patterns of intermittent proteinuria may persist in any individual or may be transient. Some of the factors known to be associated with intermittent proteinuria are summarized in

Table 2.2   Causes of proteinuria classified by type and mechanism

Intermittent proteinuria
Postural proteinuria
Non-postural
  Random finding: no known cause
  Contamination of urine: vaginal secretions
  False positive test: penicillins, sulphonamides, tolbutamide, radiological contrast agents, etc.
  Non-renal causes: fever, stress such as exercise or exposure to cold, congestive heart failure
  Glomerular lesions: focal glomerulonephritis, Berger's disease
  Anatomical abnormalities of urinary tract: obstruction, etc.

Persistent proteinuria
Glomerular causes
  Damage to glomerular basement membranes: acute or chronic glomerulonephritides (GN) such as post-infectious GN,
    membranoproliferative GN or that associated with systemic lupus erythematosus, Henoch–Schoenlein purpura, etc.;
    systemic diseases such as diabetes mellitus
  Loss or reduction of glomerular polyanion: minimal change nephrotic syndrome, congenital nephrotic syndrome
  Increased permeability in residual nephrons: end-stage renal disease, postnephrectomy
  Haemodynamic alterations: increased filtration fraction – hyper-reninaemia/angiotension; hyperfiltration in nephrons –
    early stages of diabetes mellitus
  Cause unknown: isolated asymptomatic proteinuria
Non-glomerular causes
  Decreased tubular reabsorption of filtered protein, Fanconi's syndrome, oculocerebrorenal (Lowe's) syndrome,
    galactosaemia, hepatolenticular degeneration, vitamin D intoxication, heavy metal poisoning, analgesic abuse,
    pyelonephritis, acute tubular necrosis, postrenal transplantation
  Overflow proteinuria
    Normal renal function
      Large plasma proteins (albumin) after repeated albumin or blood transfusions
      Smaller plasma proteins or protein fragments with myeloma or macroglobulinaemia
    Decreased renal threshold: albumin infusions in nephrotic syndrome
  Secretory proteinuria
    Tamm–Horsfall proteinuria: neonatal period, pyelonephritis
    Kidney-specific antigens: rapidly progressive glomerulonephritis, analgesic nephropathy
    Other: diseases of prostate and other accessory sex glands
  Histuria
    Tissue-specific antigens: diseases affecting collagen
    Organ-specific antigens: urothelial carcinoma, melanoma, neuroblastoma

Table 2.2. In most instances the cause for the intermittent proteinuria is never determined.

Postural proteinuria

The presence of abnormally increased amounts of protein in urine formed when the patient is in an upright position, but not in urine formed with the patient supine, is referred to as orthostatic or postural proteinuria. Sometimes the terms benign and orthostatic proteinuria are used synonymously. This is not correct. In one study of children in whom benign proteinuria was proven by both renal biopsy and follow-up observations,[27] fewer than half of the children had the classical orthostatic pattern. Some became proteinuric in response to orthostasis but failed to clear the proteinuria during an ensuing recumbent period.

There are other misconceptions about orthostatic proteinuria. It is fixed and reproducible in only 15% of cases. In the remaining patients it is referred to as being variable since not every orthostatic challenge results in proteinuria. Nor is orthostatic proteinuria necessarily mild in amount. Urinary protein concentrations in excess of 1000 mg/dl have been documented in subjects with the classical orthostatic pattern.[27]

The mechanisms responsible for orthostatic proteinuria remain unclear. Alterations in renal or glomerular haemodynamics, renal vein entrapment and an immune-mediated renal parenchymal process have all been postulated to play a role.[27]

Significance

Postural proteinuria was believed to be benign until a systematic study of young males with fixed orthostatic proteinuria demonstrated that

45% of the subjects had subtle alterations in glomerular architecture and that 8% had more severe morphological evidence of renal disease. These observations resulted in a more guarded prognosis for patients with postural proteinuria. Fortunately, a 20-year follow-up of these subjects has indicated that they had a good outcome despite the earlier biopsy findings.[28] None of the subjects had any evidence of significant or progressive renal disease, all had normal renal function, the incidence of hypertension in this population was not different from that in a comparably aged group of the general population, and many of the subjects no longer showed significant proteinuria. Thus, all available evidence indicates that orthostatic proteinuria as an isolated finding is benign.

It is important to emphasize that most patients with glomerular disease will have an orthostatic component to their proteinuria. Protein excretion in these patients is greater when they are active or upright than when they are resting. Thus, it is essential that orthostatic proteinuria should *not* be diagnosed unless the urine which is collected with the subject at rest has *no* protein detectable by routine methods.

Non-postural, intermittent proteinuria

Frequently, intermittent proteinuria cannot be related to posture. It may be found after exercise or in association with some other event such as stress or fever, but often appears to occur on a random basis for which there is no obvious cause.

Significance

It is clear that a high proportion of healthy children have an occasional urine sample which contains protein in detectable concentrations. Although such proteinuria can be indicative of serious disease of the urinary tract, this is the exception rather than the rule. The vast majority of observations have indicated that the intermittent occurrence of protein in the urine, as an isolated finding, does *not* indicate the presence of such disease.

Persistent proteinuria

Persistent proteinuria indicates that protein is found in every urine sample. Typically, in these patients the amount of protein present in individual urine samples may vary considerably. Such proteinuria may continue indefinitely or it may resolve as in acute glomerulonephritis.

Significance

Patients who have persistent proteinuria, especially if this is associated with additional evidence of renal disease, such as microscopic haematuria, are the ones most likely to have significant pathology in the kidney urinary tract. Thus, it is the patient with this type of proteinuria who should be identified by the clinician, so that a detailed diagnostic evaluation can be undertaken.

Causes

In the vast majority of cases, persistent proteinuria is of glomerular origin. However, nonglomerular mechanisms can cause marked proteinuria too. Thus, proteinuria can be classified logically according to the pathophysiological mechanism responsible, as shown in Table 2.2.

Glomerular mechanisms

Any disease which damages the glomerular basement membrane increases glomerular permeability to plasma proteins and typically results in proteinuria. The increased filtered load of protein that results, overwhelms the tubular reabsorptive mechanisms so that the increment in the filtered load of protein cannot be reabsorbed and the majority will appear in the urine.

The acute and chronic glomerulonephritides, irrespective of their aetiology or the type of histological abnormality found, are thought to produce proteinuria by this mechanism. As a group, the glomerulonephritides represent the most common cause for persistent pathological proteinuria. All of these diseases have obvious, severe histological damage in the glomeruli, including abnormalities in the glomerular basement membrane. It is postulated that such injury increases the 'effective pore size' in the glomeruli.[29,30] This increases the permeability of the mechanical barriers to the filtration of proteins and permits an increase, not only in the filtration of albumin, but also of larger proteins such as globulins. In consequence, the clearance of globulins is relatively high and the proteinuria is defined as being non-selective.

A second major mechanism for glomerular proteinuria is loss, or reduction, of the glomerular charge barriers which, in health, contribute to the low permeability of the glomeruli to selected proteins. This results primarily in albuminuria. There is little or no increase in glomerular permeability to globulins, so that the proteinuria is highly selective. The classical cause for this kind of proteinuria is MCNS. For many years it was of great concern that the glomerular histology of this disease showed no pathological abnormalities to explain the proteinuria. It is now known that, during relapses of the disease, the glomeruli show decreased or absent staining for glomerular polyanion, and it has been calculated that such changes would account for the albuminuria.[31] More recently, reduction of glomerular charge sites has been documented in congenital nephrotic syndrome, too, and has been proposed as the mechanism responsible for the proteinuria in this entity.[32] A decrease in glomerular charge sites could also contribute to the albuminuria observed in the glomerulonephritides.

A reduction in nephron mass results in increased glomerular permeability and in increased proteinuria from the residual nephrons. This mechanism probably accounts for the increased proteinuria observed in renal transplant donors and may be responsible for the proteinuria observed in some patients with progressive renal disease such as that due to cystic kidney diseases.

Any increase in filtration fraction will increase plasma protein concentrations at the distal end of the glomerular capillaries to a level above threshold. Such a mechanism has been postulated to explain the proteinuria observed with stress and that associated with high levels of angiotensin.

Some experimental evidence and considerable concern has been expressed recently that the increased transglomerular passage of protein may be responsible for producing permanent glomerular damage and contribute to the development of glomerulosclerosis. If this thesis is proven, efforts to minimize the transglomerular passage of protein in patients with glomerular disease will assume an even greater importance in the management of these patients in the future.[33]

Non-glomerular mechanisms

Since the proximal convoluted tubule normally reabsorbs most of the filtered protein, it is not unexpected that any damage to this segment of the nephron can result in proteinuria. Typically, the amount of protein in the urine resulting from tubular damage is not marked, but cases have been reported in which such proteinuria was sufficient to result in the nephrotic syndrome. Examples of diseases which may induce tubular proteinuria are shown in Table 2.2.

Overflow proteinuria results when the plasma level of a protein exceeds the renal threshold for that protein. This can occur even when kidney function is normal. The protein may or may not be a normal constituent of the blood. For example, plasma albumin concentration may increase sufficiently to cause albuminuria after repeated transfusion of either albumin or whole blood. Alternatively, in multiple myeloma the appearance in the plasma of Bence-Jones protein will result in loss of that protein in the urine and in clinically detectable proteinuria. Similarly, the release of free haemoglobin into the plasma causes the rapid appearance of this protein in the urine, probably because the haemoglobin tetramer dissociates readily into smaller dimers. The haemoglobin is identified as protein when turbidometric methods are used to measure proteinuria. This can represent a diagnostic problem if proteinuria and haemoglobinuria occur simultaneously, for example when haemolysis and renal disease coexist. In such situations, urinary protein electrophoresis can be most useful since haemoglobin migrates as a β_2-globulin. Other tests to quantitate haemoglobin in the urine are available also.

The increased excretion of tissue proteins into the urine may result in proteinuria too, and is referred to as 'secretory proteinuria'. In the neonatal period, losses of Tamm–Horsfall protein account for the higher levels of proteinuria typically seen at this age. Some of the proteinuria observed with the passage of renal stones and with urinary tract infections may result from irritation of the lower urinary tract and the increased secretion of tissue proteins. Inflammation of the accessory sex glands may also cause secretory proteinuria by increased addition to the urine of tissue proteins.

In the future, histuria, or loss of certain antigenic tissue proteins in the urine, may provide important diagnostic information about non-renal diseases. Although the amount of protein lost is not sufficient to be readily identified by screening methods, the topic is referred to here because of its potential importance. Non-specific antigens may be found in diseases which cause damage to basement membrane or collagen. Tissue-specific antigens have been described with endothelial carcinoma, melanoma or neuroblastoma.

Consequences of proteinuria

Proteinuria does not necessarily result in altered levels of protein in the plasma. The liver has considerable reserve capacity for increased production of new proteins and often can compensate for urinary losses. If proteinuria is heavy and protracted and exceeds the patient's ability to synthesize new protein, it will result in hypoproteinaemia and, on occasion, in the nephrotic syndrome.

Evaluation of the patient found to have proteinuria

Since isolated proteinuria is benign in the vast majority of children who have been studied, it is inappropriate to extensively evaluate all children found to have proteinuria. The cost would be prohibitive, the returns small and a great deal of unnecessary anxiety would be generated in many of these children and their families. Conversely, proteinuria may be the presenting abnormality of a serious renal disease in a small proportion of proteinuric children. The challenge facing the physician is to identify this subgroup. Indeed, algorithms have been developed for this purpose.[34] The following outline presents a logical step-by-step approach to address this task. Steps 1–3 can be accomplished at the patient's initial encounter with the physician; steps 4–6 require a return visit or admission to hospital (Figure 2.2).

Step 1: Exclude false positives

Common reasons for false positive results are given in Table 2.1. If it is concluded that the test was positive for one of these reasons, a repeat urine should be tested and shown to be negative.

Cleansing agents used for cleaning the genitalia and detergents in the urine containers are particularly important sources of error.

Step 2: Exclude non-renal causes of proteinuria

Proteinuria can arise in response to *stress* from causes such as pyrexia, exposure to cold or strenuous exercise. *Overflow proteinuria* arises when plasma protein levels increase as a result of protein infusion or disease or states such as multiple myeloma. Proteinuria can occur in *non-renal diseases*, such as congestive cardiac failure.

With the exception of stress, these are not common causes of proteinuria in children.

Step 3: Determine whether the patient has any other evidence of a disease of the kidney or urinary tract

History
A history of oedema, haematuria, polyuria, nocturia, dysuria or colicky abdominal pain may be elicited. Proteinuria may have been demonstrated at a previous examination. There may be a family history of renal failure or deafness.

Examination
Examination may reveal growth failure, hypertension, anaemia, renal tenderness or enlargement, or evidence of renal osteodystrophy.

Urinalysis
Urinalysis may show a concentrating defect (urine specific gravity 1.010). A fresh urine sample should be examined for abnormalities of sediment. Microscopic haematuria is the most common indicator of a glomerular lesion in a proteinuric patient, and the existence of haematuria with proteinuria carries a poorer prognosis than does proteinuria alone. Urine should be examined for blood both with dipstick and microscopy.

If any of the results in this stage suggest the presence of disease of the urinary tract, especially if haematuria is found, the patient requires a more detailed evaluation as outlined in step 5. If the history and physical examination are all negative, then one should proceed to step 4.

Step 4: Further documentation of the proteinuria

The family is provided with a supply of dipsticks and instructed in their use. The urine is tested twice a day for one week. The two urine samples to be checked each day are the first sample passed in the morning as soon as the patient arises, and the last sample of the day voided just before the patient retires to bed. It is important that the patient remains supine throughout the night so that the early morning

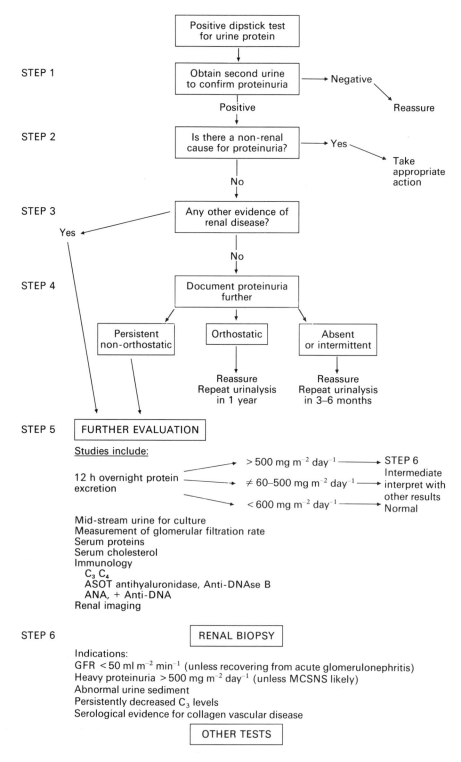

Figure 2.2 Evaluation of proteinuria

urine sample consists of urine formed when the patient was recumbent; in contrast, the evening samples represent urine formed when the patient was upright and active. These records may show:

(a) *Intermittent proteinuria* (or no further proteinuria). There is no evidence that such proteinuria is associated with severe or progressive renal disease. The patient and family are reassured but as a precaution a complete urinalysis is repeated in 3–6 months' time.

(b) *Orthostatic proteinuria* with morning samples *negative* for protein and varying concentrations of protein present in the evening samples. The patient and family are reassured and given an optimistic prognosis. The urine is rechecked in one year to ensure that the initial studies were not misleading.

(c) *Persistent proteinuria* is present if all the urine samples contain protein even though the levels may vary. This does *not* necessarily imply the presence of severe renal disease but it does require that the patient is investigated in more detail as outlined in step 5.

If the family is unable to carry out the dipstick tests in a reliable fashion, two further early morning urine samples are tested for protein. If these are both negative, the patient is reassured but a further sample is tested in 3–6 months.

If one or both of these tests show a positive, the protein excretion rate is measured in a 12 h urine sample collected overnight with the patient at rest. If the value is below 60 mg m^{-2} day^{-1} (i.e. 36 mg/m^2 in the 12 h collection period) the family is reassured. Patients with higher values should be studied and counselled as outlined in step 5. This approach assumes that only persistent proteinuria is associated with a significant increase in urine protein excretion in a 12 h urine collected with the patient supine.

Step 5: The initial further evaluation of patients with persistent proteinuria or those with intermittent proteinuria and other evidence of renal disease

Any patient who reaches this stage of study warrants a thorough evaluation. Too often when a patient has been subjected to a less detailed series of tests than those outlined below, the physician is not able to make authoritative recommendations or to provide adequate reassurance. This is quickly sensed by the family which loses confidence in the physician and requests a second opinion. The recommended tests and their rationale are summarized below.

Urine collection
If not already obtained, an overnight urine collection with the patient supine should be collected to quantitate the proteinuria. Values below 60 mg m^{-2} day^{-1} are normal. Levels above 500 mg m^{-2} day^{-1} are cause for concern and usually indicate the need for a more advanced study, as outlined in step 6. Intermediate values can only be interpreted in conjunction with the remaining test results. Measurement of the protein to creatinine ratio in a random urine sample is obtained as a baseline measurement only. This initial value should not be used to determine the management of the patient at this stage of evaluation.

Urine culture
In at least one series of children with proteinuria, occult urinary tract infections were the most common cause for proteinuria. Thus, collection of a clean-catch urine sample should be a routine part of the evaluation.

Measurement of glomerular filtration rate
A reduction in GFR usually is one of the most important indicators that a renal biopsy is required. Values for serum urea nitrogen and serum creatinine provide useful information from which GFR can be estimated and are measured as a part of our routine evaluation. They are, however, too imprecise for determining the need for a renal biopsy, so that we supplement these values by measuring GFR using one of the clearance methods. We prefer the clearance of inulin, but alternative methods are available and are equally suitable (see Chapter 8).

Even a normal value for GFR provides important information. It represents a useful baseline value that is helpful in monitoring the patient's progress. By measuring GFR, serum urea nitrogen and serum creatinine simultaneously, it permits subsequent monitoring of the patient's renal function by measurements of the latter two tests only. Repeat clearances are necessary only if the blood values indicate that a change in GFR has occurred.

Blood chemistries
Proteinuric subjects do not necessarily have al-

tered levels of protein in their blood. Hypoproteinaemia usually indicates that the patient has had heavy proteinuria for a significant period of time. Such a finding may be an important indicator for a renal biopsy. Total serum protein and serum protein electrophoresis which allows calculation of the serum albumin concentration are measured. This is more reliable than albumin measurements determined by the 'salting-out' methods. Immunological measurements are most accurate but are not always available in a routine laboratory. In addition, serum cholesterol is measured as an indicator of the presence or absence of hyperlipidaemia and the nephrotic syndrome.

Serum levels of the third and fourth components of complement (C3 or β-1-c-globulin and C4) may provide valuable indirect evidence for the existence of a glomerulonephritis. They are measured routinely at this stage of the evaluation.

Serology
Antistreptolysin-O (ASO) and antihyaluronidase titres, antinuclear antibodies (ANA) and anti-DNA antibodies are measured in all of the patients at this stage of study. Indirect evidence is being looked for that the patient may have glomerulonephritis and, based on the authors' experience, the tests are still performed even though the patient may have proteinuria without haematuria. The former two tests provide evidence for a preceding streptococcal infection, but do not indicate whether or not the strain was nephritogenic. Systemic lupus erythematosus may present in such a variety of ways that it was found worth while to look for serological evidence of a collagen vascular disease in any patient with either isolated proteinuria or haematuria or with a combination of these abnormalities.

Radiology
One is attempting to identify an anatomical abnormality of the kidneys or urinary tract. High-resolution ultrasonography provides an excellent non-invasive screening test that will document most abnormalities. However, excretory urography may be required to identify the subtle abnormalities that are often present in the type of patient being discussed here.

Protein selectivity
These measurements have not been found to help

sufficiently in management of proteinuric children to justify routine performance of this test.

Interpretation

If the results of the studies in step 5 are all normal, it is most unlikely that the patient has a serious renal disease responsible for the proteinuria. In reassuring the family, it is emphasized that proteinuria will disappear in many such children and in others proteinuria may persist for protracted periods without any evidence for progressive renal failure developing. The patient is typically seen again in 3 months' time, at which outpatient visit the urinalysis, the measurements of serum urea nitrogen and serum creatinine are repeated and a repeat measurement of the urinary protein to creatinine ratio may be useful. This visit also gives an opportunity to answer the many questions which the family has thought about in the interval. If these repeat test results are satisfactory, it provides another opportunity to give further reassurance. The patient's progress is then monitored twice during the subsequent year and thereafter at yearly intervals.

If all the screening test results are not normal, the subsequent approach to the patient's management represents a matter of judgement. If the documented abnormalities at this stage of study are relatively minor, the patient is usually watched and the abnormal study or studies repeated in 1 or more months' time before making a decision about further investigation. If, on the other hand, the abnormal finding is cause for concern, further evaluation is appropriate. The more common considerations in this advanced testing are analysed in step 6.

Step 6: More advanced evaluation of selected patients: approach and interpretation

Renal biopsy
Not all proteinuric patients warrant a renal biopsy. Indeed, there is a current trend to obtain a renal histological diagnosis in fewer patients. This is based on the argument that the biopsy does not influence management of many of the patients. We do not agree totally with this argument. Knowledge of the underlying disease process may not affect the immediate recommended therapy, but it can be most beneficial in discussing prognosis with the family. Thus,

our guidelines for renal biopsy are more liberal than some found elsewhere.

The findings on urinalysis are important when determining the need for a biopsy. Renal histology is more likely to be diagnostic when proteinuria is associated with urinary sediment abnormalities than when either proteinuria or haematuria are isolated abnormalities. Other test results also provide important indications for the need for a histological diagnosis. A reduction in GFR below 50 ml m^{-2} min^{-1} surface area usually indicates the need for this procedure. The exception is the patient who is recovering from an acute glomerulonephritis. In such patients, GFR should be remeasured in approximately 1 month to confirm the initial clinical diagnosis of an acute resolving glomerular disease.

The heavier the proteinuria, the more likely a tissue diagnosis will be established from the biopsy. Thus, we usually recommend biopsy for patients with heavy proteinuria, especially that in excess of 500 mg m^{-2} day^{-1}. Again, there is an exception. Patients under the age of 6 years who have typical features of MCNS may have heavy proteinuria, but do not need to have this diagnosis confirmed by biopsy unless a trial of steroids has shown them to be resistant to this therapy. Other patients with MCNS who require a biopsy include those who have frequent relapses or those who are steroid dependent (see Chapter 18).

Other potential indications for a renal biopsy include a persistent decrease below normal in C3 levels or serological evidence for a collagen vascular disease. We have found, as have others, that the severity or type of renal involvement in systemic lupus erythematosus (SLE) does not always correlate with the findings on urine sediment. Thus, the absence of haematuria or red cell casts does not exclude a serious glomerulonephritis due to SLE.

Occasionally the family of a proteinuric child can be reassured only if the renal histology is known. This can be an important indicator for performing renal biopsy.

Trial of steroids

If the screening evaluation shows the typical laboratory picture of MCNS and the patient is under 6 years of age, it may be appropriate to institute a therapeutic trial of steroids. A renal biopsy would be performed only if the proteinuria does not resolve within 28 days of starting treatment with oral prednisone in a daily dose of at least 2 mg/kg body weight.

The authors have cared for several children who had isolated proteinuria which persisted for several years. Mild hypo-albuminaemia was the only associated abnormality. The renal biopsy showed no histological abnormality other than a moderate degree of fusion of podocytes. A trial of steroids was followed by a protracted or apparently permanent remission of proteinuria in approximately half of these cases.

Tubular disorders

If it is suspected from the history or from the findings of eosinophils in the urine that proteinuria results from an interstitial nephritis or from some other disease process that modifies proximal tubule function, measurement of the urinary excretion of β_2-microglobulin (β_2M) can be most helpful. The fractional excretion of β_2M normally is considerably less than 0.5%. With tubular disorders, values may increase to more than 50%. Similar high values are not seen with glomerular disease even when renal function is markedly decreased. From a practical viewpoint, urine concentrations of β_2M correlate well with the fractional excretion of this protein. A urine β_2M concentration above 1 mg/litre strongly suggests proximal tubule dysfunction.

Other tests

The presence of a urinary tract infection or abnormalities on the excretory urogram may indicate the need for more extensive evaluation of the lower urinary tract. The existence of severe hypertension may justify further study, too. Similarly, evidence of tubular dysfunction may warrant an evaluation to determine the cause and whether other abnormalities of tubular function exist.

Conclusions

It is important to re-emphasize that the majority of patients with isolated proteinuria do not have progressive renal disease. However, once it is determined that a proteinuric patient warrants further study, we recommend that this investigation be thorough. This is especially so since the degree of proteinuria correlates with outcome[35] as well as the rate of progression of the underlying renal disease.[36] Thus, current efforts are concentrating on ways to reduce proteinuria using drugs such as inhibitors of angiotension converting enzyme[37] or of prostaglandin synthesis.[38] At the end of the studies, the physician must be able to answer in an authoritative manner the multitude of questions that will be posed by the typical family. If the results of the tests indicate no cause for concern, reassurance should include a discussion about 'folk-remedies' and some of the common misconceptions advised by well-meaning but usually poorly informed friends or relatives. For example, a proteinuric patient who had had a partial evaluation 1 year earlier was referred to the authors. The physician had not been able to assuage the family's fear and the child was kept on bed rest for a year on the advice of a friend who told them such bed rest would reduce the degree of proteinuria. Complete evaluation indicated no cause for concern and the patient was able to return to a normal life style.

References

1. Robson A.M. Proteinuria and the nephrotic syndrome. In: Klahr S. (ed.) *The Kidney and Body Fluids in Health and Disease*, 2nd ed. New York, Plenum Medical Book Company, 1984: 369–398
2. Brenner B.M., Hostetter T.H. and Humes H.D. Molecular basis of proteinuria of glomerular origin. *N. Engl. J. Med.* 1978, **298**, 826–833
3. Cotran R.S. and Rennke H.G. Anionic sites and the mechanisms of proteinuria (Editorial). *N. Engl. J. Med.* 1983, **309**, 1050–1052
4. Ryan G.B. and Karnovsky M.J. Distribution of endogenous albumin in the rat glomerulus. Role of hemodynamic factors in glomerular barrier function. *Kidney Int.*, 1976, **9**, 36–45
5. Renkin E.M. and Gilmore J.P. *Renal Physiology*. Washington, D.C., American Physiological Society, 1973: Chapter 9
6. Ginevri F., Mutti A., Ghiggeri G.M., Alinovi R., Ciardi M.R., Bergamaschi E., Verrina E. and Gusmano R. Urinary excretion of brush border antigens and other proteins in children with vesico-ureteric reflux. *Pediatr. Nephrol.*, 1992, **6**, 30–32
7. Barratt T.M. Proteinuria (Editorial). *Br. Med. J.* 1983, **287**, 1489–1490
8. Buffone G.J. Specific protein measurements in pediatric laboratory medicine. In: Hicks J.M. and Boecky R.L. (eds) *Pediatric Clinical Chemistry*. Philadelphia, W.B. Saunders, 1984: 447–481
9. Davies A.G., Postlethwaite R.J., Price D.A., Burn J.L., Houlton C.A. and Fielding B.A. Urinary albumin secre-

tion in school children. *Arch. Dis. Child.* 1984, **59**, 625–630
10. Brem A.S. Neonatal haematuria and proteinuria. *Clinics Perinatol.* 1981, **8**, 321–332
11. Ginsberg J.M., Chang B.S., Matarese R.A. and Garella S. Use of single voided urine samples to estimate quantitative proteinuria. *N. Engl. J. Med.* 1983, **309**, 1543–1546
12. Houser M. Assessment of proteinuria using random urine samples. *J. Pediatr.* 1984, **104**, 845–848
13. Barratt T.M., McLaine P.N. and Soothill J.F. Albumin secretion as a measure of glomerular dysfunction in children. *Arch. Dis. Child.* 1970, **45**, 496–501
14. Houser M.T., Jahn M.F., Kobayashi A. and Walburn J. Assessment of urinary protein excretion in the adolescent: effect of body position and exercise. *J. Pediatr.* 1986, **109**, 556–561
15. Yoshimoto M., Tsukahara H., Saito M., Hayashi S., Haruki S., Fujisawa S. and Sudo M. Evaluation of variability of proteinuria indices. *Pediatr. Nephrol.* 1990, **4**, 136–139
16. Mogensen C.E. and Christensen C.K. Predicting diabetic nephropathy in insulin-dependent patients. *N. Engl. J. Med.* 1984, **311**, 84–93
17. Ries M., Scharer K., Wartha R., Schmidt H. and Gehle D. Microheterogeneity of urinary albumin and tubular proteinuria in juvenile diabetes mellitus. *Pediatr. Nephrol.* 1991, **5**, 582–586
18. Donaldson M.D.C., Chambers R.E., Woolridge M.W. and Whicher J.T. Alpha$_1$-microglobulin, beta$_2$-microglobulin and retinol binding protein in childhood febrile illness and renal disease. *Pediatr. Nephrol.* 1990, **4**, 314–318
19. Brocklebank J.T., Cooper E.H. and Richmond K. Sodium dodecyl sulphate polyacrylamide gel electrophoresis patterns of proteinuria in various renal diseases of childhood. *Pediatr. Nephrol.* 1991, **5**, 371–375
20. Ellis D. and Buffone G.J. Protein clearances and selectivity determinations in childhood nephrosis: a reappraisal. *Clin. Chem.* 1981, **27**, 1397–1400
21. Vehaskari V.M. and Rapola J. Isolated proteinuria: analysis of a schoolage population. *J. Pediatr.* 1982, **101**, 661–668
22. Dodge W.F., West E.F., Smith E.H. and Bunce H. III. Proteinuria and hematuria in schoolchildren: epidemiology and early natural history. *J. Pediatr.* 1976, **88**, 327–347
23. Murakami M., Yamamoto H., Ueda Y., Murakami K. and Yamauchi K. Urinary screening of elementary and junior high-school children over a 13-year period in Tokyo. *Pediatr. Nephrol.* 1991, **5**, 50–53
24. Iitaka K., Igarashi S. and Sakai T. Hypocomplementemia and membranoproliferative glomerulonephritis in school urinary screening in Japan. *Pediatr. Nephrol.* 1994, **8**
25. Kitagawa T. Lessons learned from the Japanese nephritis screening study. *Pediatr. Nephrol.* 1988, **2**, 256–263
26. Sinniah R., Law C.H. and Pwee H.S. Glomerular lesions in patients with asymptomatic persistent and orthostatic

proteinuria discovered on routine medical examination. *Clin. Nephrol.* 1977, **7**, 1–14

27. Vehaskari V.M. Mechanism of orthostatic proteinuria. *Pediatr. Nephrol.* 1990, **4**, 328–330

28. Springberg P.D., Garrett L.E. Jr., Thompson A.L. Jr., Collins N.F., Lordon R.E. and Robinson R.R. Fixed and reproducible orthostatic proteinuria: results of a 20-year follow-up study. *Ann. Intern. Med.* 1982, **97**, 516–519

29. Robson A.M. and Cole B.R. Pathologic and functional correlations in the glomerulopathies. In: *Immune Mechanisms in Renal Disease.* Michael A.F. and Wilson C.B. (eds), New York, Plenum Medical Book Company, 1983: 109–127

30. Myers B.D., Okarma T.B., Friedman S., Bridges C., Ross J., Asseff S. and Deen W.M. Mechanisms of proteinuria in human glomerulonephritis. *J. Clin. Invest.* 1982, **70**, 732–746

31. Carrie B.J., Salyer W.R. and Myers B.D. Minimal change nephropathy: an electrochemical disorder of the glomerular membrane. *Am. J. Med. 1981,* **70**, 262–268

32. Vernier R.L., Klein D.J., Sisson S.P., Mahan J.D., Oegema T.R. and Brown D.M. Heparan sulfate-rich anionic sites in the human glomerular basement membrane. Decreased concentration in congenital nephrotic syndrome. *N. Engl. J. Med.* 1983, **309**, 1001–1009

33. Klahr S., Schreiner G. and Ichikawa I. The progression of kidney disease. *N. Engl. J. Med.* 1988, **318**, 1657–1666

34. Burke E.C. and Stickler G.B. Proteinuria in children. Review and evaluation. *Clin. Pediatr.* 1982, **21**, 741–743

35. Hisano S. and Ueda K. Asymptomatic haematuria and proteinuria: renal pathology and clinical outcome in 54 children. *Pediatr. Nephrol.* 1989, **3**, 229–234

36. Walser M. Progression of chronic renal failure in man. *Kidney Int.* 1990, **37**, 1195–1210

37. Milliner D.S. and Morgenstern B.Z. Angiotensin converting enzyme inhibitors for reduction of proteinuria in children with steroid-resistant nephrotic syndrome. *Pediatr. Nephrol.* 1991, **5**, 587–590

38. Bergstein J.M. Prostaglandin inhibitors in the treatment of nephrotic syndrome. *Pediatr. Nephrol.* 1991, **5**, 335–338

3

Oedema

K. Schärer

Oedema denotes an abnormal increase in the volume of interstitial fluid that is apparent on physical examination. It may be localized or generalized. When generalized oedema is mild, the only manifestation may be an increase in body weight, or it may be detectable only in localized areas. With more extensive fluid retention, peri-orbital oedema develops and subsequently pretibial oedema, particularly after a long period of being upright. Peri-orbital oedema is usually considered initially to be allergic in origin, and this is most often the case; it must, however, be remembered that it might be the first manifestation of generalized oedema.

Localized oedema

The sudden onset of oedema in a localized area should suggest the possibility of an insect bite, a localized infective process, or trauma. Painful swelling of the dorsa of the hands and feet can occur in sickle cell disease and Henoch–Schoenlein syndrome. Oedema of an extremity should suggest localized vascular obstruction, either venous or lymphatic, acquired or congenital in origin. Oedema of the extremities is seen in Turner's syndrome and is related to peripheral lymphoedema.

Generalized oedema

The important causes of generalized oedema are listed in Table 3.1. Rarely does the differential diagnosis of oedema present a clinical problem – the underlying disease process is usually obvious. Additionally the clinical circumstances dictate different differential diagnoses. Thus the likely causes in a well toddler presenting with mild peri-orbital oedema are different from those in the acutely sick infant in the intensive care unit. Indeed, in this latter situation the precise pathophysiological mechanisms are often difficult to define. History and physical examination, urinalysis and measurement of serum albumin are the initial assessments in a patient with oedema.

Generalized oedema can be seen in allergic reactions, where it is more properly called angio-oedema. It is seen in drug reactions, serum sickness and anaphylaxis. Recurrent angio-oedema suggests the possibility of C1 esterase deficiency. Allergic reactions are generally much less dramatic with mild peri-orbital oedema associated with common conditions such as hay fever. To avoid the embarrassment of failing to diagnose the occasional case of nephrotic syndrome in these circumstances, the urine should always be tested for protein.

A renal cause for oedema will be suggested by the presence of hypertension, cardiac enlargement, pulmonary and peripheral oedema, haematuria, proteinuria, red cell casts and elevation of blood urea and creatinine.

Congestive heart failure is recognized by a history of poor feeding, sweating, respiratory difficulty and irritability and, on examination, tachycardia, tachypnoea, congestion of the

Table 3.1 Clinical conditions associated with oedema formation in children

Renal diseases	Nephrotic syndrome
	Glomerulonephritis
	Acute renal failure
	Chronic renal failure
Heart failure	
Liver diseases	Cirrhosis
	Hepatic venous outflow obstruction
Others	Venocaval obstruction
	Hypothyroidism
	Capillary leak syndrome
In newborns	Physiological
	Hypoxia *in utero*
	Hyaline membrane disease
	Erythroblastosis fetalis
	Lymphoedema
	Congenital ascites
	Turner's syndrome
	Cystic fibrosis

lungs, enlargement of the heart with gallop, passive congestion of the abdominal organs and peripheral oedema. The urinalysis is usually normal, although the urine sodium is low and mild proteinuria may be present. The blood urea and creatinine may be elevated.

In oedema due to liver disease there is usually additional evidence of altered liver function, including reduced serum albumin, elevation in bilirubin and transaminases and bilirubin in the urine. Clinical features might include jaundice, spider naevi, emaciation, distended abdomen with ascites, collateral circulation over the abdomen and palpable liver.

Hypoproteinaemia without proteinuria would suggest severe malabsorption or protein-losing enteropathy. There may be other indications of poor nutrition such as iron-deficiency oedema.

Capillary leak syndromes may give rise to generalized oedema without proteinuria or reduced serum albumin. This may occur in generalized vasculitis (systemic lupus erythematosus, dermatomyositis, polyarteritis nodosa and mixed connective tissue disease).

Less frequent causes of oedema would include idiopathic oedema, excessive adrenocorticol steroids either exogenous or endogenous, for example, Conn's syndrome, and certain drugs.

Mechanisms of oedema formation in nephrotic and nephritic patients

The nephrotic syndrome (NS) (see Chapters 18 and 19) is the most frequent renal disorder leading to generalized oedema in children. As a result of massive protein losses by urine, changes in the extracellular fluid volume (ECFV), haemodynamic disturbances and alterations in the renal handling of sodium and calcium occur.

Under physiological circumstances sodium (Na) balance is well maintained in healthy children with a renal Na excretion adjusted closely to Na intake. High Na intake and expansion of the ECFV are associated with a high ratio of Na excretion. In contrast, low Na intake, hypovolaemia, dehydration and haemorrhage lead to Na retention. This regulating mechanism seems to work inadequately in oedematous states resulting in a rise of ECFV.

The *pathophysiological factors* involved in oedema formation have been intensively investigated in recent years.[1–49] They consist of (a) local mechanisms acting on the capillary wall, including changes in the intraglomerular haemodynamics; (b) changes in ECFV; and (c) activation of hormone systems regulating Na and water retention.

Capillary mechanisms leading to interstitial fluid accumulation are based on a disturbance of Starling forces which determine the distribution of fluid between the intravascular and interstitial fluid compartments. Physiologically these forces of the arterial end of the capillary cause a filtration pressure of about 8 mmHg, resulting in a fluid movement of the capillary into the interstitial space; at the venous end the net pressure is about 1.5 mmHg lower, which forces the movement of fluid from the interstitial tissue back to the capillary. The process of filtration and reabsorption manifests itself as the net effect of capillary and tissue hydraulic pressure and of plasma and tissue osmotic pressures which determine the direction of fluid through the capillary.

According to the classical concept of transcapillary fluid exchange, the balance of Starling forces favours the filtration of plasma at the arterial end of capillaries, while at the venous side these forces favour the uptake of fluid from the interstitial space. This concept of balanced filtration/reabsorption has been challenged by the finding that transcapillary

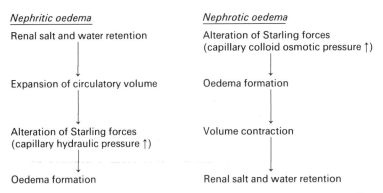

Figure 3.1 Proposed scheme of oedema formation in patients with glomerular disease

hydraulic pressure physiologically exceeds the opposing colloid osmotic pressure through the whole length of certain capillary beds. Consequently, filtration may occur along the entire capillary length.[5]

The *increase in lymphatic drainage* and the ability of lymph vessels to expand and proliferate in response to increased amounts of fluid in the interstitial space plays an important role in the removal of accumulated fluid. In addition, the increased lymph flow leads to a 'wash-out' of interstitial protein and thereby lowers the colloid osmotic pressure, which reduces fluid filtration.[6] The low compliance of the interstitial tissue contributes to the defence against oedema formation, since fluid accumulation in its space increases tissue pressure and thereby opposes capillary filtration. Nephrotic oedema develops only when fluid accumulation reaches a critical point where tissue becomes compliant and lymphatic drainage is no more effective.

The above concept is supported by the finding that the protein content of the tissue fluid is lowered in adult patients during the recovery phase of acute nephrotic syndrome,[7] suggesting that an increased lymph flow helps to maintain intravascular volume in this condition and prevents fluid accumulation in the interstitium.

In principle, capillary oedema may develop by two mechanisms: (a) when the capillary hydraulic pressure increases as a result of constant elevation of plasma volume (nephritic oedema); and (b) when colloid osmotic pressure in plasma drops (nephrotic oedema) (Figure 3.1). Neither increased capillary filtration nor decreased plasma colloid osmotic pressure alone are suffi-

cient to produce oedema. In the presence of normal renal function, a rise in capillary filtration with subsequent expansion of ECFV results in increased natriuresis.[6] On the other hand, low plasma colloid osmotic pressure *per se* does not produce oedema as demonstrated by patients with congenital analbuminaemia. Nevertheless, the decreased plasma albumin concentration is related to oedema formation in NS because the degree of oedema correlates to some extent with the severity of hypoalbuminaemia.[8] In nephrotic children, oedema usually develops when serum albumin is reduced below 20 g/litre; pleural effusion and ascites become apparent when this level falls below 15 g/litre.[9]

Renal mechanisms

Impairment of renal sodium handling plays a major role in the development of both the nephritic and nephrotic types of oedema (Figure 3.1).

In the presence of a normal glomerular filtration rate (GFR), adaptations of tubular functions permit Na and water homeostasis to occur over a wide range of intakes. If glomerular or tubular functions are disturbed, retention of fluid and electrolytes may result in oedema formation. Although reduction of GFR is rare in idiopathic NS, it may occur as a consequence of hypovolaemia with reduced renal perfusion. Intravascular volume depletion leads to a fall in glomerular capillary hydraulic pressure and activates vasoconstrictor factors to raise efferent arteriolar resistance.[10] This activation may produce a rise in GFR in spite of hypovolaemia.

A more pronounced decrease of intravascular volume, however, is associated with a persistent fall of the glomerular capillary blood flow (QA) and a reduction of the glomerular capillary ultrafiltration coefficient (K_f).[11] As a result, profound hypovolaemia with acute renal failure may be observed in NS. A low GFR associated with normal renal plasma flow has been described in NS, suggesting that factors in addition to hypoperfusion may cause a low GFR in this syndrome.[12,13] An alternative explanation for the acute renal failure in NS is an increase in tubular hydrostatic pressure, perhaps due to tubular casts of inspissated proteins.

In rats with NS induced by puromycin aminonucleoside, *glomerular microcirculation* is altered, associated with a reduced GFR, a small reduction of QA and a pronounced decline in K_f.[11] Similar changes may play a role in man. In adults with minimal change NS, depressed GFR was reported despite elevated ECFV and mild hypertension.[12] A local generation of angiotensin II may mediate these glomerular microcirculatory changes.[11]

The exact *tubular site and mechanism* of Na retention in the nephrotic kidney is not known. Previous clinical and experimental studies demonstrated an *enhanced proximal tubular* Na reabsorption in the nephrotic state. In children with minimal change NS, proximal Na reabsorption seems to be enhanced during relapse as opposed to remission.[14] According to micropuncture studies in nephrotic rats, this may be secondary to impaired tubular fluid flow.[15]

More recently, *enhanced free water clearance* was observed in adults with NS in response to head-out water immersion,[16] which is consistent with the data that a low solute free water clearance during relapse increased during remission of nephrotic children.[14] According to these authors, impaired water excretion reflects increased Na reabsorption in the proximal portion of the nephron, with a diminished distal delivery.

In contrast, other authors reported that *proximal Na reabsorption was decreased* in experimental animals and adult patients with NS,[11] which might be explained by changes of peritubular Starling forces. This view is supported by the observation that peritubular plasma protein concentrations and hence colloid osmotic pressure were significantly depressed in nephrotic rat kidneys, while peritubular capillary hydraulic pressure did not differ from controls.[11] The net effect of these changes would inhibit proximal Na reabsorption. Evidence for decreased proximal Na reabsorption has also been obtained in children with minimal change NS.[17]

In general, most studies show a well-preserved glomerulotubular balance in NS, so that Na retention could not be attributed exclusively to disturbed proximal fluid reabsorption. Therefore, progressive sodium retention appears to result rather from a reduced filtered load with constant or increased fractional fluid reabsorption in distal nephron segments.

In fact, some authors have suggested that antinatriuresis in NS may primarily be due to changes in the *distal tubule* or the collecting duct.[11] Bohlin and Berg demonstrated an increase of the fractional Na excretion to normal values after administration of furosemide in children with minimal change NS and concluded that Na retention is related to intrarenal mechanisms located in the distal parts of the nephron.[18]

It seems that the site of Na retention in NS may depend on the alteration of intravascular volume.[4] In the case of volume depletion, which is usually encountered in minimal change NS, changes in peritubular Starling forces may enhance proximal tubular sodium reabsorption to maintain body fluid volume, and thus GFR, adequately.[6,14] In contrast, in the presence of normal or elevated plasma volume, increased sodium reabsorption at the more distal part of the nephron may predominate.[11]

Alteration of intravascular volume

According to the classical concept, *reduced intravascular volume* is essential for oedema formation and sodium retention (Figure 3.2).[19] Urinary loss of protein results in a fall of plasma colloid osmotic pressure and thereby leads to an imbalance of Starling forces at the level of peripheral capillaries, which in turn entails a movement of plasma, water and electrolytes into the interstitial space. If the continuously produced fluid cannot be removed by exaggerated lymph flow, plasma volume becomes contracted and the circulation 'underfilled'.

In general, clinical data have supported this traditional concept of the afferent mechanism leading to Na and water retention. Total plasma volume (PV) was found to be reduced in about half of the nephrotic patients.[20,21] Meltzer *et*

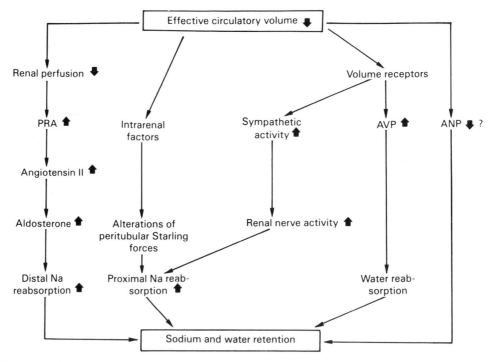

Figure 3.2 Proposed mechanisms involved in the pathogenesis of oedema formation in nephrotic syndrome (PRA, plasma renin activity; AVP, arginine vasopressin; ANP, atrial natriuretic peptide; Na, sodium)

al.[22] described a low PV in adult NS patients mainly in presence of a high plasma renin activity (PRA), which in turn was associated with minimal change lesions, whereas patients with membranous or membranoproliferative glomerulonephritis tended to have suppressed PRA and normal or elevated PV. A review of 10 studies from the literature revealed that PV in minimal change NS was reduced in 38% and elevated in 14% of patients.[12]

The 'overflow' concept postulates a primary defect in renal Na excretion, resulting in an increased ECFV, whereas according to the 'underfilling' theory a decrease in the effective PV triggers vasoconstrictor and sodium-retaining hormone activity. The failure to demonstrate that the vascular compartment is underfilled in the early stages of nephrotic oedema does not exclude the hypothesis of underfilling. It is the nature of homeostatic regulation that the regulated value is kept nearly constant; regulatory changes may well have occurred before patients could be investigated.

It should be stressed that all clinical studies are hampered by the fact that the *exact measurement of PV is difficult*, mainly for two methodological reasons: (a) postural changes – in normal men in upright posture, the true PV is 5% less than the measured PV, and in the hypoalbuminaemic state up to 15% less;[23] (b) a rapid transcapillary escape of injected iodinated albumin may lead to falsely elevated values, although this technique would account for an overestimation of only 3%.[24] The divergent opinions on these methodological problems cannot be solved at present.[25,26] By measuring total PV and blood volume with current methods during various stages of oedema formation in NS, it cannot be decided whether hyopovolaemia is in fact present. However, from studies of vasoactive hormones (Figure 3.3), there is good evidence for reduced ECFV,[27] defined as a state of fullness of the arterial compartment in relation to its holding capacity.

Humoral factors, able to mediate an increased reabsorption of tubular fluid and sodium, have been explored in a number of studies. The *renin–angiotensin–aldosterone system* has been investigated most extensively. Activation of this system depends on the maintenance of intravascular volume. If the latter is depleted, as frequently found in patients with steroid-sensitive

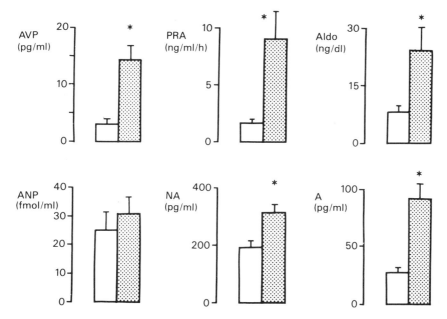

Figure 3.3 Plasma concentrations of arginine vasopressin (AVP), renin activity (PRA), aldosterone (Aldo), atrial natriuretic peptide (ANP), noradrenaline (NA) and adrenaline (A) in children with nephrotic syndrome during oedema formation (stippled bars, *n* = 17) and in healthy age-matched controls (open bars, *n* = 15). Plasma ANP was studied in 9 patients and 9 controls only. Mean ± SEM is given. *P < 0.01 (After Rascher and Tulassay[27])

NS, the activated renin–angiotensin–aldosterone system may contribute to renal Na retention. Elevated levels of PRA and of aldosterone in plasma and urine have indeed been observed in many clinical and experimental studies on the NS, including children (Figure 3.3).[28–31] Other investigations have reported low or normal PRA in the presence of sodium retention.[22,32] Although PRA correlates inversely with plasma albumin concentration, there is no significant relationship between PRA and either sodium retention or GFR. PRA also fails to correlate with blood volume.[33] The excretion of aldosterone and its metabolites as well as of 18-hydroxycorticosterone is increased in about half of the children with NS even in the absence of oedema, and a significant correlation is found between aldosterone and Na excretion.[28] Aldosterone seems, therefore, to have a limited role in the sodium retention of NS.[22,28,34] Spironolactone caused an increased sodium excretion in NS in the absence of any changes in blood pressure or GFR despite similar levels of plasma aldosterone before and after drug administration.[34] It is assumed that in this situation tubular sensitivity to aldosterone is enhanced in NS patients.

Noradrenaline, another vasoactive hormone, has been found to be elevated in the plasma of oedematous children with minimal change NS.[27] As an indicator of increased sympathetic activity, the high noradrenaline levels are interpreted as the result of volume depletion. If the plasma volume of nephrotic children is expanded by albumin infusion or by head-out water immersion, the elevated plasma noradrenaline levels are normalized.[30,31] Noradrenaline may enhance proximal tubular Na reabsorption either directly, by stimulation of renin release, or by vasoconstriction predominantly on the efferent arteriole.[4]

In the past few years special attention has been directed towards the *renal dopaminergic system* in the regulation of Na metabolism.[35] Dopamine blockade was found to reduce natriuresis induced by water immersion in normal man.[36] However, the exact role of the renal dopaminergic system in the regulation of sodium homeostasis in NS is not yet defined.

Hypovolaemia is the most important non-osmotic stimulus for *vasopressin* release in man. Rascher and Tulassay[27] observed that in children with NS, mean basal vasopressin levels in plasma are markedly elevated during oedema formation, but not after remission. In the nephrotic state these children were slightly hypo-osmolar and hyponatraemic compared with values during remission, indicating that the stimulus for vasopressin secretion is of non-osmotic nature. The higher haematocrit values during relapse of children with NS indicate that reduction of the effective circulatory blood volume may be responsible for the elevated vasopressin secretion in these patients. This is supported by studies in children with active NS using albumin infusion and water immersion to expand central blood volume. These manoeuvres result in a drop in plasma vasopressin to near normal levels and a reduction of haematocrit without any changes of plasma osmolality.[30,31] Although earlier studies have given contradictory results,[21] it may be concluded that at least in children with steroid-sensitive minimal change NS, vasopressin contributes to the impaired water excretion.[27]

Renal prostaglandins play an important role in the maintenance of renal haemodynamics and in urinary sodium excretion.[37] During the active stage of NS when vasoconstrictive hormones are stimulated, renal perfusion is maintained by renal prostaglandins. In children with NS, a slightly elevated excretion of urinary PGE_2 has been reported.[31] The concept of renal hypoperfusion in NS is supported by the findings that inhibition of prostaglandin synthesis in NS causes a significant decrese in GFR.[38]

For many years, attempts have been made to prove that a *natriuretic factor* is missing in NS.[39] The role of atrial natriuretic peptide (ANP) in the maintenance of sodium and water homeostasis is now well established. In nephrotic children, albumin infusion caused a five-fold increase in plasma ANP with a simultaneous decrease in PRA, vasopressin and noradrenaline. In addition the albumin-induced changes in Na and water excretion and GFR correlated with changes in ANP, but not with plasma aldosterone. These and other findings suggest the conclusion that ANP plays an important role in mediating changes of sodium homeostasis in NS.[31,40]

The common mechanism which triggers all the hormonal changes described in children with NS is a *reduced effective circulatory volume*. A low central blood volume and central venous pressure reduces renal perfusion and activates volume receptors, thereby stimulating vasoconstrictor hormones. Na and water retention in NS are the results of both these hormonal changes and the intrarenal factors described above (Figure 3.2). This view is supported by the fact that central volume expansion induced either by headout water immersion or by infusion of concentrated albumin solution is able to correct elevated plasma hormone levels and to induce diuresis and natriuresis in children with idiopathic NS.[30,31] Besides the suppression of vasoconstrictor hormones, the release of ANP following albumin infusion appears to be the *major trigger* for the therapeutic induction of diuresis and natriuresis in these patients.

Treatment of oedema

Each kilogram of oedema fluid represents about 140 mmol of accumulated Na. Reduction of Na intake by dietary restriction and augmentation of Na excretion by administration of diuretics are obviously the preferred modes of oedema treatment. It is usually impossible to reduce Na intake to less than 1 mmol kg^{-1} day^{-1}. A mild Na restriction corresponds to a Na intake of about 1–2 mmol kg^{-1} day^{-1}, which is often difficult to adhere to over longer periods. In chronic cases the help of a dietitian whose advice is based on a 3-day protocol of actual dietary intake should be sought. In severe cases associated with sudden oliguria, e.g. in acute renal failure or in the nephrotic state, fluid intake should be restricted. In most children with renal oedema, however, the use of diuretics is indicated.

Since the bulk of Na reabsorption occurs in the proximal renal tubule, it seems that proximally acting diuretics such as acetazolamide would be most effective in promoting diuresis. In fact, the high capacity of the distal tubule to increase solute reabsorption largely negates the effect of proximally acting drugs. The most potent diuretic agents block Na reabsorption in the ascending limb of the loop of Henle, although this segment normally accounts for only 15–20% of the filtered load. The more distal parts of the nephron are not able to increase Na reabsorption considerably as the delivery from the loop increases.

Furosemide and *ethacrynic acid* are the most frequent loop blockers. Furosemide is a weak organic acid which acts not only by augmenting Na transport but also by intrarenal haemodynamic effects (increased prostaglandin synthesis), explaining its reduced natriuretic effect when administered together with non-steroid anti-inflammatory drugs. At low excretion rates there is little natriuretic effect; at medium ranges, natriuresis increases markedly as drug excretion increases, but at higher drug excretion rates a plateau phase is observed.[41] The dosage of furosemide is therefore best determined by a progressive increase (titration on an individual basis) until the effective dose is established. Subsequently, this dose should be repeated up to four times daily as needed.[41] In adults, the plateau dosage is reached at a dose of about 4–5 mg kg^{-1} day^{-1} and sometimes as low as 2.5 mg kg^{-1} day^{-1}.

As the incidence of gastrointestinal side effects and ototoxicity of furosemide increases with dosage, more than 5 mg kg^{-1} day^{-1} should not be given as a single dose. The high potency of the drug is expected to be due to the fact that the maximal fractional Na excretion after an oral dose rises dramatically (to about 20–30% of the filtered load). The effect lasts for 6–8 h after oral, but only for 2–3 h after intravenous administration.

Thiazides are also acting primarily on the distal tubules but have a proximal effect, too. They are safe and inexpensive and should be the first choice in patients with *normal* renal function. If serum creatinine is above 200 μmol/litre they have little effect and should be replaced by furosemide. The effect of *hydrochlorothiazide* is of relatively short duration. This drug should be given twice a day (1–3 mg kg^{-1} day^{-1}), whereas *chlorthalidone* should be given only once (0.5–1 mg kg^{-1} day^{-1}). With both drugs the course of action is 2 h after an oral dose and the maximal fractional Na excretion is about 5–8% of the filtered load. *Metolazone*, a drug with a similar action to thiazides, should only be given once per 24 h and has the further advantage of retaining efficacy in the presence of a markedly reduced renal function.

Spironolactone is an agent which acts by blocking potassium-linked Na reabsorption in the late distal tubule and collecting duct. It is a competitive inhibitor of aldosterone and may therefore be indicated in case of hyperaldosteronism in nephrotic syndrome. It is usually started at an oral dose of 2 mg kg^{-1} day^{-1} up to 6 mg kg^{-1} day^{-1} in 2 doses. Its diuretic effect becomes maximal only after several days.

It may be combined with hydrochlorothiazide or furosemide. In renal failure it is contraindicated. *Triamterene* and *amiloride* are further diuretics which block potassium secretion in the distal tubule independent of the aldosterone status, but little information is available on their use in children. All these agents have a limited efficacy because maximal fractional Na excretion attained is only 2–3% of the filtered load. Their use in renal failure is generally contraindicated.

Multiple side effects have been described with the various diuretic agents mentioned above. Most of them are related to electrolyte homeostasis. Excessive volume depletion and hyponatraemia by excessive diuresis followed by collapse may be observed with all these drugs. The decrease in PV may be associated with reduced GFR and (non-osmotic) ADH release. Alkalosis and hypokalaemia are seen after application of furosemide and thiazides; in such instances, potassium supplements should be given routinely, except in cases of severe hyperaldosteronism.

Diuretic 'resistance' may occur by non-compliance or by a concomitant increase in salt intake, less frequently by diminished bioavailability of the drug following bowel oedema (e.g. in nephrotic syndrome). In congestive heart failure, where proximal Na reabsorption may be markedly increased, the distally acting diuretics lose their action. When GFR is markedly reduced, diuretic therapy becomes ineffective. Extrarenal drug metabolism may then become important for elimination.[42]

In the case of diuretic resistance, combination therapy may be useful, e.g. by giving a proximally acting agent (e.g. acetazolamide) with a loop diuretic (e.g. furosemide) or metalazone which has also proximal effects and is effective even in advanced renal failure.

Intravenous hypertonic albumin (20%) should be reserved to patients with truly resistant oedema, in order to increase plasma oncotic pressure, thereby mobilizing fluid from the interstitial to the intravascular space. Albumin will inhibit Na proximal reabsorption, although an antinatriuretic effect has also been described by some authors.[6] By the elevated intravascular volume, GFR will increase after albumin infusion and thereby stimulate Na excretion.

The treatment of oedema present in acute and chronic renal failure is treated in Chapters 21 and 22.

References

1. Moe G.W., Legault L. and Skorecki K.L. Control of extracellular fluid volume and pathophysiology of edema formation. In: Brenner B.M. and Rector F.C. (eds) *The Kidney*, 4th ed. Philadelphia, W.B. Saunders, 1991: 623–676

2. Strauss J., Freundlich M. and Zillernelo G. Nephrotic edema, ethupathogenic and therapeutic considerations. *Nephron* 1984, **36**, 73–75

3. Mavichak V. and Dirks J.H. Pathophysiology of the nephrotic syndrome: mechanisms of edema. In: Cameron J.S. and Glassock R.J. (eds) *The Nephrotic Syndrome*. New York, Dekker, 1988: 251–283

4. Tulassay T., Rascher W. and Schärer K. Intra- and extrarenal factors of oedema formation in the nephrotic syndrome. *Pediatr. Nephrol.* 1989, **3**, 92–100; Dixon B.S. and Berl T. Pathogenesis of edema in renal disease. In: Edelmann C.H. (ed) *Pediatric Kidney Disease*, 2nd edn. Little Brown Co. 1992: 565–580

5. Intaglietta M. and Zweifach B.W. Microcirculatory basis of fluid exchange. *Adv. Biol. Med. Phys.* 1974, **15**, 111–115

6. Seifter J.L., Skorecki K.L., Stivelmen J.G., Haupert G. and Brenner B.M. Control of extracellular fluid volume and pathophysiology of edema formation. In: Brenner B.M. and Rector F.L. (eds) *The Kidney*. Philadelphia, Saunders, 1986: 343–384

7. Koomans H.A., Kortlandt W., Geers A.B. and Dorhout Mees E.J. Lowered protein content of tissue fluid in patients with the nephrotic syndrome: observations during disease and recovery. *Nephron* 1985, **40**, 391–395

8. Zilleruelo G. and Strauss J. Management of nephrotic edema. In: Strauss J. (ed.) *Hypertension, Fluid-electrolytes and Tubulopathies in Pediatric Nephrology*. The Hague, Martinus Nijhoff, 1982: 189–205

9. Kaloyanides G.J. Edema. In: Massry S.G. and Glassock R.J. (eds) *Textbook of Nephrology*. Baltimore, Williams and Wilkins, 1983: 430–440

10. Dworkin L., Ichikawa I. and Brenner B.M. Hormonal modulation of glomerular function. *Am. J. Physiol.* 1983, **244**, F95–F104

11. Ichikawa I., Rennke H.G., Hoyer J.R., Badr K.F., Schor N., Troy J.L., Lechene C.P. and Brenner B.M. Role of intrarenal mechanism in the impaired salt excretion of experimental nephrotic syndrome. *J. Clin. Invest.* 1983, **71**, 91–103

12. Dorhout Mees E.J., Roos J.C., Boer P., Yoe O.H. and Simatupang T.A. Observations on edema formation in the nephrotic syndrome in adults with minimal lesions. *Am. J. Med.* 1979, **67**, 378–384

13. Berg U. and Bohlin A.B. Renal hemodynamics in minimal change nephrotic syndrome in childhood. *Int. J. Pediatr. Nephrol.* 1982, **3**, 187–192

14. Kuroda S., Aynedjian H.S. and Bank N. A micropuncture study of renal sodium retention in nephrotic syndrome in rats: evidence for increased resistance to tubular fluid flow. *Kidney Int.* 1979, **16**, 561–571

15. Krishna G.G. and Danovitch G.M. Effects of water immersion on renal function in the nephrotic syndrome. *Kidney Int.* 1982, **21**, 395–401

16. Gur A., Adefuin P.Y., Siegel N.J. and Hayslett J.P. A study of renal handling of water in lipoid nephrosis. *Pediatr. Res.* 1976, **10**, 197–201

17. Bohlin A.B. and Berg U. Renal water handling in minimal change nephrotic syndrome. *Int. J. Pediatr. Nephrol.* 1984, **5**, 93–98

18. Bohlin A.B. and Berg U. Renal sodium handling in minimal change nephrotic syndrome. *Arch. Dis. Child.* 1984, **59**, 825–830

19. Hollenberg N.K. and Schuhmann G. Renal perfusion in sodium-retaining state. In: Seldin D.W. and Giebisch G. (eds) *The Kidney: Physiology and Pathophysiology*. New York, Raven Press, 1985: 1119–1136

20. Metcoff J. and Janeway C.A., Studies on the pathogenesis of nephrotic edema. *J. Pediatr.* 1961, **58**, 640–685

21. Usberti M., Federico S., Meccariello S., Cianciaruso B., Balletta M., Pecoraro C., Sacca L., Ungaro B., Psanti N. and Andreucci V.E. Role of plasma vasopressin in the impairment of water excretion in the nephrotic syndrome. *Kidney Int.* 1984, **25**, 422–429

22. Meltzer J.I., Keim H.J., Laragh J.H., Sealey J.E., Jan K.M. and Chien S. Nephrotic syndrome: vasoconstriction of hypovolemic types indicated by renin-sodium profiling. *Ann. Intern. Med.* 1979, **91**, 688–696

23. Eisenberg S. Postural changes in plasma volume in hypalbuminemia. *Arch. Intern. Med.* 1963, **112**, 544–549

24. Geers A.B., Koomans H.A., Boer P. and Dorhout Mees E.J. Plasma and blood volumes in patients with the nephrotic syndrome. *Nephron* 1984, **38**, 170–173

25. Geers A.B., Koomans H.A., Roos J.C. and Dorhout Mees E.J. Preservation of blood volume during edema removal in nephrotic patients. *Kidney Int.* 1985, **28**, 652–657

26. Masuda H., Ito H., Hayashi S., Honda M., Hasegawa O. and Koga M. Blood volumes in children with nephrotic syndrome. *Pediatr. Nephrol.* 1987, **1**, C41

27. Rascher W. and Tulassay T. Hormonal regulation of water metabolism in children with nephrotic syndrome. *Kidney Int* 1987, **32** (Suppl. 21), S83–S89

28. Ammenti A., Müller-Wiefel D.E., Schärer K. and Vecsei P. Mineralocorticoids in the nephrotic syndrome of children. *Clin. Nephrol.* 1980, **14**, 238–245

29. Kumagi H., Onoyama K., Iseki K. and Omae T. Role of renin angiotensin aldosterone in minimal change nephrotic syndrome. *Clin. Nephrol.* 1985, **23**, 229–235

30. Rascher W., Tulassay T., Seyberth H.W., Himbert U., Lang U. and Schärer K. Diuretic and hormonal response to head-out water immersion in nephrotic syndrome. *J. Pediatr.* 1986, **109**, 609–614

31. Tulassay T., Rascher W., Lang R.E., Seyberth H.W. and Schärer K. Atrial natriuretic peptide and other vasoactive hormones in nephrotic syndrome. *Kidney Int.* 1987, **31**, 1391–1395

32. Brown E.A., Markandu N.D., Sagnella G.A., Squires M., Jones B.E. and MacGregor G.A. Evidence that some mechanism other than the renin system causes

sodium retention in nephrotic syndrome. *Lancet* 1982, **II**, 1237–1239

33. Brown E.A., Markandu N.D., Sagnella G.A., Jones B.E. and MacGregor G.A. Sodium retention in nephrotic syndrome is due to an intrarenal defect: evidence from steroid-induced remission. *Nephron* 1985, **39**, 290–295

34. Shapiro M., Hasbargen J., Cosby R., Yee B. and Schrier R. Role of aldosterone in the Na retention of patients with nephrotic syndrome. *Kidney Int.* 1986, **29**, 203

35. Krishna G.G., Danovitch G.M., Beck F.W.J. and Sowers J.R. Dopaminergic modulation of the natriuretic response to volume expansion. *J. Lab. Clin. Med.* 1985, **105**, 214–218

36. Corruzzi P., Biggi A., Musiari L., Ravanetti C., Vescovi P.P. and Novarini A. Dopamine blockade and natriuresis during water immersion in normal man. *Clin. Sci.* 1986, **70**, 523–526

37. Seyberth H.J., Leonhardt A., Tönshoff B. and Gordjani N. Prostanoids in paediatric kidney diseases. *Pediatr. Nephrol.* 1991, **5**, 639–649

38. Kleinknecht C., Broyer M., Gubler M.C. and Palcoux J.B. Irreversible renal failure after indocin in steroid-resistant nephrosis. *N. Engl. J. Med.* 1980, **302**, 691

39. Bourgoignie J.J., Hwang K.H., Ipacki E. and Bricker N.S. The presence of a natriuretic factor in urine of patients with chronic uremia. The absence of the factor in nephrotic uremic patients. *J. Clin. Invest.* 1974, **50**, 303–311

40. Hwang S.J., Tsai J.H., Lai Y.H. and Chen J.H. Plasma atrial natriuretic peptides and response of natriuretic peptide to water immersion in patients with nephrotic syndrome. *Nephron* 1991, **58**, 330–338

41. Greenberg A. and Puschett J.B. Edematous states. In: Suki W.N. and Massry S.G. (eds) *Therapy of Renal Diseases and Related Disorders.* Boston, Kluwer, 1991: 27–44

42. Brater D.C., Anderson S.A. and Brown-Cartwright D. Response to furosemide in chronic renal insufficiency. Rationale for limited dose. *Clin. Pharmacol. Ther.* 1986, **40**, 134–139

4

Disorders of growth and renal disease

D.A. Price

There has always been considerable interest in the growth patterns seen in children and adolescents with renal problems, and the subject has been well reviewed.[1-4] Increased research activity has been stimulated by the availability of recombinant human growth hormone (rhGH) and its experimental use in chronic renal failure.[5,6] This chapter briefly reviews how growth should be assessed and some of the interrelationships with renal disease.

Evaluation of growth

In any child or adolescent with a chronic disease the basic auxological measurements which should be made are of standing height and sitting height (or total and crown-to-rump length in a child under 2 years of age), weight, head circumference, pubertal staging, testicular volumes, and triceps and subscapular skinfold thicknesses. Sufficient care must be given to each of these measurements for the data to be meaningful and of clinical use.

The greatest inaccuracies in standing height arise from incorrect mounting or poor maintenance of the stadiometer,[7] the accuracy of which should be checked before each clinic. Errors are reduced by using a single trained observer. The patient is also a source of error[7] and a note should be made of the child who is particularly difficult to measure.

If growth standards are out of date the degree of short stature will be underestimated, which is relevant both clinically and to research proto-

cols. There is evidence that in the UK the 1966 charts of Tanner and Whitehouse[8,9] are no longer applicable[10] and this must be borne in mind until other charts are available. Correction of height standard deviation scores (SDS) for target height SDS (the mean of the height SDS of the parents)* will minimize the problem of inappropriate standards.

Measurements of height should be supplemented by estimations of height velocity over year intervals which can be compared with Tanner and Whitehouse standards in the prepubertal age range (up to 10 and 12 years in girls and boys, respectively). However, in the pubertal age range there are problems of comparison and standardization. The adolescent with chronic renal failure has an average delay in onset of puberty of $2\frac{1}{2}$ years[11] and simple estimations of height velocity SDS using the above standards would be misleading. In this situation a number of strategies are possible, including the use of standards for adolescents with delay,[12] or extrapolating the mean and standard deviations from the childhood component of the growth curve as analysed by Karlberg,[13] or, in study protocols, using a control group with delay in growth and adolescence.[11] Alternatively one can simply express the height velocity without standardization. The issue of expression of height velocity is of particular

---

*To calculate corrected ht SDS, subtract parents' mean ht SDS from that of the child, e.g. if actual ht SDS is −2.0 and target SDS is −1.5, then corrected ht SDS is -0.5.

Table 4.1   Factors related to poor linear growth and failure to thrive

Group A
Reduced glomerular filtration
Malnutrition
Hormonal imbalance
Uraemic toxins
Renal bone disease
Anaemia

Group B
Acidaemia
Glucocorticoid therapy
Tubular dysfunction
Hyperosmolality
Sodium depletion
Potassium depletion
Protein loss
Hypertension
Urinary tract infection
Psychosocial factors

importance in conditions where the amount of pubertal growth may be compromised.[11] Skeletal maturity should be assessed annually using a reliable method such as that described by Tanner *et al.*[14]

Poor growth in renal disease

Adult height

In a report from the European Dialysis and Transplant Association[15] adult heights of individuals dialysed or transplanted before the age of 15 years were below the normal adult range in 41% of males and 62% of females, with greater degrees of deficit in males, those who were only dialysed and not transplanted, and those who had congenital renal disease.

Delay in growth and pubertal development

In any chronic disease of childhood a major component of the associated growth problem is a slow tempo of linear growth, by implication reversible, but in reality difficult to separate from loss of growth potential. Such delay is often associated with delay in the onset of puberty and the pubertal growth spurt. Schaefer *et al.*[11] studied adolescents who developed end-stage renal failure before or during puberty and observed a mean delay in the onset of puberty of 2½ years. However, the intensity and duration of the growth spurt was decreased, resulting in

a reduction of pubertal growth of 58% in boys and of 48% in girls compared to normal children with growth delay.

Growth patterns

Individual children with renal dysfunction show a wide range of growth patterns from normality to severe impairment, and are affected by the severity of the disease, the timing of its onset, the effectiveness of treatment, and the growth retarding properties of treatment received. The infantile component (up to 2 years of age) and the pubertal component of growth[13] seem to be most vulnerable. Congenital renal insufficiency, as in renal hypoplasia, dysplasia and obstructive uropathies, have a profound influence on growth. Betts and Magrath[16] showed that such children grew very poorly in the first 2 years and then grew more steadily along a new but low trajectory. Poor pubertal growth as reported by Schaefer *et al.*[11] leads to the concept that it is important to maximize height before the onset of puberty.

Pathogenesis

Many factors may play a role in the pathogenesis of poor growth and failure to thrive in children with renal disease (Table 4.1). Factors listed under group A often coexist as part of chronic renal failure or deficient glomerular function, whereas factors listed in group B may occur in isolation or have a dominating adverse effect on growth. It is however essential to identify and correct each potentially adverse factor at every stage of the disease and treatment.

The exciting development of stimulating growth further by the use of pharmacological doses of recombinant human growth hormone will be described in Chapter 22.

Reduced glomerular filtration

A glomerular filtration rate (GFR) of 25–30 ml min^{-1} 1.73 m^{-2} has been reported as a threshold under which growth begins to be stunted, though some patients escape growth problems until the GFR falls below 10–20 ml min^{-1} 1.73 m^{-2}.[16] This observation begs the question as to how the decrease in renal function affects the growth retardation.

Malnutrition

Children with chronic renal failure can be anorexic and may have a grossly deficient energy intake which is correlated to their growth rate.[16] Nutritional supplementation, however, only improves the growth of some children.[17] This is reflected in the behaviour of rats with chronic renal failure which when supplemented still grow less well than pair-fed controls.[18]

Acidaemia

Renal conditions producing chronic acidaemia also lead to severe impairment of growth and biochemical correction can improve growth rate. This feature is often seen in the developmental anomalies itemized above, hypoplastic or dysplastic kidneys, obstructive uropathies and chronic pyelonephritis. Renal tubular acidosis most commonly presents with growth failure, and evidence of acidaemia, even in the presence of acid urine, should be sought. This subject is fully dealt with in Chapters 9 and 24.

Hormonal imbalance

The interpretation of hormonal changes in chronic renal failure is complex, partly due to changes in metabolic clearance rates of hormones and their binding proteins. Most attention has been centred on the growth hormone–insulin-like growth factors (IGFs) axis. Growth hormone (GH) is secreted in a pulsatile manner and linear growth is best correlated to the amplitudes of the pulses. The extracellular domains of GH receptors form a GH binding protein, presumably after transmitting GH stimulation. GH directly affects target organs and stimulates local and hepatic (circulating) IGF-1 and IGF-2 production. Although IGF-1 is essential in stimulating linear growth, the relative importance of local and circulating IGF-1 is as yet unproven. IGF binding proteins (IGFBPs), of which IGFBP-1 and IGFBP-3 have been best characterized and studied, circulate in the plasma (their physiological role is as yet unproven).

In CRF, GH levels are normal or raised,[19] metabolic clearance rates for GH are reduced,[20] and GH binding protein activity is low.[21] Bioassayable IGF activity is low[22] and rises after haemodialysis and transplantation.[23,24] Radio-immunoassayable IGF-1 is lowered and IGF-2 is high, although changes in IGFBPs may interfere with the estimations. There is evidence that IGFBPs are elevated, especially IGFBP-3, which may be the source of inhibition of IGF bioactivity.[25]

It has been hypothesized that, although GH levels can be high, due to reduced receptor activity insufficient IGF is generated and in the presence of excess IGFBP there is even lower bioavailability of IGF.[25]

Uraemic toxins

Phillips *et al.*[26] identified a circulating inhibitor of cartilage metabolism in the serum of uraemic adults. It is possible that IGFBPs or their subunits might inhibit IGF-1 activity.

Anaemia

Treatment of chronic anaemia of renal failure with erythropoietin will enable clinicians to determine the influence of anaemia on growth as well as on energy levels and wellbeing.

Renal bone disease

The term 'renal bone disease' could be used in a wide sense to include renal glomerular osteodystrophy, the rickets associated with tubular disorders and the more specific vitamin-D-resistant rickets and vitamin-D-dependent rickets. They have in common the ability to produce short-limbed short stature with limb deformities, and the property of responding to appropriate but differing therapy with improved growth. The upper segment is estimated from sitting height or crown–rump length and the lower segment by subtracting the former from total height or length. Careful examination and measurement of the parents is particularly indicated in the X-linked dominant condition of vitamin-D-resistant rickets (or familial hypophosphataemic rickets). This subject is fully dealt with in Chapters 5 and 24.

Glucocorticoid therapy

Immunosuppression with glucocorticoids has long been implicated in growth retardation. Interference with growth can be at the hypothalamopituitary level, in IGF-1 generation, or on the response of cartilage to growth factors. Alternate day regimens are known to be growth sparing and with the advent of cyclosporin doses can be reduced or even stopped, resulting in improved growth.[27]

Renal tubular disorders

Growth retardation is a particularly prominent feature of these disorders, perhaps partly because several of the factors mentioned above combine to worsen growth. In Fanconi's syndrome, the problem is often congenital and is associated with acidaemia, sodium and potassium deficiencies and phosphaturic rickets. Growth retardation often appears by 6–9 months of age in such congenital forms and may be impossible to treat effectively. Fanconi's syndrome secondary to cystinosis is associated with extreme short stature: the heights of individuals are often below − 4 or − 5 SDS. This subject is dealt with fully in Chapter 24.

Hyperosmolality

Chronic hyperosmolality due to excessive renal water loss is a feature of both nephrogenic diabetes insipidus and familial nephronophthisis and is associated with poor growth. As with other reversible metabolic derangements, such as acidaemia, and sodium and potassium loss, correction may result in catch-up growth to some degree.

Sodium depletion

The inability of the renal tubules to respond to aldosterone in the early months of life, pseudohypoaldosteronism, causes failure to grow, anorexia and vomiting. Adequate salt replacement allows normal growth. A similar picture, though not renal in origin, is seen in congenital adrenal hypoplasia, isolated aldosterone biosynthetic defects and inadequately treated 21-hydroxylase deficiency. Mineralocorticoid treatment, ineffective in pseudohypoaldosteronism, allows salt retention and good growth is restored.

Potassium depletion

Failure to thrive is often the presenting clinical feature in Bartter's syndrome, characterized by hypokalaemia, alkalosis, hyper-reninaemia, hyperaldosteronism, and normotension. Potassium loss may be complicated by sodium loss, and replacement of both may be necessary to restore a normal growth rate. Pseudohyperaldosteronism, is distinguished from Bartter's syndrome by hypertension and normal adrenal function. Potassium loss may also feature in other renal tubular disorders and be implicated in the associated poor growth.

Excessive protein loss

Nephrosis associated with heavy, permanent protein loss also produces extreme short stature. Only reduction in the loss of protein will allow improved growth.

Hypertension

Hypertension, a feature of many renal problems, has been implicated in growth retardation, and associated anorexia may be involved in the pathogenesis.

Urinary tract infection

Recurrent urinary tract infections may be associated with generalized failure to thrive.

Psychosocial factors

The burden of illness and continued treatment on children and their families is a particular characteristic of chronic renal disease and frequently has an impact on the psychological wellbeing of the child or adolescent. Whether in competition with all the other factors inhibiting good growth this makes an extra effect is difficult to prove in the individual child. However, emotional stress can have a profound effect on the growth of a child without renal disease.

Structural renal abnormalities in syndromes of abnormal growth

In children with recognizable syndromes where poor growth is a major feature, developmental renal anomalies are common but do not necessarily lead to compromised renal function. Nevertheless investigation of renal structure and function is indicated in children with these conditions where anomalies are so common, in order to achieve a more complete clinical assessment. Often growth-promoting agents such as growth hormone are considered for these children and treatment should be preceded by urinalysis, blood pressure measurement, estimated creatinine clearance, and ultrasound examination. A girl with Turner's syndrome has a 60% chance of having a renal or ureteric abnormality, such as horseshoe kidney, and may also be or become hypertensive. Recombinant human growth hormone treament is now frequently used in girls with Turner's syndrome and knowledge of baseline renal function is of value in the search for adverse events associated with therapy.

More than 350 dysmorphic syndromes are recorded to have associated renal tract anomalies or renal dysfunction and the reader would be well advised to consult a computerized database such as the London Dysmorphology Database[28] or the POSSUM database[29] when faced with a child with a recognized dysmorphic syndrome, in order to ascertain previously recorded renal tract abnormalities.

Investigation of failure to thrive to exclude renal disorder

This review of associations between growth failure and renal disorders allows for systematic investigation of a child with growth problems to exclude a renal aetiology. Clues should be sought in the history: a family history of renal disease, disorders of urinary stream, recurrent urinary symptoms, polyuria or polydipsia, recurrent pyrexias and recurrent vomiting are among the features that might suggest a renal aetiology. Further assessment of the urinary tract is indicated if there are such symptoms or if the cause of growth failure is obscure. This assessment should include the following:

Clinical	Anthropometric measurements
	Blood pressure
	Abdominal palpation
	Recognition of syndromes of growth failure/renal problems
Biochemical	Measurement of GFR (not simply blood urea)
	Serum creatinine
	Creatinine clearance
	^{51}Cr-EDTA clearance
	Blood gases
	Concentrating ability and serum osmolality
	Sodium status
	Potassium status
	Calcium, phosphorus, alkaline phosphatase (and X-rays) to exclude renal bone disease
	Estimation of urine protein
Infection	Exclusion of urinary tract infections

References

1. Chantler C. and Holliday M.A. Growth in children with renal disease with particular reference to calorie malnutrition: a review. *Clin. Nephrol.* 1973, **1**, 230–242

2. Scharer K. Growth in children with chronic renal failure. *Kidney Int.* 1978, **13** (Suppl. 8), 68–71

3. Broyer M. Growth in children with renal insufficiency. *Ped. Clin. North. Am.* 1982, **29**, 991–1003

4. Schaeffer F. and Mehls O. Endocrine, metabolic and growth disorders. In: Holliday M.A., Barratt T.M. and Avner E.D. (eds). *Pediatric Nephrology*, 3rd edn. Baltimore, Williams and Wilkins. 1994: 1241–1286

5. Rees L., Rigden S.P., Ward G. and Preece M.A. Treatment of short stature in renal disease with recombinant human growth hormone. *Arch. Dis. Child.* 1990, **65**, 856–860

6. Fine R.N. Recombinant human growth hormone treatment of children with chronic renal failure: update 1990. *Acta Paed. Scand.* 1990, **370** (Suppl.), 44–48

7. Voss L.D., Bailey B.J.R., Cumming K., Wilkin T.J. and Betts P.R. The reliability of height measurement (The Wessex Growth Study). *Arch. Dis. Child.* 1990, **65**, 1340–1344

8. Tanner J.M., Whitehouse R.H. and Takaishi M. Standards from birth to maturity for height, weight, height velocity and weight velocity: British children, 1965 – I. *Arch. Dis. Child.* 1966, **41**: 454–71

9. Tanner J.M., Whitehouse R.H., Takaishi M. Standards from birth to maturity for height, weight, height velocity and weight velocity: British children, 1965 – II. *Arch. Dis. Child.* 1966, **41**, 613–635

10. Chinn S., Price C.E. and Rona R.J. Need for new reference curves for height. *Arch. Dis. Child.* 1989, **64**, 1545–1553

11. Schaefer F., Seidel C., Binding A., Gasser T., Largo R.H., Prader A. and Scharer K. Pubertal growth in chronic renal failure. *Pediatr. Res.* 1990, **28**, 5–10

12. Tanner J.M. and Whitehouse R.H. Clinical longitudinal standards for height, weight, height velocity, weight velocity, and stages of puberty. *Arch. Dis. Child.* 1976, **51**, 170–179

13. Karlberg J. A biologically-orientated mathematical model (ICP) for human growth. *Acta Paed. Scand.* 1989, Suppl. 350, 70–94

14. Tanner J.M., Whitehouse R.H., Marshall W.A. *et al. Assessment of Skeletal Maturity and Prediction of Adult Height (TW2 Method)*. London, Academic Press, 1975

15. Rizzoni G., Broyer M., Brunner F.P. *et al.* Combined

report on regular dialysis and transplantation of children in Europe. *EDTA* 1985, 82–88

16. Betts P.R. and Magrath G., Growth pattern and dietary intake of children with chronic renal insufficiency. *Br. Med. J.* 1974, **2**, 189–193

17. Betts P.R., Magrath G. and White R. Role of dietary energy supplementation in growth of children with chronic renal insufficiency. *Br. Med. J.* 1977, **1**, 416–418

18. Chantler C., Lieberman E. and Holliday M.A. A rat model for the study of growth failure in uraemia. *Pediatr. Res.* 1974, **8**, 109–113

19. Czernichow P., Sellem C., Bailly Du Bois M. and Rappaport R. Variation des taux plasmatiques de somatonorme au cours du sommeil chez l'enfant normal et dans les rétards satraux avec insufisance rénale chronique ou avec somatotrophique. *Arch. Franc. Pediatr.* 1972, **29**, 1033–1041

20. Cameron D.P., Burger H.G., Catt K.J., Gordon E. and Watts J.M. Metabolic clearance of human growth hormone in patients with hepatic and renal failure. *Metabolism* 1972, **21**, 895–904

21. Postel-Vinay M.C., Tar A., Crosnier H., Broyer M., Rappaport R., Tonshoff B., and Mehls O. Plasma growth hormone binding protein activity is low in uraemic children. *Pediatr. Nephrol.* 1991, **5**, 545–547

22. Schwalbe S., Betts P., Rayner P.H.W. and Rudd B. Somatomedin activity in growth disorders and chronic renal insufficiency in children. *Br. Med. J.* 1977, **i**, 679–682

23. Stuart M., Lazarus L. and Hayes J. Serum somatomedin and growth hormone levels in chronic renal failure. *IRCS Med. Sci.* 1974, **2**, 1102–1104

24. Saenger P., Wiedemann E., Scwartz E. *et al.* Somatomedin and growth after renal transplantation. *Pediatr. Res.* 1974, **8**, 163–169

25. Mehls O., Tonshoff B., Blum W.F., Heirich U. and Seidel C. Growth hormone and insulin-like factor 1 in chronic renal failure – pathophysiology and rationale for growth hormone treatment. *Acta Pediatr. Scand.* 1990: **370** (suppl.), 28–34

26. Phillips L., Fusco A., Unterman T. and Del Greco F. Somatomedin inhibitor in uraemia. *J. Clin. Endocrinol. Metab.* 1984, **59**, 1091–1095

27. Ettenger R.B., Blifield C., Prince H., Gradus D.B., Cho S., Sekiya N., Salusky I.B. and Fine R.N. The pediatric nephrologist's dilemma; growth after renal transplantation and its interaction with age as a possible immunologic variable. *J. Pediatr.* 1987, **111**, 1022–1025

28. Winter R.M. and Baraitser, M. London Dysmorphology Database (computer program). Oxford Electronic Publishing, Oxford University Press, 1990

29. Bankier A. Pictures of Standard Syndromes and Undiagnosed Malformations (computer program). Melbourne, Computer Power Ltd, 1990

5

Disorders of mineral metabolism as a presenting feature of renal disease

Z. Mughal

The kidney plays a central role in calcium and phosphate homeostasis by regulating their urinary excretion and through its effect on vitamin D metabolism. It is, therefore, not surprising that abnormalities of mineral metabolism resulting in bone disease and skeletal deformities commonly accompany chronic renal failure in childhood. In addition, abnormalities of renal tubular function may result in hypophosphataemia with or without renal tubular acidosis, either of which may cause rickets.

In order to have a logical approach to diagnosis and treatment of a child with disorders of mineral metabolism it is necessary to understand the endocrine and nutritional factors which regulate plasma concentrations of calcium and phosphate as well as the underlying disease mechanisms. Because of the many interrelationships between renal disease and mineral metabolism this is discussed in some detail.

Calcium and phosphorus homeostasis

Normal vitamin D metabolism

In man, vitamin D is either produced endogenously in the skin upon exposure to ultraviolet light, or derived exogenously from dietary sources. Unlike other vitamins, vitamin D is not present in significant amounts in naturally occurring foods, with the exception of oily fish and eggs. In the skin, 7-dehydrocholecalciferol, an intermediate of cholesterol metabolism, is converted to previtamin D_3 by ultraviolet radia-

tion (290–320 nm wavelength), which undergoes thermal isomerization into vitamin D_3 (cholecalciferol). Vitamin D_3 is released from the skin into the circulation bound to vitamin-D-binding protein (VDBP) for transport to liver for further metabolism and to adipose and muscle tissues for storage. An equivalent system in plants and fungi yields vitamin D_2 (ergocalciferol). Both vitamin D_2 and vitamin D_3 are biologically inert, and in humans they undergo identical metabolic transformations (Figure 5.1).

Vitamin D is hydroxylated to 25-hydroxyvitamin D (calcidiol) in the liver, and subsequently released into plasma tightly bound to the VDBP, where it constitutes the most abundant metabolite of vitamin D. The synthesis of 25OHD is not tightly regulated and is dependent on the availability of vitamin D. Measurement of plasma 25OHD thus provides an index of an individual's vitamin D status. There is a seasonal variation in the plasma concentrations of 25OHD with high levels in summer (10–43 ng/ml) and low levels in winter (7–25 ng/ml).[1]

In the proximal convoluted tubule of the kidney, 25OHD is further hydroxylated into 1,25-dihydroxyvitamin D (calcitriol), the most active metabolite or the hormonal form of vitamin D. The concentrations of calcitriol in healthy children range from 19 to 69 pg/ml.[2] The production of 1,25-dihydroxyvitamin D [1,25 $(OH)_2D$] is strictly regulated by the renal 1α-hydroxylase enzyme whose activity is stimulated by hypocalcaemia via parathyroid hormone and hypophosphataemia. When the

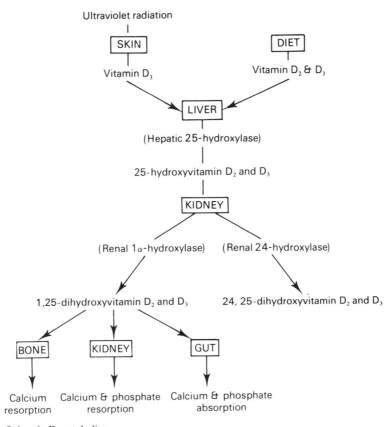

Figure 5.1 Pathways of vitamin D metabolism

supply of 1,25 (OH)$_2$D is sufficient, 1α-hydroxylase activity is inhibited and 25OHD is converted in the kidney to 24,25-dihydroxyvitamin D [24,25(OH)$_2$D] by the 24-hydroxylase enzyme. The biological significance of 24,25(OH)$_2$D in humans is uncertain.

The principal role of 1,25(OH)$_2$D is to stimulate calcium and phosphorous absorption from the small intestine. The direct action of 1,25(OH)$_2$D on bone is to produce osteoclastic resorption, and thus its antirachitic may result from maintenance of normal plasma concentrations of calcium and phosphate. In addition to its crucial role in calcium homeostasis, 1,25(OH)$_2$D also plays an important role in cell growth and differentiation.

Parathyroid hormone

Parathyroid hormone (PTH) is a polypeptide composed of 84 amino acids which is synthesized and secreted by the chief cells of the parathyroid glands. It acts by binding to specific receptors on target cells leading to activation of membrane-bound adenylate cyclase enzyme system. This activation results in intracellular conversion of adenosine triphosphate to cyclic adenosine monophosphate (cAMP) which ultimately is responsible for its biological actions. Since most cAMP resulting from the renal action of PTH is excreted in urine, renal excretion of cAMP can be used as an index of PTH function.

The principal role of PTH is to maintain plasma ionized calcium concentration within the tightly regulated normal range. PTH secretion is stimulated by hypocalcaemia, whereas hypercalcaemia has the opposite effect. PTH acts on the kidney to increase calcium reabsorption in the distal tubule and decrease phosphorous reabsorption in the proximal tubule. It also stimulates the synthesis of 1,25(OH)$_2$D in the proximal tubule, which in turn increases the dietary calcium absorption. PTH also leads to

Table 5.1   Causes of hypercalcaemia in childhood

Increased intestinal calcium absorption
Idiopathic infantile hypercalcaemia (Williams syndrome)
Vitamin D intoxication
Vitamin A intoxication
Granulomatous disorders, e.g. sarcoidosis

Decreased renal calcium excretion
Hyperparathyroidism
Familial hypocalciuric hypercalcaemia
Thiazide diuretics

Increased bone resorption
Immobilization
Hyperparathyroidism
Malignancy

Uncertain mechanism
Hypophosphatasia
Subcutaneous fat necrosis
Blue diaper syndrome
Dietary phosphate deficiency

osteoclastic bone resorption, thus causing an increase in plasma calcium and phosphorous concentration.

Calcitonin

Calcitonin is a 32 amino acid polypeptide hormone which is produced by the parafollicular or C-cells of the thyroid gland. Its principal action is to inhibit osteoclastic bone resorption. However, in humans, its physiological importance remains unclear as bone mineral metabolism is unperturbed in athyreotic patients who produce very low levels of calcitonin and in patients with medullary carcinoma of the thyroid who produce very high levels of calcitonin.

The regulation of plasma calcium concentration

In the plasma, calcium exists in three different forms: 50% as ionized or the biologically active form, 45% bound to plasma proteins (mainly albumin), and 5% complexed to phosphate and citrate. The ionized fraction of calcium is required for important biological functions such as nerve conduction, muscle contraction, blood coagulation, hormone secretion and cellular differentiation. Thus, as already discussed, PTH, $1,25 (OH)_2D$ and possibly calcitonin act in concert to maintain plasma calcium concentration within tight limits (2.15–2.65 mmol/litre total or 1.1–1.3 mmol/litre ionized) by acting at the gut, bone and the kidney. Outside the neonatal period, there is no age-related variation in the plasma calcium concentration.

Hypercalcaemia

Hypercalcaemia develops when the rate of calcium entry into the extracellular body water exceeds the kidneys' capacity for its excretion. Thus, it may occur when there is increased absorption of calcium from the gastrointestinal tract, increased release of calcium from the skeleton, decreased excretion of calcium from the kidneys or from a combination of these mechanisms. Detailed description of causes of hypercalcaemia in childhood (Table 5.1) is beyond the scope of this book; suffice to say that they are relatively rare problems in a general paediatric setting.

Symptoms of hypercalcaemia may be nonspecific, including feeding difficulties, vomiting, constipation, hypotonia and failure to thrive. Older children may present with neuropsychiatric symptoms. Hypercalcaemia results in an impaired renal concentration ability, thus leading to polydipsia and polyuria which in turn may lead to dehydration and fever. Chronic hypercalcaemia and accompanying hypercalciuria may predispose to nephrocalcinosis and nephrolithiasis.

Principles of treatment of hypercalcaemia

The approach to treatment of symptomatic hypercalcaemia consists of general supportive measures to lower plasma calcium concentration and specific treatment of the underlying cause, where possible.

Hydration and sodium diuresis
Impaired ability to concentrate urine, nausea and vomiting in severe hypercalcaemia invariably leads to dehydration. Since urinary sodium excretion results in concomitant calcium excretion, sodium diuresis is effective in lowering plasma calcium concentration. Thus, correction of dehydration with appropriate volume of intravenous isotonic saline solution (e.g. starting at twice the daily fluid allowance for age, in the absence of abnormal cardiac and renal function) and administration of a loop diuretic (e.g. 2 mg of frusemide/kg per body weight, 6 hourly) is effective short-term treatment of hypercalcaemia. Thiazide diuretics must be avoided since

they impair urinary calcium excretion and may thus exacerbate the problem. It is important to keep up with increased urinary losses of water, potassium, sodium, phosphate and magnesium during this therapy.

Mobilization

Immobilization, especially during adolescence, increases bone resorption and thus aggravates hypercalcaemia. Therefore, when possible, weight-bearing mobilization of a hypercalcaemic patient should be encouraged.

Reduction of gastrointestinal calcium absorption

Reduction of dietary calcium and vitamin D intake is effective in treating hypercalcaemia due to increased intestinal calcium absorption, for example in idiopathic infantile hypercalcaemia (Williams syndrome). In vitamin D toxicity or extrarenal synthesis of $1,25(OH)_2$ Vit D (e.g. in sarcoidosis), prednisolone 2 mg kg^{-1} day^{-1}, orally in 4 divided doses, may help to reduce plasma calcium levels by reducing intestinal calcium absorption.

Inhibition of bone resorption

Synthetic or salmon calcitonin, injected subcutaneously at a dose of 4–8 iu kg^{-1} day^{-1}, lowers the plasma calcium concentration by inhibiting bone resorption. It is the drug of choice in treatment of hypercalcaemia due to increased bone resorption. Some patients may 'escape' from the calcium-lowering response of calcitonin during prolonged and continuous administration. This 'escape' may be delayed or avoided by addition of corticosteroids.

Biphosphonates are a group of drugs which inhibit osteoclastic bone resorption and are effective in the treatment of hypercalcaemia due to conditions causing increased bone resorption and malignancy-related hypercalcaemia. One such preparation, ethane-1-hydroxy-1, 1-diphosphonate or disodium etidronate (7.5 mg kg^{-1} day^{-1}), is given in saline or 5% dextrose infusion over 4 h for 2 or 3 consecutive days for malignancy-related hypercalcaemia. An oral preparation of the drug is also available but its absorption is poor.

Dialysis

Peritoneal or haemodialysis against calcium-free dialysis solution is highly effective in lowering plasma calcium concentration.

Hypocalcaemia

As shown in Table 5.2, hypocalcaemia in childhood may occur as a consequence of inadequate calcium supply, acute increase in plasma phosphate concentration and when PTH secretion is impaired (e.g. hypoparathyroidism) or when there is resistance to its action at target sites (e.g. in pseudohypoparathyroidism). Children with hypomagnesaemia may present with signs and symptoms of hypocalcaemia since it leads to decreased PTH production and end organ resistance to its action.

Treatment of hypocalcaemia

Tetany or convulsions associated with hypocalcaemia, for whatever reason, should be treated with an intravenous infusion of 4 mg (0.1 mmol) of elemental calcium kg^{-1} h^{-1} until the symptoms cease. Ten per cent calcium gluconate solution (9.4 mg elemental calcium/ml) diluted to 2% solution is suitable for intravenous infusion; however, great care must be taken to avoid rapid injection as this can cause cardiac arrhythmias, or extravasation into subcutaneous tissues as this may lead to tissue necrosis and permanent scarring. Once the patient is asymptomatic, oral calcium supplements providing 75–100 mg kg^{-1} day^{-1} of elemental calcium in 4 divided doses may be necessary.

Hypocalcaemia secondary to magnesium deficiency is treated with deep intramuscular injections of 0.2 ml/kg of 50% magnesium sulphate solution at intervals of 8–12 h, until normal plasma magnesium concentrations are achieved. In the absence of magnesium malabsorption, 2–3 doses are generally sufficient to correct the hypomagnesaemia. Correction of hypomagnesaemia normally leads to prompt rectification of the hypocalcaemia.

Chronic hypocalcaemia resulting from hypoparathyroidism and pseudohypoparathyroidism are treated with 1,25-dihydroxyvitamin D (calcitriol), or its analogue 1α-hydroxyvitamin D (alfacalcidiol). Treatment with calcitriol or alfacalcidiol is started at the initial oral dose of 20 ng/kg body weight, and in the presence of hypocalcaemia this dosage is gradually increased to maximum dose of 50 ng/kg body weight or 2 μg/day. The aim of the treatment is to maintain plasma calcium concentration in the low normal range (2.0–2.25 mmol/litre) because in the absence of PTH or resistance to its

Table 5.2   Causes of hypocalcaemia in childhood

Inadequate calcium supply
Early neonatal hypocalcaemia – abrupt fall in placental calcium supply at birth
Severe malabsorption (short bowel syndrome)
'Hungry bone syndrome' – rapid healing of severe vitamin-D-deficiency rickets

Decrease in ionized calcium concentration
Chelation – citrate in donor blood chelates calcium, lowering the ionized calcium concentration, e.g. during exchange transfusion and respiratory or metabolic alkalosis

Phosphate overload
Excessive phosphate intake (e.g. from ingestion of unmodified cow's milk in the neonate), acute renal failure, crush injuries and rhabdomyolysis

Hypoparathyroidism
Transient – from suppression of fetal parathyroid glands secondary to maternal hypercalcaemia
DiGeorge syndrome – congenital absence of parathyroid glands. Associated with congenital heart disease, thymic aplasia and T-cell dysfunction
Idiopathic hypoparathyroidism
Autoimmune polyglandular endocrinopathy – associated with mucocutaneous candidiasis and Addison's disease
Post-thyroidectomy
Haemosiderosis (e.g. secondary to thalassaemia major treated with blood transfusions)

Hypomagnesaemia
Magnesium deficiency leads to reduced PTH secretion and end-organ (bone) refractoriness to the effects of PTH
Primary hypomagnesaemia – genetic defect of intestinal magnesium absorption
Secondary hypomagnesaemia – infants of diabetic mothers, increased gastrointestinal losses (e.g. via ileostomy), diabetic ketoacidosis

Pseudohypoparathyroidism (PHP)
PHP is characterized by hypocalcaemia, hyperphosphataemia and elevated plasma PTH concentration due to an end-organ resistance to PTH:

PHP type 1 – absent urinary cAMP and phosphaturic response to exogenous PTH administration. Phenotypic features include short stature, round face, short metacarpal and metastatic calcification
PHP type 2 – normal cAMP but absent phosphaturic response to exogenous PTH administration

Table 5.3   Normal plasma inorganic phosphate concentrations

Age (years)	*Plasmic inorganic phosphate* (mmol/litre)
Birth	1.65–2.52
0–2	1.36–2.26
2–5	1.13–2.20
5–8	1.00–2.03
8–12	0.97–1.94
12–16	0.81–1.61

Based on Cheng *et al.*[3]
Adapted from *Pediatric Clinical Chemistry*.[4]

phate absorbed from the gut is relatively constant, although it is enhanced by $1,25(OH)_2D$. The plasma concentration of phosphate is primarily regulated by the rate of renal tubular reabsorption of filtered phosphate. The rate of renal phosphate reabsorption is decreased by PTH, phosphate overload and in inherited or acquired renal tubular disorders. It is increased by dietary phosphate deprivation and growth hormone.

In assessing phosphate handling by the kidney, it is important to take account of the filtered load of phosphate as well as of the amount of phosphate reabsorbed by the tubules. Thus, a 24 h urinary phosphate measurement alone is uninterpretable since it does not take into account the filtered load of phosphate. The simplest measurement of renal phosphate handling is the percentage of tubular reabsorption of phosphate (TRP), which is easily calculated from the phosphate and creatinine concentrations on a random urine and plasma sample:

$$\text{TRP}\% = \left[1 - \frac{[UPO_4] \times [PlCr]}{[PlPO_4] \times [UCr]} \right] \times 100$$

where $[UPO_4]$ = urine phosphate concentration, $[PlPO_4]$ = plasma phosphate concentration, $[UCr]$ = urine creatinine concentration and $[PlCr]$ = plasma creatinine concentration.

Normally, more than 85% of the filtered load of phosphate is reabsorbed, but it approaches 100% during dietary phosphate deprivation.

biological action, renal tubular calcium absorption is reduced and hypercalciuria and nephrocalcinosis may occur at high-normal plasma calcium concentrations.

The regulation of phosphorous metabolism

In contrast to calcium, the plasma inorganic phosphate concentration is not tightly controlled and it is influenced by age (Table 5.3), sex and dietary intake. The amount of dietary phos-

Rickets

Rickets is a disorder of the growing child in which there is a failure of mineralization of the epiphy-

Table 5.4 Classification of rickets

Vitamin-D-related rickets
Vitamin D deficiency
   Inadequate exposure to sunlight
   Low dietary vitamin D intake
Vitamin D malabsorption
   Malabsorption syndromes, e.g. coeliac disease
   Liver disease
Abnormal vitamin D metabolism
   Anticonvulsants
Congenital 1α-hydroxylase deficiency
   Vitamin-D-dependent rickets (type 1)
Acquired 1α-hydroxylase deficiency
   Renal osteodystrophy
End-organ resistance to 1.25(O$_2$H)$_2$-D$_3$
   Vitamin-D-dependent rickets (type 2)

Hypophosphataemic rickets
Familial hypophosphataemic rickets
Fanconi's syndrome
Dietary phosphate deficiency
Tumour rickets (acquired renal phosphate wastage)

seal growth plate and newly formed bone matrix. There are many causes of rickets, but they can be classified into two broad groups (Table 5.4): (a) vitamin-D-related rickets – these conditions arise from deficiency or abnormalities of vitamin D metabolism, and (b) hypophosphataemic rickets.

This chapter only deals with vitamin-D-related and hypophosphataemic rickets. Rickets also forms an important part of bone disease associated with chronic renal failure (renal osteodystrophy), which is also discussed. The treatment of renal osteodystrophy and hypophosphataemic rickets are dealt with in Chapters 22 and 24, respectively.

Vitamin-D-related rickets

Rickets may arise as a result of vitamin D deficiency and acquired or inherited abnormalities of its metabolism. Vitamin-D-deficiency rickets is a rare problem in the UK except among children of Asian immigrants in whom it remains an important health problem. The aetiology of vitamin D deficiency in this group includes limitation of ultraviolet radiation due to skin pigmentation and sunshine avoidance for religious and cultural reasons, together with dietary deficiency.

An increased incidence of vitamin D deficiency is also seen in gastrointestinal diseases associated with fat malabsorption and liver disease. Chronic treatment with anticonvulsants, such as phenytoin, causes hepatic microsomal

enzyme induction, leading to formation of inactive vitamin D metabolites.

Type I vitamin-D-dependent rickets is a rare autosomal recessively inherited disease in which there is a specific defect in the renal 1α-hydroxylase enzyme system and this results in a failure of 1,25(OH)$_2$D synthesis.[5] Type II vitamin-D-dependent rickets is also a recessively inherited condition caused by a point mutation affecting the structure or function of the calcitriol [1,25(OH)$_2$D] receptor.[6] It is often associated with alopecia, and unlike type I vitamin-D-dependent rickets, the plasma concentration of 1,25(OH)$_2$D is high.

Clinical features

Vitamin-D-related rickets occurs more commonly during periods of rapid growth in infancy and the adolescent growth spurt. Clinical features vary with severity and the age of onset of rickets – florid skeletal deformities are more common in infancy. Infants with rickets tend to develop deformities of their weight-bearing limbs. Thus, a crawling child develops deformities in the forearms, whereas a toddler who is walking develops bow legs (genu varum) or knock knees (genu valgum). Other features of rickets include growth retardation, frontal bossing, swelling of the wrists, knees, ankles and of costochondral junctions, giving rise to a 'rachitic rosary'. Rachitic infants are often floppy, due to myopathy associated with vitamin D deficiency. Tetany and generalized convulsions may occur in patients with hypocalcaemia. Dentition may be delayed and development of tooth enamel may be impaired.

An adolescent with rickets commonly presents with vague symptoms such as aches and pains in lower limbs, especially when walking or playing games. They may also complain of weakness and difficulty in climbing up the stairs due to the proximal myopathy. Florid signs of rickets, such as swollen ends of the long bones, are rare, but patients with severe vitamin D deficiency at this age may develop genu varum.

Biochemical findings

In the early stages of vitamin D deficiency, plasma calcium concentration is low with normal plasma phosphate concentration. Hypocalcaemia leads to secondary hyperparathyroidism, which in turn results in an increase in plasma 1,25(OH)$_2$D concentration, normalization of plasma calcium concentration and a

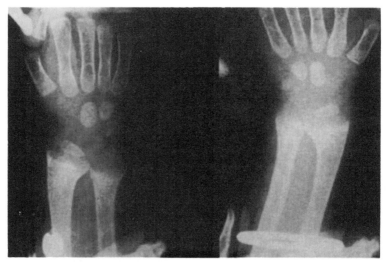

Figure 5.2 Wrist X-ray of an Asian child with rickets, showing cupping, fraying and widening of the metaphyses

decrease in serum phosphate concentration. At this stage of the rickets, plasma 25-(OH)D concentration is low and that of 1,25(OH)$_2$D normal or even high. Long-standing vitamin D deficiency eventually leads to recurrence of hypocalcaemia. Thus the plasma calcium concentration may be normal or low depending on the duration and severity of rickets. Plasma alkaline phosphatase activity is raised above the upper limits of normal for the age. Aminoaciduria due to decreased renal tubular absorption of amino acids is usually present.

Biochemical features in types I and II vitamin-D-related rickets are similar to those in vitamin-D-deficiency rickets, except that plasma 1,25(OH)$_2$D concentration is low in type I vitamin-D-related rickets and high in type II vitamin-D-related rickets.

Radiological features
The characteristic radiological signs of rickets include cupping, widening and fraying of the distal ends of the long bones with generalized osteopenia (Figure 5.2). The radiological features of secondary hyperparathyroidism such as subperiosteal erosions are rare, except in severe and long-standing cases of vitamin D deficiency.

Treatment

Oral vitamin D$_2$ or D$_3$ in therapeutic doses (1000–3000 iu/day) for 6–8 weeks is the mainstay

of treatment of vitamin-D-deficiency rickets. Healing of rickets is monitored by observing clinical and radiological improvement, a fall in plasma alkaline phosphatase activity and normalization of plasma calcium and phosphate concentrations. It is important to check the biochemistry at least once a month so that the dose of vitamin D can be adjusted according to the response, and to guard against inadvertent vitamin D toxicity.

Type I vitamin-D-dependent rickets is usually cured with physiological doses of 1,25(OH)$_2$D. Treatment of type II vitamin-D-dependent rickets is unsatisfactory; however, some patients appear to have benefited from treatment with nocturnal intravenous calcium infusions.[7]

Hypophosphataemic rickets

Rickets may be associated with disorders which result in chronic hypophosphataemia (see Table 5.4). Hypophosphataemia in the majority of these disorders arises from increased urinary phosphate excretion.

Familial hypophosphataemic rickets

The majority of patients with familial hypophosphataemic rickets have an X-linked dominant mode of inheritance (XLH), and in these patients the gene has been localized to a position on the short arm of the X-chromosome. Males tend to be more severely affected, as females carry a normal gene on the other X chromosome.

The onset is characterized by development of genu varum or lateral bowing of the legs at the time of weight-bearing. The affected child often walks with a waddling gait due to coxa vara, and an 'in-toeing' gait due to medial tibial torsion. Short stature with disproportionate shortening of the lower limbs is an important clinical feature in an untreated child. In contrast to vitamin-D-deficiency rickets, hypotonia, myopathy and tetany are absent in patients with XLH. Dental abnormalities include globular malformation of dentine with numerous accessory channels from the dental pulp to the dento-enamel junction, creating open pathways for entry of micro-organisms. Thus, patients with this condition often develop spontaneous dental abscesses in the absence of dental caries. Craniosynostosis of sutures may lead to distortion of the cranium, and premature closure of the tibial epiphysis has also been reported.

Radiological features are usually worse in the lower limbs, showing cupping, widening and fraying of metaphyses with thickened cortices and coarse trabeculation of the diaphysis of long bones. Changes of hyperparathyroidism are usually absent.

The primary defect in this condition is one of defective proximal renal tubular phosphate transport, which leads to excessive renal phosphate wastage and chronic hypophosphataemia. The plasma concentration of calcium is normal and alkaline phosphatase activity is moderately raised. The plasma concentration of PTH in untreated patients is usually normal. Thus, the TRP is < 85% in the face of low plasma phosphate and normal PTH concentrations. Plasma concentrations of 25OHD and 1,25(OH)$_2$D are usually within the normal range. Normally, hypophosphataemia is a potent stimulator of the renal 1α-hydroxylase enzyme which is responsible for the conversion of 25OHD to 1,25(OH)$_2$D. Thus, plasma 1,25(OH)$_2$D concentrations in patients with XLH are inappropriately low in the face of chronic hypophosphataemia, suggesting either defective production or increased degradation rate of 1,25(OH)$_2$D in this condition. Optimal treatment is controversial[8] and is discussed further in Chapter 24.

Hypophosphataemic rickets with hypercalciuria

This is a recessively inherited condition of hypophosphataemic rickets with hypercalcaemia.[9] Unlike XLH, plasma concentrations of 1,25(OH)$_2$D are elevated, as expected from the low plasma phosphate concentrations. Thus, these patients have increased intestinal calcium absorption, which in turn results in increased urinary calcium excretion. Treatment with oral phosphate supplements alone results in healing of rickets and normalization of hypercalciuria. Unlike XLH, these patients have muscle weakness.

Fanconi's syndrome

This term refers to a heterogeneous group of conditions characterized by proximal tubular dysfunction resulting in renal phosphate wastage, hypokalaemia, renal tubular acidosis, aminoaciduria and glycosuria. These conditions are discussed in more detail in Chapter 24. The management of hypophosphataemic rickets in this situation is identical to that recommended for XLH.

Tumour-induced hypophosphataemic rickets

Rarely, hypophosphataemic rickets may be associated with benign fibrous or mesenchymal tumours and with generalized conditions such as the linear sebaceous nevus syndrome.[10] It is likely that these tumours secrete a hormone which causes increased renal phosphate loss and reduced 1,25(OH)$_2$D synthesis. Excision of the offending tumour leads to dramatic cure of the bone disease. When this is not possible, as in generalized conditions such as the linear sebaceous nevus syndrome, the associated bone disease is treated in the same manner as XLH (see Chapter 24).

Renal osteodystrophy

Renal osteodystrophy is a frequent and potentially disabling complication of chronic renal failure in childhood. The incidence of clinically and radiologically apparent renal osteodystrophy among children with chronic renal failure ranges from 47% to 79%.[11,12] Severe and symptomatic renal osteodystrophy is particularly common among infants with congenital and obstructive renal disorders, in whom the bone disease occurs during the period of rapid skeletal growth and remodelling or when the life of patients with end-stage renal failure is prolonged by long-term haemodialysis.

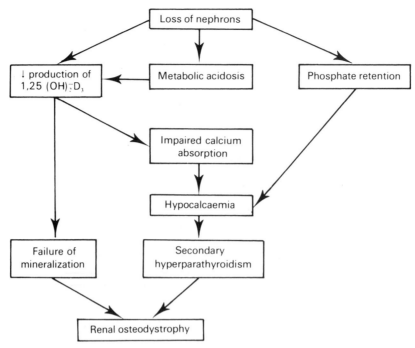

Figure 5.3 Pathways which contribute to renal osteodystrophy

Table 5.5 **Clinical and biochemical features of vitamin-D-deficiency rickets, hypophosphataemic rickets and renal osteodystrophy**

	Vitamin D deficiency	*Hypophosphataemic (XLH)*	*Renal osteodystrophy*
GENETICS		X-linked dominant	
ONSET OF SYMPTOMS AND SIGNS	Variable – infancy or adolescence	12–18 months	Variable
MUSCLE WEAKNESS	Present	Absent	Present
TETANY	Irritability, tetany, convulsions	Absent	Usually absent
DENTAL INVOLVEMENT	Delayed dentition and enamel hypoplasia	Interglobular dentine Large pulp spaces leading to spontaneous dental abscesses	
RADIOGRAPHS	Cupping, widening and fraying of metaphyses. Features of hyperparathyroidism usually absent	Changes of rickets worse in legs. Thickened cortices and trabaculation of diaphysis. Features of hyperparathyroidism usually absent	Changes of rickets and hyperparathyoidism.
BIOCHEMISTRY			
Plasma concentration			
Ca	Decreased or low normal	Normal	Normal or decreased
PO$_4$	Decreased or normal	Marked decrease	Increased
Alkaline phosphatase	Increased	Moderate increase	Increased
PTH	Increased	Normal	Marked increase
25OHD	Decreased	Normal	Normal or decreased
1,25(OH)$_2$D	Decreased, normal or increased	Normal	Decreased
Urinary excretion			
Amino acid	Increased	Normal	Normal or slightly increased

Pathophysiology

Some of the important mechanisms of renal osteodystrophy are summarized in Figure 5.3.

One consequence of falling glomerular filtration rate is an inability to excrete inorganic phosphate ingested in the diet, thus leading to

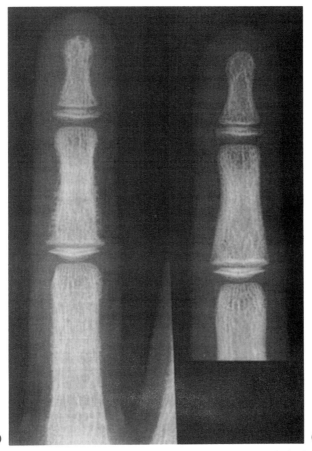

(a)   (b)

Figure 5.4 Radiograph of a finger in a patient with renal osteodystrophy showing (a) marked subperiosteal changes indicating hyperparathyroidism, with (b) resolution after treatment with $1\alpha(OH)-D_3$

hyperphosphataemia. Another consequence of declining renal function is reduced production of $1,25(OH)_2D$ which leads to impaired mineralization of bone (rickets) and decreased intestinal calcium absorption. Hyperphosphataemia and malabsorption of dietary calcium due to $1,25(OH)_2D$ deficiency cause a fall in plasma ionized calcium concentration which in turn stimulates parathyroid glands, thus resulting in secondary hyperparathyroidism.

Some patients with chronic renal failure develop a particularly severe form of bone disease which has been attributed to accumulation of aluminium in bone.[13] The sources of aluminium are from dialysis water and from oral phosphate binders, such as aluminium hydroxide. Deposition of aluminium in bone further interferes with bone mineralization and is associated with a high incidence of fractures.

Thus renal osteodystrophy is a complex metabolic bone disorder resulting from secondary hyperparathyroidism and impaired bone mineralization.

Clinical features
Renal osteodystrophy may be asymptomatic but bone pain, muscle weakness, pathological fracture, slipped epiphysis, avascular necrosis and crippling deformity, such as genu valgum or genu varum, may occur. It is also an important contributing factor to growth failure in children with chronic renal failure. Extraskeletal calcification, associated with a high plasma calcium and phosphate concentration product, is rare in children.

Patients with aluminium bone disease have a higher incidence of fractures and a tendency to hypercalcaemia, particularly in patients treated with vitamin D or its metabolites.

Biochemical features

Biochemical features of renal osteodystrophy depend on the severity of the chronic renal failure. As mentioned previously, hyperphosphataemia is almost invariably present in patients with renal osteodystrophy. This is in contrast to hypophosphataemia characteristically observed in children with vitamin-D-related and hypophosphataemic rickets (Table 5.5). The plasma calcium concentration may be normal or slightly low. The circulating concentration of parathyroid hormone is elevated and that of 1,25 $(OH)_2D$ decreased. The secondary hyperparathyroidism in renal osteodystrophy is usually severe and frequently expressed radiologically (Figure 5.4). This is usually not the case in secondary hyperparathyroidism associated with vitamin-D-related rickets, where it is usually only a biochemical finding. The plasma alkaline phosphatase activity is usually raised and is a useful biochemical index of bone disease. As the plasma alkaline phosphatase activity varies with age and methodology, it is important to use the normal range for the particular laboratory.

Radiological features

Radiological features of renal osteodystrophy vary according to the age of the child and the severity of the bone disease. In the growing child, in addition to classical radiological features of rickets with widening, cupping and fraying of the ends of the long bones, features of secondary hyperparathyroidism are usually present. The principal radiological feature of secondary hyperparathyroidism is subperiosteal erosions, which are best seen in the middle phalanges (Figure 5.4).

References

1. Stamp T.C.B. and Round J.M. Seasonal changes in human plasma levels of 25-hydroxyvitamin D. *Nature* 1974, 563–565
2. Chesney R.W., Rosen J.F., Hamastra A. and DeLuca H.F. Serum 1, 25-dihydroxyvitamin D levels in normal children and in vitamin D disorders. *Am. J. Dis. Child.* 1980, **134**, 135
3. Cheng M.H, Lipsey A.I., Blanco V., Wong H.T. and Spiro S.H. Microchemical analysis for 13 constituents of plasma from healthy children. *Clin. Chem.* 1979, **25**, 693–698
4. Meites S. (Editor in Chief) *Pediatric Clinical Chemistry*. American Association for Clinical Chemistry Inc., Washington D.C. 1981: 357
5. Fraser D., Kooh S.W., Kind H.P., Tanaka Y. and De Luka H.F. Pathogenesis of hereditary vitamin D metabolism involving defective conversion of 25-hydroxyvitamin D to 1 25-dihydroxyvitamin D. *N. Engl. J. Med.* 1973, **289**, 817–822
6. Hughes M.R., Malloy P.J, Kieback D.G., Kesterson R.A., Pike J.W., Feldman D. and O'Malley B.W. Point mutation in the human vitamin D receptor gene associated with hypocalcemic rickets. *Science* 1988, **242**, 1702–1705
7. Balsan S., Garabedian M., Larchet M., Gorski A., Cournot G., Tau C., Bourdeau A., Silve C. and Ricour C. Long-term nocturnal calcium infusions can cure rickets and promote normal mineralization in hereditary resistance to 1,25-dihydroxyvitamin D. *J. Clin. Invest.* 1986, **77**, 1661–1666
8. Latta K., Misano S. and Chan J.C.M. Therapeutics of X-linked hypophosphataemic rickets. *Pediatr. Nephrol.* 1993, 744–748
9. Tieder M., Modai D., Samuel R., Arie R., Halabe A., Bab I., Gabizon D. and Liberman U.A. Hereditary hypophosphatemic rickets with hypercalciuria. *N. Engl. J. Med.* 1985, **312**, 611–617
10. Carey D.E., Drezner M.K., Hamadan J.A., Mange M., Ahmad M.S., Mubarak S. and Nyhan W.L. Hypophosphatemic rickets/osteomalacia in linear sebaceous nevus syndrome: a variant of tumor-induced osteomalacia. *J. Pediatr.* 1986, **109**, 994–1000
11. Fine R.N., Isaason A.S., Payne V. and Grushkin C.M. Renal osteodystrophy in children. The effect of haemodialysis and renal transplantation. *J. Pediatr.* 1972, **80**, 243–249
12. Hsu A.C., Kooh S.W., Fraser D., Cumming W.A. and Fornasier V.L. Renal osteodystrophy in children with chronic renal failure: an unexpectedly common and incapacitating complication. *Pediatrics* 1982, **70**, 742–750
13. Salusky I.B., Coburn J.W., Brill J., Foley J., Slatopolsky E., Fine R.N. and Goodman W.B. Bone disease in pediatric patients undergoing dialysis with CAPD or CCPD. *Kidney Int.* 1988, **34**, 840–844.

6

Disorders of micturition

J.D. van Gool

Introduction

Definitions: enuresis vs incontinence

Because, around school age, wetting one's pants or bed more than once a week is considered abnormal, the acquired skill of being dry is synonymous with normal bladder function. As a consequence, once a child has confirmed that he or she is 'dry' during the daytime, specific questions about voiding, urge, urine flow and bladder capacity often are not asked. This polarity between wet and dry gives rise to another simplification: labelling children who wet as 'enuretics', with the concept of maturational delay as causal to their wetting, implying a self-limiting nature to the condition. This implication warrants a much more narrow definition for 'enuresis' than the all-encompassing 'maturational delay'[1] or 'no apparent organic cause'.[2]

In this chapter, enuresis is defined as a normal voiding, at a socially less acceptable place and time; the enuresis may take place primarily during sleep (enuresis nocturna), in the daytime (enuresis diurna), or both. Isolated enuresis nocturna occurs only during sleep, whereas classical enuresis diurna may occur at both daytime and night-time. All other forms or types of wetting belong to the realm of urinary incontinence, which is wetting, also at awkward times and places, in the form of involuntary loss of small amounts of urine – never a complete voiding. In children with enuresis *sensu stricto*, the voiding appears to occur uncontrolled, often even unnoticed, during sleep or during normal daytime activities. In incontinent children, the wetting is uncontrollable, however hard the child tries to prevent it, and bladder emptying is usually incomplete.

Children with classical enuresis diurna appear to be lackadaisical about their being wet. The actual moment of voiding may surprise them, but their inability to control or prevent bladder emptying is so obvious that they soon give up attempts at remedying the problem, in favour of less frustrating daytime activities. They try to live with the wetting, often with the help of some camouflage, or simply deny the existence of the problem. The wetting is usually part of a complex of behavioural problems, closely resembling an attention deficit disorder. Depending on the child's individual typology, the pressures from peers and parents to become dry will result in either 'acting out' or 'withdrawal' – to compensate for social isolation or even outright social rejection.

Incontinent children, on the other hand, tend to keep on fighting their uncontrollable leaks. Instead of resignation or denial, they adopt ingenious camouflaging schemes, and typical hold-manoeuvres, to counter the urge to void. Even after years of trying to cope with the problem, each new occurrence of wetting may still be experienced as very frustrating. Inevitably, the wetting will also be subject to parental or peer review, resulting in some reactive behaviour.

This makes it mandatory, for anybody whom the parents or the child turn to for help, to assess very carefully the layering of sets and subsets of complaints. Presenting symptoms or complaints are never specific enough to separate enuresis from incontinence: they have to be translated into specific signs and symptoms first. Translation of subjective complaints to objective signs is often confounded by the fact that the wetting can be a primary or secondary problem. Secondary wetting is usually defined as wetting occurring after a period of 6 consecutive months of being dry. In enuresis, the occurrence usually can be linked to a stressful event in the child's personal life. In functional incontinence, a urinary tract infection often offers the link. It is important to keep in mind that organic incontinence due to anatomical causes always is primary in onset.

Intake: structuring of medical history

Intake and assessment of a child with a wetting problem has to focus first on the distinction between enuresis and incontinence.[3] To be able to translate complaints about wetting, urge or voiding into concise signs and symptoms, a structured medical history is needed. Questions should be asked about bowel habits and constipation, often an associated problem in children with urge syndrome. Drinking habits are important to know too: polyuria has to be ruled out as a rare cause for the wetting problem, while, on the other hand, many children with daytime wetting tend to drink substantially less than normal. Urinary tract infections, diagnostic tests and imaging procedures, and therapeutic interventions, should be charted.

Obvious topics for specific questioning are the pattern of wetting, urge to void and reactions to urge, and micturition itself. Here a checklist can be helpful, as described later. The child should be asked to keep a chart, recording all voidings and incidents of wetting over a period of 2 weeks. The chart is best organized as a timetable, to record not only the frequency of voiding and wetting, but also the distribution over time of day or night. The motivation of a child to follow any therapeutic regimen can be greatly enhanced by making the child personally responsible for the charts – not the parents.

The physical examination should include the lumbosacral area, in search for signs of spinal dysraphism and neuropathic bladder dysfunction, and the external genitalia, to rule out epispadias, hypospadias, meatal stenosis and ectopic ureter.

Assessment of the child's behaviour is an essential part of history and examination, and should be aimed at discriminating between primary behavioural problems and subsets of problems secondary to the wetting.

The adequacy of history-taking and examination of the child who wets will be enhanced by structuring, but the intake has to be based first and foremost on a conceptual understanding of bladder/sphincter function, and of the pathophysiology of bladder/sphincter dysfunction. These principles form the topic for the next section.

Neurophysiology of bladder/sphincter function

Neuroanatomical substrate[4]

Urinary bladder and urethra form a functional unit, with opposed and alternating functions: storage and evacuation. These functions are mutually exclusive, and they are co-ordinated at roughly three levels of the central nervous system: cerebral cortex, brainstem and sacral spinal cord.

The peripheral reflex circuits involved in bladder/sphincter function are far more complex than suggested by the concept of a 'sacral micturition centre' with monosynaptic spinal reflexes. This concept is gradually being replaced by that of a supraspinally organized polysynaptic reflex, in which multiple supraspinal loops have a net inhibitory effect on the spinal reflex arcs, and also help to co-ordinate visceromotor and somatomotor responses to a reflex stimulus. All regulatory supraspinal loops – inhibitory or facilitory to the spinal reflexes for smooth detrusor and striated urethral muscles – are influenced by cortical inhibition or facilitation: the cortical pathways connect with the supraspinal loops at brainstem level.

Detrusor

Functionally, the detrusor muscle is a syncytial unit, allowing for changes in shape in three dimensions. The compliance of the bladder wall (change in intravesical pressure with increasing volume) depends mainly on the properties of the lamina propria, between mucosa and detrusor muscle: collagen fibres here are randomly orientated, each fibre crimped at low volumes and stretched when the bladder is full. Only the trigonal area has a relatively rigid shape, funnelling down as the origin of the bladder outlet with each detrusor contraction. Histologically, the smooth muscle in the region of the bladder neck is different from detrusor smooth muscle: the bladder neck can be considered as a separate functional unit, with sex differences in structure and innervation.

The human detrusor has a rich and uniform supply of postganglionic cholinergic nerve endings, originating from parasympathetic ganglion cells in the bladder wall proper and in the pelvic plexus. Preganglionic pathways to these peripheral cholinergic ganglion cells are supplied by visceromotor neurons in the intermediolateral columns of the sacral spinal cord.

Postganglionic α-adrenergic nerve endings are very sparsely distributed in the detrusor muscle, except for the trigonal area and bladder neck in the male. Adrenergic synapses on cholinergic intramural ganglion cells in the detrusor have been described: they provide for modulation of release of neurotransmitter at the cholinergic nerve endings. Postganglionic adrenergic nerve endings originate from sympathetic ganglion cells in the pelvic plexus; the preganglionic pathways to these ganglia are in the hypogastric nerve, supplied by sympathetic neurons in the intermediolateral columns of the thoracolumbar spinal cord.

Urethra

The closure mechanism of the urethra operates at three anatomical levels: urethral mucosa and submucosa, urethral smooth muscle, and striated muscle, both intrinsic and extrinsic to the urethra. Urethral mucosa and submucosa have an abundant blood supply, sympathically innervated: this vascular cushion is important in maintaining a watertight seal in the closed urethra.

Next to the submucosal sheath is the smooth muscle layer, in the male urethra continuous with the circularly orientated smooth muscle of preprostatic urethra and bladder neck, in the female urethra extending, longitudinally orientated, from bladder neck to external meatus. The nerve supply to urethral smooth muscle is presumed to be mainly cholinergic, except for the sphincteric smooth muscle in the preprostatic urethra.

Where the urethra passes through the pelvic floor, the para-urethral part of the striated pelvic floor musculature joins the intrinsic striated sphincter. This part of the pelvic floor constitutes the extrinsic external urethral sphincter, made up of both 'slow-twitch' and 'fast-twitch' striated muscle, as opposed to the intrinsic external urethral sphincter, which contains mainly slow-twitch striated muscle, capable of sustained contraction.

Most researchers agree that the pudendal nerve supplies the extrinsic part of the striated external sphincter, with axons originating from somatomotor neurons in the anterior horns of the sacral spinal cord. There is histochemical evidence that this also applies for the intrinsic striated urethral muscle. The clinical importance of structural and neurological differences between intrinsic and extrinsic striated urethral muscles is still subject to discussion. (The pathophysiology of the neuropathic bladder is discussed in Chapter 26.)

Development of voluntary control

A child first learns to control voiding with voluntary contraction of the pelvic floor: this evolutionarily important emergency brake is used to counteract and inhibit a detrusor contraction with urge – once urge is experienced and recognized as such. Actual voluntary control over detrusor and/or urethral reflex activity requires cognitive capacities: in most children this does not develop before the age of 2 years, in some it takes much longer, up to the age of 4–6 years. Development of central inhibition and facilitation of voiding is a slow process, subject to interference. Pain, discomfort or negative experiences associated with voiding will force the child to use emergency manoeuvres to prevent or postpone micturition as long as possible. Some children postpone voiding only in special situations, e.g. at playgrounds. The net result of 'emergency inhibition' is idiosyncratic use of voluntary pelvic floor contraction to inhibit urge to void, instead of normal central inhibition. Whenever emergency inhibition becomes a habit, bladder/sphincter dysfunction and incomplete bladder emptying will follow, and habitual postponement of defaecation usually also follows, with some obstipation and faecal soiling as obvious results.

Development of central control over voiding and urge is also subject to sociocultural influences, creating astounding transcultural differences in toilet training and voiding habits.[5] When being or becoming dry is made into a big issue for a child, every little failure in the slow process of acquiring full control becomes a big frustration. In the farmlands of central China and in rural Africa – and historically in the rural south of Europe – most children wear no underpants, and whenever they want they can void outdoors, girls squatting down and boys standing up. It should be interesting to compare the incidences of non-neuropathic bladder/sphincter dysfunction and recurrent urinary tract infections in such a population with those in our present-day preschool- and school-age children: they have to wear clean underpants, subject to inspection any time, and whenever they have to void, they have to go inside the house, and lock themselves into a Victorian contraption called a water-closet.

Therapeutic implications

The peripheral nerve supply to bladder and urethra is made up of three components, cholinergic, adrenergic and somatomotor, each of which can be manipulated pharmacologically.

Alpha-adrenergic drugs will increase urethral resistance, either by direct action on urethral smooth muscle or by increasing the blood supply to the urethral submucosa. These drugs are mainly used as adjuvants in the treatment of adult female stress incontinence.

Alpha-adrenergic receptor blockade with drugs like phentolamine will have the reverse effect, a marked decrease in urethral resistance. Alpha-receptor blockade with clonidine or phenoxybenzamine (0.1 mg kg^{-1} day^{-1} in 3 doses) will also have a central effect, because these drugs cross the blood-brain barrier: α-adrenergic receptors in the central nervous system regulate the tone of striated urethral muscle. The central effect can be used to counteract spasticity or dyssynergic activity of the striated urethral muscles.

Anticholinergic drugs seem a logical choice to treat detrusor overactivity: the number of detrusor contractions will reduce, which restores functional capacity to normal values and normalizes voiding frequency. Anticholinergics also alleviate pain and discomfort associated with detrusor overactivity. However, results are far less consistent and predictable in (non-neuropathic) urge syndrome or urge incontinence, than in the treatment of detrusor overactivity associated with infravesical obstruction or neuropathic detrusor hyperreflexia. Currently, the most widely used drug is oxybutinin (0.3 mg kg^{-1} day^{-1} in 3 doses). Oxybutinin may, very rarely, induce acute unrest in children, resembling psychotic states; otherwise, the margin between effect and side effect is reasonably large.

Cholinergic drugs are used less and less in paediatrics. Urinary retention or incomplete bladder emptying are much easier to treat with short periods of clean intermittent catheterization than with unpredictable drugs like betanechol chloride.

Cognitive training, bladder re-education, bladder rehabilitation – and even conditioning to some extent – require on the part of the child a developmental stage heralded by conscious, voluntary control, on the level of the cerebral cortex, over autonomous functions. Signals from bladder or urethra have to be felt and perceived as such, in order to respond in a normal, physiological way. Once non-physiological responses have become habitual, (re)learning the normal responses is a logical way to regain central inhibition and facilitation of the voiding reflexes: (re)learning bladder control is a cognitive process, with perception of the signals reinforced by biofeedback. This type of treatment may benefit from anticholinergics, as adjuvants to the training programme.

Wetting with normal bladder/sphincter function

Isolated enuresis nocturna

A child with enuresis nocturna has difficulty acquiring the skill of being dry at night – an inborn skill that usually emerges regardless of training.[6] Enuresis nocturna is one of the best known 'low-severity high-prevalence' conditions in paediatrics; it is neither a disease nor a disorder. Not every current opinion on night wetting deals with isolated enuresis nocturna: some publications include children with classical enuresis diurna who also wet at night, or even children with functional incontinence whose daytime wetting has a nocturnal component.[1,2,7] Restriction of the use of the term enuresis nocturna to children with just typical bedwetting, and nothing else, will prevent unnecessary investigations and interventions in a population with an anatomically and functionally normal lower urinary tract. A nocturnal component in any other form of wetting has nothing to do with enuresis nocturna: it has the same characteristics as the daytime component of the wetting, and should be diagnosed accordingly.

Typically, isolated enuresis nocturna is defined as bedwetting for 3 or more nights per month, or one night per week.[8] The wetting occurs as a normal voiding, with normal bladder emptying (the bed will be soaking wet), without the child noticing the urge to void or the actual voiding (a few children wake up to the wet bed, to find a dry place to sleep). Only a small proportion of children with enuresis nocturna wet the bed every night. An ample discussion of this condition is warranted, because of its high prevalence and continuous interference with normal activities in school-age children.

Prevalence vs age

Depending on sociocultural circumstances, help for enuresis nocturna will be sought when the wetting remains at 3 nights or more per month, with the child reaching school-age, or, typically, in the autumn term of the first grade. The prevalence of night wetting at age 5–6 years reportedly is 8–10%; it becomes a more serious problem at age 7–10 years, with a prevalence of 7%. Up to that age, it is reported to be more common in boys than in girls, with a ratio of up to 2:1; after age 11–12 years, this difference in prevalence between boys and girls gradually disappears.[9,10] Because of a reduction in prevalence with increasing age, about 13–15% per annum, and because of differences in definition of night-time wetting in epidemiological studies, all incidences quoted for a given age will have wide margins. Despite this inaccuracy, de Jonge's epidemiological survey of 1969[11] still serves best to illustrate the relation between age and prevalence of night wetting. Figures 6.1 and 6.2 are based on de Jonge's original survey of night- and daytime wetting in an unselected population of 9991 Dutch children. From these it can be seen that in night-time wetting, prevalence and age have an exponential relation, in marked contrast with the bimodal curve for daytime wetting, which shows the effects of toilet training. De Jonge's criteria for night- and daytime wetting are comparable to the

rather strict criteria listed in the revised 3rd edition of the Diagnostic and Statistical Manual of Mental Disorders (DSM-III-R): (1) repeated involuntary or intentional voiding during the day or night in bed or clothes; (2) at least 2 such events per month for children between the ages of 5 and 6, and at least 1 event per month for older children; (3) chronological, age of at least 5 and mental age of at least 4; (4) not due to a physical disorder such as diabetes, urinary tract infection, or seizures.

Of all cases of enuresis nocturna, 20–30% are judged to be secondary in onset, starting after a period of full night-time control of at least 6 months.[9] Secondary enuresis nocturna, however, belongs to the long list of regressive symptoms that any child might exhibit when exposed to unusual stress. It tends to disappear spontaneously whenever the stressful event has been coped with. It is debatable to include children with secondary enuresis nocturna in the population of primary isolated bedwetting: in the literature, however, most reports favour this inclusion.

The incidence of primary isolated enuresis nocturna almost doubles when the father or the mother of a child has had enuresis nocturna; when both father and mother have been bedwetters, there is a 70% chance that the offspring will have enuresis nocturna also.[10] From this, the conclusion is made that hereditary factors play an important part.

Aetiological factors

In the past, many factors have been described as contributory, or even causal, to isolated enuresis nocturna: socioeconomic class and behavioural or emotional problems are but a few. Moffat, in reviewing the available literature, found no evidence whatever for any abnormality in emotional or behavioural status in children with isolated enuresis nocturna: children with enuresis nocturna are normal children, with a problem that may induce reactive emotional or behavioural symptoms.[12] In a retrospective analysis of 153 teenagers with persistent enuresis nocturna (age 14.2 ± 2.2 years), we could only find an association between unsuccessful treatment and extreme 'fear to fail'.[13] Self-concept or behaviour did not deteriorate with treatment failure, but clear evidence could be seen of positive behavioural effects with

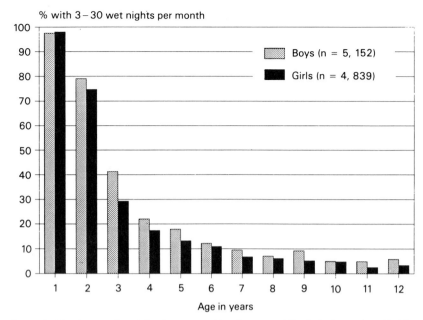

Figure 6.1 Prevalence of night-time wetting, defined as repeated involuntary voiding in bed on at least 3 nights per month, in healthy Dutch children. The difference in prevalence between boys and girls[9,10] becomes apparent only in subjects who wet the bed 21–30 nights per month (After de Jonge[11])

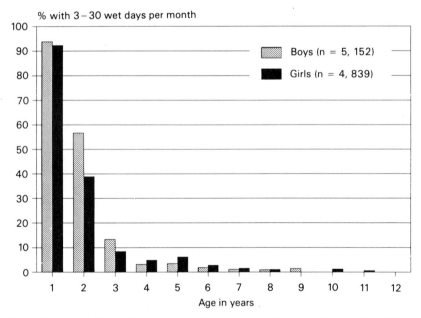

Figure 6.2 Prevalence of daytime wetting, defined as repeated involuntary voiding in clothes on at least 3 days per month, in healthy Dutch children. From age 4 on, the prevalence in girls is significantly higher than in boys: inevitably, in 1969, girls with functional incontinence and a history of recurrent UTIs will have been included in the survey (After de Jonge[11])

successful treatment. Moffat[12] also points out that enuretic children seeking treatment do not differ from those who do not, and that – after succesful treatment – no symptom substitution will occur. These findings indicate that therapeutic modalities aiming at correction of or changes in behaviour are inappropriate. Therapy should be at the same level as the condition: unperceived and uncontrolled but normal voiding during sleep.

Disturbances in sleep have been offering an attractive hypothesis for explaining enuresis nocturna. Children and parents almost invariably state the depth of sleep as causal to not noticing the urge to void – most parents claim that the children do not wake up when they take them out of bed to have them void, and many enuretics do not perceive the sound of enuresis alarms. Recent studies in sleep research could not confirm the hypothesis that enuresis nocturna is an 'arousal disorder': the actual wetting occurs in all non-REM sleep stages, while wetting during REM sleep is uncommon, and dreams with wet themes are more likely to be stimulated by the wet sheets than vice versa.[10,14]

Another circadian phenomenon has been described as causal to enuresis nocturna: 20–30% of children with enuresis nocturna lack the normal increase in endogenous antidiuretic hormone (ADH) during sleep. Consequently, substitution therapy with synthetic desamino-D-arginin-vasopressin (DDAVP) can alleviate the wetting effectively, reportedly in up to 80% of treated subjects – often only to resume after discontinuation of the ADH analogue.[15,16] In view of recent research on circadian events related to sleep, trackable by charting the output of melatonin metabolites in the urine versus time,[17] it seems worth while to reinvestigate the correlation between sleep structure and isolated enuresis nocturna.

Detrusor instability has been thought to be a factor in enuresis nocturna, as well as small-for-age values for functional bladder capacity. These associations have spurred therapeutic trials with anticholinergics, but they have never been proven. In isolated enuresis nocturna, urodynamic investigations to diagnose detrusor overactivity, or aggressive measures to treat it, are not indicated.

Strategies for management

Most therapeutic strategies are aimed at teaching the child to recognize the signals from a contracting bladder – urge at normal capacity – as being important enough to wake up to. Three strategies will be discussed, in order of their reported effectiveness. However, the doctor listening to the child with enuresis nocturna, and to the parents, and paying careful attention to the problem, is a very important part of management, whatever the strategy.

Conditioning with detector and alarm

The modern variants of the old-fashioned bell-and-pad* method, arouse the child with an audible alarm as the first drops of urine passed, still have the highest success rate reported. The detector, worn in the pants, is triggered by a change in resistance to an electrical current, whenever urine electrolytes make contact with the detector. Modern mini-alarms are battery-operated, easy to use, and usually leased or sold on prescription. However, many enuretic children simply do not wake up to the alarm: this problem may be solved by increasing the volume of the sound, or by changing the beeper or buzzer to vibrator.

Important requirements are progress reports, given by the child personally, on a monthly basis. The therapy may have to be continued for up to 3 months, and an equally long follow-up is essential for success. The method is ideally suited for children from 7 years of age on, and cure rates are reported from 55% (bell and pad) to 68% (mini-alarm), with a relapse rate of 5–10%.[18,19]

Changing sleep with central stimulants

Central stimulants such as imipramine have a frame of action on the reticular formation of the brainstem – they have been, and are still being, used extensively in the treatment of depression. Evidence for anticholinergic properties of tricyclic antidepressants such as imipramine is very weak. Given at the hour of sleep only, in a dose of 25–75 mg, they change sleep to the extent that the enuretic child may perceive again the first sensation of urge, and react to it by waking up to void. Keeping track of progress and reporting back to the prescribing physician are elementary parts of therapy, to be taken care of by the child, not by the parents. A period of 2 weeks of medication with imipramine will tell if the drug will work.

---

*In Egypt, around 1500 BC, a frog was tied to the toe of the sleeping child with enuresis nocturna. Reflex movements, associated with bladder activity, would alarm the frog to wake up the child and prevent wetting.

If it does, a total period of 4–6 weeks on imipramine should be followed by a gradual decrease in dose, over another 2–4 weeks, to consolidate the confidence regained. Abrupt discontinuation will result in a high relapse rate.[10]

Therapy with imipramine is suited for children from 9 to 11 years of age. Great care has to be taken to explain the potentially lethal hazards of the drug for toddlers and young children: fatal accidents have been reported in this age group, and many parents believe the drug to be as harmless as the condition it is prescribed for. Very rarely, a child may over-react to imipramine, with erratic behaviour right from the start of medication: these adverse effects disappear promptly after discontinuation of the drug.

Imipramine may also be used as an adjunct to therapy with the enuresis alarm, if the child does not wake up to the sound of the alarm.

Dry-bed training
The essence of this method, described by Azrin and Thienes,[20] is to wake up the enuretic child, at or just before the first urge to void arises, in order to teach him again how to perceive this signal. For two nights, the child is aroused from sleep every hour on the hour, as long as it takes to reach the goal. Dry-bed training can be done at home by the parents, with coaching by the doctor or the nurse: the intensity of this form of behavioural therapy should not be underestimated. For teenagers with persistent bed-wetting, Messer modified Azrin's method by hospitalizing the children, expanding the number of nights with forced arousals to 9, and by adding a detector to signal the slightest inadvertent loss of urine to attending personnel.[13] Dry-bed training is usually reserved for children with persistent, isolated enuresis nocturna, 11 years or older. The success rates reported vary, according to the selection of the patients, from 40% to 20%, on a long-term basis.

ADH analogues
About 12–40% of children with isolated enuresis nocturna will become dry with 10–20 μg of DDAVP at the hour of sleep, administered by nasal spray.[21] Titrating the dose from 10 to 40 μg, and maintaining therapy for at least 4 weeks, may increase the success rate to 70%.[16]

Discontinuation of the drug almost always results in recurrence of the wetting, reportedly from 70% to 90%. Some authors advocate long-term therapy, to substitute continuously the presumed absence of higher levels of endogenous ADH during sleep; others combine DDAVP treatment with the enuresis alarm.[22] Clearly, more insight is needed to clarify why circadian rhythm in endogenous ADH secretion is lost in a substantial proportion of children with enuresis nocturna, but not in all.

Treatment with DDAVP has obvious merits as a short-term measure (summer camp, holiday), and it is worth while doing a trial with DDAVP in every child with isolated enuresis nocturna. Side effects are rare, and hardly dose-related: some retention of water may occur.

As with any medication prescribed for enuresis nocturna, overdosage by the patient, on the assumption, 'the higher the dose, the quicker the cure', will occur.[23]

Classical enuresis diurna

Clinically, classical enuresis diurna is characterized by the obvious presence of primary behaviour problems. With this in mind, the common nocturnal component should not be confused with enuresis nocturna.

The wetting in children with enuresis diurna is a problem of priorities: it is never an isolated problem, but usually part of a complex of behavioural problems that result from an innate inability of the child to structure the jumble of activities and demands engulfing him every day. Most children with enuresis diurna try to live with uncontrolled voiding, deny or avoid sensations of urge, and make little effort to postpone an impending micturition – sometimes, that goes for defaecation too. This complex of behavioural problems resembles an attention deficit disorder, and children with enuresis diurna are often labelled 'chaotic', 'unstructured', are said to have a short attention span, and often need special schooling or remedial teaching. It could be postulated that the inability to fully control urge, micturition and defaecation is part of such a primary complex.[24] However, in enuresis as well as in functional incontinence, daytime wetting itself also may induce a subset of secondary behavioural problems.

The prevalence of classical enuresis diurna is unclear, as most reports include it with functional incontinence in the category of day wetting. Day wetting, defined as noticeable wetting once per week or more, has a prevalence of 5% in school-age children;[8] in any group of children with day wetting, the ratio between classical enuresis diurna and functional incontinence is roughly 1:4. The prevalence in boys is much higher than in girls, with a ratio of about 4:1.[24]

The wetting in classical enuresis diurna occurs as a complete, normal voiding: bladder/sphincter function is normal, and there is no increased prevalence of urinary tract infections, in contrast with functional incontinence. Isolated urinary tract infections (UTIs) may occur in children with enuresis, as in any population of young children, but recurrences will be rare. Nocturnal wetting is common in classical enuresis diurna, but it lacks the sleep characteristics of isolated enuresis nocturna. Encopresis is usually present, at least in the history, but without constipation.

Apart from urinalysis, and imaging of the urinary tract with ultrasound, no further studies are indicated. However, there may be a doubtful item on the checklist for urge syndrome and urge incontinence (see Figure 6.3), warranting a urodynamic study or cysto-urethrography: for instance, anatomical obstruction of the bladder outlet has to be kept in mind as a possible cause for enuresis diurna in boys, as it usually causes detrusor instability and some urge incontinence.

Strategy for management

Psychological assessment of children with classical enuresis diurna is mandatory, because of the primary behavioural problems. This assessment will help to decide whether to treat the behavioural complex as such, or to opt for treatment of the wetting alone, creating better conditions for coping with the behavioural complex. The latter will have to be organized as a training course with rigid supervision and professional coaching, aiming to (re)institute some structure to all events and demands related to micturition and defaecation.

Voiding postponement

Toddlers and school-age children occasionally have the habit of postponing micturition as long as possible, in special situations such as at playgrounds. Characteristically, micturition is postponed and postponed, until urge is so imperative that voiding irrevocably takes place, usually in the pants. Occasionally, this may grow into a permanent habit, with very infrequent voiding, incomplete bladder emptying and urinary tract infections as obvious results. This stage resembles the lazy bladder syndrome (see later): fractionated and incomplete voiding, overflow incontinence, and large residual volumes, caused by detrusor decompensation due to chronic overdistension.

Wetting with bladder/sphincter dysfunction

Prevalence and incidence

Not many publications have appeared, over the past 10 years, on the complex of non-neuropathic bladder/sphincter dysfunction and recurrent UTIs in children – surprisingly, because these patients can comprise up to 20% of the outpatient population of any paediatric nephrology service. The available literature has been written mostly by paediatric urologists, and often dealt with subgroups: symptoms such as urgency, frequency and daytime wetting were blamed on either the detrusor muscle or the urethral closure mechanism, resulting in different concepts of diagnosis and treatment. Cystometric findings of detrusor overactivity in children with recurrent UTIs were interpreted as persistent infantile bladder, occult neuropathic bladder, or isolated or subclinical neurogenic bladder. Accordingly, treatment consisted of rehabilitation programmes and anticholinergic drugs. Cystoscopy and voiding cystourethrography, on the other hand, showed abnormalities that were labelled as wide bladder neck anomaly, spinning top urethra, distal urethral stenosis, external sphincter spasticity, or sphincter dyssynergia, popularizing the concept of urethral dysfunction and stenosis, and of urethral dilatation or urethrotomy as methods of treatment.

The urodynamic window, wide enough to show the interaction between bladder and sphincter muscles by simultaneous registration of bladder pressure and urethral sphincter activity (both during bladder filling and emptying), supports the idea that most labels can be brought down to patterns of bladder/sphincter overactivity.[25,26] These clinical patterns – urge

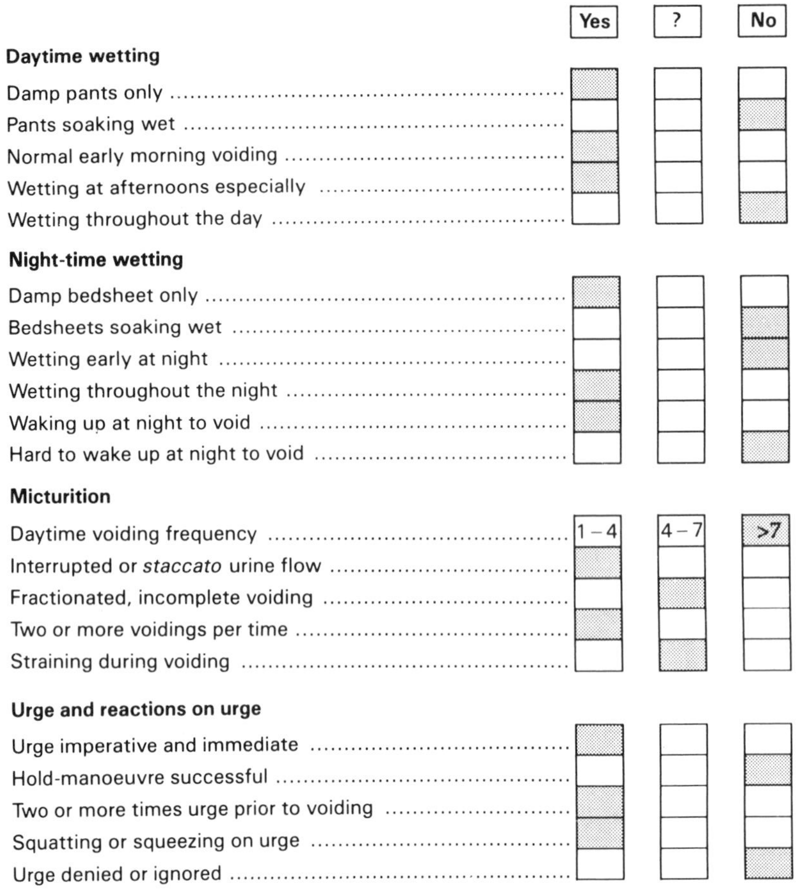

	Yes	?	No
Daytime wetting			
Damp pants only	▨		
Pants soaking wet			▨
Normal early morning voiding	▨		
Wetting at afternoons especially	▨		
Wetting throughout the day			▨
Night-time wetting			
Damp bedsheet only	▨		
Bedsheets soaking wet			▨
Wetting early at night	▨		
Wetting throughout the night	▨		
Waking up at night to void	▨		
Hard to wake up at night to void			▨
Micturition	1 – 4	4 – 7	>7
Daytime voiding frequency			
Interrupted or *staccato* urine flow	▨		
Fractionated, incomplete voiding	▨		
Two or more voidings per time	▨		
Straining during voiding		▨	
Urge and reactions on urge			
Urge imperative and immediate	▨		
Hold-manoeuvre successful	▨		
Two or more times urge prior to voiding	▨		
Squatting or squeezing on urge	▨		
Urge denied or ignored			▨

Figure 6.3 The questionnaire, used to detect covert signs and symptoms (shaded squares) of bladder/sphincter dysfunction[26]

syndrome, staccato voiding, fractionated and incomplete voiding, lazy bladder syndrome and the Hinman syndrome – may not be the distinct entities they seem to be at presentation: in all probability they represent different stages in the natural history of non-neuropathic bladder/sphincter dysfunction.[24]

With the pathophysiology of the patterns of bladder/sphincter dysfunction elucidated by urodynamic investigations, it also becomes clear how to make the clinical distinction between functional incontinence and enuresis in children with wetting: the medical history is crucial. Pertinent questions and answers can be organized in a questionnaire,[26] in four groups: daytime wetting, night-time wetting, micturition, and urge with reactions to urge (Figure 6.3).

Wetting, daytime or night-time – the pattern of wetting in functional incontinence consists of small amounts of urine, causing just wet spots. Wetting usually starts in the afternoon: during school hours, most children manage to remain dry. Children who void infrequently (fractionated and incomplete voiding, 'lazy bladder syndrome') have a similar pattern of wetting, but they tend to skip the early morning voiding. A nocturnal component in functional incontinence also consists of the loss of small amounts of urine (some children wake up at night to void), quite in contrast with nocturnal enuresis, where the wetting is a complete voiding, not noted by the child until the morning.

Micturition – daytime voiding frequency should be charted by the child, for at least 2 weeks, on a timetable. Children with urge syndrome usually void more than 7 times a day. Children with infrequent voiding keep it down to 1–3 times a day, and then have to help out with abdominal straining or manual pressure to obtain a complete voiding: this causes the urine flow to be fractionated. A staccato flow is a tell-tale sign of 'dyssynergic' urethral overactivity during voiding.

Urge and reactions to urge – sudden and imperative sensations of urge, numerous times a day, are characteristic of urge syndrome. Most children with urge syndrome have adopted typical hold-manoeuvres to prevent wetting with each uncontrollable attack of urge, but they never succeed completely. Children with classical diurnal enuresis tend to deny – when asked – that they feel urge: they try to live with uncontrolled voiding by ignoring urge.

Urinary tract infections are also an important point of distinction between enuresis and incontinence, especially when the infections are recurrent: they point to bladder/sphincter dysfunction, with incomplete bladder emptying as the underlying cause for the infections. In children with functional incontinence, a strong correlation exists with recurrent UTIs, reportedly from 50% to 90%.[2,25–27] It occurs mostly in girls, with a long history of antibiotic courses, long-term chemoprophylaxis, diagnostic procedures such as cystoscopy or voiding cysto-urethrography (VCUG), and surgical interventions such as urethral dilatation or urethrotomy.

Sometimes, stress incontinence is a feature in the medical history, usually denoting leakage of some urine in association with jumping or skipping. In urge syndrome, the sudden increase in abdominal pressure prior to the reported loss of urine provokes a detrusor contraction (with or without urge), which causes the leakage. In genuine stress incontinence, leakage is caused directly by the increase in abdominal pressure, because of structural incompetence of the urethral closure mechanism. Urethral dilatation and urethrotomy, often still performed in children with urge syndrome, may cause structural damage to the urethra and bladder neck, thereby adding genuine stress incontinence to urge incontinence.

Clinical patterns of functional incontinence

Urge syndrome and urge incontinence
Characteristic are the frequent attacks of imperative urge to void, countered by hold-manoeuvres such as squatting.[28,29] Urge incontinence, when present, usually peaks in the afternoon, and consists of slight urine loss only:

the children need two or more pairs of underpants per day. Many children do not express their urge spontaneously: they learn on their own how to cope without running the risk of being exposed as a 'wetter', by developing a host of camouflaging techniques, and only admit any sensation of urge after close questioning. Urge incontinence is also present during the night, again in the form of a slight loss of urine, which may or may not wake up the child. The urine loss at night never takes the form of a complete bladder emptying, so characteristic of isolated primary nocturnal enuresis. Symptoms and signs are caused by uninhibited – or, rather, uninhibitable – detrusor contractions, countered by the emergency brake of voluntary pelvic floor contraction. Hold-manoeuvres, such as squatting on one heel, aimed at external compression of the urethra, are added to this. Functional bladder capacity is small for age, resulting in a high voiding frequency. Micturition itself is essentially normal, with complete relaxation of the pelvic floor during actual urine flow. However, urine flow may be stopped too soon, by pelvic floor contraction, resulting in incomplete bladder emptying.

The habit of inhibiting urge with the emergency brake of pelvic floor contraction inevitably leads to inappropriate postponement of defaecation too: constipation and faecal soiling are very common symptoms, not to be confused with the encopresis in children with classical diurnal enuresis.

Giggle incontinence
Urge syndrome and urge incontinence may occur at provocation only, as in sudden increases of abdominal pressure such as jumping or laughing (detrusor instability), without the characteristic sex distribution and the strong association with UTIs. Giggle incontinence is an example, and as such is different from the occasional loss of urine induced by hilarious laughing. In giggle incontinence, actual detrusor overactivity can be provoked, regardless of the filling state of the bladder, by making the child laugh. This peculiar condition is extremely hard to cure, and most children tend to avoid laughing.

Daytime urinary frequency syndrome
Exceptionally high voiding frequencies, up to 5 times an hour, are occasionally noted in school-age children, mainly boys. This compulsory

daytime voiding can be very disturbing for parents and physicians, generating a host of diagnostic and therapeutic exercises, followed by a gradual improvement in symptoms. This condition does not relate to detrusor over-activity or any functional abnormality, nor does it react to anticholinergics. It may last up to several weeks, occasionally months, and it occurs predominantly in the winter. It disappears completely with just reassurance: it appears to be a benign self-limited condition that does not require extensive urological evaluation.[30]

Staccato voiding

Staccato voiding is often termed 'dyssynergic voiding', in analogy to the true detrusor–sphincter dyssynergia in neuropathic bladder dysfunction. Sometimes it is combined with urge syndrome; sometimes, children with stac-cato voiding only have a history of urge syndrome. The peculiar voiding pattern is caused by bursts of pelvic floor activity during voiding, resulting in peaks in bladder pressure coinciding with dips in flow rate. Flow time is prolonged, and bladder emptying is often incomplete.

The almost rhythmic pelvic floor activity during urine flow accounts for a distinct 'spin-ning top' configuration of the proximal urethra at voiding cystourethrography: the proximal ure-thra is momentarily dilated by the detrusor contracting against a closed external urethral sphincter (see later).

Fractionated and incomplete voiding

Fractionated, incomplete voiding is character-ized by a low voiding frequency, and micturi-tion occurs in several small fractions, with in-complete bladder emptying and considerable residual volumes. The detrusor muscle is hypo-active, urge is inhibited easily – when felt at all – and usually without hold-manoeuvres, and functional bladder capacity is large for age. Micturition consists of a small series of detrusor contractions, each with its own flow. Very often, abdominal pressure is exerted to speed up the voiding; in extreme cases, abdominal pressure will be the only driving force behind micturition, secondary to detrusor decompensa-tion. The flow rate is highly irregular, due to reflex activity of the pelvic floor muscles, trig-gered by each increase in abdominal pressure. Wetting in this pattern of bladder/sphincter dys-

function is intrinsically a form of overflow incontinence.

Lazy bladder syndrome

The lazy bladder syndrome is the net result of long-standing fractionated and incomplete void-ing. Abdominal pressure is the main driving force for voiding, and detrusor contractions are usually absent: large residual volumes and recurrent urinary tract infections are the rule. Occasionally children may have a low voiding frequency without fractional voiding: in typical situations (voiding postponement), or because of extreme dysuria during a urinary tract infection, micturition is postponed as long as possible, until urge is so imperative that voiding irrevocably takes place, usually in the pants.

The Hinman syndrome

Transitional phases between urge incontinence and fractional voiding do occur, as well as different grades of severity within each pattern. It may be postulated that the complex of functional incontinence and recurrent UTIs in girls starts with detrusor overactivity and hold-manoeuvres, with a gradual evolution to a lazy bladder syndrome. At the right-hand end of such a natural history is the Hinman syndrome,[31] originally described as non-neurogenic neurogenic bladder because of the striking features at cystography: thick, trabecu-lated bladder wall, functional obstruction due to 'dyssynergic' pelvic floor activity with urine flow, high-grade vesico-ureteral reflux and reflux nephropathy. Hinman postulated severe psychological disturbances as the underlying cause in his patients, and treated them with hypnotherapy.

Uroradiological findings

Not surprisingly, in children with functional incontinence VCUGs and intravenous urogra-phies show the abnormalities, characteristic for the paediatric population with recurrent UTIs: vesico-ureteral reflux (VUR), and the tell-tale signs of reflux nephropathy will be found with the prevalences known from studies on recur-rent UTIs in school-age children.[25–27,32]

A peculiar anomaly often found at VCUG is the so-called 'spinning-top' configuration of the urethra, during filling or during voiding: when-ever a girl with urge syndrome tries to inhibit imperative urge by contraction of the pelvic floor, the full force of the detrusor contraction will dilate the proximal urethra down to the level of the forcefully closed striated urethral sphincter. The resulting 'spinning-top' configuration during micturition is often still regarded as a sure sign of meatal stenosis – which is extremely rare in girls.

The detrusor muscle, contracting against a tightly closed urethra, will generate high pressures, and this explains the variability in grade of VUR in children with urge syndrome and recurrent UTIs. Traditionally, VUR is graded on the appearance of the refluxing urinary tract on one or more static images, taken during retrograde filling of the bladder and/or micturition. Peaks of high bladder pressure during filling, caused by detrusor and pelvic floor muscles contracting against each other, will momentarily dilate a refluxing urinary tract. These rapid changes in appearance make the occurence of VUR a very dynamic event, difficult to catch – let alone grade consistently – with a static imaging technique such as VCUG.[25,26,31–33]

Treatment strategies

Only a proportion of children with functional incontinence will become free of symptoms with traditional methods of treatment: careful explanation of the problem, voiding instructions and control of recurrent UTIs. Long-term chemoprophylaxis has a definite place in the management of children with functional incontinence:[34] if recurrences of UTIs can be avoided for a period of 6–9 months, symptoms and signs will diminish appreciably – in mild cases they may even disappear. However, even with a fully structured approach, in which explanation and instructions, backed up by precise history-taking and comprehensive diagnostic procedures, are organized in an outpatient programme delivered by trained 'urotherapists'[35] to both the children and the parents, a proportion of children will not respond to the treatment and continue to be incontinent.

Pharmacological treatment with anticholinergic drugs, aimed specifically at reducing the number of overactive detrusor contractions and restoring the reduced functional bladder capacity, seems to offer an advantage in children with urge syndrome. However, results are unpredictable and inconsistent, and positive effects are not always lasting. The best results with anticholinergic treatment are obtained in combination with a well-organized traditional treatment programme and it might be postulated that the general measures of the programme itself are essential for success of the treatment plan, not the anticholinergics. Even with the best possible combination of diagnostics and treatment plans, and despite enormous investment of time and energy, both by the children and the therapists, a hard core group of patients will remain refractory to treatment.

Many symptoms and signs of the urge syndrome, and of other forms of functional incontinence, are rooted in a faulty perception of signals from the bladder, and, accordingly, in habitual non-physiological responses to these signals.[29] Not surprisingly, symptoms and signs of the complex of functional incontinence and recurrent UTIs have a tendency to start at toddler age, when most children learn for the first time how to remain dry.

Children with urge syndrome have to learn again how to recognize the first sensations of urge, and how to suppress these by normal central inhibition instead of emergency procedures like urethral compression. Children with staccato voiding also have to relearn how to void with a completely relaxed pelvic floor, instead of interrupting urine flow by bursts of pelvic floor activity. The same goes for children with fractionated and incomplete voiding: they have to relearn how to void with detrusor pressure as the driving force, and how to get rid of their habit of emptying the bladder by abdominal pressure.

A programme for 'bladder (re)training' would seem a logical choice for the management of children with bladder/sphincter dysfunction, provided that the children have the cognitive capacity to understand what they are learning, and provided that an element of feedback can be incorporated into the (re)training, or (re)learning, process.[26,29] Feedback during training has been coined as 'biofeedback' by Miller[36]: 'The use of modern instrumentation to give a person better moment-to-moment information about a specific physiological process, that is under control of the nervous system, but not clearly or accurately perceived.' Urodynamic signals such as urine flow rate, pelvic floor electromyogram or detrusor pressure are perfectly suited as biofeedback.[26,35,37,38]

The success rate of such programmes – 60–

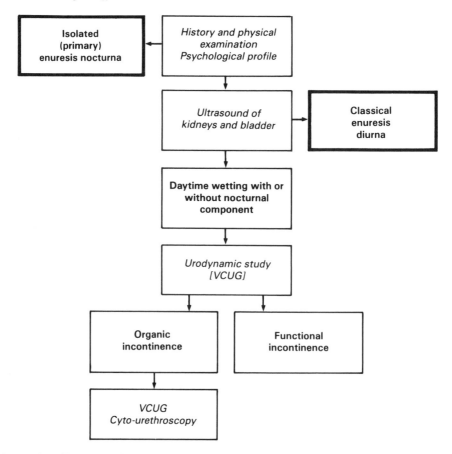

Figure 6.4 Structuring of intake and diagnostic steps in children who wet, leading to a clear distinction between enuresis and incontinence

70% in uncontrolled studies – underlines the importance of the pathophysiological concept behind the clinical complex of bladder/sphincter dysfunction and recurrent UTIs: in the children cured of incontinence and dysfunction, UTIs will not recur, often after years of persistent wetting, repeated diagnostic and therapeutic procedures such as cystoscopy, urethral dilatation or urethrotomy, and numerous patient months of antibiotic and chemotherapeutic regimens.

Diagnostic steps in children who wet

The boxes with heavy borders in Figure 6.4 denote the two forms of wetting, where bladder/sphincter function is essentially normal: all other forms of wetting imply bladder/sphincter dysfunction, and are termed incontinence. Following the steps, starting with history and physical examination, will lead to a clear distinction between enuresis and incontinence, without having to resort to a comprehensive imaging programme in every child who wets, 'just to be on the safe side'. The diagnostic steps, necessary to move down to the next decision level, are italicized in the diagram; diagnostic tests considered optional for a certain level are between brackets.

Renal imaging with ultrasound is not really necessary to arrive at the diagnosis of isolated nocturnal enuresis, but it is very helpful in the distinction between enuresis and incontinence: duplex kidneys, bladder wall thickness and post-void residual can point the way.

Voiding cysto-urethrography (VCUG) is mandatory whenever organic incontinence is suspected, but it is also indicated in the work-up of a child with functional incontinence and recurrent UTIs.

When available, urodynamic studies should be performed in all children with daytime wetting who clearly do not belong to the category of classical diurnal enuresis: these studies point the way, not only to the diagnosis but also to the right therapeutic modality. In difficult cases, with a long-standing history, urodynamics is often needed as a complement to history, physical examination and cysto-urethrography, to arrive at the distinction between organic incontinence and functional incontinence.

References

1. Järvelin M.R., Moilanen I., Kangas P., Moring K., Vikeväinen-Tervonen L., Huttunen N.-P. and Seppänen J. Aetiological and precipitating factors for childhood enuresis. *Acta paediatr. Scand.* 1991 **80**, 361–369

2. Meadow S.R. Day wetting. *Pediatr. Nephrol.* 1990, **4**, 178–184

3. McLorie G.A. and Husmann D.A. Incontinence and enuresis. *Ped. Clin. North. Am.* 1987, **34**; 1159–1174

4. Gool J.D. van. *Spina Bifida and Neurogenic Bladder Dysfunction – A Urodynamic Study*. Utrecht, Impress, 1986

5. deVries M.W. and deVries M.R. Cultural relativity of toilet training readiness: a perspective from East Africa. *Pediatrics* 1977, **60**, 170

6. MacKeith R.C., Meadow S.R. and Turner R.K. How children become dry. In: Kolvin I., MacKeith R.C. and Meadow S.R. (eds), *Bladder Control and Enuresis*. London, Heinemann, 1973

7. Editorial. Diurnal enuresis. *Lancet* 1987, **ii**, 314–315

8. Hellström A.-L., Hanson E., Hansson S., Hjälmås K. and Jodal U. Micturition habits and incontinence in 7-year-old Swedish school entrants. *Eur. J. Pediatr.* 1990, **149**, 434–437

9. Jonge G.A. de. Epidemiology of enuresis: a survey of the literature. In: Kolvin I., MacKeith R.C. and Meadow S.R (eds). *Bladder Control and Enuresis*. London, Heinemann, 1973

10. Mikkelsen E.J. and Rapoport J.L. Enuresis – psychopathology, sleep stage, and drug response. *Urol. Clin. North Am.* 1980, **7**, 361–377

11. Jonge G.A. de. *Children With Enuresis – An Epidemiological and Clinical Study*. Assen, van Gorcum, 1969

12. Moffat M.E.K. Nocturnal enuresis – psychologic implications of treatment and nontreatment. *J. Pediatr,* 1989, **114**, 697–704

13. Messer A.P. and de Jong T.P. Dry bed training and diagnosis in nocturnal enuresis. *Ned. Tijdschr. Geneeskd.* 1991, **135**, 1724–1725

14. Ferber R. Sleep-associated enuresis in the child. In: Kryger M.H., Roth Th. and Dement W.C. (eds). *Principles and Practice of Sleep Medicine*. Philadelphia, Saunders, 1989

15. Nørgaard J.P., Pedersen E.B. and Djurhuus J.C. Diurnal anti-diuretic hormone levels in enuretics. *J.Urol,* 1985, **134**, 1029–1031

16. Rittig S., Knudsen B., Nørgaard J.P., Pedersen E.B. and Djurhuus J.C. Abnormal diurnal rhythm of plasma vasopressin and urinary output in patients with enuresis. *Am.J.Physiol.,* 1989, **256**, F664–671

17. Armstrong S.M., Cassone V.N., Chesworth M.J., Redman J.R. and Short R.V. Synchronisation of mammalian circadian rhythms by melatonin. *J.Neural. .Trans.S.* 1986, **21**, 375–394

18. Forsyth W.I. and Butler R.J. Fifty years of enuretic alarms. *Arch.Dis.Child.* 1989, **64**, 789–885

19. Fordham K.E. and Meadow S.R. Controlled trial of standard pad and bell alarm against mini alarm for nocturnal enuresis. *Arch.Dis.Child.* 1989, **64**, 651–656

20. Azrin N.H. and Thienes P.M. Rapid elimination of enuresis by intensive learning without a conditioning apparatus. *Behav.Ther.* 1978, **9**, 342

21. Evans J.H.C. The efficacy of DDAVP in the treatment of nocturnal enuresis. In: Meadow S.R. (ed). *Desmopressin in Nocturnal Enuresis – Proceedings of an International Symposium*. London, Major Communications, 1989

22. Sukhai R.N., Mol J, and Harris A.S. Combined therapy of enuresis alarm and desmopressin in the treatment of nocturnal enuresis. *Eur. J. Pediatr.* 1989, **148**, 456–467

23. Herson V.C., Schmitt B.D. and Rumack B.H. Magical thinking and imipramine poisoning in two school aged children. *J. Am. Med. Ass.* 1979, **241**, 1926–1927

24. Gool J.D. van, Vijverberg M.A.W. and Jong T.P.V.M. de. Functional daytime incontinence: clinical and urodynamic assessment. *Scand. J. Urol. Nephrol.* 1992 (Suppl. 141), 58–69

25. Koff S.A. Bladder-sphincter dysfunction in childhood. *Urology* 1982, **19**, 457–461

26. Gool J.D. van, Kuijten R.H., Donckerwolcke R.A., Messer A.P. and Vijverberg M. Bladder-sphincter dysfunction, urinary infection and vesicoureteral reflux – with special reference to cognitive bladder training. *Contr. Nephrol.* 1984, **39**, 190–210

27. Gool J.D. van and Tanagho E.A. External sphincter activity and recurrent urinary tract infection in girls. *Urology* 1977, **10**, 348–53

28. Vincent S.A. Postural control of urinary incontinence: the curtsey sign. *Lancet* 1966, **ii**: 631–632

29. Gool J.D. van and Jonge G.A. de. Urge syndrome and urge incontinence. *Arch. Dis. Child.* 1989, **64**, 1629–1634

30. Koff S.A. and Byard M.A. The daytime urinary frequency syndrome of childhood. *J. Urol.* 1988, **140**, 1280–1281

31. Hinman F. Jr. Nonneurogenic neurogenic bladder (the Hinman syndrome) – 15 years later. *J. Urol.* 1986, **136**, 769–777

32. Allen T.D. Vesicoureteral reflux as a manifestation of dysfunctional voiding. In: Hodson C.J. and Kincaid-Smith P. (eds). *Reflux Nephropathy*. New York, Masson, 1979

33. Nielsen J.B., Djurhuus J.C. and Jörgensen T.M. Lower urinary tract dysfunction in vesicoureteral reflux. *Urol. Int.* 1984, **39**, 29–31

34. Smellie J.M., Grüneberg R.N., Bantock H.M. and Prescod N. Prophylactic co-trimoxazole and trimethoprim in the management of urinary tract infection in children. *Pediatr. Nephrol.* 1988, **2**, 12

35. Hellström A.-L., Hjälmås K. and Jodal U. Rehabilitation of the dysfunctional bladder in children: method and 3-year follow up. *J. Urol.* 1987, **138**, 847–849

36. Miller N.E. Learning of visceral and glandular responses. *Science* 1969, **163**, 434–437

37. Wear J.B., Wear R.B. and Cleeland C. Biofeedback in urology using urodynamics: preliminary observations. *J. Urol.* 1979, **121**, 464–468

38. Sugar E.C. and Firlit C.F. Urodynamic feedback: new therapeutic approach for childhood incontinence/infection (vesical voluntary sphincter dyssynergia). *J. Urol.* 1982, **128**, 1253–1258

7

Symptoms and signs of childhood renal tract disease

J.M. Savage, R.J. Postlethwaite

The symptoms of childhood diseases are often non-specific, testing the diagnostic skills of the paediatrician. In the most common renal disease, urinary tract infection (UTI), presentation may be with jaundice in the neonate, febrile convulsion in late infancy or failure to thrive in the toddler. Indeed throughout childhood UTI may remain totally asymptomatic. Many other urinary tract anomalies also remain asymptomatic for years, while silent deterioration in renal function can occur. The advent of antenatal ultrasound diagnosis for such conditions affords a major preventative opportunity in this situation. Similar problems arise with glomerular disease where presentation with puffy eyes is not uncommon, but most family doctors would suspect allergic conjunctivitis as a cause before eventually performing urinalysis. These diagnostic problems may be compounded by the younger patients' lack of language to express their symptoms lucidly. The names children commonly employ for the external genitalia are hardly anatomical and their use when talking to strangers may the subject of a social taboo. The clinician must, therefore, be alert to the possibility of underlying renal disease even when complaints are non-specific,[1] lest a chance for effective intervention is lost at an age when the long-term benefits are greatest.

Major manifestations

Certain symptoms and signs are strongly suggestive of renal tract pathology in children. This chapter will discuss these major manifestations, unless they are extensively covered elsewhere.

Pain of urinary tract origin

Pain can arise from the kidney, the collecting system or the bladder in childhood renal disease. Careful attention to the history may help to distinguish the site of the problem, but confusion with back pain and other causes of abdominal pain is frequent. It is worth remembering that pain of gastrointestinal origin is characteristically midline because intra-abdominal organs, including the ovaries, are bilaterally innervated in contrast to the upper urinary tract structures.[2]

Most diseases of the urinary tract are painless. Additionally, conditions that typically produce severe abdominal pain in adults may give rise to non-specific symptoms in children. Despite this, pain is an important symptom of urinary tract disease and urinary tract disease is the commonest cause of abdominal pain in children. Ten per cent of children suffer from recurrent abdominal pain. In only about 10% can an organic cause be identified for this recurrent pain, but urinary tract disease is the commonest organic cause.[3] Measurement of blood pressure, urinalysis and urine microscopy should be carried out in all children with recurrent abdominal pain.[3] It is not clear if the recommendation that a plain abdominal X-ray be obtained, preferably during the bout of pain,[3] is still appropriate, and certainly from a renal point of view ultrasonography is likely to be much more informative.

Guidelines have been evolved for identifying children with recurrent abdominal pain who require more extensive investigation,[4] and there are useful rules of thumb.[5]

- The more localized the pain, the more likely it is to have an organic origin.
- The more vague and diffuse the abdominal pain, the less likely an organic aetiology.
- The nearer to the umbilicus the pain occurs, the less likely a pathological explanation (Apley's sign).

In addition to these general guidelines when considering the possibility of a renal aetiology, a family history of relevance should be sought and the following patterns of pain would suggest a renal aetiology:

Flank pain

This arises from stretching of the renal capsule. Nausea and vomiting may precede this pain or may remain the only apparent symptom in younger children and infants. The most common cause in children is infection, where the oedema secondary to the inflammation is the cause. Swelling of the kidney also occurs in immunological processes such as acute post-infective glomerulonephritis or IgA nephropathy. Loin pain is the second most common symptom of Wilms' tumour, occurring in 20–30%, but there is almost always an easily palpable mass. In all these lesions the pain is usually localized in the flank with little radiation; it is described as a dull ache and there is usually loin tenderness on palpation.

Flank pain due to distension of the collecting system may arise with acute hydronephrosis caused for example by pelvi-ureteric junction obstruction or renal calculi. This pain may be sharper and/or colicky in character. Such pain, if brought on by excessive drinking, is very suggestive of pelvi-ureteric junction obstruction. It is more usual, however, for patients with even severe hydronephrosis to have no pain and present with non-specific symptoms or infection.

Ureteric pain

This is characteristically sharp, in the loin, radiating into the groin and usually severe and colicky. Only 16% of children with renal calculi have abdominal pain and then it is more commonly generalized abdominal pain rather than classical 'renal colic'. Anorexia, nausea, vomiting and symptoms of infection are a more usual presentation of renal calculi in children.[6] Blood clots are another important cause of ureteric pain in children. They may arise from trauma, either accidental or iatrogenic. Any cause of haematuria (see Chapter 1) may give rise to clots, but structural lesions such as cysts are more usual.

Patients with lateralized abdominal pain, particularly if this is colicky, should be screened for causes of renal calculi. Idiopathic hypercalciuria is an important cause of ureteric or flank pain in children and may occur without obvious stone formation.[7]

Abdominal pain in Henoch–Schoenlein syndrome may be difficult to distinguish from renal colic and in the absence of a typical rash, the presence of haematuria makes for further confusion. There are some reports that severe ureteric reflux may cause abdominal pain, but Smellie *et al.*[9] found no difference in the incidence of pain in urinary tract infection, with or without ureteric reflux.

Pain originating from the bladder

This is characteristically suprapubic and is generally caused by distension or inflammation. Inflammatory pain may cause severe spasms and is often accompanied by nausea, vomiting and local tenderness. Distension of the bladder in childhood is often of neurogenic origin and pain is dull or absent.

Pain in the scrotum

In children, this pain should always be assumed to be due to torsion of the testis. Orchitis is less common and is usually associated with UTI. Mumps orchitis is generally confined to adults.

Dysuria

Pain on micturition is known as dysuria and can be sharp, stinging or burning in character. A classification of causes is given in Table 7.1. The most likely pathological cause in children is UTI, but there may be no serious underlying problem. Many normal babies cry and even

Table 7.1 Causes of dysuria

Normal behaviour in young infants
Attention-seeking in toddlers
Urinary tract pathology
    urinary tract infection
    passage of stone
    bladder neck irritation by stone
    acute nephritis
Local external factors
    napkin dermatitis
    meatal ulcer
    balanitis
    vulvovaginitis
Drugs
    amitriptyline
    chlordiazepoxide
    imipramine
    isoniazid
    cyclophosphamide
    sulphonamide

scream on micturition[10] and it is impossible to be sure whether the sensation of passing urine has been painful or has merely woken the infant up. A scalding sensation is more likely when the concentration of the urine is increased, but such discomfort may be external rather than arising in the urethra, particularly if a napkin rash is present.

Increased concentration of the urine occurs in babies who are pyrexial, or who are not feeding well for any reason, possibly including teething. In the infant and toddler age group, dysuria should only be attributed to urinary infection on the basis of an associated significant colony count of organisms cultured from a mid-stream or bladder aspiration urine sample. Parental reaction to complaints of painful micturition in young children may on occasions lead to its use for attention-seeking.

Thorough examination of the external genitalia and perineal area is imperative when dysuria occurs. Napkin dermatitis and balanitis will be obvious, but a more careful examination will be needed to detect vulvovaginitis or a meatal ulcer.

The persistence or troublesome recurrence of dysuria with frequency in the absence of clear evidence of UTI is often referred to as the frequency-dysuria syndrome. This diagnosis does not exclude a pathological cause. In older children with dysuria, the syndrome presents a diagnostic problem in up to 20% of hospital referrals screened for causes of renal calculi (see Chapter 32).

Sulphonamide crystalluria is a historical cause of dysuria; other drugs more recently associated with the symptom include imipramine, which is often prescribed for enuresis, and cyclophosphamide, used in the treatment of nephrotic syndrome.

Haematuria and urine discoloration

When the urine is abnormally dark the presence of *infection, blood* or *urobilinogen* should be suspected. To exclude these possibilities midstream urine microscopy and culture should be combined with chemical 'stick' testing. Haematuria is exhaustively discussed in Chapter 1. In practice the urine is more likely to darken as a result of concentration, e.g. during a pyrexial illness. Placing urine samples in a refrigerator while awaiting specimen collection may cause *crystal formation*. Phosphate crystals merely make the sample appear cloudy, but urates may produce a reddish-brown precipitate or an overall pink tinge. Such crystals will dissolve on boiling. *Food dyes* only rarely affect urine, making it red. Beetroot, blackcurrant juice, blackberries and rhubarb contain anthocyanins, but vegetable dyes are added to many commercial food preparations. Alcaptonuria and tyrosinosis are *rare inborn metabolic errors* causing dark/black urine. There is a long list of *drugs* which may discolour urine[11] (see Table 1.1). Those likely to be administered to children include laxatives containing cascara, dantron (Dorbanex) or senna which produces a red colour. Antimicrobials incriminated are sulphonamides (yellow), rifampicin (red) and nitrofurantoin (red). Pyridium (phenazopyridine hydrochloride) and quinine or pamaquin may render urine orange to brown.

Many normal pre-school children pass urine 10 times per day and some parents will mistakenly regard this as too frequent. The rate of voiding varies with age and so an obvious *increase* in frequency is a more significant symptom.

Frequency resulting from bladder irritation is often accompanied by a feeling of urgency. This may occur in UTI, the presence of a bladder stone and on rare occasions with pelvic appendicitis or inflammation. Detrusor muscle instability causing these symptoms may be seen with a mild neurogenic bladder or may be a familial condition, but both cause symptoms throughout life and are associated with small volume bladders or cystogram.

An increase in the volume of urine passed (polyuria) may also result in frequency. In this situation, urgency is uncommon. Toddlers are the most difficult group to assess clinically because of the normal high frequency of micturition and further because toilet demands may be employed to gain attention. Rarely in older children polyuria and frequency may result from psychogenic polydipsia. We have seen several children with habitual frequent micturition but no underlying pathology. These children did not drink excessively but frequently passed small volumes of urine. Lack of nocturia was often a clue.

A useful screening test of urine-concentrating ability is estimation of early morning urine osmolarity; a value of < 800 mosmol/litre is normal. In these difficult situations admission to hospital to assess frequency and volume may be required, with use and access to toilet facilities carefully monitored.

Abnormalities of voiding and urinary stream

Any infant or child suffering from urinary retention or difficulty in starting to pass urine, or who exhibits a poor stream, requires urological investigation to exclude obstruction, neurogenic bladder and UTI. All neonates should pass urine within the first 48 h of life and 90% will do so within 24 h. Poor urinary stream in the newborn male is traditionally associated with posterior urethral valves, but routine antenatal ultrasound scanning means obstructive uropathy presenting after birth should become historic. Small children with UTI may refuse to pass urine because of dysuria and develop significant retention, and this situation may also be precipitated by the discomfort of a bladder stone. For a full discussion consult Chapter 6.

Daytime and night-time wetting, urgency and frequency, and dysfunctional voiding

These problems are discussed in more detail in Chapter 6.

Polyuria and polydipsia

Polyuria is defined as the passage of large volumes of urine, and as a general guide the volume should exceed 1 litre in pre-school children, 2 litres in school-aged children and 3 litres in adults. *Polydipsia* is abnormally increased water intake and thirst. Normal urine volumes are ill-defined in childhood and the range will depend on (a) the volume ingested and resulting water requiring excretion, (b) the amount of solute requiring excretion, and (c) the ability of the kidney to dilute and concentrate. All these factors vary with maturity, age and size. In early infancy beyond the first week, water intake is about 150 ml kg^{-1} day^{-1}; of this, 25 ml/kg is incorporated in growing tissue and 25 ml/kg is accounted for by insensible loss. Thus the urine output is approximately 100 ml kg^{-1} day^{-1}. Intake and output of fluid per kg body weight fall with age and increasing ability of the kidney to concentrate and excrete a solute load. *Normal daily urine volume*[12] at 1 year is of the order of 500 ml/day, reaching 600 ml by 3 years, 700 ml by 5 years, 1 litre at 7–8 years and adult volumes of 1.5 litres by 15 years of age.

Frequency of micturition and nocturia should not be confused with polyuria. In the former, small amounts of urine are passed repeatedly but the total daily volume is normal. By the age of 5, most if not all urine is passed by day, although this diurnal pattern is absent in enuretic children. Nocturia is the passage of urine at night in the absence of enuresis and while it can occur in polyuric patients, it may also be associated with frequency in UTI, with congestive heart failure, and with renal or hepatic failure when the total urine volume is not increased.

Aetiology of polyuria

An exhaustive list of causes of polyuria is given in Table 7.2, but in practice only a few of these will be seen with any significant frequency. *Abnormal feeding habits* in toddlers may result in the diet being totally fluid. This may be part of a more general behaviour problem and parents will often complain that the child has a poor appetite for solids (which is hardly surprising). These small children do not seek drinks at night. A similar but more difficult problem to manage is *psychogenic polydipsia* in older children. *Diabetes mellitus* is distinguished by high urine osmolarity due to the presence of glucose. Glycosuria also occurs in some tubular disorders such as the Fanconi syndrome, but aminoaciduria and cystinuria are then also likely to be present. Following the relief of an *obstructive uropathy*, e.g. posterior urethral valves, polyuria occurs, initially due to the osmotic load of the

Table 7.2 Causes of polyuria in children

Increased fluid intake
   Primary polydipsia – behavioural/psychogenic
   Hypothalamic polydipsia
   Hyperreninaemia including Wilms' tumour

Increased osmotic load
   Glucose – diabetes mellitus
            – total parenteral nutrition
            – enteral tube feeding
   Urea   – relieved obstructive uropathy
            – hypercatabolic states (burns)
            – chronic renal failure
            – following transplantation
   Mannitol – infusion

Central diabetes insipidus – failure of ADH production
   Idiopathic   – congenital or familial type
   Post-traumatic – basal skull fracture
   Neoplasia   – infra- or suprasellar
                – leukaemia
                – craniopharyngioma
                – histiocytosis X
   Post-hypophysectomy
   Infections – encephalitis, meningitis, post-tuberculous
   Vascular – aneurysm or thrombosis

Nephrogenic diabetes insipidus – tubular unresponsiveness
                             to ADH
   Acquired – obstructive uropathy
           – potassium depletion
           – hypercalcaemia
           – sickle cell disease
           – chronic renal failure
             (polycystic disease, etc.)
           – drugs: amphotericin, methoxyflurane, tetra-
             cycline
   Sex-linked inherited

Drugs
   Diuretics including theophylline
   Drugs causing nephrogenic diabetes insipidus
     (above)
   Mannitol infusion

Physiological diuretic syndromes
   Nephrotic syndrome remission
   Recovery phase of acute tubular necrosis

high blood urea, but often persisting because of permanent functional tubular damage. In the diuretic phase of *acute tubular necrosis*, polyuria may lead to volume depletion and diuresis is typical of the onset of a remission in steroid-treated minimal change *nephrotic syndrome*. *Drugs* may increase urine volume and, although an obvious effect of diuretics, this may be overlooked when for example a slow-release theophylline preparation is used in the treatment of asthma. *Central diabetes insipidus* (DI) is due to

failure of ADH production. Such failure is likely to be a secondary phenomenon related to intracranial neoplasia, infection, trauma or surgery. It can be congenital in association with structural brain abnormality and very rarely familial, with either dominant or recessive inheritance. *Nephrogenic DI* is due to end-organ unresponsiveness to ADH which results in a complete or partial urine concentrating defect. The familial form is classically sex-linked recessive affecting males, but the females may have slight reduction in concentrating ability if investigated. Hypokalaemia and hypercalcaemia interfere with the cellular action of ADH, but like obstructive uropathy also affect the renal medullary solute concentration to disrupt tubular function and produce polyuria. *Sickle cell disease* produces tubular polyuria which initially is reversible by exchange transfusion, but becomes permanent when recurrent sickling leads to ischaemic renal papillary damage. As in more obvious polyuric states, reduced urine-concentrating ability in children, for example in *polycystic disease*, becomes hazardous should they develop vomiting or diarrhoea when severe dehydration and collapse can develop rapidly.

Diagnosis in polyuria and polydipsia

A careful clinical history and simple baseline renal function tests will enable differentiation into the major groupings in Table 7.2. Blood for electrolytes, urea, creatinine and calcium can be determined by auto-analyser screening and the first urine passed in the morning should be tested for glucose, specific gravity and osmolality. The results will determine the direction of further investigations and radiology. The distinction between psychogenic polydipsia (PP), central DI and nephrogenic DI is often a problem which can only be solved by a carefully supervised *water deprivation test*,[12,13] with subsequent administration of vasopressin. This is a potentially hazardous test in patients with DI. *In infancy, an initial screening procedure should be first undertaken*, as follows, since PP is unlikely. Urine and blood samples are collected for osmolality estimations prior to a feed, i.e. after a 3–4 h fast. When plasma osmolarity is high in the presence of hyposthenuria, water deprivation should be avoided and instead response to vasopressin assessed. In older children, free fluids are allowed overnight until 8.00 h when the bladder is emptied and blood taken for osmolality. If the fasting plasma osmolarity is > 295 mosmol/kg H_2O, then DI is invariably the diagnosis, but if < 285 mosmol/kg, the diagnosis is most likely PP. Unless the plasma osmolarity is convincingly raised, water is withheld for up to 8 h or until 3% body weight is lost should this occur first. Each hour urine is collected for volume and osmolality measurement and the patient weighed. At the end of the test, plasma osmolality is again estimated. In PP there will be no significant change in plasma osmolality, whereas an obvious rise, often to > 300 mosmol/kg, occurs in DI. Distinction between central and nephrogenic DI can now be achieved by observing the response to subcutaneous lysine vasopressin (5 iu per m² surface area), or to nasal DDAVP (desmopressin 20 µg/m² SA). Urine osmolality should exceed 800 mosmol/kg after adequate fluid deprivation in PP, but only after vasopressin in central DI. Measurement of plasma ADH level when available may aid diagnosis; it is generally raised in nephrogenic DI, but undetectable in central DI and PP (discussed further in Chapter 10).

Anaemia

This is a feature of chronic renal impairment and is normochromic and normocytic in nature. Anaemia is not a feature of acute renal failure unless there has been acute blood loss or haemolysis. A mild normocytic normochromic anaemia may occur in acute nephritic syndrome, but is a dilutional phenomenon due to fluid overload. The major mechanisms which contribute to the anaemia of CRF are shortened red blood cell survival, decreased erythropoietin production and blood loss due to platelet dysfunction, e.g. from the gastrointestinal tract. Iron and folate deficiency due to poor appetite and nutrition may compound these effects, so that iron, ferritin and folate levels should always be checked in these patients. A degree of anaemia on a similar nutritional basis may be encountered in small children with untreated recurrent or chronic urinary tract infection.

Abdominal masses

Sixty-five per cent of abdominal masses in the newborn period are retroperitoneal in location and 55% are renal in origin. The main renal lesions are hydronephrosis (25%) and multicystic dysplastic kidney (15%).[14] These lesions are now usually identified by antenatal ultrasound.

Beyond the newborn period, the percentage of abdominal masses that are retroperitoneal increases to 78%. This is largely due to the increase in malignant masses of both the kidney (Wilms' tumour 28%) and the adrenals (neuroblastoma 21%).[14]

In approaching the paediatric patient with an abdominal mass, a careful history and examination are important. There are various clues which might suggest a renal cause. A history of oligohydramnios with possibly mild postural deformities at birth is suggestive of an antenatal renal lesion. A family history of renal problems, hypertension and renal failure should be sought. Abdominal pain, symptoms suggestive of urinary infection, preceding poor feeding with or without polyuria, unexplained vomiting, haematuria and abnormal urinary stream are all suggestive of underlying urinary tract abnormalities. Examination should include the spine, external genitalia, blood pressure and bladder assessment.

A distended bladder may result from voluntary urinary retention and should be examined after the bladder has been emptied. Pathological bladder enlargement may be due to bladder outlet obstruction (see Chapter 28) or neuropathic bladder (see Chapter 26). Tumours of the lower urinary tract in children are uncommon and are usually sarcomas or embryonal tumours. They present with abnormalities of micturition or an abdominal mass rather than haematuria. The tumour may be palpable abdominally or there may be a distended bladder. They are always palpable rectally and this examination must be performed to exclude this possibility. Genital and other pelvic masses such as haematocolpos or teratomas are important, not only because they may be mistaken for bladder lesions but because there may be an associated obstructive uropathy.

Table 7.3 lists the common causes of renal masses. Ultrasonography has enormously simplified the approach to the diagnosis of renal masses in children. On the basis of the history, clinical and ultrasound examination, the mass can usually be confidently identified as being renal in origin. The age of the patient, whether or not the lesion is bilateral, the presence or absence of bladder abnormalities and the appearances on ultrasound suggest a provisional diagnosis in the majority of cases. The main

Table 7.3 Common unilateral and bilateral renal tract masses

	Unilateral	Bilateral
Hydronephrosis	Obstructive hydronephrosis	Obstructive hydronephrosis
	Non-obstructive hydronephrosis	Non-obstructive hydronephrosis
Cystic	Multicystic dysplasia	Cystic dysplasia
	Cystic dysplasia	Autosomal dominant polycystic kidney disease
	Simple cyst	Cysts with syndromes
Bright echo pattern		Autosomal recessive polycystic kidney disease
Solid diffuse		
Miscellaneous:	Compensatory hypertrophy	Infection in the newborn
	Duplication	Beckwith–Weidemann syndrome
	Fused crossed ectopia	Acute renal failure
		Storage disorders
Infection:	Acute pyelonephritis	Acute pyelonephritis
	Pelvinephric abscess	
	Xanthogranulomatous pyelonephritis	
Immunological:		Glomuerulonephritis
		Nephrotic syndrome
Vascular:	Arterial or venous thrombosis	Arterial or venous thrombosis
	Acute cortical necrosis	Acute cortical necrosis
Tumours		Leukaemia/lymphoma
Solid focal		
Tumours:	Wilms' tumour	Wilms' tumour
	Mesoblastic nephroma	
	Renal carcinoma	
Infection:	Renal abscess	Multiple renal abscesses

patterns seen on ultrasound are hydronephrosis, cystic lesions, bright echo pattern and solid lesions which may be focal or diffuse (Table 7.3). Accurate diagnosis generally requires further imaging. Imaging in paediatric kidney disease is discussed in Chapter 11 and many of the specific lesions are discussed in other chapters (particularly Chapters 25, 26 and 28). Figure 7.2 gives an indication as to which further imaging techniques are generally useful in the different situations.

In our view, however, apart from the first-level investigation, the further investigation of renal masses in children is a specialized task which should be individualized after discussion between the paediatric radiologist, surgeon, nephrologist and, if a tumour is a possibility, the oncologist.

Identification of a mass as hydronephrosis does not usually present any problems. Micturating cystography, to exclude reflux as a cause

of the hydronephrosis and to assess the bladder, and diuresis renography to assess differential function and to distinguish obstructive from non-obstructive hydronephrosis, are almost always the next line of investigation. The further investigation of the dilated urinary system is discussed in Chapter 28.

A congenital hydronephrosis must be distinguished from a multicystic dysplastic kidney since hydronephrosis may be corrected surgically. In hydronephrosis, the 'cystic areas' should be seen to communicate and there is almost always function on the radionuclide scan. With multicystic dysplasia, the multiple hypoechoic cysts should be seen to be non-communicating and there will be no function on the radionuclide scan. Rarely, a non-functioning kidney on radionuclide imaging might not convincingly be shown to have non-communicating cysts. In this instance, antegrade pyelography will be required to distinguish the two lesions.

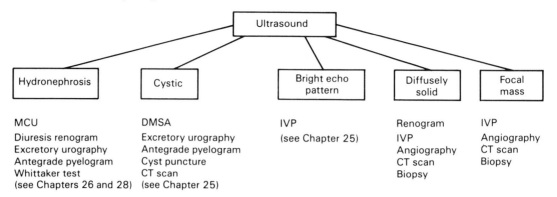

Figure 7.1 Diagnostic evaluation of renal masses

Whether this is actually necessary is a controversial point, as the successful surgical rescue of a non-functioning congenital hydronephrosis is unlikely.

Cystic lesions are discussed in detail in Chapter 25. It is important to realize that in autosomal recessive polycystic kidney disease the cysts are microscopic and produce a characteristic bright echo pattern rather than discrete cysts on ultrasonography.

Many solid renal lesion masses should present no diagnostic problems. The kidneys are often palpable in the normal neonate and enlargement of the kidneys may be a sign of generalized infection in this age group. Compensatory hypertrophy, duplication, fused crossed ectopic, and acute pyelonephritis should easily be identified. Beckwith–Wiedemann syndrome (macroglossia, omphacele, organomegaly) is a rare but important cause of bilaterally enlarged kidneys. Seven per cent of affected individuals develop Wilms' tumor and 6-monthly ultrasound is required to monitor for this. Bilateral renal enlargement occurs in most cases of acute renal failure and in immunological conditions such as glomerulonephritis and nephrotic syndrome.

Xanthogranulomatous pyelonephritis[15] presents with non-specific symptoms of infection, anaemia and a palpable renal mass. It is an unusual complication of infection, typically *Proteus* urinary tract infection. Previously it was usually identified at operation and nephrectomy was curative. The histology is characteristic. We have recently treated 3 children in whom the diagnosis was suspected on ultrasonography, confirmed by percutaneous renal biopsy, and following treatment with antibiotics useful

renal function has been preserved in 2 of the 3 cases.

Renal vein thrombosis usually presents with a flank mass, haematuria and sometimes hypertension. Ultrasonography shows renal enlargement with increased echogenicity of the involved kidney obscuring the normal central echo complex.[14] Renography, either with a dynamic or static renogram, usually shows no function. This pattern on imaging plus the clinical presentation and predisposing factor (see Chapters 21 and 30) should allow for confident diagnosis.

In acute leukaemia and lymphomas, both kidneys may be infiltrated by malignant deposits. The generalized disease is likely to be obvious and diagnostic difficulties are unlikely.

Wilms' tumour represents 10% of malignant tumours in the paediatric age group and 22% of all abdominal masses.[14] Peak age of diagnosis is 2–3 years and more than 75% present before 5 years. The tumour is bilateral in 8–12% of cases, most commonly in the younger age group and with familial cases. The most common presentation is with an abdominal mass which is firm, non-tender and rarely crosses the midline. Additional features include hypertension, haematuria and less frequently fever and abdominal pain.[14] Rarely, polycythaemia from increased erythropoietin production may be present.

There are a large number of recognized associations of Wilms' tumour, including hemihypertrophy, aniridia and Beckwith–Wiedemann syndrome. In Drash syndrome, different combinations of ambiguous genitalia, nephropathy and Wilms' tumour which is often bilateral are found.[16]

The diagnosis of Wilms' tumour is usually

Table 7.4   Non-specific symptoms occurring with increased frequency in childhood urinary tract disease

Neonatal jaundice
Colic/irritability in infancy
Pyrexia
Convulsion
Abdominal and back pain
Pallor/anaemia
Nausea, anorexia and vomiting
Failure to thrive/growth retardation
Offensive-smelling urine
Facial swelling
Tachypnoea
Deafness
Perineal discomfort

suspected on clinical grounds. The characteristic imaging finding is that of a solid, intrarenal mass. Ultrasound demonstrates an intrarenal mixed echogenic mass. Haemorrhage or necrosis appear as sonolucent areas. Excretory urography shows stretching and distortion of the pelvicalyceal system without renal displacement. In 10% of cases, the affected kidneys are non-functioning. Calcification is rare (3–5%) and is much more likely with neuroblastoma.[14] The further evaluation of Wilms' tumour, histology and treatment, falls within the province of paediatric oncology rather than nephrology. Treatment consists of a combination of surgery, irradiation and chemotherapy. The prognosis is excellent with favourable histology (80–90%). Approximately 10% are sarcomatous and have a poor prognosis.[14]

Mesoblastic nephroma (fetal renal hamartoma, benign congenital Wilms' tumour) is the most common neoplasm found in the first few months of life. It is usually large at birth. Imaging shows an intrarenal mass. This lesion is cured by nephrectomy and no distant metastases have been reported. Rarely the histology will reveal a more invasive lesion which requires more aggressive therapy.

Renal adenocarcinoma is predominantly a tumour of adulthood, although it can be seen rarely in childhood. Differentiation from Wilms' tumour is only usually possible on histological grounds.

Non-specific manifestations

Non-specific symptoms occurring with increased frequency in childhood urinary tract disease are listed in Table 7.4. In many instances, such as *neonatal jaundice* or *irritability in infants*, urinary problems are not common causes but it is important to consider the possibility in differential diagnoses and include urine cultures and simple plasma renal function tests in the basic investigative work-up. Both symptoms can result from UTI in which pyrexia is not a constant feature. When *pyrexia* does occur in UTI, although there may be no specific symptoms, a febrile *convulsion* can be precipitated. Renal disease is the commonest cause of severe hypertensive encephalopathy in children and seizure is a frequent presentation of accelerated hypertension. *Abdominal and back pain* have been discussed earlier in this chapter. *Pallor* may result from chronic infection, from anaemia associated with poor appetite or with chronic renal impairment. The combination of *nausea, vomiting and anorexia* is perhaps the most common presenting symptom complex of illness in the young child. It is frequently seen in the presence of urine infection, in renal tubular acidosis and when uraemia develops either acutely or as a result of chronic renal insufficiency.

Vomiting alone does not always indicate illness since many babies ruminate and regurgitate small volumes of food. Nausea is a symptom of older children. Simple precipitants such as travel sickness, or dislikes for specific foods and gastroenteritis, should be excluded. If anorexia is added to the history the chances of an organic basis is extremely high, although all three occur in migraine and the periodic syndrome.

There are three major aetiological groups:

- Infections – foremost are the frequent acute viral conditions of childhood, otitis media, UTI, meningitis and hepatitis.
- Gastrointestinal problems including appendicitis, bowel obstruction, inflammatory bowel disease and coeliac disease.
- A miscellaneous group of disorders remains including diabetic acidosis, raised intracranial pressure, uraemia and some metabolic disorders such as galactosaemia.

For clinical purposes, division of patients into those with acute symptoms from those with persistent problems aids logical investigation.

Although only 20% of children who *fail to thrive* are likely to have organic disease,[17] it is a common feature of chronic renal insufficiency when *growth retardation* as measured by height is most obviously affected. The phenomenon is seen in tubular disorders which cause acidosis, salt wasting or polyuria even in the absence of uraemia. It may also be related to disturbed vitamin D, calcium and phosphate metabolism leading to rickets and osteodystrophy. Children with these groups of renal problems frequently have anorexia causing calorie deficiency and poor weight gain.

Failure to thrive has been associated with chronic urinary infection. This is most likely a secondary effect due to loss of appetite, since the majority of patients with chronic pyelonephritis thrive normally.

There is end-organ resistance to growth hormone in childhood uraemic states delaying growth. Long-term prednisolone therapy in glomerular disease or following transplantation may result in *growth retardation*. These latter children may however be overweight for their height because of steroid appetite stimulation. Acute nephritis and nephrotic syndrome may present with *facial swelling*. In the early stages when oedema is confined to the periobital area, these conditions may be mistaken for allergic reactions.

Parents on occasions suspect UTI because their child has *offensive-smelling urine*. The smell of urine is most likely to be related to its concentration, to the presence of enuresis or poor hygiene. Nappies worn overnight smell particularly strongly when urea-splitting organisms are presented to produce ammonia. *Pseudomonas aerogenes* has an associated foul smell which may be detectable from infected urine, especially at first voiding in the morning or from neurogenic bladders which are extremely susceptible to this organism.

Tachypnoea

When a metabolic acidosis develops, compensatory mechanisms produce faster, deeper breathing in an effort to blow off carbon dioxide. Although this is characteristically seen in chronic renal failure and in distal renal tubular acidosis, other causes include diabetic ketoacidosis, dehydration associated with diarrhoea and reduced renal perfusion, drugs such as salicylate and certain inborn errors of metabolism. Tachypnoea is also seen in the absence of acidosis in hypoxaemia, encephalopathy and hyperthermia.

Deafness

There is a genetic basis for one-third to one-half of childhood deafness. The best known association with renal disease is the autosomal dominant hereditary nephritis of the Alport syndrome. Males are more severely affected than females by both components. Affected males develop sensonineural deafness in mid-childhood and renal failure in late teenage years. Cases account for 2–3% of chronic renal failure and 1% of deafness. Deafness also is more frequent in patients with renal tubular acidosis and renal hypoplasia. Potter's syndrome of renal agenesis is the most dramatic association between renal disease and external ear malformation.[18] This has led to the presence of any external ear malformation or pre-auricular pit or tag becoming an indication for renal ultrasound in the neonate to exclude renal malformation.

Perineal discomfort and vulvovaginitis

Inflammation of the vulval area produces a symptom pattern of local pain, burning or itch and external dysuria. Parents often complain of a strong or unpleasant smell from the area or from the child's pants. Differentiation of these symptoms from those of UTI is difficult, especially in younger and inarticulate children who fail to localize the problem, and there is a symptomatic overlap with the frequency/dysuria syndrome.

Thorough examination of the child and the pants is essential, but time must first be spent winning the patient's confidence and allowing her to relax. This may readily reveal vulval inflammation, swelling and discharge. The pants may be too tight and of a potentially irritant material such as nylon. Evidence of sexual trauma must not be overlooked. Gentle separation of the labia is usually all that is required. Vaginal examination is usually unnecessary unless a foreign body is suspected, and can usually be achieved using a simple auroscope and perhaps a fine blunt metal probe. When a gentle tactful approach fails to win a child's co-operation, adequate sedation is important before a second attempt is made but a general anaesthetic is rarely required.

The skin and epithelium of the child's vulval area is delicate and sensitive, and easily irritated by many agents. Once inflammation occurs there is a high risk of secondary infection. *Poor hygiene* is the most common initiating factor and the organisms commonly found on the perineum are likely to be implicated.[19] *Chemical irritants* are also commonly involved. Antiseptic creams for nappy rash and bubble bath solutions may set up chemical contact or allergic reactions. *Trauma* is most likely to be accidental, but examination should ensure the hymen is intact. Foreign body trauma occurs in the summer from sand particles and may also be due to trapped scraps of toilet tissue. The actual insertion of foreign bodies in the vagina is rare in children. *Threadworms* are known to cause vulval irritation and the characteristic night itch may give the clue. Itch may also be due to local *skin conditions* including atopic or seborrhoeic eczema, scabies or fungal infection. Measles and other childhood exanthemas such as chickenpox and scarlet fever can involve the vulva and cause transient symptoms.

When secondary infection is suspected, swabs and wet smears should be taken to identify the organism. Pus in the vagina can on occasions be milked down by a finger in the rectum. *Candida, Trichomonas* and gonorrhoeal infections are rare in children. Pre-existing eczema and diabetes predispose to monilial infection, but it is more likely to follow a course of antibiotics. When *Trichomonas* infection is found outside the neonatal period the suspicion of sexual contact becomes high and such contact is inevitably the basis for gonorrhoea.

Careful counselling of parents is important, as many mothers will be upset by the diagnosis. Parents should be assured the condition is minor. The psychological effect on the child of too meticulous attention to hygiene may need to be emphasized, particularly where a sensitivity reaction to antiseptic creams has precipitated or perpetuated the problem.

The approach to management depends on the severity of the inflammation, the presence of infection and the initiating factors. When the child is still in nappies, ammoniacal irritation and possible maceration of skin by moisture should be minimized. Where enuresis is a precipitating factor in older children, efforts directed at resolving this problem should be initiated. General advice to the older age group should include daily baths or washing of the genital area, wiping from front to back after using the toilet, wearing loose-fitting cotton pants, avoiding tight-fitting clothes, and avoiding topical ointments, antiseptics and deodorants.

When secondary infection is present, antibiotics should be prescribed systemically because of the risk of skin sensitization from topical application. Metronidazole and nystatin should also be given orally.

On occasions, patient's symptoms are resistant to the treatment prescribed or persist in recurring despite what seems adequate preventative measures. Usually it is inflammation or discomfort which persists rather than overt infection. In this situation only, one may resort to a local oestrogen application.

The adult vagina is under endogenous oestrogen stimulation and has an epithelium 40–50 cells thick containing glycogen which is acted on by lactobacilli to produce a local pathogen-resistant acid medium. The child's vaginal epithelium in contrast is thin, perhaps 5 cells thick since there is no oestrogen effect. The lack of glycogen results in a neutral pH vaginal bacterial culture medium. If 0.01% dienoestrol cream is applied sparingly 3 times daily for 2–3 weeks, the change in vaginal pH to acid with thickening of the epithelium generally achieves a cure.

Labial adhesions can form as a result of vulval inflammation or be present from birth. Gentle separation of the labia and treatment as above with 0.01% dienoestrol cream is all that is required and will prevent recurrence.

Balanitis

Inflammation and infection of the foreskin causes local pain, tenderness, swelling and dysuria. On occasions difficulty in micturition results from sealing of the meatus by coagulated purulent debris under the prepuce. If examination of the penis is not routinely performed in boys with dysuria, UTI can be falsely diagnosed due to gross contamination of specimens taken for culture.

The problem is usually seen in infants and toddlers still wearing nappies and is associated with poor local hygiene. Forced retraction of the foreskin in the first 2 years of life when the prepuce is normally adherent to the glans may play a role. Tearing of the natural adhesions may result in bleeding and secondary infection. Poor hygiene and self-manipulation are factors in older children.

Balanitis responds promptly to oral antibiotics. Local topical antibiotic or antiseptic creams may also be used but carry a risk of skin sensitization. Symptomatic relief can be achieved by frequent warm baths and simple analgesics.

Provided that response to an antibiotic is rapid, careful attention to hygiene may be the only further treatment required. Circumcision is indicated for resultant phimosis or recurrence. Where possible this may be delayed until the child is out of nappies because of the increased risk of a complicating meatal stenosis.

Urinary symptoms and sexual abuse

Recurrent urinary infection and dysuria are said to occur with increased frequency in girls subjected to sexual abuse. When dysuria is found to be secondary to vulvovaginitis or when a vaginal discharge is present, this possibility must be considered and the doctor will have to ask questions of the mother and perhaps the child.[20,21] The mother should be asked if she has any idea how the child got the discharge and whether anyone could have touched her in the vaginal area where she has the problem. It is likely that the child should also be questioned with the parents' permission. Depending on the family reaction to the initial interview, and the clinical and culture findings, the paediatrician must decide on involvement of specialists skilled in the area of child abuse and of social agencies. It is suggested that 10% of children are sexually abused[22] and that where vulvovaginitis is present the evidence of abuse is found in 20%[23] Any clinical evidence of bruising or trauma in the genital area in boys or girls carries a high index of suspicion.

Early clinical diagnosis in paediatric renal disease

It is possible to live a normal life and normal lifespan with one kidney. With two kidneys there is obviously an enormous functional reserve when disease strikes. Because of this, progressive renal damage often remains undetected for a long time. Identification of the problem in this silent period should be a major preventative aim for the paediatrician. This can be achieved in several ways:

- Family screening in genetic conditions, e.g.

Table 7.5   Factors which increase the risk of associated renal anomaly

Raised α-fetoprotein
Oligohydramnios
Large placenta[24]
Large fontanelles, separation of suture[24]
Congenital postural deformity[25]
Urinary ascites
Single palmar crease
Single umbilical artery[26]
Auricular abnormalities[27]/deafness
Branchial fistulae
Polydactyly
Supernumerary nipples[28]
Gut abnormalities
  Tracheo-oesophageal fistula
  Gut atresia
  Anal/rectal anomalies
Vater association
Spinal cord defects
Scoliosis/vertebral abnormalities
Absent abdominal muscles
Ambiguous genitalia/cloacal abnormalities
Hemihypertrophy
Congenital heart disease
Partial lipodystrophy
Nail hypoplasia/absent patellae
Cutaneous lesions
  Cafe au lait patches
  Chagran patches
  Adenoma sebaceum
  Depigmented patches
  Lesions of Fabry's disease
Eye problems
  Keratoconus
  Coloboma
  Cataracts
  Microphthalmia
  Retinal dysplasia/tapetoretinal degeneration
  Retinitis pigmentosa
  Aniridia

polycystic renal disease, Alport's syndrome and vesico-ureteric reflux.
- Referral for diagnostic imaging of all children with UTI.
- Renal ultrasound antenatally or of all neonates to detect obstructive uropathy.
- Recognition of clinical associations with renal disease.

Factors with an increased risk of associated renal abnormality/disease

An increasingly bewildering array of syndromes with renal involvement, both inherited and

Table 7.6 **Malignant disease associations**

Wilms' tumour – Isolated hemihypertrophy
  – Beckwith–Wiedemann
  – Neurofibromatosis
  – Wilms', aniridia, genito-urinary abnormalities, mental handicap
  – Drash syndrome[16]
von Hippel–Lindau disease[29]

non-inherited, are described. The use of a computer database, such as the POSSUM database, to identify these syndromes is discussed in Chapter 23. In addition, there are a number of non-specific associations of renal disease. Consequently, a number of clinical features should alert one to the possibility of an associated renal tract problem. Some of the more common associations are listed in Table 7.5. The presence of one of these features should prompt appropriate investigation for a possible renal association. The most frequently indicated investigation would be an ultrasound, but the investigations should be directed by interrogation of the database for the likely association.

There are a number of associations which indicate an increased risk of malignancy (Table 7.6). Regular monitoring in the Beckwith–Wiedemann syndrome has already been discussed. The Wilms' tumour, aniridia, genito-urinary abnormality and mental handicap association represents a contiguous gene complex.

References

1. James J.A. Important clinical manifestations of renal disease. In: *Renal Disease in Childhood*, 3rd edn. St Louis, Mosby, 1976: 33–50
2. Bruskewitz R. Urinary tract signs and symptoms. In: Franklin S.S. (ed.) *Practical Nephrology*. New York, Wiley, 1981: 3–22
3. Apley J. *The Child with Abdominal Pains*, 2nd edn. Oxford, Blackwell Scientific, 1975
4. Levine M.D. and Rappaport L.A. Recurrent abdominal pain in schoolchildren; the loneliness of the long distance physician. *Pediatr. Clin. North Am.* 1984, **31**, 969–991
5. Schechter N.L. Recurrent pains in children: an overview and an approach. *Pediatr. Clin. North Am.* 1984, **31**, 949–968
6. Walther P.L., Lamm D. and Kaplan G.W. Paediatric urolithiasis: a ten year review. *Paediatrics* 1980, **65**, 1068–1072
7. Heiliczer J.D., Canonigo B.B., Bishof N.A. and Moore E.S. Noncalculi urinary tract disorders secondary to idiopathic hypercalciuria in children. *Pediatr. Clin. North Am.* 1987, **34**, 711–718
9. Smellie J. *et.al.* Children with urinary tract infection. A comparison of those with and without ureteric reflux. *Kidney Int.* 1981, **20**, 717–722
10. Illingworth R.A. *Common Symptoms of Disease in Children*, 6th edn. Oxford, Blackwell, 1979: 290–302
11. Shirkey H.C. Drugs causing discolouration of the urine and faeces. In: *Paediatric Therapy*, 6th edn. St Louis, Mosby, 1980: 163–166
12. Forfar J.O. and Arneil G.C. (eds) Biochemical and physiological tables. In: *Textbook of Paediatrics*, 3rd edn. London, Churchill Livingstone, 1983: 1985
13. Perheentupa J. The neurohypophysis and water regulation. In: Brook, C.G.D. (ed.) *Clinical Paediatric Endocrinology*. London, Blackwell Scientific, 1981: 315
14. Merten D.F. and Kirks D.R. Diagnostic imaging of paediatric abdominal masses. *Pediatr. Clin. North Am.* 1985, **32**, 1397–1425
15. Hughes P.M., Gupta S.C. and Thomas N.B. Xantho-granulomatous pyelonephritis in childhood. *Clin. Radiol.* 1990, **41**(5), 360–362
16. Drash A., Sherman F., Hartmann W. and Blizzard R.M. A syndrome of pseudo-hermaphroditism, Wilms' tumour and degenerative renal disease. *J. Pediatr.* 1970, **76**, 585–593
17. Sills R.H. Failure to thrive. The role of clinical and laboratory investigation. *Am. J. Dis. Child.* 1978, **132**, 967–969
18. Crawford M.d'A. *The Genetics of Renal Tract Disorders.* Oxford, Oxford University Press, 1988: 541
19. Altehek A. Vulvovaginitis, vulvar skin disease and pelvic inflammatory disease. *Pediat. Clin. North Am.* 1981, **28**, 397–411
20. Altchek A. *Vaginal Discharges in Difficult Paediatric Diagnosis.* Philadelphia, W.B. Saunders, 1990: 383
21. Read L. What to ask when sexual abuse is suspected. *Arch. Dis. Child.* 1987, **62**, 1188–1195
22. Zeitlin H. Investigation of the sexually abused child. *Lancet* 1987, **ii**, 842–847
23. Emans S.J., Woods, E.R., Flagg, N.T. and Freeman, A. Genital findings in sexually abused symptomatic and asymptomatic girls. *Pediatrics* 1979, **79**, 778–785
24. Rapola J., Huttunen N.-P. and Hallman N. Congenital and Infantile Nephrotic Syndrome. In: Edelmann C.M. (ed.), *Pediatric Kidney Disease.* 2nd ed. Boston, Little Brown, 1992, 1291–1305
25. Morgan G., Postlethwaite R.J., Lendon M. *et. al.* Postural deformities in congenital nephrotic syndrome. *Arch. Dis. Child.* 1981, **56**, 959–961
26. Leung A.K.C. and Robson W.L.M. Single umbilical artery. A report of 159 cases. *Am. J. Dis. Child* 1989, **143**, 108–111
27. Lachiewicz A.M., Sibley R. and Michael A.F. Hereditary renal disease and preauricular pits. Report of a kindred. *J. Pediatr.* 1985, **106**, 948–950

28. Varsano I.B., Jaber L., Garty B.Z., *et al.* Urinary tract abnormalities in children with supernumerary nipples. *Pediatrics* 1984, **73**, 103–105

29. Maher, E.R., Yates, J.R.W., Harries, R. *et al.* Clinical features and natural history of von Hippel–Lindau disease. *Q.J. Med.* 1990, **283**, 1157–1163

8

Assessment of the glomerular filtration rate

C.M. Taylor

Estimation of the glomerular filtration rate (GFR) is the most commonly used indicator of overall renal performance. However, to apply this appropriately one needs a clear understanding of the dynamic physiological processes involved, the mechanisms by which GFR is regulated and the limitations of the clinical and laboratory techniques used to deduce it. In many of these areas there have been valuable recent advances which provide the clinician with new insights into this long-established investigation.

Physiology

Glomerular filtration rate refers to the bulk flow of solvent (water) from plasma across the glomerular capillary membrane into the urinary space. The rate at which solutes travel with the water depends upon their molecular size, shape and charge, as well as the properties of the filter membrane. GFR cannot be measured directly in clinical practice, but as small solute molecules are filtered with the same freedom as water, GFR can be estimated from their clearance rate from plasma. Substances used to measure clearance must be accurately quantifiable in blood and urine and neither absorbed nor secreted by the tubule. The amount cleared in a given time (urine concentration × volume, UV) will be proportional to the amount presented to the glomerulus in the plasma. As the plasma concentration (P) is known, the least volume of plasma water which contained the marker

can be derived from the standard formula UV/P.

The net efflux of water from any capillary is dependent upon the hydrostatic and oncotic pressure gradient across the membrane – Starling's forces (Figure 8.1). A major distinguishing feature of glomerular capillaries is that they are derived from the arterial vasculature and

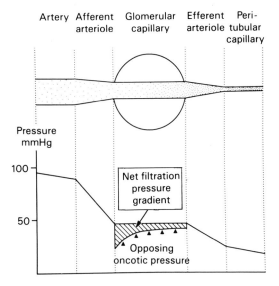

Figure 8.1 A representation of Starling's forces in the glomerulus, showing the hydrostatic pressure in plasma and the opposing oncotic pressure gradient across the capillary. The effect of hydrostatic pressure of the filtrate has been omitted for simplicity, and the oncotic pressure of filtrate is regarded as zero. The shaded area shows the net filtration pressure gradient along the capillary (After Lote,[46] by kind permission of the author)

operate at higher intraluminal pressures than peripheral capillaries. The forces favouring filtration are the intracapillary hydrostatic pressure ($P_{capillary}$) and the extracapillary oncotic pressure ($\pi_{filtrate}$), whereas those opposing it are the intracapillary oncotic pressure (π_{plasma}), which is mostly comprised of plasma albumin, and the hydrostatic pressure outside the capillary ($P_{Bowman's\ capsule}$). Thus:

Filtration pressure =
$$(P_{capillary} - P_{Bowman's\ capsule}) - (\pi_{plasma} - \pi_{filtrate})$$

In health, very little protein escapes into the glomerular filtrate and the component $\pi_{filtrate}$ can be disregarded. A further complex variable consists of the hydraulic conductivity and the effective surface area of the glomerular filter. These two components, which cannot be distinguished in practice, are together known as the filtration coefficient (K_f). And so for practical purposes:

GFR =
$$K_f(P_{capillary} - P_{Bowman's\ capsule} - \pi_{plasma})$$

In physiological terms the oncotic pressure of arterial plasma and the hydrostatic pressure in the urinary space of Bowman's capsule are relatively constant. GFR is therefore regulated by changes in intracapillary pressure and K_f. As water escapes from the capillary, leaving the plasma proteins behind, the oncotic pressure of plasma rises towards the distal end of the capillary. In some species this is sufficient to balance the hydrostatic forces so that the filtration gradient is abolished in the distal capillary. Such equilibration probably does not occur in adult man, so that filtration continues along the whole length of the capillary. This being the case, alteration of either $P_{capillary}$ or K_f will induce proportional changes in GFR. By contrast, in situations where equilibration does take place, perhaps in infancy where the intracapillary hydrostatic pressure is lower, changes in K_f will have a much attenuated effect. Mechanisms by which K_f might be controlled are poorly understood. The anatomical arrangement of contractile elements within the mesangial cells suggests that the surface area of the capillary may be adjusted in part by mesangial activity. However, at present it is uncertain that GFR is regulated by changes in K_f.[1] More is known about renal

blood flow and the regulation of capillary pressure.

In health, renal plasma flow remains constant over a wide physiological range of systemic arterial blood pressure. Reduction of renal perfusion pressure is met with a rapid fall in vascular resistance upstream from the glomerulus. In some mammals this response includes changes in the interlobular arteries, although the principal site of both renal resistance and autoregulation is the afferent arteriole. With a more profound pressure reduction, efferent arteriolar tone increases. The net effect of these changes is the preservation of both plasma flow and intracapillary pressure. The following hypotheses are helpful in explaining control of renal blood flow and GFR, respectively.

Myogenic theory

The myogenic theory requires that afferent arteriolar wall tension is held *constant* by smooth muscle function. From Laplace's law, tension is proportional to the product of radius and pressure. It follows that if the latter is reduced radius must *increase*, thus lowering resistance and preserving flow. (The difficulty one has in visualizing this is because one usually thinks of pipes as rigid vessels in which case wall tension *falls* in proportion to pressure reduction.) The theory is supported by experiments in which the interstitial pressure surrounding the glomerulus could be manipulated to alter the gradient across the arteriolar wall.[2] Reducing the pressure gradient across the vessel caused the afferent arteriole to dilate, but no change in efferent diameter was seen. The rapidity of these responses gives further support to the myogenic theory.[3]

Tubuloglomerular feedback theory

For salt and water homeostasis to be achieved there needs to be a balance between glomerular filtration and the reabsorptive function of the tubule. From anatomical studies more than 50 years ago, Goormaghtigh first suggested that tubular function might regulate GFR. The vascular pedical of the glomerulus is in intimate contact with the distal tubule of the *same* nephron at the juxtaglomerular apparatus (JGA). The JGA consists of the macula densa cells of the distal tubule (which have functional similarities to the cells of the thick ascending limb) and extraglomerular mesangial (Goormaghtigh) cells, some of which are intimately associated with the arterioles and contain renin granules. Between these there is a fluid-filled cleft. It is probable that the ionic content of fluid in the cleft is related to the delivery of sodium and chloride to the distal nephron at the level of the macula densa, and is the signal for mesangial cell response. Micropuncture studies, in which fluid and electrolyte delivery to the distal nephron can be separated from proximal function, confirm the phenomenon of tubuloglomerular feedback control, although details of the mediation of these effects remain to be evaluated.[4]

Physiological variation in GFR

In individuals of some mammalian species, glomerular filtration rates fluctuate over a wide physiological range. It is by no means constant in man. There is a well-defined circadian rhythm of both GFR and renal plasma flow (RPF), the GFR in the daytime being approximately a third greater than in the night.[5] Moreover, an increase of GFR and RPF of similar magnitude is observed in the 3h following a protein-rich meal,[6] an effect which is mimicked by an intravenous infusion of amino acids.[7] The mechanisms involved are incompletely known but glucagon, released postprandially from the pancreas, plays an important role, not directly within the kidney but via an intermediate hepatic product.[8] The increase of GFR appears to require both the presence of growth hormone[9] and intact prostaglandin synthesis.[10] The circadian rhythm is independent of the regulatory changes brought about by dietary protein load.

The magnitude of these changes demands that GFR estimation should be standardized wherever possible to a fixed time in the day, and the dietary intake known or preferably controlled. The difference between the basal GFR and that occurring after stimulation by a dietary protein load is known as the 'renal functional reserve'. Its measurement has not found a place in clinical practice as yet, and it must not be confused with the increase in single nephron GFR which accompanies renal hypertrophy in patients who have sustained a reduction of renal mass.[11]

Developmental changes and standardization for body size

It is convenient that the GFR is proportional to body surface area (BSA) from about 3 years

of age until middle adult life. Although consistent, the relationship between GFR and BSA does not imply functional interdependence. However, by expressing GFR per BSA, useful comparisons can be made both between patients of dissimilar size, and in the same individual at different times during growth from middle childhood onwards. Exceptions to this include the observation that after puberty GFR/BSA in males exceeds that in females by about 10%, and that disturbances of growth caused by disease may affect the denominator BSA independently from GFR.

Profound changes in renal function occur at birth as part of the adaptation to extra-uterine life. The total complement of nephrons is present at 36 weeks' gestation and thereafter glomeruli grow to more than double their diameter by adulthood. In absolute terms the GFR increases approximately ten-fold from birth to 3 years of age, the steepest change being in the first days of life. Even if GFR is expressed per body surface area, one finds a 50% increase in the first 3 days, a doubling at 2 weeks and a six-fold rise at 3 years.[12,13] The maturational change in the kidney and the rapid physical growth of the child in the first 3 years makes any relationship between GFR and body dimension complex. In clinical practice it is permissible to extrapolate from Figure 8.2 to obtain guidance as to the normality or otherwise of GFR/BSA estimations in normally grown

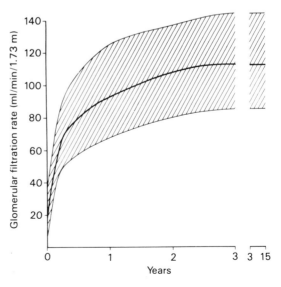

Figure 8.2 GFR (ml min^{-1} 1.73 m^{-2}) in childhood (Data compounded from References 12, 13, 14, 18 and 45)

children below 3 years of age. In neonates, however, there is good reason to relate GFR to body weight. Coulthard and Hey[14] found that in healthy babies in the first week of life the variation in inulin clearance was halved when expressed per weight rather than surface area. For example, GFR ranged between 4.5 and 22.6 ml min^{-1} m^{-2} which could be reduced to 0.6 to 1.6 ml min^{-1} kg^{-1}. It is noteworthy that unlike postnatal age, gestational age has negligible effect on GFR/BSA[13] or GFR/weight[15] in the perinatal period.

GFR estimation in clinical practice

Inulin clearance

Inulin is a polysaccharide of plant origin and consists of a chain of approximately 30 β-1:2 linked fructofuranose units. The molecular weight varies between 5000 and 5500 dalton, depending on its preparation. It is a larger molecule than others used to estimate GFR such as iothalamate (613 dalton), and the chelates ^{51}Cr-edetic acid (EDTA) and ^{99m}Tc-diethylene triamine penta-acetic acid (DTPA) (both approximately 400 dalton). After an intravenous bolus injection, inulin is quickly distributed into a volume which equates to the extracellular fluid space. In anephric individuals the plasma concentration then remains constant, confirming that it is not metabolized and is dependent on the kidney for excretion. Trace amounts are lost into bile, but this can be discounted. As it is not bound to plasma proteins, is freely filtered at the glomerulus, and is neither secreted nor reabsorbed by the tubule, inulin is an ideal marker for estimating GFR and it remains the 'gold standard' by which other methods are judged. Inulin (as fructose) is measured in biological fluids by a reaction with β-indolyl acetic acid in the presence of concentrated hydrochloric acid to give a purple colour which is read by photometry.[16] Naturally, patients must avoid drinks containing fruit juices from which fructose can be absorbed. There is negligible cross-reaction from other sugars and although the method is somewhat tedious it can be adapted to run on an autoanalyser and provide accurate results.[17]

The standard clearance method requires the measurement of both the plasma and urine concentrations of inulin, and the urine volume over a given time. Because the amount of inulin excreted into the urine is directly proportional to the plasma concentration, the formula UV/P gives the clearance rate in ml/min. Prior to the study the patient's height and weight are carefully measured so that surface area can be deduced and the clearance expressed in ml min^{-1} m^{-2}, or conventionally in ml min^{-1} 1.73 m^{-2}, the latter being the surface area of the average adult man. A cannula is placed into a freely flowing peripheral vein, and a bolus of inulin given over 2 min followed by a continuous infusion delivered by a syringe pump. A typical priming bolus dose is 50 mg/kg body weight. The infusion rate is calculated to give a constant plasma concentration in the region of 20 mg/100 ml. Thus for a child with a surface area of 1 m^2 and a GFR of about 100 ml min^{-1} m^{-2}, the desired steady-state plasma level would be achieved by giving inulin at 20 mg/min. After an equilibration period of 45 min, timed urine collections are obtained (e.g. two consecutive 1 h periods), a plasma sample being taken from a separate vein at the beginning and end of each. The mean plasma inulin concentration for each period can be calculated arithmetically if the difference between beginning and end measurements is small, or interpolated from a semilogarithmic plot of plasma inulin over time.

Formal inulin clearances are rarely performed in paediatric practice. This is partly because the precision is not essential for making clinical decisions and simpler alternatives exist. More importantly, the test depends heavily on the accuracy of timed urine collections and, as infants and young children neither void to command nor void to completion, bladder catheterization becomes obligatory. However it is possible to dispense with urine collection altogether using the constant infusion technique. If the plasma inulin concentration is steady, the term UV must be equal to the amount of the marker infused. With an accurately calibrated syringe pump giving a constant infusion, GFR can be derived from the formula:

$$\text{GFR} = \frac{\text{Dose administered per unit of time}}{\text{Plasma concentration}}$$

The equilibration time needed to achieve a constant plasma level depends on the plasma half-life, which in turn relates to the volume of distribution and the GFR. In infants, the pro-

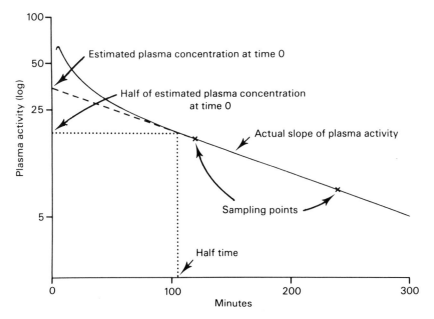

Figure 8.3 Plasma activity curve following the bolus injection of ^{51}Cr-EDTA

portionately greater extracellular fluid volume and the low clearance rate is such that it takes 24 h to achieve a steady state.[18]

^{51}Cr-EDTA slope clearance

Although ^{51}Cr-EDTA can be used for clearance studies by the continuous infusion technique, it is more often used for the single injection, slope clearance method. This method has been extensively evaluated in adults and children.[19–21] However, the validity of slope clearance remains unconfirmed in neonates and young infants. The isotope chromium-51 (^{51}Cr) emits beta-radiation, has a half-life of 28 days and can be readily quantified in a scintillation counter. The chelate meets all the requirements of a marker for GFR estimation in that it is stable, does not become protein bound, and is cleared in the kidney in a similar way to inulin.

Following the bolus injection of ^{51}Cr-EDTA (time 0), the plasma activity rises abruptly and then declines as indicated in Figure 8.3. In the initial phase of a two-compartment model, the chelate diffuses from the vascular to the larger non-vascular extracellular space until equilibration occurs. However, as the vascular compartment is cleared by glomerular filtration, plasma activity then falls below that of the extracellular fluid. The chelate returns to the plasma at a

rate determined by the concentration gradient between the two compartments. In practice, the intercompartmental equilibration following injection occurs within 90 min, and by 2 h plasma activity declines as a single component exponential. Using mannitol as a marker, Newman *et al.*[22] showed that clearance could be derived from the formula:

$$\text{Clearance} = \frac{\text{Theoretical volume of distribution} \times 0.693}{\text{Half time}}$$

(0.693 is the natural logarithm of $\frac{1}{2}$)

The mono-exponential part of the plasma activity curve is obtained from two blood samples, the first being drawn 2 h after injection and the second at 3 h. There is no advantage in taking additional samples, but in patients expected to have impaired function the second should be delayed to 4 or 6 h after injection. From this the plasma half-life of the chelate is derived. The theoretical volume of distribution is calculated from the estimated plasma concentration at time 0, extrapolated from the linear part of the curve, and the dose given. Where glomerular filtration rates are greater than 10 ml min^{-1} 1.73 m^{-2}, slope clearance of ^{51}Cr-EDTA exceeds simultaneously performed formal (UV/P) clearance and it is conventional to apply a correction factor of 0.77. Two further corrections are required to estimate GFR. The first allows for the difference in activity between the venous plasma which is tested and the arterial plasma which is filtered; the second accommodates the observation that the clearance of ^{51}Cr-EDTA is about 5% less than inulin. Together a correction of 0.87 is needed.[20]

[51]Cr-EDTA slope clearance is a reliable method of GFR estimation, the coefficient of variation of repeated measurements in individuals being less than 4%, and a change of 11% predicting a significant difference with 95% probability. The dose of ^{51}Cr-EDTA is 1.0 μCi/kg body weight, which gives very little radiation exposure to the subject – less than 1 week's natural background radiation. The uroepithelium is the target organ and so diuresis and frequent voiding helps to minimize risks.

The syringe containing the EDTA is weighed before and after the injection so that the exact dose can be calculated. Sources of error usually occur on injecting, so that the dose given is inaccurate. This can be overcome by ensuring that the intravenous cannula is well sited, does not have side ports and is thoroughly flushed through with saline after the bolus. It must be noted that the slope clearance method will prove inaccurate in patients who are either dehydrated or oedematous.

^{99m}Tc-DTPA and single kidney GFR

Technetium-99 m is a short-lived radioisotope emitting only gamma radiation at an energy of 140 keV, and is therefore well suited to gamma camera imaging techniques. The chelate ^{99m}Tc-DTPA fulfils many of the criteria for a marker of GFR, although up to 6% becomes bound to plasma proteins[23] and the tracer exhibits some instability.[24] Nevertheless it has been found to give similar slope clearance results to ^{51}Cr-EDTA.[25] Products from different manufacturers give dissimilar performance and in our experience Pentetate (Amersham International) proved the most reliable.[26]

The advantage of ^{99m}Tc-DTPA is that renography can be performed at the same time as a two-point slope clearance and the individual kidney function derived. This is done by dividing the overall clearance in proportion to the activity observed from each kidney during the second phase of the renogram – between 1 and 3 min after bolus injection. Deconvolutional analysis, a mathematical programme which simulates the effect of the isotope bolus arriving instantaneously at the renal artery, can be applied to further improve the prediction of single kidney GFR.[27] The dose of ^{99m}Tc-DTPA required for imaging is in the order of 50 μCi/kg body weight, and the radiation exposure to the subject is 40–200 times that of a ^{51}Cr-EDTA slope clearance.

Methods using creatinine

Creatinine continues to be the most widely used and best researched endogenous marker for GFR estimation. It is produced by the irreversible non-enzymatic dehydration of creatine phosphate in muscle, the daily excretion of creatinine being constant in the individual and proportional to muscle bulk. Creatinine has a molecular weight of 113 and is therefore freely filtered at the glomerulus. There is, however, a small but significant component of tubular secretion.[28] The ability to measure creatinine with precision in biological fluids has improved in recent times, which is important because at normal levels of renal function the plasma concentration of creatinine is low, especially in the young. Because this term appears as the denominator of the clearance formula, UV/P, a small error in plasma measurement has a disproportionately large effect on the calculation of GFR.

Techniques of creatinine measurement

The Jaffé technique, which is the basis for many automated assay methods, involves a colorimetric reaction with alkaline picrate. Interference from other chromogens causes overestimation, particularly at low concentrations of true creatinine. Attempts to avoid this have included an initial step of adsorption with Fuller's earth or sample dialysis, and kinetic rather than endpoint analysis of the reaction. The latter has the advantage that small volume samples can be processed, and results accord well with reference techniques, but some variation remains at low range.

Automated enzymatic methods are increasingly popular and have the attractions of speed and good specificity. For example, Kodak Ektachem produce multi-layered analytical slides onto which 10 μl samples are spread. Reagents are contained in the layers beneath, and the

Table 8.1 Constants for various age groups

	Constant k [creatinine μmol/litre (mg/dl)]
Low birth weight infants (< 2.5 kg)	30 (0.33)
Normal infants 0–18 months	40 (0.45)
Girls 2–16 years	49 (0.55)
Boys 2–13 years	49 (0.55)
Boys 13–16 years	60 (0.70)

coloured end-product is read from the obverse of the slide. One method uses creatinine imino-hydrolase to generate ammonia, which in turn gives rise to a blue dye with bromphenol blue. A control slide without the enzyme measures ammonia alone and this is subtracted to derive creatinine concentration. Unlike the Jaffé reaction, sample haemolysis, bilirubin, cephalosporins and ketoacids do not interfere, although 5-fluorocytosine gives an artefactually high result. A single slide Kodak method enzymatically hydrolyses creatinine to creatine and thence to sarcosine. Hydrogen peroxide is then released by sarcosine oxidase, and in the presence of peroxidase a colour is developed from a leuco dye. It has to be emphasized that these newer techniques give lower measurements of (true) creatinine, and that the widely quoted comparisons between creatinine clearance and other standardized methods of GFR estimation have usually been made with the earlier picrate methods.

Plasma creatinine as an estimate of GFR

A major obstacle to formal creatinine clearance studies is the need to have accurate, timed urine collections, which in young children requires bladder catheterization. Even in the best hands the variation between clearances is wide. However, in practice GFR can be estimated from the plasma creatinine concentration alone with greater precision, thus making conventional creatinine clearance in children an obsolete investigation. The theoretical background is as follows. For an individual in the steady state, the production rate of creatinine by muscle balances urinary excretion ($U \times V$). GFR is then proportional to the reciprocal of plasma creatinine concentration ($1/P$), i.e. a doubling of plasma creatinine implies a halving of GFR. However, if muscle mass can be related to an anthropometric measurement this could replace the numerator in the equation ($U \times V$) and

be applied to patients of differing size. Two authors simultaneously showed that body height fulfilled this relationship where GFR is expressed per body surface area.[29,30] Thus:

$$GFR/BSA = k \times Height/Plasma\ creatinine$$

where height is in cm, creatinine in μmol/litre and GFR is factored to 1.73 m². The constant k for children between the age of 3 and 15 years is in the order of 40, and where creatinine is in mg/dl, k is about 0.5. The exact value of k depends on the technique used to measure plasma creatinine and reference method for GFR. Below the age of 3, where the relationship between GFR and BSA is not constant, and in adolescent males whose muscle bulk is increased, different values of k are needed. Schwartz and co-workers have produced the following constants given in Table 8.1.[31]

The value and the limitations of this approach to GFR estimation have been fully reviewed by Haycock,[32] and this is recommended further reading. It is clear that the formula can only be applied to children who are somatically normal, and that errors will occur if used in anorexic or obese patients in whom the ratio of muscle mass to BSA is abnormal. The loss of muscle which occurs in some patients with chronic renal failure implies that the constant k for them will not only differ from normals but will change further with time. Also, estimation of GFR by this method cannot be used if there is rapidly changing renal function such as may occur in acute renal failure.[33]

At normal levels of renal function there is a poorer correlation between the formula estimate and standard clearance methods. This is partly due to the difficulty of measuring low concentrations of plasma creatinine with accuracy. However, in children over 2 years of age, a height/creatinine ratio of >2.1 cm μmol^{-1} litre^{-1} indicates a normal GFR, and a ratio <1.5 predicts abnormal renal function with 95% confidence.[34,35] There is no doubt that the sequential estimation of GFR by this formula in an individual patient with renal disease gives the clinician the most useful information for the least inconvenience to the child, or cost to the service. Morris *et al.*[35] showed that a difference of 19 ml min^{-1} 1.73m^{-2} between two estimates using the formula indicated a real change of GFR with 95% confidence. In following a patient with renal disease, repeated results should be plotted semilogarithmically against

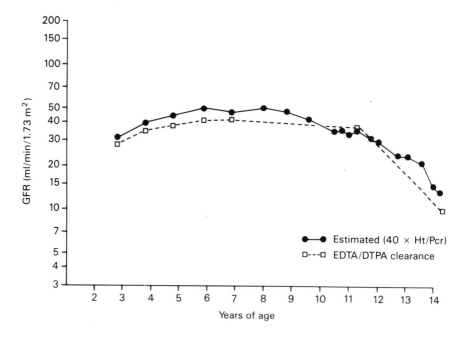

Figure 8.4 Example of GFR monitoring in a child with renal dysplasia

time to illustrate rates of change, as shown in the example (Figure 8.4). It is axiomatic that occasional radionuclide clearances are performed for comparison. The changes of height/creatinine usually track well with the infrequent clearance studies, although the increasing tubular secretion of creatinine that occurs with chronic renal failure means that the formula overestimates true GFR once low levels of renal function are reached.[36]

Urea clearance

Although it is a small, freely filtered molecule which is easily measured, urea is of negligible value in the estimation of GFR. Plasma urea concentrations are strongly influenced by changes in protein catabolism, and as much as 50% of filtered urea may be reabsorbed by the tubule. One should not guess levels of renal function from blood urea.

The clinical interpretation of GFR measurement

GFR and reduced renal mass

The GFR is the sum of the function of the whole population of nephrons. Unfortunately clinicians do not have a test of how many nephrons a patient has. Given the very great reserve capacity of the normal kidney (that is, the ability of individual nephrons to hyperfunction and hypertrophy), GFR measurements alone are a poor guide to the extent of kidney destruction by disease processes. An obvious illustration of this is that following uninephrectomy for live kidney donation, the contralateral kidney increases its GFR by a third within hours. Alternatively, in a disorder such as idiopathic focal glomerular sclerosis, where the nephron population is being steadily depleted, GFR will remain in normal range until late in the disease when the last remaining glomeruli, already filtering maximally, start to succumb (Figure 8.5). A similar situation exists in any patient with chronic renal impairment secondary to reduced renal mass. Here the increased perfusion and capillary hypertension in individual hypertrophied glomeruli cause accelerated focal segmental sclerosis and further nephron loss.[37] This is a vicious circle which leads remorselessly to end-stage failure, although dietary and pharmacological interventions appear to slow this process in some experimental studies.

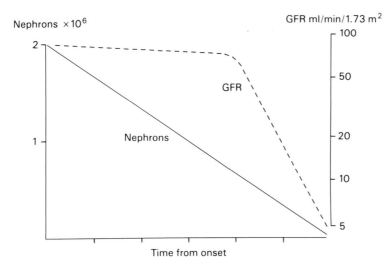

Figure 8.5 Hypothetical relationship between GFR and nephron population in a progressively destructive glomerular disease such as focal glomerular sclerosis

In the absence of a measure of nephron numbers, the interpretation of GFR is helped by having an assessment of the patient's overall renal mass. These days this is simply and non-invasively achieved with ultrasound, although similar information can be gained from the renal parenchymal area on a urogram or even a plain radiograph. The clinical question then becomes, 'Is the estimated GFR appropriate to the amount of kidney tissue present?'

It has been shown, for example, that in patients with the coarse scarring of reflux nephropathy who have sustained various degrees of nephron loss, renal parenchymal volume correlates well with the overall GFR and renal plasma flow.[38] The same is true for size and GFR of individual kidneys. The proviso is that there must be no active parenchymal inflammation at the time of the test which would cause a further fall of filtration rate. In practice, the scarring of reflux nephropathy has to be extensive and bilateral if renal impairment is to occur. By contrast, unilateral renal scarring is not expected to lead to a reduction of overall function.[39] To find a subnormal GFR in this situation would suggest an undisclosed problem with the contralateral 'normal' kidney. Solitary kidneys usually hypertrophy in early childhood and achieve near normal function, although the markedly increased GFR per nephron may be disadvantageous in the long run.

Reduced GFR with normal renal mass

With normal renal function, both children and adults filter and reabsorb the equivalent of their entire plasma volume every 25 min or so. It is therefore important that in this dynamic process glomerular filtration and tubular reabsorption are held in precise balance. Moreover, for terrestrial animals in whom water conservation is paramount, there is a strong teleological argument for fail-safe mechanisms to down-regulate filtration if the tubular recovery of salt and water should fail. The reduced GFR and oliguria of acute renal failure can be thought of in terms of acute renal success![40] This goes beyond the theory of physiological tubuloglomerular feedback (see above) and into the realm of pathological processes. As tubular performance governs glomerular function it is not surprising that, as a generalization, tubulo-interstitial disorders induce a more profound fall of GFR than glomerular lesions alone.[41-43]

From the above, one can draw the following broad but useful conclusions. Where kidneys are of normal size and unobstructed, but GFR is impaired, a diffuse parenchymal disease is present. The more profound the renal failure, the more likely it is that the disorder affects the tubules or interstitium. Examples of the latter include drug-induced tubulopathies, inflammatory interstitial disease such as renal transplant rejection or infiltrative lesions. However, the most common cause in paediatric practice is acute 'vasomotor' oliguric renal failure induced by hypovolaemic shock. In vasculopathies such as the haemolytic uraemic syndrome, the mechanism for the abrupt switching-off of filtration is not clear, but tubular ischaemia certainly occurs and may contribute to the event.

Drug effects on GFR

In normal adults and older children, angiotensin-converting enzyme (ACE) inhibitors and prostaglandin synthetase inhibitors have negligible effect on GFR. However, in situations where filtration is being supported by increased angiotensin-induced efferent arteriolar constriction, ACE inhibitors will cause a fall in GFR. Renal artery stenosis is a good example of this. The normal newborn has a physiologically increased renin–angiotensin axis[44] and is also at risk of GFR reduction by these drugs.

Vasodilatory prostanoids, PGE_2 and PGI_2, are important in preserving renal blood flow when systemic blood pressure falls. Hypotensive episodes are therefore more likely to result in reduced renal function where prostaglandin inhibitors are used. Moreover, these effects have been exploited therapeutically to reduce GFR, for example in certain patients with nephrotic syndrome who have life-threatening proteinuria.

Elevated GFR

In some clinical situations the filtration rate may be pathologically elevated. An example of this is the steroid-responsive nephrotic syndrome of childhood. It is apparent from the formula for GFR that a reduction in plasma oncotic pressure and a rise in filtrate protein concentration will increase filtration. This may be an adequate explanation for the phenomenon, which in the short term is not harmful. Sustained hyperfiltration occurs in some patients with type 1 diabetes mellitus, the mechanism for this being incompletely understood. In this situation the GFR increase *per nephron* is not as great as that which occurs after extensive renal ablation, and the hyperfiltration is probably unrelated to the later development of diabetic nephropathy.

Key points

- In that tubular and glomerular functions are interrelated, the GFR provides a valuable guide to overall renal performance.
- Interpretation of GFR in children must take account of age-related physiological development, especially in the first months of life.
- Height/creatinine estimates of GFR are superior to formal creatinine clearance as long as the limitations of the formula are observed. Ratios > 2.0 cm μmol^{-1} litre^{-1} fairly predict normal function, whereas ratios < 1.5 cm μmol^{-1} litre^{-1} in children over 1 year of age indicate renal impairment. Plasma creatinine is relatively insensitive in elucidating change of GFR within, or near to, the normal range. Nevertheless, *height/creatinine is the method of choice in general paediatric practice* and nearly all clinical decisions can be made without resorting to additional methods.
- Inulin clearance remains the gold standard for clinical research.
- Radionuclide slope clearance methods agree well with formal inulin clearance and are reproducible. Compared to creatinine-based methods, they are better able to identify subtle changes of function close to the normal range, and remain accurate at low levels of GFR. Using ^{99m}Tc-DTPA and simultaneous renography, individual kidney GFR can be deduced.
- Always consider whether GFR is proportional to renal mass. With a decreased GFR there are either too few nephrons or the normal complement of nephrons have their function down-regulated.
- To visualize the change in a patient, plot the GFR on semilogarithmic graph paper.

References

1. Oken D.E. Does the ultrafiltration coefficient play a key role in regulating glomerular filtration in the rat. *Am. J. Physiol.* 1989, **256**, F505–515
2. Gilmore J.P., Cornish K.G., Rogers S.D. and Joyner W.L. Direct evidence for myogenic autoregulation of the renal microcirculatioin in the hamster. *Circ. Res.* 1980, **47**, 226–230
3. Stein J.H. Regulation of the renal circulation. *Kidney Int.* 1990, **38**, 571–576
4. Blantz R.C., Thomson S.C., Peterson O.W. and Gabbai F.B. Physiologic adaptations of the tubuloglomerular feedback system. *Kidney Int.* 1990, **38**, 577–583
5. Koopman M.G., Koomen G.C.M., Krediet R.T., de

Moor E.A.M., Hock F.J. and Arisz L. Circadian rhythm of glomerular filtration rate in normal individuals. *Clin. Sci.* 1989, **77**, 105–111

6. Hostetter T.H. Human response to a meat meal. *Am. J. Physiol.* 1986, **250**, F613–618
7. Braenale E., Kindler J. and Sieberth H.G. Effects of an acute protein load in comparison to an acute load of essential amino acids on glomerular filtration rate, renal plasma flow, urinary albumin excretion and nitrogen excretion. *Nephrol. Dial. Transplant* 1990, **5**, 572–578
8. Friedlander G., Blanchet F. and Amiel C. Renal function reserve. *Toxicol. Lett.* 1989, **46**, 227–235
9. Kleinman K.S. and Glassock R.J. GFR fails to increase following protein ingestion in growth hormone deficient adults. *Kidney Int.* 1985, **27**, 296
10. Brouhard B.H. and LaGrone L. Effect of indomethacin on the glomerular filtration rate after a protein meal in humans. *Am. J. Kidney Dis.* 1989, **13**, 232–236
11. Zuccala A. and Zucchelli P. Use and misuse of the renal functional reserve concept in clinical nephrology. *Nephrol. Dial. Transplant* 1990, **5**, 410–417
12. McCrory W.W. *Developmental Nephrology.* Massachusetts, Harvard University Press, 1972
13. Guignard J.P., Torrado A., Da Cunha O. and Gautier E. Glomerular filtration rate in the first three weeks of life. *J. Pediatrics* 1975, **87**, 268–272
14. Coulthard M.G. and Hey E.N. Weight as the best standard for glomerular filtration in the newborn. *Arch. Dis. Child.* 1984, **59**, 373–375
15. Heijden A.J., Grose W.F.A., Ambagtsheer J.J., Provoost A.P., Wolff E.D. and Sauer P.J.J. Glomerular filtration rate in the preterm infant: the relation to gestational and postnatal age. *Eur. J. Pediatr.* 1988, **148**, 24–28
16. Heyrovsky A. A new method for the determination of inulin in plasma and urine. *Clin. Chim. Acta* 1956, **1**, 470–474
17. Dawborn J.K. Application of Heyrovsky's inulin method to automatic analysis. *Clin. Chim. Acta* 1965, **12**, 63–66
18. Coulthard M.G. Comparison of methods of measuring renal function in pre-term babies using inulin. *J. Pediatr.* 1983, **102**, 923–930
19. Chantler C., Garnett E.S., Parsons V. and Veall N. Glomerular filtration rate measurements in man by the single injection method using ^{51}Cr-EDTA. *Clin. Sci.* 1969, **37**, 169–180
20. Chantler C. and Barratt T.M. Estimation of glomerular filtration rate from plasma clearance of 51-chromium edetic acid. *Arch. Dis. Child.* 1972, **47**, 613–617
21. Winterborn M.H., Beetham R. and White R.H.R. Comparison of plasma disappearance and standard clearance techniques for measuring glomerular filtration rate in children with and without vesico-ureteric reflux. *Clin. Nephrol.* 1977, **7**, 262–270
22. Newman E.V., Bordley J. and Winternitz J. The interrelationships of glomerular filtration rate (mannitol clearance), extra cellular fluid volume, surface area of the body and plasma concentration of mannitol. A definition of extracellular fluid clearance determined by following the plasma concentration after a single injection of mannitol. *Bull. Johns Hopkins Hosp.* 1944, **75**, 253–268
23. Klopper J.F., Hansen W., Atkins H.L., Eckelman W.C. and Richards P. Evaluation of ^{99m}Tc-DTPA for the measurement of glomerular filtration rate. *J. Nucl. Med.* 1972, **13**, 107–110
24. Blaufox D.M., Chervu L.R. and Freeman L.M. Radiopharmaceuticals for quantitative study of renal function. In: Subramanian G., Rhodes B.A., Cooper J.F. *et al.* (eds) *Radiopharmaceuticals.* New York, Society of Nuclear Medicine, 1975: 389–392
25. Hilson A.J.W., Mistry R.D. and Maisey M.N. ^{99m}Tc-DTPA for the measurement of glomerular filtration rate. *Br. J. Radiol.* 1976, **49**, 794–796
26. Griffiths P.D., Doole Z., Green A., Taylor C.M. and White R.H.R. Comparison of ^{51}Cr-EDTA and ^{99m}Tc-DTPA slope clearances in children with vesicoureteric reflux. *Child. Nephrol. Urol.* 1988, **9**, 283–285
27. Kainer G., McIlveen B., Hosch L.R. and Rosenberg A. Assessment of individual renal function in children using ^{99m}Tc-DTPA. *Arch. Dis. Child.* 1979, **54**, 931–936
28. Sjostrom P.A., Odlind B.G. and Wolgust M. Extensive tubular secretion and reabsorption of creatinine in humans. *Scand. J. Urol. Nephrol.* 1988, **22**, 129–131
29. Counahan R., Chantler C., Ghazali S., Kirkwood B., Rose F. and Barratt T.M. Estimation of glomerular filtration rate from plasma creatinine concentration in children. *Arch. Dis. Child.* 1976, **51**, 875–878
30. Schwartz G.J., Haycock G.B., Edelmann C.M. and Spitzer A. A simple estimate of glomerular filtration rate in children derived from body length and plasma creatinine. *Pediatrics* 1976, **58**, 259–263
31. Schwartz G., Brion L.P. and Spitzer A. The use of plasma creatinine concentration for estimating glomerular filtration rate in infants, children, and adolescents. *Ped. Clin. North Am.* 1987, **34**(3), 571–590
32. Haycock G.B. Creatinine, body size and renal function. *Ped. Nephrol.* 1989, **3**, 22–24
33. Kwong M.B.L., Tong T.K., Mickell J.J. and Chan J.C.M. Lack of evidence that formula-derived creatinine clearance approximates glomerular filtration rate in pediatric intensive care population. *Clin. Nephrol.* 1985, **24**, 285–288
34. Davies J.G., Taylor C.M., White R.H.R., and Marshall T. Clinical limitations of the estimation of glomerular filtration rate from height/plasma creatinine ratio: a comparison with simultaneous ^{51}Cr edetic acid slope clearance. *Arch. Dis. Child.* 1982, **57**, 607–610
35. Morris M.C., Allanby C.W., Toseland P., Haycock G.B. and Chantler C. Evaluation of a height/plasma creatinine formula in the measurement of glomerular filtration rate. *Arch. Dis. Child.* 1982, **57**, 611–615
36. Walser M., Drew H.H. and LaFrance N.D. Reciprocal creatinine slopes often give erroneous estimates of progression of chronic renal failure. *Kidney Int.* 1989, **36**, Suppl. 27, S81–85

37. Brenner B.M., Meyer T.W. and Hostetter T.H. Dietary protein intake and the progressive nature of kidney disease. *N. Engl. J. Med.* 1982, **307**, 652–659

38. Troell S., Berg U., Johansson B. and Wikstad I. Comparison between renal parenchymal sonographic volume, renal parenchymal urographic area, glomerular filtration rate and renal plasma flow in children. *Scand. J. Urol. Nephrol.* 1988, **22**, 207–214

39. White R.H.R. and Taylor C.M. The non-operative management of primary vesicoureteric reflux. In: Johnston J.H. (ed) *Management of Vesicoureteric Reflux.* Baltimore, Williams and Wilkins, 1984

40. Thurau K. and Boylan J.W. Acute renal success. The unexpected logic of oliguria in acute renal failure. *Am. J. Med.* 1976, **61**, 308–315

41. Risdon R.A., Sloper J.C. and de Wardener H.E. Relationship between renal function and histological changes found in renal-biopsy specimens from patients with persistent glomerular nephritis. *Lancet* 1968, **2**, 363–366

42. Mackensen-Haen S., Bader R., Grund K.E. and Bohle A. Correlations between renal cortical interstitial fibrosis, atrophy of the proximal tubules and impairment of the glomerular filtration rate. *Clin. Nephrol.* 1981, **15**, 167–171

43. Katafuchi R., Takebayashi S., Taguchi T. and Harada T. Structural-functional correlations in serial biopsies from patients with glomerulonephritis. *Clin. Nephrol.* 1987, **28**, 169–173

44. Yared A. and Yoshioka T. Autoregulation of glomerular filtration in the young. *Sem. Nephrol.* 1989, **9**, 94–97

45. Winberg J. The 24-hour true endogenous creatinine clearance in infants and children without renal disease. *Acta Paediat.* 1959, **48**, 443–452

46. Lote C.J. *Principles of Renal Physiology.* London, Chapman and Hall, 1990

9

Acidosis and alkalosis

M.A. Lewis, J.E. Wraith

Metabolic acidosis

Definition

Metabolic acidosis is a primary reduction in plasma bicarbonate which can be due to:

- Bicarbonate loss.
- Reduced hydrogen ion excretion.
- Excess hydrogen ion load.

In many cases the cause of acidosis is obvious and no problems of diagnosis are present. Occasionally the cause is less obvious and diagnosis can be difficult, with potential causes including renal tubular acidosis, inborn errors of metabolism, toxins and poisons. Most reviews of acidosis in children concentrate on distinguishing the different types of renal tubular acidosis, whereas the more common problem in general paediatric practice is to determine if acidosis is due to an extrarenal cause or a renal cause. This chapter will concentrate on the initial evaluation of acidosis and more detailed discussion and investigation of renal tubular acidosis will be found in Chapter 24.

Physiology

Excellent reviews of acid-base physiology are available for reference.[1-4] The homeostatic mechanisms necessary for normal acid-base balance are illustrated in Figure 9.1. A number of simple tests, shown below, can usually provide a good indication of the likely causes of metabolic acidosis.

Plasma anion gap

This is a useful guide to the potential cause of metabolic acidosis.[5,6] This can be calculated:

$$\text{Anion gap} = Na^+ - (Cl^- + HCO_3^-)$$
$$\text{mmol/litre}$$

The normal positive gap of 8–16 mmol/litre represents phosphates, sulphates and other negative ions not usually measured. When bicarbonate is lost either by the gastrointestinal tract or kidney, compensatory hyperchloraemia occurs and the anion gap remains normal, giving rise to hyperchloraemic acidosis with normal anion gap. When there is accumulation of acids, e.g. lactate, these are buffered against bicarbonate giving rise to a normochloraemic metabolic acidosis with raised anion gap. The anion gap in this situation is usually increased to above 20 mmol/litre.

Urine pH

The urine pH measures the small amount of free hydrogen ions in the urine. In the presence of a significant metabolic acidosis, if the distal renal tubular function is intact the urine pH should be < 5.5 at all ages and < 5.0 in older children. To measure urine pH it is essential to use a pH meter.

Urine anion gap

Measurement of the urine anion gap has been

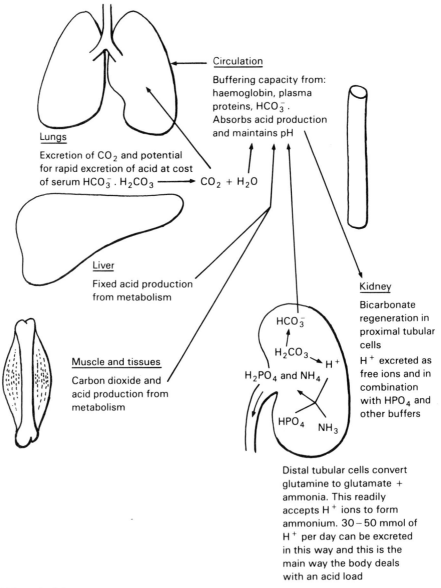

Figure 9.1 Acid-base physiology

proposed as an indirect index of urinary NH_4^+ excretion,[8] and has largely superseded measurement of the urine pH. The capacity of the distal tubule to general NH_4^+ ions in response to acidosis is much greater than its ability to produce free hydrogen ions; thus measurement of the urine NH_4^+ should be more sensitive than measurement of the urine pH. NH_4^+ is not easily measured directly but can be estimated from the urine anion gap:

$$\text{Urine anion gap} = (Na^+ + K^+ + NH_4^+)$$
$$- (Cl^- + HCO_3^-)$$

In acidosis, bicarbonate is eliminated from the urine. NH_4^+ cannot be directly measured but the difference between $(Na^+ + K^+)$ and (Cl^-) will estimate it. Thus, if urine (Cl^-) is greater than $(Na^+ + K^+)$, this suggests NH_4^+ production by the kidney. The patterns of metabolic acidosis described below are then seen.

Table 9.1 Increased anion gap

Endogenous
(a) Inborn errors of metabolism
(b) Lactic acidosis
  – primary
  – secondary
(c) Ketoacidosis
  – diabetes mellitus
  – starvation
(d) Renal failure

Exogenous
Toxins and drugs

Increased plasma anion gap
Urine $(Cl^-) >$ urine $(Na^+ + K^+)$
(urine pH < 5.5)

This pattern would suggest a primary metabolic acidosis. Possible causes are given in Table 9.1. Essentially, in this circumstance there is either an endogenous or an exogenous load of acid. Clinical circumstances and age of the patient would usually give a good clue as to whether or not the acid load was likely endogenous or exogenous.

Endogenous
Inborn errors of metabolism are a group of inherited disorders that can present in the newborn period or early childhood with an overwhelming illness associated with a marked metabolic acidosis.[7] The disorder may be one of amino acid metabolism, e.g. maple syrup urine disease or organic acid metabolism, e.g. methylmalonic or proprionic acidaemia. Inherited disorders of carbohydrate metabolism may cause severe lactic acidosis, e.g. glycogen storage disease type I.

Clinical signs and symptoms are very non-specific, e.g. vomiting, lethargy, hypotonia, seizures and coma. The key to diagnosis is a high index of suspicion by the clinician. A history of a previous neonatal death in a sibling is a helpful clue. Typically the infant is normal at birth and symptoms usually develop towards the end of the first week, after milk feeds have been established. The presence of massive ketonuria is an unusual finding in the newborn period and should always suggest the possibility of an inborn error of metabolism.

With some disorders the urine has a characteristic odour, e.g. maple syrup in maple syrup urine disease or 'sweaty feet' in isovaleric acidaemia.

Plasma amino acid and urine amino and organic acid analyses should be carried out by a laboratory experienced in the diagnosis of these disorders. While awaiting results, dietary protein should be restricted and adequate calories supplied as carbohydrate and lipid emulsions. Once diagnosis is established, the offending metabolite can be reduced by dialysis, usually peritoneal, or rendered harmless by transportation into the cells by using a glucose and insulin infusion similar to the treatment of hyperkalaemia.

Lactic acidosis is an important cause of severe metabolic acidosis. It may be primary due to a defect in pyruvate metabolism or more commonly secondary to hypoxia.

Exogenous
The presence of a severe metabolic acidosis in a previously healthy child should raise the possibility of accidental or deliberate ingestion of drugs and toxins. In childhood, the classic example is due to salicylates, which disrupt Krebs' cycle and oxidative phosphorylation leading to a marked metabolic acidosis due to lactate accumulation. The other major effects of salicylates on the respiratory centre leading to respiratory alkalosis is much less evident in children as compared to adults. The finding of a positive urinary Phenistix is a clue to diagnosis and the excretion of harmful metabolites can be enhanced by a forced alkaline diuresis. Ethanol inhibits hepatic gluconeogenesis and causes under-utilization of lactate by the liver leading to lactic acidosis which can be severe in children, especially if there is pre-existing liver disease.

Breakdown products of methyl alcohol and ethylene glycol also precipitate lactic acidosis secondary to a disruption of mitochondrial function due to a direct toxic effect.

Because of the variable accumulation of metabolites in renal failure, this can produce an acidosis with either a normal or increased anion gap.

Normal plasma anion gap
Urine $(Cl^-) >$ (urine $Na^+ + K^+$)
(urine pH < 5.5)

This pattern suggests loss of bicarbonate which can either be from the gastrointestinal tract or the kidneys. Causes are listed in Table 9.2.

The small bowel, biliary and pancreatic secretions contain about five times as much bicarbonate as plasma. Any condition leading to severe

Table 9.2   Normal anion gap acidosis

Gastrointestinal
Diarrhoeal disease
Small bowel or pancreatic drainage
Bowel augmentation cystoplasty and ureteral diversion

Renal
Renal tubular acidoses
Other tubular syndromes
Renal failure

Miscellaneous
Adrenal insufficiency
Carbonic anhydrase inhibitors/deficiency
Cholestyramine
Parenteral nutrition

diarrhoea, artificial drainage and/or fistulation will lead to a considerable loss of bicarbonate. Compensatory hyperchloraemia maintains a normal anion gap. These conditions, particularly acute diarrhoeal diseases, are a very common cause of acidosis but rarely cause a diagnostic problem. The only severe diarrhoeal illness not associated with bicarbonate loss is congenital chloride diarrhoea (see later).

Urine in contact with the colon for any length of time will exchange chloride for bicarbonate and hence cause loss of bicarbonate. This was a considerable problem when ureterosigmoidostomy was a common form of urinary diversion. This problem largely disappeared when cutaneous urinary diversions were fashionable, but with the advent of bowel augmentation cystoplasty it is beginning to appear again, although it is only a small minority of such patients that experience significant disturbances in acid-base balance.

Renal loss of bicarbonate occurs in proximal tubule acidosis. In this condition there is a low renal threshold for bicarbonate. Compensatory hyperchloraemia again maintains a normal anion gap and it is important to note that when serum bicarbonate has fallen below threshold, an acid urine can be achieved. Proximal renal tubule acidosis is discussed in more detail in Chapter 24.

Normal plasma anion gap
Urine $(Na^+ + K^+) >$ *urine* (Cl^-)
(urine pH > 5.5)

These features would suggest inability to acidify the urine typical of distal renal tubule acidosis. The different types and causes of distal renal tubule acidification defects and the further investigations are discussed in Chapter 24.

Metabolic alkalosis

Definition

Metabolic alkalosis can be defined as a primary elevation of plasma bicarbonate with corresponding rise in blood pH. As a compensatory mechanism, alveolar hypoventilation leads to a rise in PCO_2 in an effort to lower the pH to normal. This can be due to:

- Excess intake of base.
- Cl^- depletion (chloride responsive).
- H^+ loss (chloride unresponsive).

Ingestion of base is rarely seen in childhood. In adults, excess bicarbonate may be obtained from anti-acid preparations, the so-called 'milk-alkali' syndrome. Healthy kidneys are well adapted to deal with excess bicarbonate; when the renal threshold is exceeded, bicarbonate leaks into the urine and normal pH is maintained.

Chloride-responsive alkalosis

By far the most common cause of metabolic alkalosis is associated with chloride depletion. The causes are shown in Figure 9.2. In vomiting, for example due to pyloric stenosis, there is H^+ and Cl^- loss. The loss of Na^+ and K^+ leads to extracellular volume contraction. The kidney responds by enhanced Na^+ reabsorption. The disproportionate loss of Cl^- as HCl, NaCl and KCl means that Na^+ can only be retained at an accelerated rate of exchange with H^+ and K^+ in the distal tubule; this maintains the alkalosis and leads to hypokalaemia. As soon as Cl^- is made available to the kidney it is retained at the expense of HCO_3^-, correcting the alkalosis; this is called 'chloride-responsive alkalosis'. Examination of random urinary electrolytes will show a very low concentration of Cl^-.

Congenital chloride diarrhoea is a rare condition in which affected infants are unable to transport Cl^- against an electrochemical gradient. Unabsorbed chloride in the ileum and colon has an osmotic effect and severe diarrhoea results. Affected infants are usually born prematurely and there is usually a history of polyhydramnios. Symptoms begin in the first two weeks of life with abdominal distension, ileus and severe watery diarrhoea. Diagnosis is established by finding a low plasma and urine Cl^- and extremely high levels in the faecal fluid.

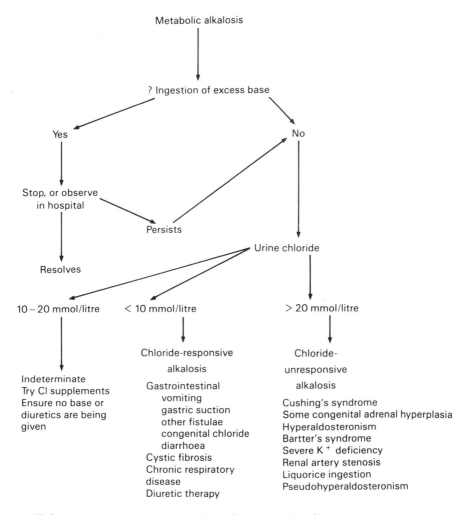

Figure 9.2 Metabolic alkalosis

Metabolic alkalosis, hyponatraemia and hypokalaemia result. Cl^- and K^+ replacement is necessary. The condition is inherited as an autosomal recessive.

Children with cystic fibrosis lose excessive amounts of Na^+ and Cl^- in their sweat and can rapidly become volume depleted and Cl^- deficient in hot weather.

In chronic respiratory failure, the kidney's response to the respiratory acidosis is to retain HCO_3^- at the expense of Cl^-, thus depleting the Cl^- pool. If the PCO_2 is returned to normal suddenly, for example, by mechanical ventilation and the patient is given insufficient Cl^- he cannot adjust renal acid excretion and the plasma HCO_3^- remains high, resulting in alkalosis. Although usually regarded as a Cl^--responsive alkalosis, the effect of diuretic therapy on tubular function can lead to both a stimulation of the renin/angiotensin system and a high distal tubular Na^+ delivery. This results in increased distal Na^+ reabsorption with K^+ and H^+ secretion. The resulting acid loss generates the alkalosis; thus diuretic therapy may be better classified as a chloride-resistant alkalosis. Although early in diuretic therapy urinary Cl^- loss is high, with chronic usage equilibration occurs and loss parallels intake.

Chloride-unresponsive alkalosis

Direct excretion of H^+ by the kidney is the second commonest cause of metabolic alkalosis in childhood. The causes are shown in Figure 9.2. In this group, Cl^- replacement does not alleviate the alkalosis and these are termed 'chloride-unresponsive alkaloses'.

Mineralocorticoids enhance distal Na^+ reabsorption at the expense of H^+ ions and thus promote urinary acidification. This activity may be a primary event, independent of renin, as seen in Cushing's syndrome, some varieties of congenital adrenal hyperplasia, primary hyperaldosteronism or excess liquorice ingestion. On the other hand, it may be secondary to high renin activity due to extracellular volume depletion (secondary hyperaldosteronism), Bartter's syndrome or renal artery stenosis. With the exception of severe K^+ depletion and Bartter's syndrome, this group is associated with extracellular fluid volume expansion and hypertension. In all cases, urinary Cl^- concentration is elevated.

The differential diagnosis of the two groups is usually not difficult, as the underlying disorders provide the major clues to diagnosis. Evaluation should include a critical assessment of hydration and careful check for hypertension. The crucial biochemical test is the urinary concentration of Cl^-

Management of severe metabolic acidosis and alkalosis

The mainstay of treatment of acid-base disorders has to be the treatment of the underlying conditions. Occasions arise where treatment with a buffer is required either as emergency management of an acute clinical state or as chronic management of a tubular disorder not amenable to specific correction. This treatment with buffer is much more commonly required in the case of acidoses than alkaloses.

Immediate treatment of an acute acidotic state is indicated in the presence of a deteriorating clinical condition while the underlying disorder is being treated, or to maintain a reasonable haemodynamic state while treatment is started for the underlying condition. This usually only applies to situations where the blood pH is below 7.10. There are good theoretical reasons for not correcting less severe acidosis that is not in itself life threatening. Acidosis causes vasodilatation and correction with bicarbonate causes vasoconstriction. Thus in the acutely sick patient, administration of bicarbonate leads to a worsening of the peripheral circulation allowing a persistence of anaerobic metabolism and lactic acid production in the tissues. Good oxygenation with vasodilatation is a much more appropriate and successful course of action. This is made more pertinent by experimental evidence showing that administration of bicarbonate worsens intracellular acidosis by the formation of carbonic acid in the cytoplasm of the cells.[9]

The usual buffer used to correct acidosis is sodium bicarbonate. Trishydroxymethylaminomethane (Tris) combines with carbonic acid to form hydroxy-Tris and bicarbonate. It has no advantage over sodium bicarbonate, although it is often used as it has a non-sodium base on the mistaken assumption that this will avoid volume overload. Giving cations in the form of Tris is no different to giving cations in the form of sodium. A disadvantage of Tris is the strong alkalinity of the solution which proves highly irritant.

The actual amount of buffer to give is at best a guess. An approximate formula which is widely used for total correction of acidosis is:

$$\text{Amount of base in mmol} = 0.3 \times \text{Base deficit} \times \text{Body weight (kg)}$$

Total correction is rarely, if ever, indicated. In addition the relationship between plasma bicarbonate and pH is far from linear, small increments in bicarbonate leading to large shifts in pH for initial pH values less than 7.20. In the severely acidotic patient, initial therapy aimed at raising the plasma bicarbonate by 5 mmol/litre will have a marked effect on pH even if the initial bicarbonate is less than 10 mmol/litre.

Assuming an effective volume of distribution of bicarbonate of 50% of body weight, to raise the bicarbonate by 5 mmol/litre involves giving an initial dosage of 2.5 mmol/kg. Using this formula, with subsequent repetition if necessary, is more appropriate than total or half-correction using the formula stated earlier and avoids potentially harmful large swings in pH.

Severe metabolic alkalosis, i.e. plasma bicarbonate greater than 50 mmol/litre, is a rare occurrence. Changes in the peripheral and central nervous system are similar to hypocalcaemia with mental confusion, predisposition to seizures, paraesthesiae, muscle cramps and cardiac arrhythmias. This situation is usually only seen in patients with long-term loss of gastric juices, excessive diuretic therapy or hyperadrenalism due to neoplasia. In such patients, corrective measures are slow and often take quite some time to correct the degree of alkalosis. The most important aspect of therapy is saline repletion. As long as renal function is good, potassium chloride infusion in a dosage of 3 mmol kg^{-1} day^{-1} is useful in the treatment of alkalosis associated with the loss of gastric secretions. More rapid correction can be achieved with ammonium chloride 5.35% solution (1 mmol/ml), infused using the same formula as for the correction of metabolic acidosis. The use of acetazolamide or other acids is not advised.

References

1. Kurtzman N.A. and Batlle D.C. (eds) Acid-base disorders. *Med. Clin. North Am.* 1983, **67**(4), 751–929

2. Brewer E.D. Disorders of acid-base balance. *Ped. Clin. North Am.* 1990, **37**(2), 429–447

3. Halperin M.L., Goldstein M.B., Steinbourg B.J. and Jungas R.L. Biochemistry and physiology of ammonium excretion. In: Seldin D.W. and Giebisch G. (eds) *The Kidney: Physiology and Pathophysiology.* New York, Raven Press, 1985: 1471–1490

4. Koeppen B., Giebisch G. and Malnic G. Mechanism and regulation of renal tubular acidification. In: Seldin D.W. and Giebisch G. (eds) *The Kidney: Physiology and Pathophysiology.* New York, Raven Press, 1985: 1491–1525

5. Oh M.S. and Carroll H.J. The anion gap. *New Engl. J. Med.* 1977, **297**, 814–817

6. Gabow P.A., Kaeburg W.D., Fennessey P.V., Goodman S.I., Gron P.A. and Shriver R.W. Diagnostic importance of an increased anion gap. *New Engl. J. Med.* 1980, **303**, 854–858

7. Wraith J.E. Diagnosis and management of inborn errors of metabolism. *Arch. Dis. Child.* 1989, **64**, 1410–1415

8. Batlle D.C., Hizon M., Cohen E., Gutterman C. and Gupta R. The use of the urinary anion gap in the diagnosis of hyperchloraemic acidosis. *New Engl. J. Med.* 1988, **318**, 594–599

9. Ritter J.M., Doktor H.S. and Benjamin N. Paradoxical effect of bicarbonate on cytoplasmic pH. *Lancet* 1990 **335**, 1243–1246

Disturbances in fluid and electrolyte balance

T.J. Beattie

Fluid and electrolyte homeostasis is an essential requirement for optimal cellular and organ function, and is maintained in the face of wide variation in input and output associated with both physiological and pathophysiological states. The kidney plays the major role in monitoring these variations and in instituting the appropriate responses.

Distribution and composition of body fluid compartments

Water is by far the most abundant component of the human body, constituting in health 65–85% of body weight. Body water can usefully be considered as distributed between two main compartments, the intracellular fluid compartment (ICF) and the extracellular fluid compartment (ECF). The ECF can be further divided into the intravascular and interstitial compartments, separated by capillary membranes. There are important age-related changes in both total body water and in its distribution (Table 10.1).[1]

Osmotic forces are important in determining the distribution of water between the ICF and the ECF. Since cell membranes are fully permeable to water, osmotic equilibrium is maintained and the volume of each compartment is determined by the concentration of osmotically active solutes or the effective osmolality (tonicity) of the compartment.

Each fluid compartment has one major osmotically active solute that, because it is largely restricted to that compartment, determines its relative volume: potassium for the ICF, sodium for the ECF and plasma proteins for the intravascular compartment. This differential composition is maintained by molecular size and charge or by active membrane pumps. Solutes such as urea, however, which permeate cell membrane freely have no influence on transcellular water movement.

The standard biochemical technique for the measurement of osmolality in plasma is by freezing point depression. This technique measures the solute content of the water contained in the specimen, but provides no information about the tonicity of the plasma as it measures all solutes whether permeant or impermeant. When the water content of the plasma is normal (93%) the osmolality of the plasma, and therefore by deduction of the ICF, may be approximated by the following formula, which has been shown to fall within 5–10 mosm/kg of the measured value:

Plasma osmolality (mosm/kg) = 2 × Plasma sodium (mmol/litre) + Plasma glucose (mmol/litre) + Plasma urea (mmol/litre)

Control mechanisms for extracellular and intracellular fluid volume and composition

The kidney is central to the control of ECF volume and tonicity via the integrated mechanisms of sodium and water excretion. The

Table 10.1 Body water and age

	Pre-term	*Term*	*1–3 years*	*Adult*
Total body water (% of body wt)	85%	80%	65%	65%
Extracellular fluid (% of body wt)	55%	45%	25%	25%
Intracellular fluid (% of body wt)	30%	35%	40%	40%

afferent stimuli for the regulation of sodium and water excretion are the effective intravascular volume and the tonicity of the arterial blood supplying the supraoptic and paraventricular nuclei of the hypothalamus.

Changes in sodium and water excretion in health and disease occur by alteration in renal and intrarenal haemodynamics, GFR and tubular reabsorption, and are induced by a variety of effector mechanisms (Figure 10.1).

The ICF volume is dependent on the ECF tonicity and the intracellular ionic concentrations, the most important being potassium, which is determined by cell membrane pump action.

Although the biological mechanisms for thirst and urine concentration are present in early infancy, they are limited by the totally dependent state of the infant with respect to intake and by a submaximal urine concentrating ability. The combination of high-energy expenditure and high water turnover per unit mass, in addition to the use of non-human milk, providing an excess of solute for excretion, makes the infant particularly vulnerable to disturbances in fluid and electrolyte balance following brief insults.

Water and electrolyte requirements

Unfortunately for the busy clinician, calculations of water requirements do not easily relate to mass. Water turnover relates directly to energy expenditure, since most of the energy output of the body is dissipated as heat. This heat loss carries water with it directly by insensible losses through skin and lungs and indirectly by the requirement for excretion of waste products of metabolism in the urine. This is the only

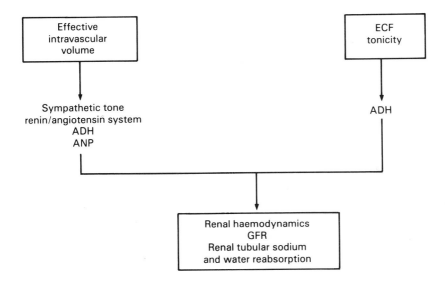

Figure 10.1 Control of ECF volume and tonicity

relationship which remains constant throughout infancy and childhood.[3]

Maintenance water requirements

Maintenance water requirements consist of water normally lost through the skin and respiratory tract (insensible water loss), the kidney (obligatory urine volume) and a small amount in the stool. Assuming that water turnover and therefore requirement bears a strict relationship to energy expenditure, and in the absence of renal functional impairment and abnormal losses, the relationship between water requirement and calorie expenditure may be stated in the following way:[2]

Insensible water loss: 45 ml/100 cal expended
Obligatory urine volume: 50–55 ml/100 cal expended
Stool water: 0–5 ml/100 cal expended

The allowance for urine volume is based on the production of isotonic urine (osmolality 300 mosm/kg). This may be seen as a rather generous allowance, but importantly allows solute excretion without taxing renal concentrating ability.

The best assessment of calorie expenditure is that of the computed average daily expenditure of the hospitalized patient[3] and may be calculated as follows: 100 cal/kg up to 10 kg; 50 cal/kg for each additional kg between 10 and 20 kg, and 20 cal/kg for each additional kg above 20 kg. Using this formula, the total maintenance intravenous water requirement is 1 ml/cal expended per day (Table 10.2)

Recommendations for the perinatal period and for the low birth weight infant are somewhat different and readers are referred to recent reviews on this subject.[4]

Oral maintenance requirements are 20–25% higher because of the associated increase in solute load with the accompanying diet.

Modifications to the above formula are required in certain situations. An increase in water requirements is necessary in the following circumstances:

- In the presence of abnormal water and electrolyte losses.
- In persistent pyrexial illnesses, the requirements should be increased by 12% for each °C above 37.5°C.
- The presence of sweating requires an increase of 10–25% in water requirement, and in patients with cystic fibrosis electrolyte requirements should be doubled.
- In conditions associated with sustained hyperventilation or excessive muscular activity, an increase of 25–50% may be required.
- In hypermetabolic states, e.g. severe thermal injury, salicylate intoxication and thyrotoxicosis, an increase of 25–75% may be required.
- In the newborn and young infant whose temperature is maintained by radiant heat or who is nursed under a phototherapy unit, the requirement will increase by 25%.

In addition, the circumstances below dictate a reduction in maintenance water requirements:

- In oedematous and antidiuretic states.
- In those infants and children nursed in high environmental humidity or during treatment with nebulized gas therapy.
- In the sedated or paralysed patient, a 40% reduction will be required because of the reduced energy expenditure
- In the presence of compromised renal function and oligoanuria.

In the presence of oligoanuria, calculation of maintenance water requirements should take into account two additional sources of water normally of no relevance. First, the water of oxidation, a product of metabolism of fat and carbohydrate which amounts to 12 ml/100 cal expended. Secondly, preformed water derived from tissue catabolism which amounts to 3 ml/100 cal expended. In oligoanuria, therefore, the maintenance water requirement should be:

Table 10.2   Maintenance fluid and electrolyte requirements

	Weight (kg)	*Daily requirement*
Water	3–10	100 ml/kg
	11–20	1000 ml plus 50 ml/kg for each additional kg above 10 kg
	>20	1500 ml plus 20 ml/kg for each additional kg above 20 kg
Sodium, potassium and chlorine	3–10	2.5 mmol/kg
	11–30	2 mmol/kg
	>30	1.5 mmol/kg

[Insensible water loss − (Water of oxidation + Preformed water)] + Measured urine volume

Maintenance electrolyte requirements

Obligatory electrolyte loss is small and the kidney has a wide range of latitude in electrolyte excretion. It is the aim of normal maintenance, therefore, to provide an amount (Table 10.2) which will neither induce maximal renal conservation nor require excretion or a large unwanted excess. Electrolyte deficits are seen mainly in association with excess gastrointestinal or urinary loss, but sweating may also lead to considerable loss of electrolytes.

When treating infants and children with very large electrolyte deficits, the daily requirements are essentially negligible and may be disregarded. If parenteral fluid therapy is conducted over a relatively short period, the need for calcium, phosphate and magnesium supplements is negligible unless there are documented abnormalities in the plasma levels of these electrolytes. If the infant or child subsequently requires total parenteral nutrition, full electrolyte replacement will be necessary.

Disorders of sodium and water balance

Introduction

Disturbances of sodium and water balance are a frequent occurrence in paediatric clinical practice, both as primary and secondary manifestations of disease processes. Dehydration is a well-accepted but inaccurate term used to describe situations in which invariably there are combined water and electrolyte deficits, and in practice is used interchangeably with saline depletion.

The evaluation of a water deficit is by necessity a clinical one (Table 10.3), and in practice the accuracy of the evaluation reflects the experience of the clinician.[5]

In addition there is a tendency for inexperienced clinicians to equate changes in plasma sodium with changes in total body sodium status, e.g. a low plasma sodium is automatically assumed to indicate sodium deficiency and treated with the administration of saline. Interpretation of changes in plasma sodium requires information on the presence or absence of a fluid deficit and in particular assessment of the effective intravascular volume.

Table 10.3   Symptoms and signs of ECF volume contraction

Symptoms
Thirst
Restlessness
Confusion

Signs of reduced interstitial fluid (dehydration)
Dry mouth
Sunken eyes
Loss of skin turgor
Sunken fontanelle

Signs of reduced intravascular volume (hypovolaemia)
Increased core peripheral temperature difference
Poor peripheral venous filling
Tachycardia
Oliguria
Low central venous pressure
Hypotension
Peripheral circulatory failure

Urinary electrolyte (sodium and chloride) concentrations are of value, particularly in the patient with an obvious fluid deficit and also as confirmation of a low effective intravascular volume in patients with expansion of the ECF, e.g. cardiac failure, hepatic failure and nephrotic syndrome.[6]

A word of warning, however, is necessary against the slavish use of urinary electrolyte measurements, since both random measurements and excretion rates generally reflect intake.

The evaluation of the patient with a complex fluid and electrolyte problem not only requires serial biochemical monitoring, but equally importantly serial clinical evaluation, body weight and sodium and water balance recordings. It must be stressed that it is the combination of these clinical and biochemical data which allows successful management.

Hyponatraemia

Pure sodium deficiency is very rarely observed in paediatric practice, the occurrence in association with a fluid deficit being the norm. In the presence of sodium deficiency, a reduction in ECF volume is invariably present and the symptoms and signs reflect this (Table 10.3).

Complex classifications of hyponatraemic states may be produced (Table 10.4) but are unhelpful in assessing the clinical problem. It is intended here to give some practical guidelines on the assessment of hyponatraemic states

Table 10.4   Causes of hyponatraemia

Factitious hyponatraemia
Hyperglycaemia
Impermeant solutes:
   Mannitol
   Ethylene glycol
   Alcohol
   Methanol

Pseudohyponatraemia
Hyperlipidaemia
Hyperproteinaemia

True hyponatraemia
1. Loss of sodium in excess of water
   Gastrointestinal loss:
      Diarrhoea
      Vomiting
      Aspiration
      Fistulae
      Stoma
   Skin loss:
      Heat stress
      Cystic fibrosis
      Adrenal insufficiency
   'Third space' loss:
      Thermal injury
      Intestinal obstruction
      Ascites
      Muscle trauma
   Renal loss:
      Osmotic diuresis
      Diuretic therapy
      Post-obstructive diuresis
      Recovery phase of ATN
      Salt-losing CRF
      Renal tubular disorders
   Adrenal disease:
      Congenital and acquired adrenal insufficiency
2. Gain of water in excess of sodium
   SIADH
   Excessive water intake
   Glucocorticoid deficiency
   Hypothyroidism
   Antidiuretic drugs
   Reset osmostat
   Oedematous states:
      Nephrotic syndrome
      Hepatic failure
      Cardiac failure
      Renal failure

without necessarily being comprehensive (Figure 10.2).

Prior to undertaking the assessment of hyponatraemia it is important, first, to ensure that the blood sample has not been improperly drawn, e.g. at a site proximal to a hypotonic saline or dextrose infusion, and secondly to measure the plasma osmolality. The plasma osmolality may be high, normal or low (Figure 10.2).

Factitious hyponatraemia

Factitious hyponatraemia occurs as a result of fluid shifts between the ICF and ECF compartments due to the presence of abnormal relatively impermanent solutes in the ECF compartment. Examples of such solutes are glucose, mannitol or low molecular weight toxins, e.g. alcohol, methanol and ethylene glycol. In factitious hyponatraemia, the measured plasma osmolality is high despite the low plasma sodium and, with the exception of hyperglycaemia, the deficit between the measured and calculated plasma osmolalities will be > 10 mosm/kg.[7]

Pseudohyponatraemia

Many clinical biochemical laboratories report plasma sodium concentrations in mmol/litre of plasma and not in mmol/litre of plasma water. If there is an increase in the non-aqueous phase of plasma, as in hyperlipidaemia or hyperproteinaemia, the reported sodium concentration will be artificially low. The aetiology of the hyponatraemia is usually obvious in these cases and if the protein or lipid is extracted, and the estimation repeated, the plasma sodium concentration will be normal. In pseudohyponatraemia, the measured plasma osmolality is usually within normal limits and the deficit between the measured and the calculated osmolalities will again be > 10 mosm/kg.[7]

True hyponatraemia

In this circumstance, the measured plasma osmolality will be subnormal (< 285 mosm/kg). This occurs when either there is a loss of sodium in excess of water or a gain of water in excess of sodium (Figure 10.2). In order to allow further evaluation, a clinical assessment of hydration and in particular of intravascular volume is essential (Table 10.3).

Loss of sodium in excess of water
Extrarenal loss
Gastrointestinal – Diarrhoea
                 Vomiting
                 Fistulae
                 Aspirate
                 Ileostomies

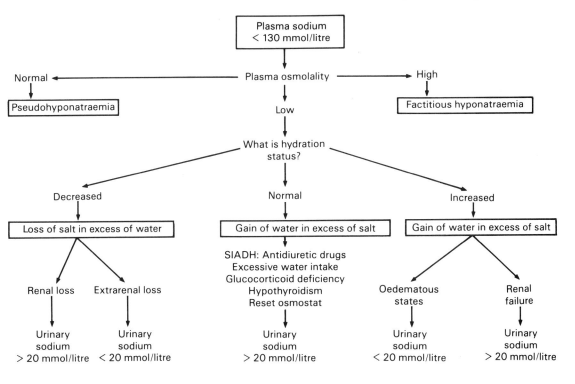

Figure 10.2 Assessment of hyponatraemia

Skin   – Excessive normal sweating (cystic fibrosis, adrenal insufficiency)

Third space losses – Thermal injury
Intestinal obstruction
Ascites
Muscle trauma, etc.

These conditions will all give rise to the classical signs of dehydration and hypovolaemia (throughout this discussion the term hypovolaemia is taken to indicate the presence of a reduced effective intravascular volume). The kidneys respond appropriately with production of a small volume of concentrated urine with a urinary sodium concentration of < 20 mmol/litre on a random sample, and frequently < 10 in the older child with normal renal function. In addition, the urine osmolality will be high, as discussed in Chapter 21. All the above conditions may result in isotonic losses, i.e. equivalent losses of sodium and water, and in this circumstance the plasma sodium will remain within normal limits (130–150 mmol/litre). In addition, the urine biochemical findings will remain unchanged.

Hyponatraemic states are increasing in incidence and now may account for up to 25% of infants with diarrhoeal dehydration.[8] The clinical signs of hypovolaemia/dehydration may present with a correspondingly smaller fluid deficit than in isonatraemic/isotonic dehydration. As well as the effect on ECF volume, the rapid drop in sodium concentration leads to a drop in ECF osmolality. If hypotonic replacement fluid is given, symptomatic water intoxication (see below) may occur despite the total body fluid deficit.[8]

Salt-losing states
Renal   – Osmotic diuresis
Diuretic therapy
Post-obstructive diuresis
Recovery phase of acute tubular necrosis
Salt-losing chronic renal failure
Renal tubular disorders
Non-renal – Mineralocorticoid deficiency/resistance

In the above conditions the clinical signs of hypovolaemia/dehydration will be present, but

Table 10.5   Causes of SIADH

CNS disorders
Infection
Malignancy, primary or secondary
Trauma
Hypoxic–ischaemic encephalopathy
Vascular accidents
Guillain–Barré syndrome
Cerebral malformation

Pulmonary disorders
Infection, acute and chronic
Malignancy
Cystic fibrosis
Positive pressure ventilation

Post-surgery
Anaesthetic or premedication
Abdominal, cardiothoracic and neurosurgery

Miscellaneous
Acute intermittent porphyria
Leukaemia
Lymphoma

the kidney will not respond appropriately. Urine sodium concentration remains high (> 20 mmol/litre) and urine volume will be maintained to a relatively late stage, thereby enhancing the risk of significant salt and water loss. The association of hyponatraemia and significant hyperkalaemia should always suggest the possibility of adrenal insufficiency.

Gain of water in excess of sodium
Syndrome of inappropriate ADH secretion. Physiological regulation of ADH secretion involves both osmotic and non-osmotic stimuli.[9] In certain pathological states, continued secretion of ADH in the presence of ECF hypo-osmolality may either be appropriate, in the presence of non-osmotic stimuli, e.g. diminished intravascular volume, or inappropriate where no obvious stimuli are present. Since the initial description of the syndrome of inappropriate ADH secretion (SIADH), it has become clear that in some of the conditions in which it has been described (Table 10.5), notably malignant disease, ectopic production of ADH is responsible. In others, the mechanism remains unclear and the subject of ongoing debate.[10]

In SIADH, an increase in the ECF volume and reduction in osmolality fails to suppress ADH secretion and if normal fluid intake is maintained hyponatraemia develops. The sequence of events shown in Figure 10.3 will continue until a new equilibrium is achieved, when restoration of aldosterone secretion and decreased collecting duct permeability serve to limit the sodium loss and water retention, respectively. The term SIADH is frequently misused in clinical practice, since many examples of hyponatraemia may have an alternative explanation. It is therefore important that the following diagnostic criteria are followed:

- Hyponatraemia and hypo-osmolality.
- An inappropriately elevated urine osmolality. In the presence of reduced plasma osmolality, a maximally dilute urine (osmolality of < 100 mosm/kg) should be expected. A urine osmolality above this level should be viewed as inappropriate in the presence of reduced plasma osmolality. Urine osmolity therefore may be isotonic or hypotonic compared with plasma and still be considered inappropriately high in the context of this syndrome.
- Evidence of an increase in body water. This is usually shown by an increase in body weight rather than by overt oedema or a hyperdynamic circulation. It is perhaps best characterized as an absence of signs and symptoms of hypovolaemia/dehydration in the presence of hyponatraemia.
- Absence of other conditions which cause a retention of free water and hyponatraemia, e.g. renal, hepatic, cardiac failure or adrenal, pituitary and thyroid dysfunction.
- The absence of other known stimuli of ADH secretion, e.g. drugs, thermal injury, pain and nausea.

Additional findings are helpful but not essential:

- History of conditions associated with SIADH (Table 10.5).
- Decreased plasma urea and creatinine as a consequence of increased ECF volume and glomerular filtration rate (GFR).
- Urinary sodium excretion, as in normal subjects, is a reflection of sodium intake in these patients and the urine concentration is usually > 20 mmol/litre, but shows a normal response to sodium restriction.

This variety of hyponatraemia may be acute or chronic and is primarily due to water retention in the absence of sodium retention, with the retained water being distributed equally be-

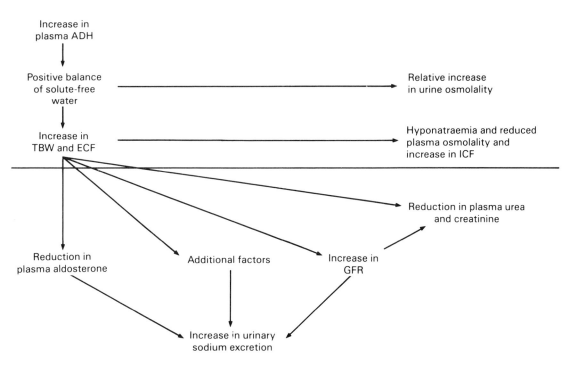

Figure 10.3 Mechanisms of SIADH. Events above the line are always present in this syndrome; events below the line usually but not invariably accompany the syndrome

tween the ICF and ECF spaces. The symptoms of SIADH are predominantly neurological as a result of the increase in intracerebral water and rarely present until the plasma sodium falls below 120 mmol/litre, but may develop at higher levels of plasma sodium if the rate of fall has been rapid. The early signs are lethargy, irritability, leading to stupor and disorientation and later to convulsions, and signs of raised intracranial pressure.

Reset osmostat. Chronic, asymptomatic hyponatraemia may occasionally be seen in children with chronic infection or malnutrition. In these patients the level of ECF osmolality at which ADH is released is < 285 mosm/kg.[10,11] Since these patients respond appropriately to both salt and water loading, specific therapy is not indicated.

Antidiuretic drugs. A number of drugs are capable of causing hyponatraemia secondary to renal water retention (Table 10.6).

Excessive water intake. Compulsive water drinking as a cause of hyponatraemia is rare in children. It is occasionally seen in adolescents, particularly girls with emotional or psychiatric disturbance. Other examples of excessive water intake occur with the use of hypotonic intravenous and oral fluid and enema therapy and following the absorption of water through the respiratory tract in patients treated with nebulized gas therapy or in a humidified atmosphere.

As with SIADH, the retained water is distributed between the ICF and ECF spaces so that oedema and hypervolaemia (cardiac failure, hypertension) are rarely seen. Symptoms again are neurological in severe cases. Urine volume will be increased in an attempt to eliminate the increased water intake, and urinary sodium excretion will reflect sodium intake (and the concentration will further be affected by the high urine flow). Urine will be maximally dilute (osmolality < 100 mosm/kg). The haematocrit will be reduced, and both haemodilution and the increased GFR reduce the plasma urea.

Table 10.6   Drugs associated with hyponatraemia

Promote ADH release
Chlorpropamide
Clofibrate
Carbamazepine
Vincristine
Vinblastine
Cyclophosphamide
Opiates
Histamine
Isoprenaline
Nicotine
Colchicine
Barbiturates

Potentiate ADH action
Chlorpropamide
Tolbutamide
Phenformin

Impair renal water excretion independent of ADH
Oxytocin
Thiazide diuretics

Oedematous states. In the nephrotic syndrome and in patients with hypoproteinaemia secondary to malnutrition, the reduction in plasma oncotic pressure allows a movement of fluid from the intravascular to the interstitial space. This reduction in effective circulating volume produces an increase in renal tubular reabsorption of sodium and water by a variety of mechanisms. This may be viewed as an attempt to correct the hypovolaemia, but because of the reduced plasma oncotic pressure the sodium and water retention leads to an expansion of the interstitial space and the production of oedema. Other oedematous states such as hepatic and cardiac insufficiency act through similar mechanisms consequent upon on a reduction in the effective intravascular volume.[12] Hyponatraemia develops in these conditions if more water than sodium is administered. Provided that the renal function is normal, the kidneys will respond appropriately, producing small volumes of concentrated urine with a urine sodium < 20 mmol/litre.

Renal failure (with salt and water retention). Salt and water retention may occur in both acute and chronic renal insufficiency. In the presence of a hypo-osmolar intake, more water than sodium will be retained, resulting in hyponatraemia. Retention of sodium and water results in expansion of the ECF, so that oedema and

hypervolaemia dominate the clinical picture. The urine volume is usually reduced and the urine sodium concentration will be > 20 mmol/litre. Urine osmolality will be similar to the plasma osmolality which should be maintained despite the hyponatraemia, because of the elevation in the plasma urea.

Therapy of hyponatraemia

The management of hyponatraemia is dependent on the severity and duration of the hypotonic state as well as on the underlying pathogenesis. It is beyond the scope of this review to describe in detail disease-specific therapies, but a summary of the approach to the correction of hyponatraemia based on the above diagnostic categories will be outlined.

When considering therapy of extrarenal losses of salt and water and salt-losing states of renal and non-renal origin, it is useful to realize the extent of the sodium as well as the fluid deficit. The sodium deficit may be approximated in the following manner:

$$(140 - \text{Plasma sodium}) \times 0.65 \times \text{Body weight in kg}$$

As clinical evidence of hypovolaemia develops early in hyponatraemic dehydration, a resuscitation phase is commonly required and the fluid should be given as plasma or isotonic saline at a volume of 20 ml/kg over 30–60 min. If the possibility of a hypoadrenal state is considered, intravenous hydrocortisone should be given concomitantly with the intravenous fluid replacement. When the resuscitation phase has been completed, the fluid deficit should be replaced with 0.9% saline and the maintenance fluids should be appropriate to the age of the child. The aim should be to achieve the correction of the fluid and sodium deficit within a 24 h period. Throughout the period of rehydration, routine clinical monitoring should be carried out, in particular of urine output and weight and potassium replacement given when the urine output is satisfactory.

In the infant who is not shocked and able to tolerate oral fluids, the use of an oral rehydration solution is justified. The deficit replacement solution should contain 60–90 mmol/litre of sodium and the maintenance fluid, 40 mmol/litre of sodium.

Hyponatraemia in the presence of clinically obvious fluid overload should be treated primarily by salt and water restriction with diuretic therapy. In hypoproteinaemic states, in order to preserve the intravascular volume a concomitant infusion of salt-poor albumin may be advisable. Guidelines on the management of salt and water retention in renal failure are given in Chapters 21 and 22.

The management of water retention in SIADH is related to the severity of the neurological symptoms and the basis is the creation of a negative water balance at the same time as attempting to remove or correct the underlying cause of the impaired water excretion. In an asymptomatic patient, water should be restricted to 25% of daily maintenance requirements. If severe water restriction is not successful, intravenous loop diuretics may be used in order to increase free water excretion. Sodium and potassium losses in the urine should be measured and replaced while holding water replacement to a minimum.

When symptoms of water intoxication are present, the objective is to correct the severe cerebral overhydration. This may be accomplished by rapidly increasing the effective osmolality of the ECF by the use of mannitol or hypertonic saline either alone or in combination with loop diuretic therapy. Plasma electrolytes must be monitored frequently during this phase of therapy and urinary electrolytes should be measured and replaced in a low volume of intravenous fluid as above.[13] If the syndrome of inappropriate ADH secretion is felt to warrant prolonged therapy, certain pharmacological agents may be considered, e.g. lithium or demeclocycline.

Attention has been focused in recent years on the possible relationship between the treatment of patients with hyponatraemia and water retention and the neurological outcome. Concern exists that some patients, particularly those with chronic hyponatraemia, do well initially and then suddenly develop significant neurological deterioration leading to death or permanent sequalae. Brain histology in fatal cases shows both central pontine myelinolysis and demyelination of extra pontine myelin-bearing neurons.[14] In a typical case, fluctuating levels of consciousness, behavioural disturbances or convulsions are the prodromal signs. Despite some experimental data supporting the relationship of this complication to the rapidity of

correction of the hyponatraemia there are few clinical data, especially in children, to support this notion.

However, in view of the possibility that the correction of the hyponatraemia is responsible for demyelination, it would seem sensible first in symptomatic patients, after the plasma sodium has been corrected to approximately 125 mmol/litre, and secondly in asymptomatic patients, to aim for a slow correction over 24–48 h.[15]

Hypernatraemia

Hypernatraemia is by definition a plasma sodium > 150 mmol/litre. It reflects a deficiency of water relative to salt, but importantly does not reflect total body sodium which may be high, normal or low.

Since sodium is the principal extracellular osmole, hypernatraemia leads to hypertonicity of the ECF. The volume of this compartment is therefore relatively well maintained and the intracellular compartment bears the brunt of the fluid deficit. The classical signs of dehydration/hypovolaemia are therefore relatively less evident for any given fluid deficit. The physiological responses to hypernatraemia are first an increase in ADH secretion when the plasma osmolality increases above 285 mosm/kg. If the plasma tonicity remains high, despite ADH secretion, the second and more important response mechanism – that of thirst – comes into play. The awake and alert patient will then increase his water intake to order to maintain normal ECF tonicity.

There are several conditions (Table 10.7) but only two major mechanisms which result in hypernatraemia (Figure 10.4):

- loss of water in excess of sodium.
- gain of sodium in excess of water.

Loss of water in excess of sodium

Extrarenal loss

Gastrointestinal
Hyperventilation
Pyrexia

The commonest presentation of hypernatraemia in clinical practice is in association with a fluid

Table 10.7   Causes of hypernatraemia

Loss of water in excess of sodium
Extrarenal loss:
    Diarrhoea
    Vomiting
    Hyperventilation
    Pyrexia
Inadequate intake
Renal loss
    Diabetes insipidus
    Hyperglycaemia
    Osmotic diuretics

Gain of sodium in excess of water
Excess oral ingestion:
    Erroneous reconstitution of milk / NG feeds
    Sea water ingestion
Excessive intravenous administration:
    Sodium bicarbonate
    Hypertonic saline
    Sodium citrate
Saline enemas
Mineralocorticoid excess:
    Cushing'ᶜ syndrome
    Conn's syndrome

deficit – the syndrome of hypernatraemic dehydration. When a hypernatraemic state develops, the pathogenetic mechanisms differ from that of isotonic and hypotonic constriction in that water loss has been proportionately greater than sodium loss. This picture is most frequently seen in acute viral gastroenteritis second-ary to hypotonic stool fluid loss and poor/absent free water intake, perhaps exacerbated by inappropriate high-solute feeding.

The relative incidence of hypernatraemic diarrhoeal dehydration, however, has fallen significantly over recent years,[8] and this is probably related to changes in feeding practices.[16]

Less commonly, hypernatraemic dehydration may occur in association with an acute respiratory infection due to an increase in insensible water loss through the lung and in febrile illnesses through increased insensible skin water loss. Again this may be aggravated by the simultaneous ingestion or administration of a hypertonic fluid or diet.

In hypernatraemic dehydration, because the ECF volume is relatively sustained, signs of hypovolaemia / dehydration are less evident and shock is an infrequent occurrence. Classically the infant or child has periods of irritability interspersed with lethargy progressing to a diminished conscious level, hypertonia, convulsions and eventually coma.

These findings prior to a plasma sodium estimation should strongly suggest a hypernatraemic state. Neurological complications in this syndrome are thought to be induced by two main mechanisms. First, prior to institution of therapy intracranial haemorrhage may occur when the osmolar gradient develops rapidly. This reflects the fact that the brain acts as a

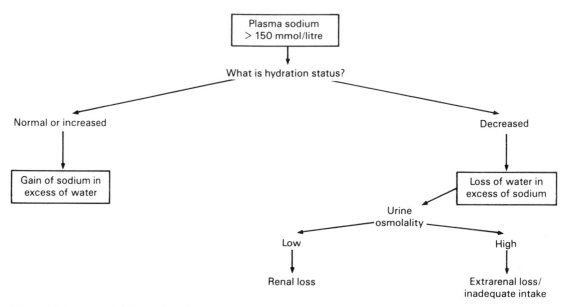

Figure 10.4 Assessment of hypernatraemia

single cell in response to osmotic changes in the ECF space. Both intra- and extracerebral bleeding may occur and thrombosis often follows and may extend the neurological insult.[17]

The second neurological problem occurs during therapy, and again reflects the rapid fluid shifts which may occur across the blood–brain barrier. The problem develops because of the existence of 'idiogenic' osmoles within the brain cell which are amino acids, particularly taurine. These 'idiogenic' osmoles may develop as a result of cellular damage secondary to dehydration or as a protective mechanism. The latter suggestion is perhaps more appropriate in that when the hypernatraemic state is chronic, the brain water content may return to normal or near normal levels.[18]

The relevance of these complications relates to the attractiveness of the brain for water during rehydration, thus when rehydration is rapid the development of cerebral oedema is inevitable. In hypernatraemic dehydration the renal response will be appropriate, with production of small concentrated volumes of urine with a sodium concentration < 20 mmol/litre. Another biochemical feature of this syndrome is hypocalcaemia, which is rarely associated with frank tetany and is of obscure aetiology. In addition, hyperglycaemia is also a frequent occurrence in hypernatraemic states and again is of obscure aetiology but importantly does not require insulin therapy.

Inadequate intake

Inadequate water intake secondary to lack of availability, or to a disturbed thirst mechanism, presents the same clinical picture as excessive unreplaced extrarenal loss of water. Infants who cannot obtain water for themselves, comatose patients and patients with hypodipsia, but with intact osmoregulation, e.g. ADH secretion, either primary or secondary to a central nervous system lesion affecting the thirst centre, are most prone to recurrent episodes of hypernatraemic dehydration. In these patients the renal response will be appropriate, with production of small volumes of concentrated urine with a sodium concentration < 20 mmol/litre.

Renal water loss

Renal disease   – Congenital and acquired nephrogenic diabetes insipidus

Non-renal disease – Central diabetes insipidus, diabetic ketoacidosis, osmotic diuretics

Uncontrolled hypotonic fluid loss occurs due to impaired urinary concentration ability in two circumstances. First where there is an absent/poor response to adequate ADH levels, and secondly in the absence/reduction of ADH secretion. In both these circumstances the urine osmolality is inappropriately low in the face of increased ECF osmolality.

Diabetes insipidus, central[19] or nephrogenic,[20] is a generic term applied to a number of disorders with similar clinical features (Table 10.8). Polyuria, in the absence of an osmotic diuresis and episodic hypernatraemia is the hallmark of these disorders. Polyuria should be suspected if the age-related urine volume (Table 10.9)[21] is increased by at least a factor of 2 or 3. In the older child nocturia, nocturnal enuresis, thirst and polydipsia are the major clinical features. If the onset is in early infancy, as in severe cases, the presence of polyuria may not be appreciated. The affected infants demonstrate irritability, frequent feed requirements, unexplained fever, constipation, failure to thrive and developmental delay. These infants, in contrast to older children, are at significant risk of hypernatraemic dehydration.

Assessment of the above patients should include simple baseline renal function tests,

Table 10.8   Causes of diabetes insipidus

Central
Idiopathic
Cerebral malformation
Post head injury/intracranial surgery
Intracranial tumour, haemorrhage and infection
Granulomatous disease, e.g. tuberculosis, sarcoidosis
Histiocytosis
Sickle cell disease

Nephrogenic
Congenital
Renal disease:
   Chronic renal insufficiency
   Obstructive uropathy
   Dysplasia
   Cystic disease
   Reflux nephropathy
   Sickle cell nephropathy
   Fanconi's syndrome
Hypokalaemia
Hypercalcaemia
Drugs

Table 10.9   Normal urine volumes

Age (years)	Volume (ml/24 LM)
1	500
3	600
5	700
7–8	1000
15	1500

plasma electrolytes and calcium and urinary tract ultrasound. Assuming the foregoing investigations are normal, an assessment of the urine concentrating capacity and the response to exogenous ADH or analogue (DDAVP) is warranted.

A water deprivation test is a potentially hazardous procedure and should under no circumstances be undertaken in the presence of hypernatraemia and increased plasma osmolality. In these circumstances DDAVP should be administered at a dose of 2 $\mu g/m^2$ intravenously or 20 $\mu g/m^2$ intranasally. Urine osmolality should be repeated in 4 h and if the response is adequate the urine osmolality should be > 800 mosm/kg.

If the patient is adequately hydrated and has a normal plasma sodium a careful water deprivation test should be carried out over 6–8 h or until 3% of the body weight is lost should this occur first. Each urine passed within that period should be collected for measurement of volume and osmolality. If at any point the urine osmolality exceeds 800 msom/kg, the test can be aborted. At the end of the deprivation period the urine and plasma osmolality should be estimated. If the urine osmolality is < 800 mosm/kg, DDAVP should be given and a further urine and plasma osmolality checked after 4 h.

In central diabetes insipidus, with a complete defect in ADH secretion and in nephrogenic diabetes insipidus, there will be no change in the urine osmolality during water deprivation but the plasma osmolality often rises to > 300 mosm/kg. Following DDAVP, the urine osmolality will exceed the normal threshhold in central diabetes insipidus, but will remain unchanged in nephrogenic diabetes insipidus.

A major adavantage of the water deprivation test is in the recognition of partial defects in ADH secretion/action.

Nephrogenic diabetes insipidus refers to an ADH-resistant defect in urine concentration and may be either congenital or acquired (Table 10.8). Almost all of the patients with congenital nephrogenic diabetes insipidus are males and

most present in early infancy with marked symptomatology, although variation in clinical severity is seen. Female siblings may have a mild form of the disorder demonstrable only by fluid deprivation.

Acquired nephrogenic diabetes insipidus occurs more frequently and usually in the context of some form of instrinsic renal disease. A similar picture, however, may be present in hypokalaemia or hypercalcaemia of some duration and with certain drug therapy, e.g. lithium, rifampicin.

Adolescents with compulsive water drinking who present with polyuria may demonstrate a suboptimal response to water deprivation and DDAVP, but importantly the plasma osmolality in these patients remains normal in contrast to patients with diabetes insipidus. A period of treatment with DDAVP and fluid restriction is required to re-establish a normal urine concentrating response.

Other major causes of hypotonic fluid loss are diabetic ketoacidosis (DKA), hyperglycaemia associated with total parenteral nutrition and occasionally following excessive therapy with osmotic diuretics such as mannitol in the management of raised intracranial pressure.

In DKA, unrecognized hypernatraemia contributes to the hyperosmolality, since an increase of 5 mmol/litre in plasma glucose above normal should lower the measured plasma sodium by 2.5 mmol/litre by inducing a shift of water into the ECF. The degree of hypernatraemia may be appreciated by using the following formula: corrected plasma Na = plasma Na + 2.5 mmol/litre for every 5 mmol/litre glucose above normal.[22]

Gain of sodium in excess of water

Excess oral ingestion of sodium:	Erroneous reconstitution of milk or nasogastric feed Sea water ingestion
Excessive administration of intravenous sodium solution:	Hypertonic saline infusion Sodium bicarbonate infusion Sodium citrate
Saline enemas Mineralocorticoid excess:	Conn's syndrom Cushing's syndrome

Hypernatraemia in the absence of a fluid deficit

is an unusual clinical occurrence. It develops after administration of excessive amounts of sodium, e.g. sea water ingestion, the inadvertent use of salt rather than dextrose in preparing milk and nasogastric feeds, or the administration of intravenous sodium bicarbonate in the treatment of acidosis or cardiorespiratory arrest. It has also been described following exchange tranfusion of the preterm infant in which hypernatraemia has been attributed to sodium citrate used as anticoagulant. Occasionally patients with conditions associated with mineralocorticoid excess such as Cushing's or Conn's syndromes develop hypernatraemia and oedema.

Treatment of hypernatraemia

Most of the conditions leading to hypernatraemia noted above may be treated by identifying the cause and remedying this. In the presence of established hypernatraemia and dehydration no matter what the aetiology, rehydration therapy should follow a standard protocol. This should be instituted after correction of any circulatory deficit and the two main features of this protocol are first that normal hydration should be achieved over a period of no less than 48 h and perhaps longer and secondly that the deficit replacement fluid is relatively hypotonic to the patient. The basic principles of fluid replacement do not differ from those in hypotonic or isotonic dehydration, i.e. the calculation of the fluid deficit is based on the admission body weight and added to the maintenance fluids and any ongoing losses over the chosen period of rehydration.

In the presence of hypernatraemia and provided that there is no oliguria, the calculated deficit should be added to the maintenance fluid for a 48 h period and a total volume given over this period as 0.18% solution and 5% dextrose. If the initial plasma sodium is >170 mmol/litre, it is safer to extend this period to 72 h. There is usually coexisting potassium depletion, and potassium may be added to the infusion fluid in the presence of adequate urine flow at a concentration of 30–40 mmol/litre. In the presence of significant metabolic acidosis, the anion composition of the infusate may be altered to contain bicarbonate. A useful replacement solution is that of a combination of 1 litre of 5% dextrose and 32 ml of 8.4% sodium bicarbonate which is approximately equivalent to 0.18% sodium solution.

In DKA, if the 'corrected' plasma sodium is >150 mmol/litre the sodium concentration in the deficit replacement fluid should be 75 mmol/litre.

Plasma sodium levels should be monitored every 4–6 h and the intravenous fluid regimen should aim to produce a fall in the plasma sodium of approximately 10–15 mmol litre/day. If there is any evidence of deterioration in the neurological status, water intoxication should be suspected and the rate of the infusion must be slowed and mannitol given if there is adequate urine output. If, on initial assessment, oliguria is noted in the absence of circulatory impairment, the urinary sodium concentration should be assessed to obtain evidence that the aetiology of the oliguria is purely volume depletion, in which case the urinary sodium concentration would be <20 mmol/litre and the other parameters consistent with prerenal uraemia (see Chapter 21). In these circumstances a fluid challenge with 0.45% saline in 5% dextrose at a rate of 5–10 ml $kg^{-1} h^{-1}$ for 4 h should be given and if urine output responds, the intravenous fluid should be changed to 0.18% saline in 5% dextrose and the remaining deficit and maintenance replaced over the following 48 h.[17] If oliguria persists, a further complication of the hypernatraemia state should be suspected, that of renal venous thrombosis.[23] This is usually associated with the presence of either frank or microscopic haematuria, thrombocytopenia and renal enlargement. In the presence of continued oliguria, careful replacement should be carried out under central venous pressure monitoring and consideration for referral for renal replacement therapy should be made, since both peritoneal and haemodialysis and continuous arteriovenous haemodiafiltration are effective in lowering plasma sodium concentration.

There are limited data on the use of oral rehydration solutions in hypernatraemic dehydration. However, if the infant has no evidence of circulatory impairment and is not vomiting, careful rehydration using the above principles using a solution containing sodium of 40 mmol/litre could be undertaken.

In patients with proven central diabetes insipidus, administration of aerosolized DDAVP (Desmospray) at a dose of approximately 20 $\mu g/m^2$ will correct the urinary concentration defect. This dose, however, should be individualized and the water intake regulated to prevent the onset of hyponatraemia.

The management of congenital nephrogenic diabetes insipidus is discussed in Chapter 24 and of acquired nephrogenic diabetes insipidus associated with renal disease in Chapter 22.

Disorders of potassium balance

Introduction

Potassium is the principal intracellular cation, and is important in the regulation of a variety of cell functions. Disorders of potassium balance and distribution, especially those of rapid onset, are of clinical importance because of the effect on resting membrane potential of nerve and muscle cells. The ratio between intracellular and extracellular potassium is maintained in the face of variation in intake by a variety of control mechanisms affecting distribution and excretion.

The distribution of potassium between the ICF and ECF compartments is controlled primarily by cell membrane pump activity, but is influenced by acid-base status, hormonal (insulin, mineralocorticoids) and adrenergic (both alpha and beta) activity.[24]

The kidney is the major excretory organ for potassium but is less efficient in responding to wide variations in intake than with sodium. Urinary potassium is predominantly derived from distal nephron secretion, since over 90%

Table 10.10   Causes of hypokalaemia

Hypokalaemia associated with total body potassium deficiency
Inadequate intake
Extrarenal loss:
   Diarrhoea
   Fistulae
   Stomas
   Laxative abuse
   Excessive sweating
Renal loss:
   Diuretic therapy
   Diabetic ketoacidosis
   Renal tubular disease
   Non-diuretic drug therapy
   Excess renin production

Redistribution hypokalaemia
Metabolic/respiratory alkalosis
Hypokalaemic periodic paralysis
Insulin administration
Drugs/toxins

Table 10.11   Plasma potassium concentrations in newborns, infants and children (mean ± standard deviation)

Age	Plasma K concentration (mEq/litre)
Newborn*	
30–32	6.5 ± 0.5
33–35	5.6 ± 0.2
36–38	5.3 ± 0.3
39–41	5.1 ± 0.2
Infants,† n = 14	
1–12 months	5.0 ± 0.5
Children,† n = 22	
2–20 years	4.3 ± 0.4

*Gestational age in weeks; measurements obtained at 1 week of age (From Sulyok *et al.*[25])
†From Schwartz G.J. and Feld L.G. Unpublished observations.

of the potassium filtered at the glomerulus is reabsorbed. Potassium secretion reflects total body potassium as well as potassium intake and is enhanced by increased delivery of sodium and water to the distal nephron as well as by increased mineralocorticoid activity and ECF alkalosis.

The urinary Na/K ratio in infants and children is generally between 1 and 4, with the higher value seen in preterm infants. Estimation of this ratio may be of value in the assessment of possible renal potassium wasting.

Hyperkalaemia and hypokalaemia may result from alterations either in total body potassium or in the distribution of potassium between the ECF and the ICF compartments (Table 10.10). It is however, important to appreciate the normal age-related variation in ECF/plasma potassium levels (Table 10.11).

Hypokalaemia

Hypokalaemia associated with total body potassium deficiency

Inadequate intake
The majority of patients with hypokalaemia will have a deficiency in total body potassium. This may result from inadequate intake in association with physiological obligatory renal and gastrointestinal loss which is accentuated if the sodium content of the diet is high. Hypokalaemia and total body potassium deficiency is commonly seen in protein calorie malnutrition but may also be seen in infants fed incorrect formulae.

Extrarenal losses

Perhaps the commonest cause of hypokalaemia in infants and children, however, is secondary to either acute or chronic gastrointestinal loss. Diarrhoeal losses of potassium may be very significant and in addition upper gastrointestinal obstruction and upper and lower gastrointestinal fistula or stoma losses as well as ureterosigmoidostomies may lead to chronic potassium deficiency. In an adolescent, inappropriate laxative abuse may be relevent.

Excessive sweating or heat stress may induce potassium deficiency through a combination of exocrine gland loss and secondary hyperaldosteronism due to ECF volume contraction (see below). Patients with cystic fibrosis are particularly at risk of this complication and may present with a pseudo-Bartter's syndrome (see Chapter 24).

Excessive renal loss

Diuretic therapy
Diabetic ketoacidosis
Renal tubular disease
Non-diuretic drug therapy
Mineralocorticoid excess
Excess renin production

Excessive renal loss of potassium may occur with the long-term use of diuretic therapy, in association with the osmotic diuresis of DKA and with a variety of renal tubular disease, eg Fanconi's syndrome, renal tubular acidosis and following the use of penicillin, carbenicillin and renal tubular toxins, e.g. cisplatin, amphotericin B.

Mineralocorticoid excess occurs in non-salt-losing congenital adrenal hyperplasia, Cushing's syndrome and Conn's syndrome and similar effects may accompany high-dose corticosteroid therapy. In addition, patients who sustain thermal injury and subsequent reduction in ECF volume may develop hypokalaemia from the resulting secondary hyperaldosteronism. Finally a picture consistent with mineralocorticoid excess is seen in patients who ingest large quantities of liquorice.

Excess renin production may occur as a secondary phenomenon in accelerated hypertension, renal artery stenosis and Bartter's syndrome or may be associated with certain tumours, e.g. Wilms' tumour and haemangiopericytoma. Assessment of the urinary sodium Na/K ratio will reveal a subnormal value (< 1)

in all the conditions producing excessive renal loss.

Redistribution hypokalaemia

Metabolic/respiratory alkalosis
Familial periodic paralysis
Insulin administration
Drugs/toxins

Hypokalaemia may occur without a deficiency in total body potassium. This is most commonly seen in the context of either an acute metabolic or respiratory alkalosis. The intracellular shift of potassium is precipitated by a fall in extracellular hydrogen ion concentration. Familial hypokalaemic periodic paralysis is a rare disorder characterized by intermittent attacks of muscle weakness usually developing within the first or second decade. The plasma potassium concentration falls during the attack and returns to normal during the recovery phase. Episodes are precipitated by a high-carbohydrate and low-potassium diet, exercise, infection and alcohol ingestion.

Glucose administration or glucose and insulin given together induces a shift of potassium from the ECF to ICF compartments. The clinical setting in which this may be seen is in the management of diabetic ketoacidosis, but the effect is used therapeutically in the treatment of hyperkalaemia.

Hypokalaemia has been described in individuals who have ingested food contaminated with soluble barium salts as well as in those who are treated with various antibiotics and chemotherapeutic agents.

Clinical features of hypokalaemia

The effects of hypokalaemia depend on the extent, duration and degree of associated total body potassium deficiency and the rapidity of onset. The symptoms and signs are mainly as a result of the effect on skeletal, cardiac and smooth muscle and renal tubular function. Clinical features may therefore be a combination of polyuria and polydipsia secondary to an ADH unresponsive urinary concentration defect, muscle weakness and paralytic ileus. Characteristic ECG changes occur (lowering or inversion of the T-wave and exaggeration of the U-wave, often producing an illusion of QT lengthening) and bradyarrhythmias may develop, especially if hypokalaemia develops with concomitant digoxin therapy. Further manifestations of hypokalaemia and potassium deficiency are glucose intolerance and neuro-psychiatric symptoms, e.g depression, apathy and confusional states.

In hypokalaemic states, the obvious therapeutic measure is that of replacement in association with therapy of the primary condition. In mild to moderate deficiency, either supplementation of diet with potassium-rich foods or the use of oral potassium supplementation as the chloride or bicarbonate salt is sufficient. In conditions associated with metabolic acidosis, e.g renal tubular acidosis, the citrate salt should be used. In severely depleted patients with neuromusclar symptoms and/or ECG abnormalities, intravenous supplementation should be undertaken. It is important to remember that great care should be taken over the rate of potassium administration by the intravenous route, since the rate of potassium uptake by the cell is limited. Intravenous supplementation should be no greater than 0.25 mmol kg^{-1} h^{-1}, with potassium concentrations no greater than 60 mmol/litre in the replacement fluid. During therapy, ECG monitoring and frequent plasma potassium levels are mandatory. Potassium chloride is the usual replacement salt for intravenous use and should be the only one used in alkalotic states.

Potassium supplementation may be indicated in redistribution hypokalaemia despite the absence of a total body deficit, and in familial hypokalaemic periodic paralysis acetazolamide may be of value.

Table 10.12   Causes of hyperkalaemia

Pseudohyperkalaemia
Improper collection or handling of blood sample
In vitro haemolysis
Leucocytosis or thrombocytosis

True hyperkalaemia
Increased potassium load:
   Oral/intravenous supplementation
   Blood transfusion
   Endogenous cell breakdown
Decreased renal excretion:
   Acute renal failure
   Chronic renal failure
   Mineralocorticoid deficiency/resistance
   Potassium-sparing diuretics
Redistribution hyperkalaemia
   Metabolic/respiratory acidosis
   Mineralocorticoid and insulin deficiency
   Drug-induced
   Hyperkalaemic periodic paralysis

Hyperkalaemia (Table 10.12)

Pseudohyperkalaemia

Improper collection or handling of blood sample
In vitro haemolysis
Leucocytosis or thrombocytosis

Pseudohyperkalaemia commonly occurs from the improper collection of venous blood where too vigorous exercising of the arm or prolonged stasis induces red cell rupture and release of intracellular potassium. Similar circumstances occur when the capillary route is used for blood sampling.

True hyperkalaemia

Increased potassium load

Oral/intravenous supplementation
Blood transfusion
Endogenous cell breakdown

Extrinsic and intrinsic potassium loading may occur with excessive oral or intravenous administration, the use of old blood for transfusion and when massive cell breakdown occurs associated with thermal injury, extensive crush injury, massive intravascular haemolysis and spontaneous or chemotherapeutic-induced lysis of large tumour masses. The tolerance of the individual to this type of potassium loading depends on the level of renal function.

Decreased renal excretion

Acute renal failure
Chronic renal failure
Mineralocorticoid deficiency or resistance
Potassium-sparing diuretics

The most important clinical setting in which hyperkalaemia exists is that of acute and chronic renal failure and this will be dealt more fully in Chapters 21 and 22.

Adrenal insufficiency or Addison's disease is characterized by salt wasting and hyperkalaemia. In addition, primary hypoaldosteronism and pseudohypoaldosteronism present a similar clinical picture. Some patients with mild to moderate chronic renal insufficiency, usually secondary to interstitial nephritis, obstructive uropathy and sickle cell disease, may develop a syndrome of hyporeninaemic hypoaldosteronism. This is characterized by a degree of hyperkalaemia inappropriate to the level of glomerular filtration rate. Hyperkalaemia may result from the use of potassium-sparing diuretics, but in practice this is usually not seen unless the patient has associated renal insufficiency.

Redistribution hyperkalaemia

Metabolic or respiratory acidosis
Mineralocorticoid and insulin deficiency
Drug-induced
Familial periodic paralysis

The commonest situation in which the distribution of potassium is disturbed is metabolic acidosis. The extracellular shift of potassium is precipitated by an increase in the extracellular hydrogen ion concentration. In diabetic ketoacidosis this effect is enhanced by insulin deficiency.

Mineralocorticoid deficiency also inhibits transmembrane potassium movement, as does therapy with beta-blockers and angiotensin-converting enzyme inhibitors. Arginine used in growth hormone provocation tests has been reported to induce hyperkalaemia in patients with chronic renal failure. Patients with familial hyperkalaemic periodic paralysis are sympto-

Table 10.13 Approximate relationships between plasma potassium concentration and electrocardiographic abnormalities (From Winters,[26] by permission)

13.0	
12.0	*Arrhythmias which may occur with hyperkalaemia:*
	Terminal ventricular fibrillation — Sinus bradycardia or arrest
11.0	1° arteriovenous block
	Nodal or idioventricular rhythm
	Ventricular tachycardia,
10.0	fibrillation or arrest
	Further widening of QRS
9.0	
	No P-wave, widened QRS; S–T depression; peaked T-waves
8.0	
	Prolonged P–R interval; peaked T-wave
7.0	
6.0	
	Normal
5.0	
4.0	
	Low-amplitude T-wave; prominent U-wave
3.0	
	S–T depression; low-amplitude T-wave; prominent U-wave
2.0	*Arrhythmias which may occur with hypokalaemia:*
	Ventricular premature beats
1.0	Atrial or nodal tachycardia
	Ventricular tachycardia or fibrillation
0.0	

matic following exercise, cold exposure or following potassium ingestion.

Clinical features of hyperkalaemia

Mild elevations in plasma potassium concentration, generally speaking, are not associated with clinical signs or symptoms. With more significant increases the patient may exhibit muscle weakness, but the main features of significant hyperkalaemia are visible on ECG monitoring: the first sign occurring at a plasma level of 7 mmol/litre, being a prolongation of the PR interval and a peaked T-wave; by 8 mmol/litre the QRS complex is widening and the ST segment is depressed; with further increases there is further widening of the QRS complex until ventricular fibrillation occurs at levels of 9 mmol/litre and above. The risk of major arrhythmias is enhanced by the presence of acidosis and hypoxia and in these contexts may occur at lower plasma levels.

The priority in the treatment of hyperkalaemia is dictated by the presence of major ECG abnormalities (Table 10.13). Management of hyperkalaemia in chronic renal insufficiency is based on dietary restriction in combination with diuretic therapy and perhaps bicarbonate supplementation.

Some patients with hyperkalaemic periodic paralysis benefit from acute treatment with a beta-adrenergic agonist, e.g. salbutamol, which enhances cellular potassium uptake.

Acknowledgements

The author wishes to acknowledge the expert secretarial assistance of Mrs Lynda McCarroll.

References

1. Friis-Hansen B.J. Body water compartments in children. *Pediatrics* 1961, **28**, 169–181
2. Winters R.W. Maintenance fluid therapy. In: Winters R.W. (ed.) *The Body Fluids in Pediatrics*. Boston, Little, Brown, 1973: 113
3. Holliday M.A. and Segar W.E. Maintenance need for water in parenteral fluid therapy. *Pediatrics* 1957, **19** 823–832
4. El-Dahr S.S. and Chevalier R.L. Special needs of the new born infant in fluid therapy. *Ped. Clin. North Am.* 1990, **37** 323–336
5. MacKenzie A., Barnes G. and Shann F. Clinical signs of dehydration in children. *Lancet* 1989, **2**, 605–607
6. Kamel K.S., Ethier J.H. Richardson R.M.A. *et al.* Urine electrolytes and osmolality: when and how to use them. *Am. J. Nephrol* 1990, **10**, 89–102
7. Gennari F.J. Serum osmolality: uses and limitations. *N. Engl. J. Med.* 1984, **310**, 102–105
8. Finberg L. The changing epidemiology of water balance and convulsions in infant diarrhoea. *Am. J. Dis. Child.* 1986, **140**, 524
9. Zerbe R.L. and Robertson G.L. Osmotic and non-osmotic regulation of thirst and vasopressin secretion. In: Nairns T.G. (ed) *Clinical Disorders of Fluid and Electrolyte Metabolism*, 5th edn. McGraw-Hill, 1994: 81–100
10. Bartter F.C. and Delea C.S. Disorders of water metabolism. In: Chan J.C.M. and Gill J.R. (eds) *Kidney Electrolyte Disorders*. Edinburgh, Churchill Livingstone 1990: 107–135
11. Goldberg M. Hyponatraemia. *Med. Clin. North Am.* 1981, **65**, 251–269
12. What causes oedema? *Lancet* (Editorial) 1988, **1**, 1028–1030
13. Hantmann D., Rossier B. *et al.* Rapid correction of hyponatraemia in the syndrome of inappropriate secretion of anti-diuretic hormone. *Ann. Int. Med.* 1973, **78** 870–875
14. Laureno R. and Kamp B.I. Pontine and extrapontine myelinolysis following rapid correction of hyponatraemia. *Lancet* 1988, **1**, 1439–1441
15. Sterns R.H., Thomas D.J. and Herndon R.M. Brain dehydration and neurological deterioration after rapid correction of hyponatraemia. *Kidney Int* 1989, **35**, 69–75
16. Arneil G.C. and Chin K.C. Lower solute milks and reduction of hypernatraemia in young Glasgow infants. *Lancet* 1979, **2**, 840
17. Findberg L. Hypernatraemic (hypertonic) dehydration in infants. *N. Engl. J. Med.* 1973, **289**, 196–198
18. Trachtman H., Barbour R., Sturman J.A. *et al.* Taurine and osmoregulation *Pediatr. Res.* 1988, **23**, 35–39
19. Roberton G.L. Diseases of the posterior pituitary. *Clin. Endocrinol. Metab.* 1981, **10**, 204–210
20. Knoers N. and Monnens L.A.M. Nephrogenic diabetes insipidus. In: Holliday M.A., Barratt, T.M. and Avner A.D. (eds) *Pediatric Nephrology*, 3rd edn. Williams and Wilkins, 1993: 662–669
21. Forfar J.O. and Arneil G.C. (eds). Biochemical and physiological tables. *Textbook of Paediatrics*, 3rd edn. London, Churchill Livingstone, 1983: 1985
22. Harris G.D., Fiordalisi I and Finberg, L. Safe management of diabetic ketoacidemia. *J. Pediatr.* 1988, **113**, 65–68
23. Arnei G.C. and Beattie T.J. Renal venous thrombosis. In: Edelmann C.M. Jr (ed.) *Pediatric Kidney Disease*, 2nd edn. Boston, Little, Brown, 1992: 1905–1915
24. Schwartz G.J. and Feld L.G. Body fluids and nutrition: potassium. In: Holliday M.A., Barratt T.M. and Vernier R.L. (eds) *Pediatric Nephrology*, 2nd edn. Baltimore, William and Wilkins, 1987: 114–127

25. Sulyok E., Nemeth, M. and Tenyl I. Relationship between maturity, electrolyte balance, and the renin–
angiotensin–aldosterone system in newborn infants.
Biol. Neonate 1979, **35**, 60–65

26. Williams G.S., Klenk E.L. and Winters R.W. Acute
renal failure in paediatrics: In Winters R.W. (ed), *The
Body Fluids in Paediatrics*. Little Brown and Co. 1973:
523–557

11

Imaging of the kidneys and renal tract

I. Gordon

Introduction

Approach to renal/urological problems

The improvement in real-time abdominal ultrasound (US) has changed the face of imaging of the renal tract so that adequate non-invasive imaging is possible for all children. This is especially important in infants and for children in renal failure. Computerized tomography (CT) and magnetic resonance imaging (MRI) are newer techniques which have limited but specific indications in paediatric nephro-urology. This chapter will discuss the specific advantages and disadvantages of these techniques and the established imaging techniques such as intravenous urography (IVU).[1,2]

Whenever imaging of the renal tract is required, the guiding principle in paediatrics should be to choose the least invasive technique with the lowest radiation dose and work up to the most invasive technique which may well also carry the highest radiation burden for the child. Inevitably this means that all children should start with a US; the only exception to this rule is in the case of severe abdominal trauma.

A visit to a radiology department should be an atraumatic experience for the child and parent and a combination of factors must be taken into account to minimize the anxiety of the child and the family. The attitude of every member of the department must be positive, reassuring and sympathetic. This includes the reception staff as well as the radiographers/technicians and radiologists. Explanations to allay anxiety should be offered to the child and parent at all stages of the visit, including when an appointment is made, as well as throughout the visit for the actual examination.

The objective is to have a co-operative child who can also express his/her fear and/or anxiety. The parent frequently helps the child to overcome his/her anxiety and most parents should be positively encouraged to remain with their child throughout the examination. People working with children must be skilled in the art of blending the proper degree of gentleness and understanding with firmness to achieve excellent technical results in a child who has not suffered psychological trauma from the examination.

The radiologist's role

The term radiologist applies to all those involved in imaging, irrespective of the particular modality: US, nuclear medicine, angiography, CT and MRI are all included. The radiologist involved in paediatric renal imaging must be conversant with the advantages and limitations of each technique, so as to assist the clinician in requesting the appropriate investigation. Factors such as risk, discomfort, radiation dose, cost and timing of the procedures must be considered, as well as the skills in a particular department. Algorithms are particularly useful since they both stimulate discussion between clinician and radiologist as well as ensure a rational use of imaging resources. The radiolo-

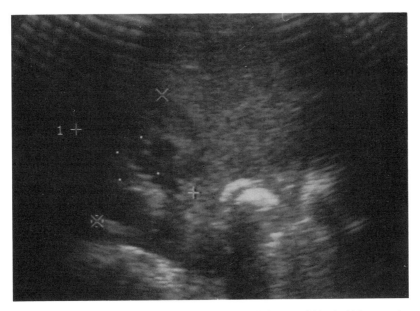

Figure 11.1 Transverse ultrasound section of the left kidney showing a bright area within the kidney, casting an acoustic shadow strongly suggestive of a calculus in a 2-year-old boy with urinary tract infection

gist, in discussion with his clinical colleagues, must ensure that the algorithm is always fitted to the individual child. One valuable forum for ensuring this co-operation is regular clinical radiological review sessions to decide on appropriate investigations and to review the results.

Imaging techniques

Abdominal ultrasound examination (US)

US is non-invasive, with no radiation burden. It should be available in all units responsible for the care of children with renal disease. The examination is independent of function, providing anatomical detail of the retroperitoneal and intra-abdominal structures. Coronal views can reliably be reproduced and allow accurate measurement of renal length, important in assessing renal growth and in the establishment of normal growth charts for US.

The ability to delineate both the normal and abnormal anatomy is directly related to the skill of the ultrasonographer, who must be experienced in examining children and fully conversant with the spectrum of diseases in childhood. Co-operation of the child is required; therefore, a skilled ultrasonographer operating in a quiet environment, geared to children, leads to good results. The major drawbacks are the problems presented by the unskilled operator and the difficulty in comparing accurately small changes in dilatation on sequential US. In addition to the kidneys, the ureters and bladder must be examined. The dilated ureter may be detected either at its upper end or at its lower end behind the bladder, especially when the latter is full. Information on the thickness of the bladder wall, the presence of ureterocele and on the completeness of bladder emptying with micturition should be part of the routine information provided. In the infant, the US should begin with the bladder since micturition may occur at any time and an empty bladder precludes a complete US. Calculi and nephrocalcinosis have a characteristic appearance (Figures 11.1–11.3).

In the presence of an abdominal mass,[3] the US can define the origin and nature of the mass, and determine whether it is cystic or solid. A solid mass on US should be considered as malignant and dissemination sought with the US, including examination of the liver and inferior vena cava (IVC). Notable exceptions are renal venous thrombosis (RVT), especially in the neonate, as well as recessive polycystic disease. The latter is usually bilateral and symmetrical and the bright echo pattern is characteristic (see Chapter 25).

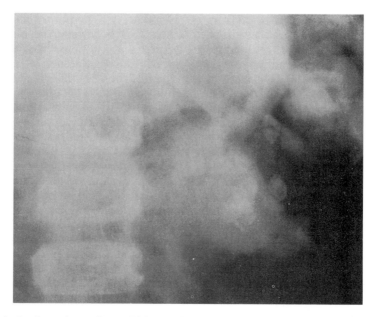

Figure 11.2 Abdominal radiograph revealing multiple calculi in the left kidney in a 2-year-old boy with urinary tract infection

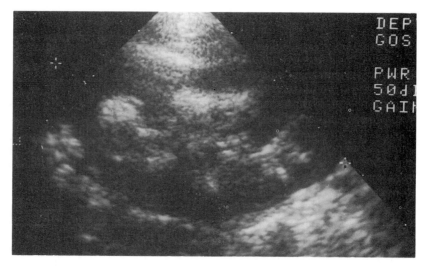

Figure 11.3 The longitudinal ultrasound section of the right kidney showing echogenic areas strongly suggestive of nephrocalcinosis in a child with distal renal tubular acidosis

The kidney in the neonate is different from the older child, since there is very clear distinction between the renal cortex and medulla in the neonate; this may be so marked that to the unskilled observer the medulla appears transonic, suggesting the diagnosis of multiple cysts when in fact it is normal. The echogenicity of the cortex and medulla must be carefully as-

sessed since certain conditions have characteristic appearances, e.g. recessive polycystic disease, acute infection, cystic dysplasia and RVT among others.

The introduction of duplex colour doppler US allows the differentiation between flow and a dilated static system. Originally there was enthusiasm to use the resistive index, i.e. the difference between the systolic and diastolic pulse divided by the diastolic pulse, in children who had undergone renal transplantation, to reach an early diagnosis of rejection, but these early results have not stood the test of time. Currently the value of the resistive index is being evaluated in the diagnosis of obstruction of the urinary tract. The limitations of each imaging modality must be known so that the clinician does not request an examination where there is a high false positive or a high false negative rate.

Radioisotopes

Renal pathophysiology can be assessed using either dynamic scans with ^{99m}Tc-diethylenetriaminepenta-acetate (^{99m}Tc-DTPA), or ^{123}I-hippuran or ^{99m}Tc-mercaptoacetyltriglycine (^{99m}Tc-MAG3), or with static scans using ^{99m}Tc-DMSA. Uptake and excretion of the dynamic isotope scan is detected by a gamma camera; probe renogram systems are obsolete in paediatrics.

Dynamic scan (^{99m}Tc-DTPA or MAG3 or ^{123}I-hippuran)

The uptake phase may be defined as the process of removal of isotope from the blood as it passes through the kidney: using ^{99m}Tc-DTPA this reflects pure glomerular filtration; using ^{99m}Tc-MAG3 or ^{123}I-hippuran this reflects proximal tubular excretion of the isotope. In the normal kidney ^{123}I-hippuran correlates with effective renal plasma flow, while ^{99m}Tc-MAG3 reflects a different aspect of proximal tubular function. Analysis of the kidney during the period 80–150 s, i.e. that part of the uptake phase prior to any isotope appearing in the renal pelvis, enables differential renal function to be assessed. In the normal kidney the excretory phase is not defined as a separate entity; in the presence of dilatation this phase becomes recognizable and inducing a diuresis (e.g. frusemide), drainage may be assessed. Good drainage, i.e. a renal curve falling to < 75% within 10 min or < 50% within 20 min of the diuretic, generally excludes an obstruction. A poor response to a diuretic stimulus may be seen in obstruction, but has also been noted with poor renal function or gross dilatation of the collecting system, or in the presence of a full bladder, i.e. a false positive result (see also Chapter 28).

Indications
^{99m}Tc-DTPA or MAG3 is indicated for differential renal function, if there is dilatation of the collecting systems, following surgery on the pelvis or ureter,[4] for indirect cystography,[5] and following renal transplantation. ^{99m}Tc-DTPA with captopril stimulation may yet prove to be a sensitive screening procedure for renovascular hypertension.

Static scan[6]

^{99m}Tc-DMSA binds to the proximal convoluted tubules; only 10% is excreted in the urine. The delayed static images after the IV injection represent functioning cortical mass. Posterior and both oblique projections should be routinely obtained. Certain centres prefer pinhole views of each kidney to the oblique projection. Anterior views including the empty bladder are essential when an ectopic kidney is to be excluded. Absolute quantification of the kidneys 6 h after injection may be undertaken. The advantage in paediatrics lies in the ability to distinguish between deterioration in the one kidney or growth in the other kidney.

Indications
The high radiation dose of this examination compared to the dynamic scans suggests that ^{99m}Tc-DMSA should not be used interchangeably with ^{99m}Tc-DTPA or MAG3. Wherever renal function is being assessed ^{99m}Tc-DTPA or MAG3 should be used unless one of the following circumstances arise which suggests that a ^{99m}Tc-DMSA is the investigation of choice. In renovascular hypertension, both ^{99m}Tc-DTPA and DMSA, pre- and post-captopril, are required to diagnose both the extrarenal and intrarenal arterial abnormalities (see Chapter 15).

In the 'wet' girl, if the US and IVU are normal then a ^{99m}Tc-DMSA scan may be the only method to detect an occult duplex kidney. In acute pyelonephritis or UTI with VUR,[7–9] the ^{99m}Tc-DMSA scan is the most sensitive technique for the detection of renal involvement which may go on to scar formation (Figures 11.4 and 11.5). In children with gross dilatation (e.g. prune belly syndrome) where only differential function may be possible, ^{99m}Tc-DMSA is more informative than ^{99m}Tc-MAG3. In chronic renal failure when differential function is required, the value of ^{99m}Tc-MAG3 is being investigated to replace ^{99m}Tc-DMSA.

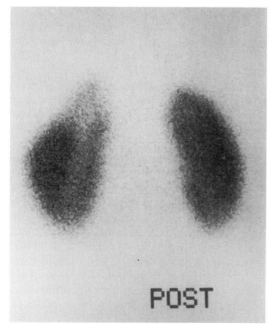

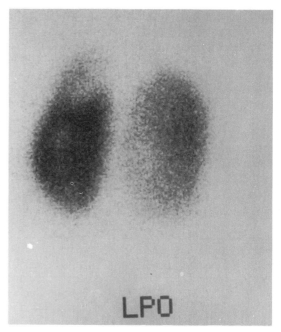

Figure 11.4 ^{99m}Tc-DMSA findings in acute urinary tract infection. The ultrasound examination was normal. Posterior view of the ^{99m}Tc-DMSA scan showing a normal right kidney. The upper pole of the left kidney shows decreased uptake of isotope with the renal outline being preserved (see also Figure 11.5)

Figure 11.5 Left posterior oblique view of the ^{99m}Tc-DMSA scan showing the defect in Figure 11.4 to better advantage

Radioisotope cystogram

Direct radioisotope cystogram (DRC)
The technique is similar to the MCU and requires bladder catheterization, draining the urine off, and instilling ^{99m}Tc-pertechnetate (500 μCi) and normal saline until the bladder is full, when micturition should occur. The entire procedure is carried out in front of, or on top of, the gamma camera linked to a computer system. Both renal areas and the bladder are kept in the field of view. The advantages are mainly the high sensitivity of this technique plus the low radiation exposure compared to a conventional MCU, the dose being reduced by a factor of 20. The disadvantage is that bladder catheterization is still required (Figures 11.6 and 11.7).

Indirect radioisotope cystogram (IRC)
Thirty to 60 min after the IV injection of ^{99m}Tc-MAG3, when 70% of the isotope is in the bladder, the child is asked to void in front of the gamma camera. The background is lower at the time of micturition using ^{99m}Tc-MAG3 since

it is cleared quicker by the kidneys than ^{99m}Tc-DTPA. Voiding views have been shown to be as accurate as the MCU in detecting reflux. The advantages of IRC are that there is no increase in radiation dose above the routine dynamic scan, it is non-invasive, does not require bladder catheterization, provides information about renal function and is physiological. The disadvantages lie in the fact that the child must be co-operative, i.e. be toilet trained, and that VUR will only be detected during the voiding phase since the filling of the bladder is from the kidneys. When there is a high urine flow rate, as seen for example after the administration of frusemide or in an over-hydrated child, VUR may not be detected. If the voided urine volume and activity are measured and correction factors applied for decay and attenuation, then quantification provides full bladder volume, residual bladder volume, urine flow rate in ml/s and, if reflux has occurred, reflux volume in cubic centimetres.[5,10,11]

Indications
When VUR has been documented by MCU, follow-up should be by isotope cystogram. In

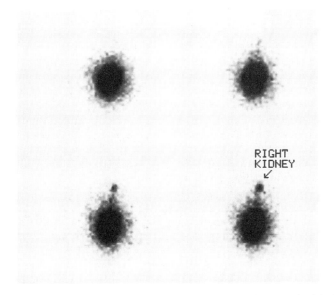

Figure 11.6 Direct radioisotope cystogram in a patient aged 15 months showing reflux into the right kidney

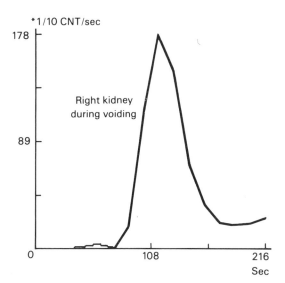

Figure 11.7 Graphical representation of the direct radioisotope cystogram showing right renal reflux. Same patient as in Figure 11.6

girls with UTI, the possibility of using this as a screening procedure to detect VUR has been suggested. Whenever the child can co-operate, then an IRC should be carried out. If no reflux is seen on IRC, then one can proceed to the DRC if one wishes to ensure that no reflux occurs during the filling phase of the cystogram.

Radiology

Plain film and IVU

The plain abdominal radiograph is essential before every IVU.[12] Nephrocalcinosis and calculi may be overlooked after IV contrast and the US may miss small calculi. The spine warrants careful observation and in the presence of chronic renal failure the femoral epiphyses may slip and renal osteodystrophy may be obvious. The IVU provides only a coarse index of renal function.

Indications
The IVU should not be the first examination of the renal tract; rather the IVU should be tailored to the specific clinical problem, resulting in few radiographs, a lower radiation dose and specific answers to the clinician. When a small kidney is discovered on US or isotope examination and no VUR is found, then an IVU to show the calyceal anatomy may prove helpful in establishing the cause. In the presence of uncommon syndromes (e.g. Laurence–Moon–Biedl) and certain diseases (e.g. dysplasia or medullary necrosis), visualization of the calyces is helpful and a high-quality IVU is required. The IVU provides a good basis for assessing renal growth, but US may provide similar information. Following acute renal failure in the

neonate, the diagnosis of medullary necrosis can only be excluded on IVU; this should be carried out at 3 months of age. Recurrent loin pain with a normal US warrants an IVU with a water load during the acute attack of pain to exclude an intermittent pelvi-ureteric junction (PUJ) obstruction. Recurrent UTI with a normal US and ^{99m}Tc-DMSA scan may require an IVU to exclude such pathology as a calyceal cyst or a bladder diverticulum. Whenever a complicated duplex kidney is suspected clinically, then an IVU is the examination of choice if the US is normal or if doubt exists as to which side the ectopic ureterocele arises. The IVU is the best examination to provide anatomical detail of the non-dilated ureter, important in exstrophy and following urinary diversion.

Contraindications
In the neonate, the kidneys may not be visualized within 48 h of birth despite normal renal function; therefore an IVU at this age is contraindicated. In acute renal failure, the contrast may aggravate the renal failure.

Technique
Fluid and food are withheld for approximately 2–3 h prior to the investigation. Excessive dehydration causes an unhappy unco-operative child and in the presence of chronic renal failure may be frankly harmful. A micro-enema may be useful. Intravenous low osmolar contrast should be used, especially in the neonate, e.g. iothalamate at a maximum dose of 3 ml/kg body weight of contrast with 300 mg iodine per millilitre. Intramuscular or subcutaneous contrast is strongly avoided. Within a minute of the end of the IV injection, children are given a gassy drink, whereas babies and toddlers are given a bottle. The radiographs taken should be tailored to the specific clinical indication. To outline calyceal anatomy best, abdominal compression should be used; coned radiographs of the renal area at 5 and 10 min may be sufficient. If ureteric anatomy is required, a full-length radiograph at 15–20 min may be more appropriate. If the diagnosis of recessive polycystic disease is suspected, coned views of the renal areas over 24 h may be required to see the contrast in the dilated collecting ducts. A renal window view, where the X-ray tube is angled 35 degrees to the feet and the X-rays are centred on the xiphisternum, may be useful when outlining the calyces; no patient movement is required. A

full-length film, including the kidney and the base of the bladder, should be obtained when a duplex kidney is suspected. When an obstruction/dilatation of the collecting system has been discovered on US and the exact level of dilatation is uncertain, delayed images may be required. Visualization of the kidney on IVU may be delayed in the neonate, and radiographs at 2, 6 and 18 h after the IV contrast may be useful. Tomography has no role when the IVU is carried out in the context of modern imaging.

Micturating cysto-urethrogram (MCU)

This is the definitive method of assessing the lower urinary tract, but may reveal upper tract detail if VUR is present.[1]

Technique
An X-ray table with an overhead X-ray tube allows free access to the child by the parent, radiologist and nurse. The child does not feel caught between the large mobile overhead image intensifier and the table top; this enhances co-operation. Dilute contrast (20% iodine) is introduced via a size 6 or 8 catheter (feeding tube). The bladder may either be filled via gravity using an inverted contrast bottle at a fixed height above the table top or slowly injected using a 50 ml syringe. The small catheter size prevents too rapid filling of the bladder. Sedation is rarely necessary and a parent should always accompany the child. Preparation of the child and parent prior to the MCU has been very useful to both the child and the professional team in having a more co-operative child. In all boys, the urethra must be demonstrated; this is best done during voiding in the oblique projection. The bladder must be visualized when full, during and after micturition; in addition, visualization in the early filling phase will permit detection of small ureteroceles as well. Oblique views to show the vesico-ureteric junction during micturition are important if VUR is noted.

Indications
The pathology which may be detected includes VUR, bladder function and anatomy, and in boys the urethra. An MCU is indicated in all children under 1 year of age with a UTI; when there is ureteric dilatation; when a small kidney is discovered; with terminal haematuria accompanied by lower urinary tract symptoms; in renal failure of undetermined cause; with cer-

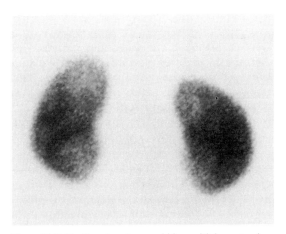

Figure 11.8 Findings in a 4-year-old boy with hypertension due to fibromuscular hyperplasia. ^{99m}Tc-DMSA scan showing focal decreased uptake of isotope and the upper pole of the right kidney. Differential function showed that each kidney contributed 50% to overall renal function (see also Figures 11.9 and 11.10)

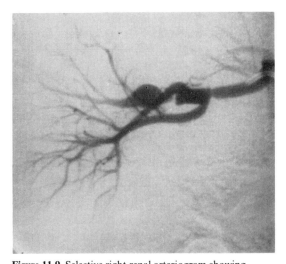

Figure 11.9 Selective right renal arteriogram showing narrowing of the renal artery immediately prior to the bifurcation. The upper pole vessel then shows a second area of narrowing immediately before the aneurysmal dilatation of the intrarenal portion of the upper pole vessel. Same patient as in Figure 11.8

tain voiding problems and when a thick-walled bladder is seen on US.

Contraindications

For the follow-up of VUR, a radioisotope cystogram can be carried out, and may be useful as a screening procedure for girls with a UTI.

Antegrade pyelogram[1]

This investigation should be carried out by an experienced operator, done either in theatre immediately prior to surgery to provide anatomical detail of pelvis and/or ureter unavailable from US or IVU, or as the basis for urodynamic studies when it is combined with pressure flow measurements to determine the physiological significance of a dilated upper urinary tract.

Retrograde pyelogram[1]

This examination has a limited role in nephrology. Rarely when the anatomy remains uncertain, despite numerous other imaging modalities, a retrograde pyelogram is helpful.

Arteriography[1]

Introduction
This invasive investigation with its high radiation dose should be reserved for special clinical situations. When used judiciously it is an invaluable asset with an unrivalled ability to demonstrate vascular anatomy. Potential complications must be borne in mind.

Technique
Arteriography should be carried out by a skilled operator with paediatric experience, using the smallest catheter compatible with obtaining adequate results. Selective renal arteriography with magnification should be part of the procedure. Small doses of non-ionic contrast should be used; this may be further aided by using digital subtraction angiography (DSA) for the aorta and main renal arteries (Figures 11.8–11.10). Cut films with a rapid changer are preferable for small intrarenal arterial anatomy. Cine-radiography is inadequate.

Indications
Hypertension; preceding conservative surgery for Wilms' tumour either in a single kidney or bilateral Wilms' tumour; trauma, complicated by persistent haematuria or hypertension; in suspected vasculitis, especially in polyarteritis, the splanchnic vessels including the hepatic arteries should also be visualized; prior to interventional procedures, e.g. embolization for arteriovenous malformations or balloon dilatation for stenosis are all indications for arteriography.

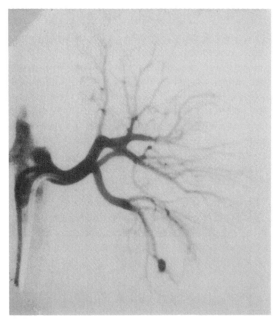

Figure 11.10 Selective left renal arteriogram showing a normal main renal vessel. There is a small aneurysm in the lower pole of the kidney arising from the 4th division vessel. Same patient as in Figure 11.8

Bone radiography

High-quality bone radiographs may monitor renal osteodystrophy in children with chronic renal failure. Magnification using a fine-focus X-ray tube provides the quality required. With high-quality biochemical parathyroid hormone assay available, the role of bone radiographs becomes questionable since there is a long lag period between the development of osteodystrophy and its appearance on the radiograph.

Computerized axial tomography (CT)

Technique
Preparation of the child ensures that minimal sedation is required. Images are taken before and after intravenous contrast; images during the injection allow assessment of the patency of the IVC. Oral and/or rectal contrast is used in pelvic tumours and neuroblastoma.

Indications
Every child with a Wilms' tumour or a neuroblastoma or a rhabdomyosarcoma in the pelvis requires a CT scan. Nephrocalcinosis is readily detected on CT, so that when doubt exists as to the nature of the US appearances of a bright medulla which suggest calcification, then a thin CT cut of the kidneys without contrast will confirm or refute the presence of calcium. CT has not been helpful in children with polycystic disease, obstructive uropathy or duplex pathology.

Magnetic resonance imaging (MRI)

Technique
Quite heavy sedation is used as a routine since this is a long procedure and a quiet, still child is required for an adequate examination. The exact image sequence depends on the information required and the strength of the magnet available.

Indications
Children with a neuropathic bladder and no obvious cause require full investigation of the spine and its contents. MRI detects mass lesions readily, but in the spinal cord intrinsic pathology of the long tracts have not been distinguished in cases of 'occult neuropathic bladder'. In children with malignant tumours, MRI has not provided any new anatomical information which was not available from CT; instead it provides the possibility of suggesting what is tumour rather than haemorrhage or necrosis.

The neonate

Introduction

The immature kidney of the neonate is different from the older child both in its US appearance and also in the handling of isotopes or contrast. At 36 weeks' gestation there is the adult complement of nephrons, i.e. 1 million; all further growth is via hyperplasia mainly in the tubules. The proximal tubule becomes more convoluted, while the loop of Henle elongates, although its position *vis-à-vis* the medulla is unchanged. The glomerular pore increases in size rapidly within the first 3 months of life. Glomerular filtration rate (GFR) and renal plasma flow are low and renal vascular resistance is high, especially in the outer cortical zones, so that there is a preferential distribution of renal blood flow to the juxtamedullary region at birth. The GFR increases three-fold by 1 year of age and reaches that of the mature kidney close to puberty. The proximal tubular function, as measured by clearance of para-amino hippurate, is low in the neonate, increasing to adult values before 2 years of age. Proximal tubular reabsorptive capacity is poorly developed, and as a consequence there is greater dependence on distal sodium reabsorption to maintain sodium balance, with a much higher plasma renin activity and aldosterone concentration than in the adult. There is difficulty in disposing of an osmotic and/or a sodium load and consequently a greater risk of volume overload with inappropriate IV therapy or with IV contrast material. In the neonate/infant there is a relatively large extracellular fluid space so that readily diffusible substances injected intravenously (e.g. DTPA or intravenous contrast for IVU) have a large volume of distribution and therefore a relatively low plasma concentration.

Imaging

A US will answer anatomical questions such as how many kidneys are present, their size and echogenicity. If dilatation is present, whether this includes the ureters and what is the state of the bladder and the bladder base. The next mode of investigation depends on the clinical problem and the result of US. In the presence of dilatation of the urinary tract, especially the ureter, an MCU is required since dilatation may be caused by VUR or obstruction.

High-quality dynamic isotope scans are generally best achieved at 4 weeks of age when some renal maturity has occurred. The young infant ^{99m}Tc-DTPA scan is characterized by poor visualization of the kidneys, a high background throughout the examination and a relatively flat renal curve even for a normal kidney. Using ^{99m}Tc-MAG3, the kidneys are readily visualized since this isotope remains in the intravascular space because of the high protein binding, and the higher renal extraction than ^{99m}Tc-DTPA. Relatively poor function as seen on the ^{99m}Tc dynamic or static scan does not imply irreversible damage and no long-term management should be planned on these results; rather the scan should be repeated either when the infant is older ($\pm$ 3 months.) or following a drainage procedure. An IVU requires an injection of up to 3 ml/kg of a contrast agent which is osmotically active and has a high sodium content. This may be detrimental to an immature kidney. An IVU in the neonatal period may aggravate

renal venous thrombosis (RVT) or medullary necrosis. Even in normal neonates an IVU may fail to outline the kidneys, especially in the first 48 h of life. These factors suggest that there is no place for an IVU within the first 2–3 days of life. When an IVU is undertaken, delayed images at 6, 12 and 18 h may be necessary to visualize the kidneys. An IVU should not be carried out in the neonate with sepsis or renal failure. The IVU should *only* be undertaken to answer specific clinical questions; the new non-ionic contrast media with 30% iodine should be used with a maximum dose of 3 ml/kg.

Clinical applications are discussed in Chapter 31. The investigations of the various clinical problems are discussed in the appropriate chapters. Hypertension and haematuria are discussed here to illustrate how a combined radiological/clinical approach is developed.

Hypertension

Aims of imaging

Since 90% of hypertension is secondary to renal disease in children over 1 year of age, the object is to discover a 'renal' or adrenal abnormality.

Imaging

A full US should include doppler US of the aorta and renal arteries. A normal US does not exclude a single particularly upper pole scar, renovascular pathology or a phaeochromocytoma. The next investigation (Figure 11.11) is a ^{99m}Tc-DMSA scan; this will detect renal scars and cystography would then be indicated. A normal US and normal ^{99m}Tc-DMSA scan do not exclude renovascular disease. The exclusion of this ultimately requires angiography, but the use of both ^{99m}Tc-DTPA and DMSA before and after captopril stimulation is currently being evaluated as a screening technique for renovascular hypertension. Arteriography demands a free flush aortic injection as well as selective renal injections in both anteroposterior and oblique projections, in order to diagnose both intrarenal and extrarenal renovascular disease.

Neurofibromatosis and fibromuscular hyperplasia are probably the two commonest vascular pathologies encountered. An IVU may be useful

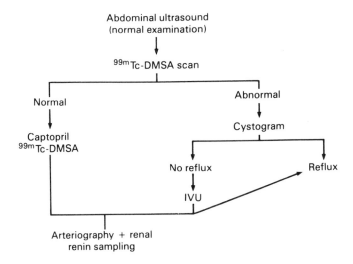

Figure 11.11 Sustained hypertension in paediatrics – normal US to detect renal scars

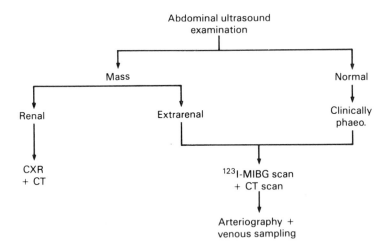

Figure 11.12 Sustained hypertension in paediatrics – abdominal US may reveal a mass

if the DMSA is abnormal, but the cystogram fails to demonstrate reflux. It may confirm the presence of pyelonephritic scarring or suggest renovascular disease.

Abdominal US may reveal a mass (Figure 11.12). If this is renal, CXR and CT scan would be the next line of investigation. If extrarenal, iodine meta-iodobenzylguanidine (MIBG) scan, followed by CT scan with specific attention focused on the areas of abnormality seen on the ^{123}I-MIBG scan, followed by arteriography and venous sampling, would be indicated. This pattern of investigation would also be followed if there was strong clinical and biochemical

suspicion of phaeochromocytoma even in the presence of a normal US.

The discovery of a small kidney on US (Figure 11.13) necessitates a ^{99m}Tc-DMSA scan and MCU; the former to assess the degree of the function of the kidney and the latter to look for VUR. In the absence of VUR, an IVU is indicated to outline the calyces in an attempt to establish the cause of the small kidney. The differential diagnosis lies between renal venous thrombosis, dysplasia, reflux nephropathy, post-obstructive atrophy and arterial pathology. The presence of normal calyces on IVU would suggest that arteriography was indicated.

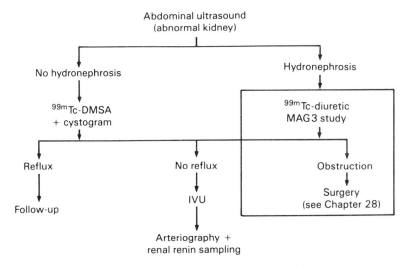

Figure 11.13 Sustained hypertension in paediatrics – abdominal US may detect a small kidney

Haematuria

The commonest cause of haematuria is urinary tract infection, which will require appropriate investigation. Although very few genito-urinary tumours present with isolated haematuria, the diagnosis is so important that some imaging should be undertaken early in the investigation of a child with haematuria. Clues which will direct the further investigation of haematuria have already been discussed in Chapter 1.

Imaging

A full US examination if normal will exclude a renal or bladder tumour and an obstructive uropathy (see Chapters 1 and 28). A plain abdominal radiograph will further exclude calculi. Only if the haematuria persists and there is a normal renal biopsy should further imaging be undertaken in the form of a CT scan. Arteriography is very rarely undertaken unless the haematuria follows trauma. A renal biopsy is a form of iatrogenic trauma and if haematuria develops or worsens, arteriography may reveal an arteriovenous fistula.

References

1. Aaronson I.A. and Cremin B.J. *Imaging Techniques in Clinical Paediatric Uroradiology.* Edinburgh, Churchill Livingstone, 1984: 17–37

2. Lebowitz R.L. Paediatric uroradiology. *Ped. Clin. North Am.* 1985, **32**, 1353–1362

3. Merten D.F. and Kirks D.R. Diagnostic imaging of pediatric abdominal masses. *Ped. Clin. North Am.* 1985, **32**, 1397–1426

4. van der Vis-Melsen M.J.E., Baert R.J.M. *et al.* Scintigraphic assessment of lower urinary tract function in children with and without outflow obstruction. *Br. J. Urol.* 1989, **64**, 263–269

5. Carlsen O., Lukman B. and Nathan E. Indirect radionuclide renocystography for determination of vesicoureteral reflux in children. *Eur. J. Nucl. Med.* 1986, **12**, 205–210

6. Bingham J.B. and Masey M.N. An evaluation of use of ⁹⁹Tcᵐ-dimercaptosuccinic acid (DMSA) as a static renal imaging agent. *Br. J. Radiol.* 1979, **51**, 599–608

7. Goldraich N.P., Ramos O.L. and Goldraich I.H. Urography versus DMSA scan in children with vesicoureteric reflux. *Paediatr. Nephrol.* 1989, **3**, 1–5

8. Stoller M.L. and Kogan B.A. Sensitivity Tc gap 99m DMSA for the diagnosis of chronic pyelonephritis: clinical and theoretical considerations. *J. Urol.* 1986, **135**, 977–980

9. Verber I.J., Strudley M.R. and Meller S.T. 99m Tc DMSA scan as first investigation of urinary tract infection. *Arch. Dis. Child.* 1988, **63**, 1320–1325

10. Bower G., Lovegrove F.T., Geijselh van der Scaff A. and Guelfi G. Comparison of direct and indirect radionuclide cystography. *J. Nucl. Med.* 1985, **26**, 465–468

11. Chapman S.J., Chantler C., Haycock G.B., Masey M.N. and Saxton H.M. Radionuclide cystography in vesico-ureteric reflux. *Arch. Dis. Child.* 1988, **63**, 650–651

12. Lucas A. The window view of the renal area in infants and children. *Radiography* 1979, **45**, 216

12

Renal biopsy

R.H.R. White

Introduction

Percutaneous needle biopsy of the kidney has been used in the investigation of children with renal disease for more than 30 years, and is a safe and effective procedure in experienced hands. The earliest attempts at renal biopsy were attended by high risks and comparatively low success rates, and its establishment as an acceptable routine procedure was largely the result of the increased anatomical precision which was a feature of the technique described by Kark and Muehrcke in 1954.[1] Its use in children was first reported three years later[2] and there followed a series of papers reporting high success rates with minimal risks.[3-5]

Several technical advances have been developed since that time, of which two in particular have had a major influence on the success of the procedure. In the original description the radiological renal outlines were related to surface landmarks and the site for insertion of the biopsy needle was marked on the skin prior to biopsy.[1] It was found from experience that this was almost invariably located 1–2 cm below the 12th rib alongside the lateral border of the paraspinal muscle bundle, which is easily palpated,[5] and for many years biopsy was carried out 'blind'. It required experience to obtain a high success rate with this method, sometimes necessitating perseverence through several unsuccessful attempts, to the patient's discomfort. The introduction of direct fluoroscopic needle guidance[6,7] enhanced the precision of the procedure, making it both safer to perform and easier for trainees to learn.

The other major advance was the development of the Travenol 'Tru-Cut' disposable biopsy needle. The original Silverman needle had a heavy hub and, after insertion, required a 360° rotation of the inner needle to remove a core of tissue, making it difficult to use in young children undergoing biopsy under sedation and local analgesia. It was modified by infilling the tips of the inner needle, making their depth of insertion adjustable, adding a depth stop and contructing the mounts from aluminium,[8] and proved adequate, despite the need for regular hand-sharpening. However, a controlled, prospective comparison of the two needles demonstrated that the White-Silverman needle caused more compression artefacts of glomeruli than the Tru-Cut needle, owing to the squeezing action of the prongs of the inner needle,[9] and the latter has now become the standard instrument.

The use of ultrasound as an alternative and less invasive imaging procedure for biopsy needle guidance has rightly been explored during the past 15 years, in both adults and children.[10,11] However, it lacks the anatomical precision afforded by direct fluoroscopy, and limits the operator's selection of sites of entry of the needle into the kidney from a single skin puncture. Thus it has not replaced fluoroscopy as the standard procedure in most paediatric renal units. On the other hand its advantage is that it is applicable in patients whose renal function is severely compromised. As ultrasonic imaging technology advances in the future, it will doubtless acquire an increasing role in the performance of renal biopsy; it is probably easier to learn the ultrasound-assisted technique from the start than to adapt to it from fluoroscopy.

The circumstances prevailing in 1959 obliged the writer to observe biopsy being performed in adults and then adapt it to children; this is not a practice to be commended today. Past personal experience of having to repeat a number of biopsies attempted unsuccessfully in young children by adult nephrologists, or by well-meaning paediatricians with limited exposure to nephrology during their training, has reinforced the absolute necessity for renal biopsy in children to be undertaken only by an experienced paediatric nephrologist, in a centre equipped with the appropriate laboratory facilities and expertise, and it is in such centres that trainees should gain their experience. The method described below has been developed and improved by the writer over a period of more than 30 years, and employs fluoroscopy. While enough detail is given to illustrate subtle differences in the approach to children, as opposed to adults, it is emphasized that the technique can only be learnt by observing an experienced operator and practising under supervision, and it requires up to a year of supervised training to achieve competence. It is not a procedure for house staff and should be reserved for career trainees.[12,13]

Performing renal biopsy

Preparation

It is important that the nephrologist who is to perform the biopsy should meet the child and parents beforehand, to explain the procedure and describe the arrangement options available. Most renal biopsies in children can be satisfactorily performed under light sedation and local analgesia, with minimal risk and inconvenience. However, an occasional child will require a general anaesthetic, necessitating endotracheal intubation, and this option should be discussed during the consultation, so that an elective decision can be made if possible. If the doctor is seen by the child to have a kindly disposition and to behave courteously towards the parents, the level of co-operation is likely to be enhanced. In our department the interview is reinforced by a two-page handout which briefly describes the procedure, preliminary precautions and postoperative management. The responsible parents, and older child patients, are expected to read this before signing a consent form.

Until November 1987 we routinely admitted children to hospital the day before biopsy and retained them until the following day. The worsening bed shortage, which frequently led to cancellation, forced upon us the need to perform biopsy on a day-case basis, to which we were agreeable in view of our good safety record. It quickly became apparent that children and parents preferred it, and were prepared to make long journeys in the early morning in order to avoid an overnight stay. This is now our routine practice, except for a minority of families obliged to travel a long distance by public transport and, of the first 200 biopsies performed in this manner, we have only had to detain a child on account of minor post-biopsy complications on nine occasions.

The preliminary consultation should also include enquiry about any familial bleeding tendency, and stress the avoidance of platelet-inhibiting drugs such as aspirin. In preparation for biopsy, a haemoglobin estimation and coagulation screen, usually comprising a platelet count and bleeding, prothrombin and partial thromboplastin times, should be undertaken. We routinely check the child's blood group even though transfusion is rarely needed.

Premedication

The patient should have no food or drink for 4 h before biopsy. If the child is to have a general anaesthetic, the anaesthetist in charge should advise on the appropriate premedication. For biopsy under local analgesia, the 'ideal' premedication will minimize apprehension without making the child too sleepy to co-operate. We have experimented with some of the newer preparations, such as ketamine, temazepam and droperidol, without much success, and recommend the following well-tried combination, which we give *orally* 1 h before biopsy:

Promazine hydrochloride, 2 mg/kg body weight up to 50 mg, then 1 mg/kg up to a total of 75 mg; and pethidine, 1 mg/kg up to a maximum of 50 mg.

For the majority of children this has proved

satisfactory. Pethidine may rarely induce vomiting and in this instance, or if the child remains apprehensive and restless, a small dose of diazepam emulsion, e.g. 0.1 mg/kg, can be given intravenously during the procedure. For young children we also apply lignocaine/prilocaine (Emla) analgesic cream to the back bilaterally in occlusive dressings, 1 h before biopsy, using the landmarks for the entry site previously described.[5] The accompanying nurse has an important role in administering what Vernier[3] described as 'vocal anaesthesia', to distract an apprehensive child. Recently we have experimented with allowing a parent to remain present throughout biopsy, in a similar role.

The procedure

The patient is placed prone on the X-ray couch, with a foam bolster or rolled towel under the abdomen, to minimize the anteroposterior mobility of the kidneys. A winged needle is inserted into an accessible vein, preferably on the back of the hand, and strapped in place. While the skin overlying both kidneys is cleansed with a suitable antiseptic such as 0.5% alcoholic chlorhexidine solution, and draped with a perforated towel, an assistant injects iopamidol-370 (Niopam, Merck), 1–1.5 ml/kg, intravenously.

On completion of the injection a nephrogram should appear, providing the opportunity to review the size and position of both kidneys by fluoroscopy before selecting one for biopsy. The majority of biopsies are performed to investigate glomerular disorders, and the choice of kidney is immaterial from the pathological aspect. In the writer's experience the left kidney is more often selected for biopsy because its outline is less frequently obscured by bowel gas. Using aseptic technique, the operator now brings a metal probe into the image-intensified field until its tip touches the skin and overlies the margin of the lower pole of the kidney. The skin is then marked with a sterile swab dipped in Bonney's blue, to indicate the needle entry site.

The skin, subcutaneous tissue and overlying muscles are next infiltrated with 5–10 ml of 1% lignocaine hydrochloride, according to the age and adiposity of the child. A 75 mm, 22-gauge spinal needle is now inserted, to locate the lower pole of the kidney; in an obese adolescent a longer needle may be needed. The kidney is screened intermittently as the needle is advanced, until it penetrates the capsule at or a little lateral to the lower pole. Penetration is recognized by a respiratory 'swing' imparted by the kidney, as well as a distinct, transmitted arterial pulsation. Sometimes the needle rotates around its axis, and this is a useful supplementary sign. Its position in the kidney is confirmed by screening, when the tip of the needle can be seen to move in parallel with the lower calyces during respiration (Figure 12.1a). Before removing the needle it can, if necessary, be withdrawn 2–3 mm and used to infiltrate further lignocaine outside the renal capsule. By grasping it with thumb and forefinger in contact with the skin, the skin-to-kidney depth will be revealed on withdrawing the needle.

A stab incision is made at the entry site, using a no. 15 scalpel blade, to facilitate insertion of the biopsy needle. The Tru-Cut needle is available in three shaft lengths, and the greatest convenience is afforded by the shortest one that can be used; it should be 3.5 cm or more longer than the estimated skin-to-kidney depth, to allow for complete penetration of the capsule and full insertion into the parenchyma. The instrument is guided along approximately the same track as the spinal needle, until penetration of the capsule is confirmed on screening (Figure 12.1b). If the tip bypasses the kidney, the needle should be completely withdrawn and reinserted at a slightly different angle. The differing textures of fat, muscle, fascia and kidney are appreciated with greater sensitivity if the needle, during insertion, is handled by its shaft than by the mount. The tip of the middle finger can be used as a rough depth guide, and the free hand can with advantage be lightly rested on the rib cage to monitor the phase of respiration. It is important to avoid manipulating the fully inserted needle during inspiration, to minimize the risk of a capsular tear. It is essential to penetrate the capsule before attempting biopsy; an attempt made from without invariably causes the child pain by stretching the capsular nerve endings, and usually results in technical failure.

The Tru-Cut needle has two components (Figure 12.2). The outer needle is provided with a cutting bevel with which a core of renal tissue is removed, and the solid inner component has at its tip a 2 cm notch, which retains the core of tissue when the instrument is in the closed position. When assembled, the two parts are interlocked by the specially designed mounts, in

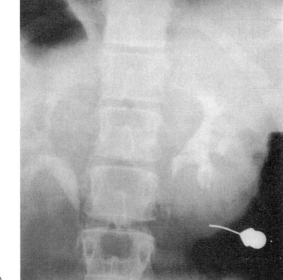

(a)

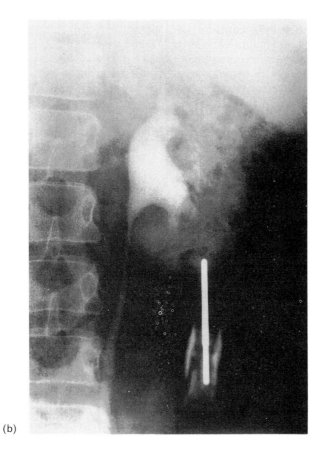

(b)

Figure 12.1 Locating the kidney by fluoroscopic imaging. (a) A 75 mm spinal needle with its tip in the lower pole of the right kidney. The slight curve on the needle is created by the caudad inspiratory excursion of the kidney. (b) A Tru-Cut biopsy needle in position ready for biopsy

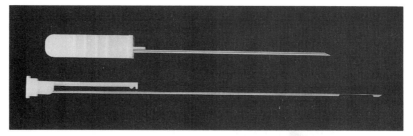

Figure 12.2 A 115 mm Tru-Cut (Travenol) biopsy needle, its two components separated (see text for description)

order to restrict their movements to exposing and covering the notch. The needle is fully inserted in the closed position until the capsule is penetrated. The inner component is then thrust vigorously into the parenchyma and held still while the outer needle is advanced to its limit, after which the instrument is withdrawn. These three movements are best made in rapid succession during the passive expiratory phase of respiration. The needle is then opened to reveal the core of tissue, which is carefully teased out of the notch and aligned on a small piece of sterilized microscope slide, to prevent it from curling in the fixative. It is our normal practice to obtain a second specimen, to ensure an adequate glomerular yield for optical, immunofluorescence and electron microscopy, and the needle may on this occasion be guided to the lower lateral part of the kidney, rather than the lower pole.

Transplant biopsy

The transplanted kidney is located extraperitoneally in the iliac fossa, is palpable abdominally and, unlike the native kidney, does not move on respiration. Because, in this situation, the kidney is less well visualized fluoroscopically, and is often functioning poorly when biopsy is indicated, a different technique must be used. After the alignment of the kidney has been checked and its depth from the surface measured ultrasonically, the Tru-Cut biopsy needle is guided into the cortex manually, while the kidney is palpated. If an adequate specimen is obtained at the first attempt, it is preferable to avoid a second insertion into a rather precarious solitary kidney.

Handling of specimens

The small cores of tissue can quickly desiccate, and it is essential to place them in fixative as soon as practicable. In childhood, light micros-

copy (LM) is not infrequently undiagnostic, and greater reliance has to be placed on immunofluorescence (IF) and electron microscopy (EM). It is therefore prudent to remove small portions of cortical tissue for preservation for IF and EM even if these are not part of the local laboratory's routine, so that they can if necessary be sent elsewhere. The ideal arrangement is for a laboratory technician to be present at biopsy, to receive each specimen into a Petri dish lined with moistened gauze, and to align them under a dissecting microscope so that cortex and medulla can be differentiated by the operator (Figure 12.3). The technician may then excise two or three 1.0 mm cubes of cortex for EM and a 3 mm piece for IF, depending upon availability.

The choice of fixatives is a matter for discussion with the histopathologist. The best results for LM are obtained, in the writer's opinion, by fixation for 5–6 h in Bouin's alcoholic picrate solution, followed by overnight fixation in 10% buffered formalin. This results in less cellular shrinkage and preserves a clear urinary space in the glomeruli, so that the morphology of the tuft and the presence or absence of adhesions can be adequately assessed. It has further advantages when glomerular morphometry is to be employed as a research tool[14,15] For IF, the small fragment of tissue is snap-frozen in liquid nitrogen, while specimens for EM are most commonly fixed in 2.5% glutaraldehyde buffered with 0.1 molar sodium cacodylate.

It is not appropriate to describe the further processing of specimens in this chapter, but the choice of embedding material for LM deserves comment. Most laboratories employ paraffin wax which, when carefully sectioned by an experienced and meticulous technician, can yield sections of 2 μm or even 1 μm thickness. It is technically easier to cut very thin sections when the tissue is embedded in glycol methacrylate.

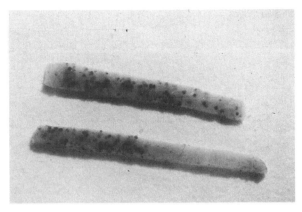

Figure 12.3 Two freshly obtained cores of renal tissue, showing the distinction between cortex and medulla. In this instance, extensive intracapillary thrombosis has made the glomeruli easily visible; usually they appear bloodless

However, in our department we experienced considerable difficulty in obtaining satisfactory trichrome stains, which are of critical importance in the evaluation of intraglomerular deposits, and we therefore abandoned methacrylate, reverting to paraffin, after 10 years' trial. Moreover, if the tissue preserved for EM contains no glomeruli, it is possible subsequently to deparaffinize the main core of tissue and reprocess part of it for EM, even though the results are less than perfect.

Postoperative management and complications

Following biopsy, the child should be kept resting quietly in bed for 5–6 h; restless toddlers are better cradled in their mothers' arms than allowed to cry in the cot. The pulse and blood pressure should be monitored. Because of the rich blood supply of the kidney, some bleeding is unavoidable. Postoperative ultrasound scans show that this usually takes the form of a small haematoma overlying the capsular punctures.[16] Such small haematomas remain asymptomatic, and routine scanning is not advocated. A more substantial haematoma will give rise to loin pain and a palpable mass and, in our experience, is very rare. A little soreness and stiffness is usually experienced in the back following biopsy, due to the trauma of lignocaine infiltration and insertion of the biopsy needle; it can be relieved with paracetamol.

Microscopic haematuria is almost invariably observed on routine urinalysis following biopsy, and need cause no anxiety. If, however, the biopsy needle has inadvertently penetrated a calyx, transient heavy haematuria is almost certain to occur. Fortunately this is a rare event, particularly when fluoroscopic guidance is employed. In order to minimize the risk of clot formation and resulting colic, a diuresis should be promoted by means of a liberal fluid intake postoperatively. In children who are actively nephrotic this is better achieved by administering a single dose of frusemide, 2 mg/kg intravenously. Prolonged haematuria is exceptional in children, provided that coagulation defects have been excluded preoperatively and care has been taken to avoid calyceal trauma. In a large adult series, 6.9% of patients had macroscopic haematuria, which persisted in 3.7% for more than 24 h.[17] The writer can recall only four occasions when, as a result of prolonged haematuria, the plasma haemoglobin fell sufficiently to necessitate transfusion, in a series exceeding 1300 biopsies.

Other rarely reported complications include arteriovenous fistula, renal capsular tear requiring exploration or nephrectomy, ureteric clot colic, penetration of the bowel (usually the colon retroperitoneally) and inadvertent biopsy of adjacent organs, notably the spleen, liver and pancreas.[12] Serious complications are less liable to occur in children than in adults, in whom the elastic recoil of divided arteries is less vigorous and the incidence of both hypertension and vasculitis is higher.[12,16] Death directly due to biopsy is fortunately very rare. Most were reported in the 1960s, and include the author's only case which was due to cardiac arrest associated with general anaesthesia, the biopsy procedure itself being straightforward.[5]

Table 12.1   Some causes of technical failure

Failure to locate the kidney
Inexperience
Obesity
Unco-operative child – local analgesia
Acute renal failure – absent fluoroscopic nephrogram
Massive splenomegaly displacing left kidney

Fibrotic renal tissue
Chronic renal failure
Dysplasia
Advanced reflux nephropathy
Polycystic kidneys

Insufficient glomeruli for diagnosis
Medullary biopsy
Small fragments of tissue
Incorrect manipulation of needle components – inexperience

Table 12.2   Contraindications to renal biopsy

Bleeding tendency
Anticoagulant/antiplatelet therapy
Severe, uncorrected anaemia
Severe, uncontrolled hypertension
Ectopia and fusion defects
Renal neoplasm
Large cysts
Gross hydronephrosis
Contracted, fibrotic kidney
Perinephric abscess
Solitary kidney (see comment in text)

Technical failure

A renal biopsy must be considered a failure if it contains no glomeruli, or insufficient to make a diagnosis. A minimum of five glomeruli is the conventional aim; however, early segmental sclerotic lesions could be absent from a superficial specimen containing 20 glomeruli. Ideally a biopsy specimen should include the corticomedullary junction (Figure 12.3).

The writer recalls a technically difficult biopsy in 1963, consisting entirely of medulla; however, a fragment of blood clot contained three glomerular tufts dislocated from their capsules, which were clearly diagnostic of mesangiocapillary glomerulonephritis. Diagnostic failure may also occur if, despite an adequate glomerular yield for LM, the tissue set aside for IF and EM contains no glomeruli, especially in a child with recurrent haematuria in whom the differential diagnosis of the IgA and Alport nephropathies requires consideration.[13] Since

employing a dissecting microscope to identify cortical tissue, we have experienced very few failures of this nature.

The main causes of technical failure are listed in Table 12.1. Inexperience is undoubtedly the commonest cause, and it is mandatory that trainees should have the immediately available assistance of an experienced operator until they have achieved competence. To obtain a tissue specimen necessitates holding the inner component of the biopsy needle in position while the outer component is advanced and this, in turn, requires opposing movements of the left and right hand. A common cause of failure in the learner is to withdraw the inner component instead of advancing the outer one.

Where biopsy is needed for diagnosis in acute renal failure, the kidney can nowadays be located ultrasonically. In the writer's personal experience, attempted biopsy of contracted kidneys associated with chronic renal failure has, in the past, been associated with such a high failure rate that this is now regarded as a contraindication. With modern imaging techniques, biopsy is today seldom indicated in the other conditions characterized by fibrosis. The remaining causes of failure are rare, though not entirely avoidable even with experience.

Contraindications

The main contraindications to renal biopsy are listed in Table 12.2. Where biopsy is mandatory for diagnosis in the presence of a coagulation defect, this should first be appropriately corrected. Likewise, anticoagulant or antiplatelet therapy should be discontinued for at least 1 week before and 1 week after biopsy. Severe hypertension should be brought under control before attempting biopsy. Ectopic kidneys are generally inaccessible to percutaneous biopsy, but it is possible, with experience, to biopsy a horseshoe kidney along its lateral border, avoiding the malrotated lower pole calyces. It is unwise to biopsy a neoplasm because of the risk of seeding tumour cells distally, while penetration of a hydronephrotic kidney may cause a urinary fistula to develop. Solitary kidney is repeatedly cited as an absolute contraindication to biopsy,[12,18,19] but if there is no other reliable means of establishing a diagnosis, it may reasonably be performed by an experienced operator, particularly in a co-operative older child who exhibits no other contraindications.[20]

Applications of biopsy

It is not intended to describe the almost innumerable applications of renal biopsy; the indications in specific clinical disorders will be found in the relevant chapters. Biopsy may play important roles in initial diagnosis, evaluation of the severity of disease processes, and assessment of progress, whether spontaneous or in response to treatment; these will be discussed in broad terms, with examples. As a by-product of these applications, biopsy can make substantial contributions to research.

Initial diagnosis

Renal biopsy should be used to reach a diagnosis when this cannot be achieved reliably by less invasive techniques. It should not be needed in, for example, uncomplicated acute nephritis, provided that an aetiological diagnosis has been reached on the basis of raised plasma streptococcal antibody titres and a reduced complement C3 level which gradually returns to normal. If, on the other hand, hypertension, heavy proteinuria or hypocomplementaemia persist for more than 4–6 weeks, biopsy would be indicated to confirm or eliminate a diagnosis of mesangiocapillary glomerulonephritis.[21]

In the 1960s, renal biopsy was a routine pretreatment procedure in children with the nephrotic syndrome. However, these early studies demonstrated the correlations between the minimal change lesion, highly selective proteinuria and steroid-responsiveness,[22] rendering it subsequently unnecessary to biopsy nephrotic children unless they were infants, had persistent microscopic haematuria in addition to proteinuria, or failed to respond to a one-month course of prednisolone in adequate dosage.

Renal biopsy is an essential diagnostic tool in a child who presents with persistent microscopic haematuria, with or without recurrent attacks of macroscopic haematuria.[13] It is useful to separate such patients into the minority with accompanying heavy proteinuria, who should be biopsied without undue delay, and those who have trivial or no proteinuria, who should first be more extensively investigated non-invasively for evidence of 'surgical' lesions

such as tumour and calculus, idiopathic hypercalciuria, and familial involvement. The importance of both IF and EM as part of the biopsy processing cannot be overemphasized, since the two commonest causes are IgA nephropathy and Alport's syndrome.

The commonest cause of primary acute renal failure in childhood is, today, the haemolytic uraemic syndrome, which does not require biopsy for diagnosis, and in which it is usually contraindicated because of the low platelet count. However, from time to time a child, usually of school age, presents with hypertension, proteinuria and rapidly failing renal function, in whom the diagnosis is unclear. After scanning the kidney ultrasonically, and correcting any coagulation defect if necessary, biopsy should be performed as a matter of urgency. This is likely to show crescentic or necrotizing glomerulonephritis of post-streptococcal aetiology[23] or due to mesangiocapillary glomerulonephritis,[24] microscopic polyarteritis nodosa, Wegener's granulomatosis, Goodpasture's syndrome or the 'idiopathic' type.[25]

There are several causes of asymptomatic, non-postural proteinuria, which include membranous nephropathy and focal segmental glomerulosclerosis, even in the absence of nephrotic oedema. Once it has been established by an ultrasound scan that the kidneys are anatomically normal and unscarred, biopsy should be undertaken to establish the diagnosis. Although biopsy is contraindicated in chronic renal failure with shrunken kidneys, it may be used, for example, to establish a diagnosis of familial juvenile nephronophthisis, in a child with moderately impaired renal function and smooth kidneys which are only slightly reduced in size.

The main indication for biopsy of the renal allograft is to diagnose the cause of deterioration or cessation of function. Parenchymal changes include immunological rejection and recurrence of the native disease. Before biopsy is undertaken, however, steps must be taken to eliminate vascular thrombosis, obstructive hydronephrosis and acute pyelonephritis as causes of dysfunction.

Evaluation of severity of disease

In systemic disorders which involve the kidneys there is usually, although not invariably, involvement of the skin, joints or alimentary tract which enables a firm diagnosis to be made. In these instances biopsy may be required to determine the severity of renal involvement and the need for treatment. A good example is that of systemic lupus erythematosus, in which the clinical presentation does not always reflect the severity of the underlying renal lesion, which ranges from minor glomerular abnormalities, through membranous nephropathy, to diffuse proliferative glomerulonephritis with or without crescents.[26] Since the latter form requires aggressive treatment, biopsy is imperative, even if urinary abnormalities are comparatively trivial.

A further example is Henoch-Schoenlein purpura, which involves the kidneys in up to 60% of cases.[27] Clinicopathological correlations derived from routine biopsy in the 1960s,[28] coupled with extended follow-up,[29] have laid the foundations for the current recommendations regarding biopsy. The majority of children whose only renal manifestation is haematuria will recover without residual renal functional impairment, and do not need biopsy. On the other hand, those with a nephritic or nephrotic onset, or with persistent heavy proteinuria, have a 10–15% chance of a more severe lesion in which 50% or more of the glomeruli are affected by epithelial crescents, while this risk rises to as much as 50% when the patient exhibits a mixed nephritic–nephrotic presentation.[27] It is these patients who should be selected for biopsy.

Assessment of progress

A repeat biopsy may be required to assess progress, and is most strongly indicated where potentially toxic therapy is being administered, so that an informed judgement can be made whether or not to continue treatment for an extended period. To appreciate the need for biopsy, as opposed to less invasive investigations, it is necessary to understand the complex relationship between glomerulosclerosis, proteinuria and the glomerular filtration rate (GFR). In chronic disorders such as focal segmental glomerulosclerosis and mesangiocapillary glomerulonephritis, as the population of glomeruli declines through sclerosis, the remnant glomeruli undergo anatomical and functional hypertrophy, and it is only when maximal hyperfunction has been achieved that continuing depopulation will lead to a fall in GFR. Before this happens, glomerular hyperfiltration will lead to increasing proteinuria and progressive segmental glomerulosclerosis, even if the native disease has become inactive.

Thus the preservation of a normal GFR and variations in the amount of proteinuria may fail to reflect adverse changes in the glomeruli, and perhaps delude the clinician into believing that prolonged treatment with, say, corticosteroid or antiplatelet therapy is beneficial. Bearing in mind the long time-scale over which such diseases evolve, it is rarely necessary to consider repeat biopsy less than 2 years from the original one, with the possible exception of systemic lupus erythematosus, whose volatile nature may demand a repeat biopsy after a year's initial treatment, and of rapidly progressive glomerulonephritis, particularly when plasmapheresis is used to treat Goodpasture's syndrome.

Research

Until the advent of a safe and satisfactory biopsy technique,[1] little was known about the early stages of various forms of glomerulonephritis except from necropsy studies, or about the changes accompanying resolution or progression. Through the pioneering of biopsy as a routine procedure in the 1960s, a whole new world of glomerular pathology was created, and much of the knowledge gained at that time, e.g. the morphological classification of the nephrotic syndrome[30] and of Henoch–Schoenlein nephritis,[28] remains relevant today.

Paraffin and methacrylate blocks can be stored indefinitely, and further sections cut when required for research purposes; in this way we were able to carry out glomerular morphometry on material obtained from nephrotic children.[14] These studies demonstrated that the glomeruli in focal segmental glomerulosclerosis (FSGS) had significantly greater mesangial cellularity than those with minimal change (MC). Furthermore, while glomerular size increased with age in MC, it did not in FSGS, suggesting that the latter disease is an entity and not a variant of MC.

During the past decade the demands of society regarding human experimentation have led to stricter ethical codes, and some of the renal biopsies performed in the 1960s would, by today's standards, be regarded as inappropriate, even though at that time they yielded crucially important information which it was subsequently possible to relate to the long-term outcome.[22,23,28] In more recent years, repeat renal biopsies, undertaken to assess progress, have contributed substantially to our understanding of the natural history of disease processes, a good example being that of FSGS.[31] Moreover, biopsies undertaken to investigate proteinuria in children with reflux nephropathy have yielded important new data concerning the vascular and glomerular changes associated with hyperfiltration.[20]

In summary, the role of biopsy in research is as a by-product of clinical investigation; the clinician must satisfy himself that it will contribute in some way to the patient's management. Obtaining 'normal' data as a baseline has always presented a dilemma; autolysis makes necropsy material generally unsuitable for comparison. However, it is reasonable, for instance, to make the assumption that the glomeruli in steroid-responsive nephrotic syndrome are essentially normal, and we used these to form the basis of measurement of normal basement membrane thickness in children.[32]

Conclusion

Care in the selection of patients for biopsy and skill in its performance are of paramount importance, as has already been emphasized. Of no less importance is the processing of the material obtained and interpretation of the results. The preparation of 1–2 μm sections is considerably more demanding than of standard 5 μm surgical biopsy sections, while the need for IF and EM increases the labour-dependency and costs of renal biopsy. To achieve satisfactory results requires special technical training, and both expertise and enthusiasm on the part of the histopathologist. It follows that, to offer an effective renal biopsy service, extensive training is necessary to provide the relevant skills, which must then be maintained by regular practice. Biopsy should never be undertaken in centres where the appropriate facilities and expertise do not exist.[12,13]

Renal pathologists, by and large, handle little material from children; at the same time, paediatric pathologists must of necessity be general. For these reasons it is prudent for at least one of a team of paediatric nephrologists to have gained some familiarity with renal pathology during training, and to maintain a lifelong interest in it. Likewise it is helpful if the pathologist has an understanding of the clinical disorders associated with glomerulonephritis. There is no doubt that the patient's interests are best served when the clinical and histological aspects are jointly reviewed by the nephrologist and pathologist, and such reviews have, in the author's experience, provided a remarkably good forum of learning for trainees.

References

1. Kark R.M. and Muehrcke R.C. Biopsy of the kidney in prone position. *Lancet* 1954, **i**, 1047–1049
2. Galan E. and Maso C. Needle biopsy in children with nephrosis. *Pediatrics* 1957, **20**, 610–625
3. Vernier R.L. Kidney biopsy in the study of renal disease. *Pediatr. Clin. N. Am.* 1960, **7**, 353–371
4. Dodge W.F., Daeschner C.W. Jr, Brennan J.C., Rosenberg H.S., Travis L.B. and Hopps H.C. Percutaneous renal biopsy in children: I. General considerations. *Pediatrics* 1962, **30**, 287–296
5. White R.H.R. Observations on percutaneous renal biopsy in children. *Arch.Dis.Child.* 1963, **38**, 260–266
6. Ginsburg I.W., Dinant J.R. and Mendez L. Percutaneous renal biopsy under direct radiology control. *J. Am. Med. Ass.* 1962, **181**, 211–213
7. Edelmann C.M. Jr and Greifer I. A modified technique for percutaneous needle biopsy of the kidney. *Pediatrics* 1967, **70**, 81–86
8. White R.H.R. A modified Silverman biopsy needle for use in children. *Lancet* 1962, **i**, 673
9. White R.H.R. and Jivani S.K.M. Evaluation of a disposable needle for renal biopsy in children. *Clin. Nephrol.* 1974, **21**, 120–122
10. Birnholz J.C., Kasinath B.S. and Corwin H.L. An improved technique for ultrasound guided percutaneous renal biopsy. *Kidney Int.* 1985, **27**, 80–82
11. Yoshimoto M., Fujisawa S. and Sudo M. Percutaneous renal biopsy well-visualized by orthogonal ultrasound application using linear scanning. *Clin. Nephrol.* 1988, **30**, 106–110
12. Gault M.H. and Muehrcke R.C. Renal biopsy: current views and controversies. *Nephron* 1983, **34**, 1–34
13. White R.H.R. The investigation of haematuria. *Arch. Dis.Child.* 1989, **64**, 159–165
14. Yoshikawa N., Cameron A.H. and White R.H.R. Glomerular morphometry I: nephrotic syndrome in childhood. *Histopathology* 1981, **5**, 239–249
15. Yoshikawa N., Cameron A.H. and White R.H.R. Glomerular morphometry II: familial and nonfamilial haematuria. *Histopathology* 1981, **5**, 251–256
16. Proesmans W., Marchal G., Snoeck L. and Snoeys R. Ultrasonography for assessment of bleeding after percutaneous renal biopsy in children. *Clin. Nephrol.* 1982, **18**, 257–262
17. Diaz-Buxo J.A. and Donadio J.V. Jr. Complications of percutaneous renal biopsy: an analysis of 1,000 consecutive biopsies. *Clin. Nephrol.* 1975, **4**, 223–227

18. Moncrieff M.W. Percutaneous renal biopsy in childhood. *Postgrad. Med. J.* 1972, **48**, 427–429

19. McGonigle R. and Sharpstone P. Kidney biopsy. *Br. Med. J.* 1980, **280**, 547–549

20. Morita M., Yoshiara S., White R.H.R. and Raafat F. The glomerular changes in children with reflux nephropathy. *J. Path.* 1990, **162**, 245–253

21. Cameron J.S., Glasgow E.F., Ogg C.S. and White R.H.R. Membranoproliferative glomerulonephritis and persistent hypocomplementaemia. *Br. Med. J.* 1970, **4**, 7–14

22. White R.H.R., Glasgow E.F. and Mills R.J. Clinicopathological study of nephrotic syndrome in children. *Lancet* 1970, **ii**, 1353–1359

23. Clark G., White R.H.R., Glasgow E.F., Chantler C., Cameron J.S., Gill D. *et al.* Poststreptococcal glomerulonephritis in children: clinicopathological correlations and long-term prognosis. *Pediatr. Nephrol.* 1988, **2**, 381–388

24. Habib R., Kleinknecht C., Gubler M.C. and Levy M. Idiopathic membranoproliferative glomerulonephritis in children. Report of 105 cases. *Clin. Nephrol.* 1973, **1**, 194–214

25. Rosen S., Falk R.J. and Jennette J.C. Polyarteritis nodosa including microscopic form and renal vasculitis. In: Churg A. and Churg J. (eds) *Systemic Vasculitides.* New York, Igaku-Shoin, 1991: 57–77

26. Adu D. and Cameron J.S. Lupus nephritis. *Clin. Rheum. Dis.* 1982, **8**, 153–181

27. White R.H.R. Henoch–Schönlein purpura. In: Churg A. and Churg J. (eds) *Systemic Vasculitides.* New York, Igaku-Shoin, 1991: 203–217

28. Meadow S.R., Glasgow E.F., White R.H.R., Moncrieff M.W., Cameron J.S. and Ogg C.S. Schönlein–Henoch nephritis. *Q.J. Med.* 1972, **41**, 241–258

29. Goldstein A.R., White R.H.R., Akuse R. and Chantler C. Long-term follow-up of childhood Henoch–Schönlein nephritis. *Lancet* 1992, **339**, 280–282

30. Churg J., Habib R. and White R.H.R. Pathology of the nephrotic syndrome in children. *Lancet* 1970, **ii**, 1299–1302

31. Morita M., White R.H.R., Coad N.A.G. and Raafat F. The clinical significance of the glomerular location of segmental lesions in focal segmental glomerulosclerosis. *Clin. Nephrol.* 1990, **33**, 211–219

32. Morita M., White R.H.R., Raafat F., Barnes J.M. and Standring D.M. Glomerular basement membrane thickness in children. *Pediatr. Nephrol.* 1988, **2**, 190–195

13

Urinary tract infections : significance, pathogenesis, clinical features and diagnosis

U. Jodal

Terminology

The terms used in this chapter are those recommended by the British Medical Research Council Bacteriuria Committee with slight modifications.

Urinary tract infection (UTI) is the common term for conditions in which there is growth of bacteria within the urinary tract. This is a heterogeneous group of disorders but of special importance is the identification of individuals with complicated UTI, i.e. those with reduced renal function, obstruction, dilating reflux or neurogenic dysfunction of the bladder.

Bacteriuria is presence of bacteria in bladder urine. Growth of $\geqslant 100\,000$ colony-forming units (cfu) in freshly voided urine usually indicates bacteriuria, as does any growth from urine obtained by suprapubic aspiration.

Symptomatic UTI can be classified into high infections localized to the renal parenchyma, *acute pyelonephritis*, with high fever as the major symptom, and low infections, *acute cystitis*, with acute voiding symptoms as the major feature. Such classification is of practical importance since renal infection carries a risk of renal scarring and requires more aggressive treatment, investigation and follow-up than an infection restricted to the lower urinary tract. Ten to twenty per cent of the symptomatic infections cannot be classified into pyelonephritis and cystitis by history, clinical findings and simple laboratory investigations and are called *unspecified UTI*. For practical purposes, children with unspecified UTI are best managed as having renal infection.

Covert (or asymptomatic) *bacteriuria* is the term used when bacteriuria is found in repeated samples from a child who does not report symptoms, usually at a health investigation or a routine check-up.

Pyelonephritic renal scarring or *reflux nephropathy* are the radiological terms used for focal or generalized damage of a kidney with reduction of the parenchyma, usually with related calyceal clubbing or blunting. There is a strong association with past or present vesico-ureteric reflux but renal scarring may develop without demonstrable reflux.

Incidence

UTI is one of the most common bacterial diseases in children. Of 7-year-old school entrants in Göteborg, 7.8% of the girls and 1.6% of the boys had had symptomatic UTI verified by urine culture.[1] In half of the children the UTI had been associated with high fever according to the original records from hospital or outpatient clinics, and in the majority of these a diagnosis of acute pyelonephritis was supported by laboratory tests.

The incidence of first-time UTI is highest during the first year of life. This is most marked for boys but also evident for girls, as seen in Figure 13.1. The high incidence of UTI in boys is representative of a non-circumscribed population. There is no similar epidemiological study of circumcised males, but it has been convincingly shown that the incidence of UTI is

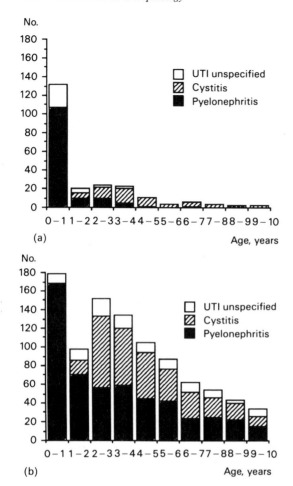

Figure 13.1 All children below 10 years of age with first-time symptomatic UTI identified at the Children's Hospital in Göteborg 1970–79 according to age and clinical classification: (a) boys, *n* = 225; (b) girls, *n* = 952

from the Aberdeen area.[3] Only 38 of 572 children referred for radiological investigation during a 10-year period were under 2 years of age; comparative figures for Göteborg with a similar child population of about 80 000 were 431 of 1177.[4]

The recurrence rate is high and 30% of the girls have a new infection within 1 year and 50% within 5 years. Some girls have a long series of recurrences. Among boys the recurrence rate is lower, 15–20%; after 1 year of age boys have few recurrences, however, and it is unusual that they have repeated infections.[5]

Consequences of childhood UTI

UTIs cause significant morbidity, suffering for the children and inconvenience and anxiety to the families. These infections also lead to a considerable consumption of medical resources. Although the majority of children with UTI have an excellent prognosis, there is risk of serious complications in a small group, especially in those with obstructive malformation and dilated vesico-ureteric reflux.

Obstructive malformations are found in some 2% of girls and 10% of boys investigated because of UTI.[5] Reflux can be demonstrated in 30–40% in both sexes and the reflux dilates the upper urinary tract in 25–50% of these, the variation depending on the selection of the patient material.

Permanent kidney damage (renal scarring or reflux nephropathy) that is identified by urography within 1–2 years after acute pyelonephritis develops in 10–15% – more often after repeated infections. This has serious implications which are discussed further in Chapter 14.

Aetiology and pathogenesis

Escherichia coli causes the majority of UTI and 80–90% of first-time infections in children.[6] Bacteria of the *Proteus* species are found in about 30% of boys with uncomplicated cystitis, and *Staphylococcus saprophyticus* in a similar proportion of adolescents of both sexes with acute UTI. Patients with stone, obstruction and neurogenic bladder disturbance may have *E. coli* in the urine but are commonly infected by bacteria such as *Proteus*, *Pseudomonas*, *enterococci* and *Staphylococcus aureus* or *Staph. epidermidis*; such infections are often difficult to treat.

reduced to approximately one-tenth in boys so treated.[2]

Figure 13.1 illustrates that infections diagnosed during the first year of life are mostly acute pyelonephritis. A first-time UTI classified as acute cystitis occurs especially in girls within the age group 2–6 years. It needs to be pointed out that to identify an epidemiological pattern as the one described, there must be a high awareness among the doctors at the primary care level of the high incidence of UTI in infants and small children. If these infections are undetected, many of the children will present with UTI later and may at that time already have pyelonephritic renal scarring. An example of a skew epidemiological pattern is given in a study

Table 13.1   Risk factors for development of pyelonephritic renal scarring (reflux nephropathy)

Obstruction

Reflux with dilatation

Low age

Delay of treatment

Number of pyelonephritic attacks

Bacteria of low virulence

In the first months following treatment with an antibiotic, the bacteria causing a recurrence are frequently resistant. The reason is not persistence of resistant bacteria within the urinary tract but a change of the normal bowel flora caused by the antibiotic. The bacteria that invade the urinary tract usually originate in the bowel of the patient. In boys there is also a reservoir under the prepuce. UTIs are ascending and as the first step there is colonization of the peri-urethral area by Gram-negative bacteria, mostly *E. coli*. Temporary ascent of bacteria into the bladder is probably not uncommon in the female, since the length of the urethra is only 3–4 cm in women and 1–2 cm in girls. Elimination of bacteria that have entered the bladder is related to regular and complete emptying, and the establishment of bacteriuria is facilitated by residual urine. Malformations and neurogenic diseases can cause impaired emptying, but the most common cause by far is functional bladder disturbances. In a recent study of children with acute cystitis, over half were shown by ultrasound measurement to have residual urine at the time of the infection as well as 6 months later. This suggests that the inability to empty the bladder was a primary defect and not a secondary phenomenon induced by the bacterial toxins.[7]

Further ascent of bacteria to the kidneys may occur through vesico-ureteric reflux. The explanation for the invasion of the upper urinary tract in the 60–70% of children with pyelonephritis without demonstrable reflux may be the capacity to adhere to uroepithelial cells that is found in some *E. coli* bacteria.

Bacterial properties

In 70% of the girls with first-time pyelonephritis, the *E. coli* isolated in the urine have adhesins that specifically bind to receptors on the surface of epithelial cells in the urinary tract. This ability facilitates the bacterial invasion, which is especially important in individuals without reflux. Turbulence in the stream of urine can carry bacteria upwards and adhesion makes it possible to avoid being washed out. Furthermore, bacterial adhesion to epithelial cells is often the first step in the initiation of inflammation through mucous membranes by making possible contact between bacterial toxins and the tissues. When this happens at the ureteral orifice, ureteritis is induced leading to a functional disturbance with impaired flow of urine and increased chances for the bacteria to ascend further and cause pyelonephritis.[8]

Bacteria thus need special virulence properties to cause pyelonephritis in children with a normal urinary tract. Such properties are found not only in some *E. coli* bacteria but also in *Staph. saprophyticus*. On the other hand, isolation of bacteria that have low virulence within the urinary tract such as *Pseudomonas*, *Haemophilus influenzae*, *Staph. aureus* or *Staph. epidermidis* means that the patient should be suspected of having major anomalies.

Development of renal scarring

Factors that have been shown to be associated with renal scarring are given in Table 13.1. The most serious type of obstruction is the urethral valve which will affect both kidneys; early detection and operation as well as long-term follow-up is essential. The grade of reflux is of importance. In children with the first UTI classified as acute pyelonephritis, scarring developed in 5% of those without reflux, 17% of those with reflux to the renal pelvis without dilatation (grade 2) and 66% of those with dilating reflux (grades 3–5 on a 5-grade scale).[4]

Young age is also of importance and the risk is especially high during the first 2–3 years of life. Scars may develop after the age of 5 years,[9] but the risk seems to be rather limited. It is essential that treatment is not delayed since inadequate therapy or delayed start of treatment markedly increases the frequency of pyelonephritic scarring. Still more serious is when acute pyelonephritis is overlooked and the child is not treated at all. The risk of such an event is highest in infants since that is the age when the diagnosis is most difficult.

The single most important factor to decrease the risk of renal scarring is probably a high awareness among primary care doctors that fever in an infant or small child can be a symptom of acute pyelonephritis. The diagnosis should be considered especially in children lacking symptoms from other organs and if there are unspecific systemic symptoms such as vomiting, abdominal pain, malaise or anorexia. A measure to decrease the risk of pyelonephritic recurrences is to give long-term low-dose antibacterial prophylaxis to high-risk patients, e.g. children with dilated reflux. Such prophylaxis may be indicated also in small children without reflux who have recurrent attacks of pyelonephritis, since the risk of scarring increases with the number of attacks.

Bacteria of low virulence are significantly more often associated with renal scarring compared to bacteria of high virulence.[10] This can be partly explained by a lower virulence being required for bacteria to invade a compromised individual. Another factor of importance may be that bacteria of low virulence cause less severe symptoms leading to a delay of diagnosis and treatment.

Clinical presentation

The symptoms of children with UTI depend on the level of the infection as well as the age of the child. In classical acute pyelonephritis the patient has high fever and other systemic symptoms together with back or flank pain and renal tenderness. Lower urinary tract symptoms may or may not be present. This clinical picture is not often encountered in children. Instead, high fever of at least 38.5°C but mostly in the range 39–41°C is often the only symptom in acute pyelonephritis. Children usually cannot localize and/or describe back or flank pain before 4–5 years old, but also older children with renal infection frequently lack such symptoms. Renal tenderness may be detected in younger children able to co-operate during the physical examination.

Symptoms from the lower urinary tract such as dysuria, frequent voiding and incontinence are usually not detected in infants but can be identified from the age of $1\frac{1}{2}$–2 years. Even in older children such symptoms are often lacking in children with acute pyelonephritis, in spite of the fact that the bladder contains bacteria. On the other hand, voiding symptoms are not equivalent with bacterial infection of the lower urinary tract; in a study in general practice, only 6 of 34 children presenting with dysuria had significant bacteriuria.[11] A careful history may reveal the use of local irritants and inspection of the genitals or a local inflammation such as a vulvitis or a balanitis. It should be kept in mind, however, that acute infections of the lower urinary tract with frequent voiding tend to result in low bacterial counts. In studies of young women with frequency and dysuria growing less than 100 000 cfu/ml in voided urine, half were shown to have low counts of bacteria in urine obtained by suprapubic aspiration or catheterization.

During the first month of life the clinical features of UTI are usually vague. Poor weight gain or failure to thrive may be the presenting symptom. Anorexia, lethargy, feeding difficulties, irritability, body tenderness and hypothermia are often encountered in septic conditions. Some neonates have high fever, although that is usually not the major symptom of renal infection until after the neonatal period.

Covert (or asymptomatic) bacteriuria

The introduction of the quantitative culture during the 1950s resulted in a marked interest in silent urinary infections. These were believed to cause renal scarring and many screening programmes were started. The concept of covert bacteriuria as a risk to the kidneys has been revised, however, and it is no longer considered indicated to screen healthy children for bacteriuria.[12–16]

Non-treatment of asymptomatic schoolgirls with bacteriuria was tested in a number of prospective studies during the 1970s. The non-treatment was shown to be associated with normal growth of the kidneys without development of new scars, provided that the urinary tract was radiologically normal.[12–15] In patients with renal scarring, non-treatment was rarely tried. However, in the Cardiff–Oxford study, girls with such findings were included in the randomization, and progression of pre-existing scarring was found to be equal among treated and untreated subjects;[14] the renal function did not differ between the groups.[17] Development of scars in previously normal kidneys was rarely seen. Thus, there was no evidence to suggest that antibacterial treatment of schoolgirls with covert bacteriuria had a beneficial effect.

Instead, further studies in Göteborg indicate that treatment increases the risk of complications.[18] Elimination of the bacteria of low virulence in asymptomatic children resulted in recurrences in 80%; these recurrences were in the form of acute pyelonephritis in 15% of the children with normal kidneys and in 30% of those with renal scarring. In girls left untreated, the original strain mostly remained in the urinary tract for many years without development of symptoms. The presence of an established bacterial strain in the urinary tract seems to prevent invasion by other bacteria, thus functioning as a kind of biological prophylaxis against colonization by other potentially virulent bacteria. It should be emphasized, however, that patients to be left untreated must not have symptoms or signs indicating renal involvement. The obtaining of a detailed history is crucial and recent febrile episodes and failure to thrive should be specifically asked for.

Although the children with covert bacteriuria had not complained of symptoms that lead to medical consultation, the majority of them did in fact give a history of such symptoms as urgency, urge incontinence and difficult micturition when given specific questions about voiding habits. This was emphasized by Savage and associates when they proposed the term covert bacteriuria as more appropriate than asymptomatic bacteriuria.[19] Bladder dysfunction is frequently found among girls with covert bacteriuria. The pathogenesis is probably multifactorial and it is difficult to know whether the bladder dysfunction is the cause of the bacteriuria or if the bacteriuria is the cause of the abnormal bladder function. However, the symptoms do not seem to be time-related to the acquisition of bacteriuria. Furthermore, there is no evidence that antibacterial treatment will affect the lower urinary tract symptomatology in these children. In a controlled study, Savage and co-workers found no improvement of enuresis, frequency or urgency after antibacterial treatment.[12] It is possible that these patients have an underlying functional disturbance of the lower urinary tract and a secondary liability to urinary infections corresponding to the situation in children with neurogenic bladder disorders. This dysfunction may have been initiated by a previous symptomatic UTI or an inflammation of the genital area such as vulvitis. Painful voiding can have started a vicious circle of lower urinary tract dysfunction and recurrent

UTI. Bladder rehabilitation programmes have been shown to be effective in this type of children.[20,21]

Mass screening for bacteriuria in infancy has been discussed as a means of preventing pyelonephritic renal scarring. In a study of 3581 healthy infants with repeated urine cultures during the first year of life, the incidence of bacteriuria verified by suprapubic aspiration was 0.9% in girls and 2.5% in boys.[22] Two infants developed pyelonephritis within 2 weeks of the verification of bacteriuria and the others remained free of symptoms. The bacteriuria cleared spontaneously within a few months in 36 of 45 untreated infants and in response to antibiotics given for infections in the respiratory tract in a further 8. Recurrences of bacteriuria were observed in 20% of the children but only one had pyelonephritis. During a 6-year follow-up period, no indications of renal damage were found; a repeat urography performed in 36 of the 50 children did not reveal development of renal scarring in any child.[16] Mass screening for bacteriuria in infancy seems to result primarily in the detection of innocent bacteriuric episodes and is not recommended. Although screening for bacteriuria in healthy children does not have a place in any age group, it is important to perform urine cultures freely in symptomatic children and especially in infants.

Diagnosis

The basis of the diagnostic procedure is analysis of urine with culture as the most important investigation. The normal bladder is sterile. There is, however, a high risk that the urine becomes contaminated by bacteria during the passage from the bladder to the sampling container, especially in infants and small children. If this leads to a false diagnosis of UTI the child will unnecessarily be subjected to antibacterial treatment, investigation and follow-up. On the other hand, failure to identify the child with UTI is associated with a risk of progressive renal damage. Therefore, *the quality of the urine sample is of crucial importance.*

Methods of urine collection

The ideal sample of voided urine has a long bladder incubation time and is collected after uncovering of the urethral orifice as a *mid-stream specimen*. A long interval between micturitions permits the bacteria to multiply and reach high counts which decreases the overlap between samples representing contamination and true bacteriuria. The mid-stream technique means that the first urine containing most of the 'loose' bacteria in the urethra and in the peri-urethral region are omitted. This method should always be used in children with adequate bladder control.

In infants and small children, urine is mostly obtained as a *bag sample*. The use of adhesive bags gives a high risk of contamination, however, and about 10% of such samples from healthy infants grow at least 50 000 cfu/ml.[22] Practical aspects are to dry the skin thoroughly after cleaning of the peri-urethral area, to keep the child in an upright position to prevent the urine from coming in contact with the skin or from entering the vagina, and to remove the bag immediately after the child has voided. A single bag specimen should not be relied upon for a diagnosis of UTI, even if there is pure growth of more than 100 000 cfu/ml urine; verification by a repeat sample is essential, preferably obtained by suprapubic aspiration or catheterization.

The best technique to obtain an uncontaminated urine specimen is by direct aspiration from the bladder by a *suprapubic puncture*. This is a simple procedure in infants since the bladder is an intra-abdominal organ during the first years of life. With the child in supine position, a thin needle attached to a syringe or to a vacuum container is inserted vertically in the midline 1–2 cm above the symphysis. Urine is usually obtained at a depth of 2–3 cm. The trick is to know when there is urine in the bladder. The chance is good when the nappy has been dry for at least 30 min and especially after the baby has been fed and the diuresis is high. With careful preparations the success rate at the first attempt is 80–90%. If an ultrasound machine is available, the urine content of the bladder is easily evaluated.

Suprapubic aspiration causes no more distress to the child than any other needle puncture. Complications are rare: macroscopic haematuria occurs in about 2%, but transient microscopic haematuria is seen in the majority. Accidental penetration of the bowel may happen but does not lead to any problems except for contamination of the sample; there will be very few if any problems of interpretation, however, since bowel aspiration will result in growth of colonies of many different types which is typical of contamination. In our hospital, suprapubic aspiration is the preferred method to obtain urine for verification of UTI in small children. In infants below 1 year of age, about 80% of the diagnoses of UTI are based on this technique; above that age, however, it is difficult to carry out needle aspirations for psychological reasons, although the anatomical prerequisites remain.

Catheterization of the bladder is another way of obtaining urine with minimal contamination. In many centres this technique is rarely used mainly because of the risk of introducing infection and of the psychological effects on children above 1 year of age. In other centres, catheterization seems to be more commonly used. We perform catheterization if suprapubic aspiration has failed, especially if the child is severely ill and a reliable urine sample needs to be ascertained before antibacterial treatment is started.

Culture of urine

Urine should always be immediately refrigerated at 4°C until cultured, to prevent growth of contaminating bacteria. It is essential that this temperature is kept also during transport. Most bacteriological laboratories use a calibrated loop containing approximately 0.002 ml of urine for routine culture. This means that growth of one colony of bacteria on the culture medium is equivalent to 500 cfu/ml. To obtain higher sensitivity, a larger volume of urine has to be cultured.

A dipslide culture has about the same sensitivity to detect live bacteria as the calibrated loop technique. With proper training it can be used and interpreted locally, provided that dipslides are used regularly to retain the skill. It is possible to perform sensitivity testing on a dipslide, but it is usually better to send a dipslide with significant growth to a bacteriological laboratory for such an analysis. There are two possible pitfalls with the dipslide that should be mentioned. The most common problem is when there is confluent growth of colonies of different types. This usually indicates contamination but may be due to massive numbers of one bacterial strain combined with only a few contaminating bacteria. Such differentiation is hardly possible on the dipslide, but is usually easy in a traditional culture. Instead of sending the positive dipslides to the laboratory for characterization of the bacteria, it is mostly better to send the urine, provided that it has been kept overnight in the refrigerator and that the transportation is easy. The other pitfall with the dipslide is that some bacteria that can cause UTI do not grow on CLED or McConkey agar which are mostly used. Such bacteria are not frequent but should be thought of in septic infants, especially during the first months of life, and in those with malformations of the urinary tract. Most of these bacteria will be identified by a laboratory using blood agar or other rich culture media.

The interpretation of the results of the cultures depends on the method of urine collection as well as on the clinical background. In urine obtained by suprapubic aspiration, any growth is considered significant. In catheter urine the level of significance is 10^3–10^4 cfu/ml, but more precise reference values are lacking. For voided specimens the traditional cut-off level of 100 000 cfu/ml is roughly valid, but the probability of true bacteriuria in a single culture is not higher than 70–80%. However, in combination with acute symptoms from the urinary tract such as marked dysuria and frequency together with pyuria, the writer would consider one urine sample adequate for a diagnosis of UTI. A similar evaluation can be made in the older child presenting with high fever and back pain together with pyuria. For all patients lacking symptoms specific for the urinary tract, two voided urine specimens should be required.

A diagnosis of covert bacteriuria requires repeated samples over a period of several days in a child without fever or acute urinary symptoms within the preceding 2 weeks.

Other urine findings

Pyuria is measured with highest precision by microscopy of unspun urine using a counting chamber; more than 10 leucocytes/μl in a boy and 50 in a girl is abnormal. A more crude but mostly adequate estimate of pyuria is obtained by analysis of urine sediment or by the use of test strips which react to granulocyte esterase activity in the urine. A colour change corresponding to a 2 + reaction means roughly 75 and 3 + 500 leucocytes/μl.

Determination of pyuria is a helpful rapid investigation in a child suspected to have symptomatic UTI. Pyuria is present in practically all episodes of symptomatic UTI; a urine sample without pyuria as an indication of inflammation within the urinary tract speaks against symptomatic UTI. In contrast, pyuria is lacking in more than half of the cases of covert bacteriuria. However, the presence of leucocytes in the urine is not diagnostic of UTI. It may be found in febrile children with infections outside the urinary tract, in inflammatory diseases of other types in or near the urinary tract and as a contamination from the vagina. Pyuria should be taken as an indication for adequate urine collection and culture.

The *nitrite test* is based on the ability of most urinary pathogens to reduce nitrate to nitrite. The reduction is time dependent and a positive test requires a long bladder time, preferably > 4 h, or significant residual urine. Therefore the sensitivity of the nitrite test is only 40–50% in infants and small children with frequent voiding. The specificity of a positive test is over 99% in girls and thus practically equivalent to bacteriuria. In boys, the nitrite test is less reliable since nitrite may accumulate under the prepuce of the normal male and thus give a false positive result. Furthermore the test must be performed on a urine sample that is fresh or has been immediately refrigerated since contaminating bacteria that grow will generate nitrite.

Haematuria occurs frequently in children with symptomatic UTI and is macroscopic in 20–25% of those with acute cystitis. To establish a diagnosis of UTI, however, determination of haematuria or albuminuria is of no value.

Level diagnosis

A number of tests have been described for the level diagnosis or localization of UTI. Some are complicated and require special facilities or skills. Some are simple but may instead not be specific. It is quite safe to state that there is no universally accepted test that is applicable in everyday practice. One of the major obstacles in the development of such a test is that we have no technique to establish the 'true' character of a UTI – no gold standard. Localization of bacteria by ureteral catheterization or bladder wash-out has been used but is difficult in infants and small children. Pitfalls include intermittent discharge of bacteria from the kidney, resulting in false negative results, and vesicoureteric reflux that may lead to false positive findings.

Another principle for level diagnosis is measurement of host reactions to renal inflammation. An example is the temporary tubular dysfunction leading to decreased renal concentrating capacity for several weeks after the infection. Determination of antibodies to the infecting bacteria has a high predictive value for renal involvement, but requires that the original bacteria are available. Antibody-coated bacteria can be visualized using fluorescein-labelled anti-immunoglobulin but this technique is unreliable in children, mainly because of the delay of several days before there is antibody production.

Renal imaging can reveal an inflammatory process in the kidney. Swelling of the kidney and dilatation of the collecting system can be seen on urography. General swelling is also seen on ultrasonography but requires measurement and comparison with age-matched reference values for volume. When used in acute UTI, kidney volume in 79 children with pyelonephritis was increased to an average of 175% of normal. In 71% of cases, affected kidneys showed an enlargement of at least 2 standard deviations above the mean of the reference value. Normalization of renal volume was seen after 1–2 months. In 96 children with lower UTI defined by clinical and simple laboratory data, the mean kidney volume was 99.7%.[23]

An interesting technique to show an inflammatory process in the kidney is DMSA scanning using a gamma-camera. Affected areas are seen as uptake defects on the scan. A problem is that it is not possible to distinguish between acute inflammatory changes and already established renal scars.[24,25] The timing of the investigation is of importance since temporary uptake defects may persist for several months. Despite many publications during the past few years, there are no long-term studies evaluating the positive as well as negative predictive value of acute changes for development of renal scarring.

In primary care, a method for level diagnosis has to be rapid and inexpensive. A classical finding indicative of renal infection is white cell cylinders in the urine sediment. However, these cylinders are easily overlooked if pyuria is massive, and they are easily dissolved, especially in alkaline urine. The sensitivity is therefore low. Serum C-reactive protein (CRP) and sedimentation rate may be high in any inflammatory reaction with significant tissue involvement.

Even though these methods lack kidney specificity, they are of value in identifying those children with UTI who have marked host reactions. In acute cystitis the infection is mostly superficial involving only the bladder mucosa, and a generalized host reaction is not elicited. These nonspecific tests are as a rule of no help in patients with diseases in several organ systems, but this is unusual in children.

In typical cases of acute pyelonephritis there is hardly any reason for performing tests for infection level in routine medical care. Such patients should be treated immediately, and most doctors would also agree that diagnostic imaging and long-term follow-up are indicated. In patients above 1–2 years of age with no or equivocal signs of renal involvement, there is uncertainty as to how extensive the investigations need to be. This is the group for which level diagnostic tests is primarily needed.

Monitoring

An early follow-up visit after 3–4 days for children managed as outpatients is of value not only to ascertain that the healing process is uneventful but to initiate imaging procedures. Furthermore, it is an optimal time to inform the patient and her family about the mechanisms of UTI and about preventative measures such as regular voiding and bowel habits. They should learn about the risk of new infections and the symptoms most commonly found in UTI, especially fever without obvious cause. Oral and written instructions are given on how a urine sample is best obtained, preferably as a mid-stream morning specimen, together with a container in which the urine should be brought to the clinic refrigerated in ice.

The further follow-up schedule is adapted to local traditions and resources. In our unit there is only one more check-up of children with an uneventful cystitis but all other children are followed for at least 1 year after the UTI. As we do not believe that detection of covert bacteriuria is of major importance, the emphasis at the controls is on repeated information of the patient and encouragement to come for extra controls whenever symptoms occur that can be caused by UTI.

Home monitoring can be useful in some children. This can be done with dipslides which the families usually learn to handle well after instruction. We use an information sheet with simple drawings on how to dip two-thirds of the agar plate in the urine or to void directly on it, and to drain off drops of urine by putting the bottom edge of the slide against tissue paper. If there is surplus urine in the dipslide container, it may run across the agar surface during the handling in the mail, thus causing secondary inoculation and difficulties of interpretation. Most uropathogens will grow at room temperature, and a count and sensitivity testing can be done on arrival at the hospital. If no growth is present the dipslide is incubated at 37°C for 24 h before disposal.

References

1. Hellström A., Hanson E., Hansson S., Hjälmås K. and Jodal U. Association between urinary symptoms at 7 years old and previous urinary tract infection. *Arch. Dis. Child.* 1991, **66**, 232–234

2. Wiswell T.E. and Roscelli J.D. Corroborative evidence for the decreased incidence of urinary tract infections in circumcised male infants. *Pediatrics* 1986, **78**, 96–99

3. McKerrow W., Davidson-Lamb N. and Jones P.F. Urinary tract infection in children. *Br. Med. J.* 1984, **289**, 299–303

4. Jodal U. The natural history of bacteriuria in childhood. *Infect. Dis. Clin. North Am.* 1987, **1**, 713–729

5. Winberg J., Andersen H.J. Bergström T., Jacobsson B., Larson H. and Lincoln K. Epidemiology of symptomatic urinary tract infection in childhood. *Acta Paed. Scand.* 1974, Suppl 252, 1–20

6. Jodal U. and Winberg J. Management of children with unobstructed urinary tract infection. *Ped. Nephrol.* 1987, **1**, 647–656

7. Lidefelt K.J., Erasmie U. and Bollgren I. Residual urine in children with acute cystitis and in healthy children: assessement by sonography. *J. Urol.* 1989, **141**, 916–917

8. Roberts J.A., Suarez G.M., Kaack B., Källenius G. and Svenson S.B. Experimental pyelonephritis in the monkey. VII. Ascending pyelonephritis in the absence of vesicoureteral reflux. *J. Urol.* 1985, **133**, 1068–1075

9. Smellie J.M., Ransley P.G., Normand I.C.S., Prescod N. and Edwards D. Development of new renal scars: a collaborative study. *Br. Med. J.* 1985, **290**, 1957–1960

10. de Man P., Claesson I., Johansson I.M., Jodal U. and Svanborg-Edén C. Bacterial attachment as a predictor of renal abnormalities in boys with urinary tract infection. *J. Ped.* 1989, **115**, 915–922

11. Dickinson J.A. Incidence and outcome of symptomatic urinary tract infection in children. *Br. Med. J.* 1979, **1**, 1330–1332

12. Savage D.C.L., Howie G., Adler K. and Wilson M.I. Controlled trial of therapy in covert bacteriuria in childhood. *Lancet* 1975, **I**, 358–361

13. Lindberg U., Claesson I., Hanson L.Å. and Jodal U. Asymptomatic bacteriuria in schoolgirls. VIII. Clinical course during a 3-year follow-up. *J. Ped.* 1978, **92**, 194–199

14. Cardiff–Oxford Bacteriuria Study Group. Sequelae of covert bacteriuria in schoolgirls. *Lancet*, **i**, 889–893

15. Newcastle Covert Bacteriuria Research Group. Covert bacteriuria in schoolgirls in Newcastle upon Tyne: a 5-year follow-up. *Arch. Dis. Child.* **56**, 585–592

16. Wettergren B., Hellström M., Stokland E. and Jodal U. Six-year follow-up of infants with screening bacteriuria. *Br. Med. J.* 1990, **301**, 845–848

17. Verrier-Jones K., Asscher A.W., Verrier-Jones E.R., Mattholie K., Leach K. and Thomson G.M. Glomerular filtration rate in schoolgirls with covert bacteriuria. *Br. Med. J.* 1982, **285**, 1307–1310

18. Hansson S., Jodal U., Norén L. and Bjure J. Untreated bacteriuria in asymptomatic girls with renal scarring. *Pediatrics* 1989, **84**, 964–968

19. Savage D.C.L., Wilson M.I., McHardy M., Dewar D.A.E. and Fee W.M. Covert bacteriuria of childhood. A clinical and epidemiological study. *Arch. Dis. Child.* 1973, **48**, 8–20

20. van Gool J.D., Kuitjen R.H., Donckerwolcke R.A., Messer A. and Vijverberg M. Bladder-sphincter dysfunction, urinary infection and vesico-ureteral reflux with special reference to cognitive bladder training. *Contrib. Nephrol.* 1984, **39**, 190–210

21. Hellström A.-L., Hjälmås K. and Jodal U. Rehabilitation of the dysfunctional bladder in children: method and 3-year followup. *J. Urol.* 1987, **138**, 847–849

22. Wettergren B., Jodal U. and Jonasson G. Epidemiology of bacteriuria during the first year of life. *Acta Paed. Scand.* 1985, **74**, 925–933

23. Dinkel E., Orth S., Dittrich M. and Schulte-Wissermann H. Renal sonography in the differentiation of upper from lower urinary tract infection. *Am. J. Roentgenol.* 1986, **146**, 775–780

24. Goldraich N.P., Ramos O.L. and Goldraich I.H. Urography versus DMSA scan in children with vesicoureteric reflux. *Pediatr. Nephrol.* 1989, **3**, 1–5

25. Smellie J.M. The DMSA scan and intravenous urography in the detection of renal scarring; editorial comment. *Pediatr. Nephrol.* 1989, **3**, 6–8

14

Management and investigation of children with urinary tract infection

J.M. Smellie

Introduction

Urinary tract infection (UTI) is a recurrent condition and important in childhood because of its symptoms which may be either troublesome or overlooked, because of the potential risk of renal involvement and as a marker for unsuspected underlying pathology. The main objectives in management are to relieve symptoms, to protect the kidneys from damage and to identify the cause of the infection in order to prevent recurrence.

Urinary infection may occur for a number of reasons and with varied consequences, although in the majority of children it is benign. The prognosis both for recurrence and for renal damage is closely related to the findings on investigation. However, clinical and experimental studies indicate that rapid recognition and treatment of urinary infection, particularly in the infant and young child in whom the non-specific symptomatology is least well recognized, are essential if renal involvement and subsequent renal scarring are to be prevented.

The coarse renal scarring of chronic atrophic pyelonephritis or reflux nephropathy is both the most common and also the most serious renal abnormality found when children are investigated for urinary infection. Vesico-ureteric reflux (VUR) is almost always found in these children, though it tends to be self-correcting with time and may have stopped in some older children.[1] The scarring is permanent and while found overall in about 12% of children with UTI the proportion increases with age and with exposure to recurrent infection. New renal scars can be acquired or extension of scarring may continue throughout childhood,[2,3] but it is in infancy and early childhood that the rapidly growing kidney appears to be most susceptible to infective damage.[4,5]

Overview

In considering plans of management, children presenting with urinary infection may be broadly grouped in a number of ways:

A *In relation to significance*
1 Those with VUR (35%) or obstruction (4–6%) in whom there is a risk of renal damage.
2 Those with frequently recurring symptomatic infection but with no significant structural defects of the urinary tract (this includes those with unstable bladders).
3 Those with bacteriuria detected on screening (covert or screening bacteriuria). They may be symptomless or have symptoms for which their parents have not sought medical advice. By school entry at 5 years or over, the renal prognosis in general is good and is related to the presence or absence of scarred kidneys rather than to VUR or bacteriuria. Even minimal symptoms should be regarded as potentially serious under the age of 5 years.

B *In relation to age*

Any serious consequences of UTI are most likely to be initiated in the first few years of life. In this age group, recognition and rapid treatment are crucial.

Among older children there are those with bladder instability who have troublesome symptoms and only a small renal risk, while others, particularly those with VUR, may have already sustained, or may be at risk of, further renal damage. It is important to identify scarring and VUR in order to prevent fresh or extending damage.

C *In relation to findings on investigation*

(a) Evidence of inflammation: those with raised C-reactive protein, ESR, WBC count.

(b) Evidence of acute renal involvement: abnormal water concentration tests (DDAVP test), diffuse impairment in renal uptake of ^{99m}Tc-dimercaptosuccinic acid (DMSA).

(c) Abnormalities predisposing to infection: obstruction, urinary tract dilatation, stones, increased residual urine, VUR, constipation and bladder diverticula, etc.

(d) Evidence of renal damage: radiological renal scars, persistent focal defects in DMSA uptake, asymmetry of renal function on a DMSA scan not due to a duplex system, raised plasma creatinine levels.

Principles of management

Each child with urinary infection deserves individual consideration. Age, past and family history and findings on clinical examination are important.

General principles include:

1 Rapid diagnosis of the presenting infection (thinking of, and collecting, a specimen of urine for microscopy and culture before starting antibacterial treatment are integral to the management).

2 Immediate antibacterial treatment while awaiting confirmation of the diagnosis if UTI is suspected and other serious infectious causes have been excluded.

3 Prevention of further infection pending investigation.

4 Adequate investigation of first known UTI.

5 Arrangement for appropriate further treatment.

6 Follow-up until symptoms are controlled or the kidneys are no longer at risk. Continuity of care is important.

Diagnosis depends upon the proper collection of a specimen of urine before the administration of antibacterial treatment and the demonstration of a significant pure growth of organisms on culture. Immediate refrigeration at 4°C to prevent growth of contaminants is as important as transfer of a freshly passed specimen to a sterile container. Methods of collection include a mid-stream in older children, a clean catch in infant boys, a perineal bag correctly applied, catheterization in the sick dehydrated infant, and suprapubic aspiration in the sick infant or young child. These have already been discussed (Chapter 13). Suprapubic aspiration, which is a simple procedure in experienced hands, can be facilitated by ultrasonography if this is available. Transfer to the laboratory should be under refrigerated conditions, or in a borate tube. Culture of a dipslide is an alternative, but a sample for microscopy is needed if antibiotics have already been started. Parents of sick infants and children are well motivated to collect urine samples, and also to take the child or the sample to hospital.

Once the sample is collected, treatment can be started. If antibacterial treatment has already, or recently, been given, urine microscopy should be specifically requested.

Treatment of the acute symptomatic infection

There should be no delay after suspecting the diagnosis of UTI in collecting a sample of urine, making a preliminary diagnosis and starting treatment. The presenting symptoms may be non-specific or misleading and the diagnosis depends on obtaining a significant pure growth of organisms on culture of a fresh sample of urine, properly collected before the start of antibacterial treatment.

Clinical history and examination

A full clinical history and examination should be carried out, attending to details of the perinatal history and antenatal scans, drinking, voiding and bowel habits (often unknown to the parents) and family history of urinary infection, VUR, renal disease or hypertension.

Examination should include palpation for bladder and kidneys, blood pressure, spinal examination and lower limb reflexes and sensation, the external genitalia and the urine stream in boys.

Management of the child with acute symptomatic UTI

1 *Eliminate infection* as rapidly as possible. Serious bacterial infection such as meningitis or acute appendicitis should be excluded in the ill child.
2 *Establish clinical and microbiological surveillance* to ensure that antibacterial treatment has been appropriate and effective.
3 *Prevent further infection* of a susceptible urinary tract by uninterrupted low-dose antibacterial prophylaxis until the cause and renal status have been determined by investigation.

Hospital admission for treatment or investigation increases the risk of colonization of the bowel flora with resistant *coliform* organisms and hence of recurrent infection with resistant organisms.

Antibacterial treatment
The choice of drug and route of administration will depend upon:
(a) The age and condition of the child, indicating the possible need for parenteral treatment.
(b) The local community or hospital antibacterial resistance pattern for urinary pathogens. Currently in Britain there is widespread amoxycillin resistance and in areas where trimethoprim (TMP) has been widely and exclusively used, high levels of TMP resistance have been reported.
(c) Any history of recent antibacterial treatment which might have affected the bowel flora resistance pattern will influence the choice of drug. Thus tonsillitis treated with amoxycillin may be followed by UTI with an amoxycillin-resistant *Klebsiella* species.
(d) The possible effect of the chosen drug on the bowel flora resistance pattern should also be considered.

Dose and duration. If there is no response to treatment within 48 h, the nature and sensitivity of the infecting organism should be checked and an appropriate change of drug made. Full-dose treatment is usually continued for 5–7 days: there is no evidence that courses of 14 days or longer are more effective in eradicating infection or in reducing the recurrence rate and they are more likely to result in the emergence of resistant strains. Suitable drugs at the present time include trimethoprim, co-trimoxazole, nitrofurantoin and cefadroxil and those currently appropriate in infancy and the newborn.

Single dose or 24 hours' treatment may be used effectively in the older child with afebrile urinary infection and lower tract symptoms, or where previous investigation has shown there is no VUR, obstruction or renal involvement. It is *not* advised in the infant or in a child presenting with their first infection, or where renal involvement is likely.

Persistent infection. If the infection persists or the original pathogen is replaced by a resistant organism, outflow obstruction should be suspected and the urinary tract investigated without delay. Repeated changes in antibacterial drugs in these children are inappropriate and will inevitably be followed by the emergence of organisms with multiple resistance.

Further management
After elimination of the presenting infection, low-dose antibacterial prophylaxis is recommended to prevent any recurrence until appropriate investigations have been carried out. For suitable drugs and dosage see Table 14.1.

Although a selective approach is sometimes adopted to the treatment of children with UTI depending upon whether they have fever or have symptoms mainly related to the lower urinary tract, it is advisable to assume that any UTI may potentially affect the kidney, particularly in the young child. In one clinical series describing the development of new scars in children with urinary infection, half the new scars followed

Table 14.1 Antibacterial drugs for the prophylaxis of UTIs given in a single evening dose

Drug	Dose $(\mathrm{mg\,kg^{-1}day^{-1}})$
Trimethoprim	1–2
Co-trimoxazole:	
Trimethoprim	1–2
Sulphamethoxazole	5–10
Nitrofurantoin	1

the delayed treatment of children whose UTI was unaccompanied by acute symptoms or high fever.[2]

Pathogenesis

An important objective in the management of these children is to discover the cause of the infection in order to prevent recurrence. Factors in its aetiology must therefore be considered briefly.

Organisms originating in the bowel gain ready access to the bladder, more easily in girls with a shorter urethra than in boys, usually after intermediate peri-urethral or preputial colonization, and the organisms will multiply in the bladder urine if conditions are favourable. Normally they are diluted by freshly formed urine and eliminated by regular, complete voiding. Imbalance of the host–pathogen relationship in childhood UTI is mainly due to breakdown of these host defences. Motility of the organism, its ability to adhere to the uroepithelium and invade the urinary tract, and its possible nephrotoxic properties are matters of importance but are of less practical significance.

Stasis

The main factor contributing to the bacterial colonization of the urinary tract is stasis with an increase in the volume of residual bladder urine. Favouring this are mechanical or neuropathic *obstruction* to flow (stones, valves, ureterocele, spinal dysraphism or injury) and, in children with VUR, the return of *refluxed urine* from the ureter to the bladder or its accumulation in the dilated atonic ureter. *Infrequent or incomplete voiding*, often associated with *constipation* (the loaded colon may impede complete bladder emptying) or the collection of urine in diverticula, will all encourage recurrence of infection. Voiding will be infrequent if the fluid intake is too low and can be hesitant if there is local soreness from chafing, threadworms or sexual abuse. The importance of *bladder instability* or detrusor sphincter dyssynergia without overt neurological deficit is now widely recognized as a cause of increased residual urine. It is often accompanied by frequency and urgency, by day wetting and squatting, by constipation and sometimes by secondary VUR.

Impairment of local antibacterial activity

This may be due for example to inflammation of the bladder mucosa, and also favours infection. It may follow bacterial or viral infection or result from mechanical or chemical irritation by stones, foreign bodies or antiseptics, such as chlorinated swimming pool water, and may be promoted by surface tension lowering agents in bath water, such as 'foam baths'.

Investigation

Purpose

Investigation of the urinary tract is undertaken

- to find the cause of the infection,
- to determine the state of the kidneys and whether there has been, or may be a risk of, renal involvement,
- to assess risk factors such as VUR or obstruction,
- to plan appropriate management and predict the prognosis.

Every child with a proven UTI should be investigated. The choice and extent of primary investigation, at present under review, depends both on the information needed and also on local facilities, interest and experience in interpretation. Consultation between the clinician and microbiologists, imagers and paediatric surgeons or urologists will help to resolve the complexities of the condition.

Clinical presentation is a poor guide to underlying abnormality of the renal tract.[6] In a retrospective analysis of children with VUR and UTI, no relationship was found between severity of presenting symptoms and grade of VUR or likelihood of renal scarring being found.[7]

Methods of investigation

1 *Microbiology.* Collection, preservation and transport of a urine sample to the laboratory is essential and has been discussed (Chapter 13). Local practice varies but by urinoscopy (the visual inspection of freshly passed urine), nitrite testing (Ames dipsticks) and microscopy if available, a provisional diagnosis can be made and treatment started. A laboratory result with organism sensitivity should be available in 48 h.

2 *Other laboratory tests.* C-reactive protein, ESR and WBC counts which indicate an inflammatory response are not routinely performed in this country for children with urinary infection. Neither is a water concentration test, which specifically indicates renal involvement during the acute process. Plasma electrolytes and creatinine should be measured in the sick child.

3 *Imaging.* This should be planned so that the relevant information can be obtained with the minimum irradiation or invasion, and as an outpatient if possible. There is a natural reluctance to subject children to unnecessary investigation, but there is a need to identify the small number at risk of renal damage as soon as possible, so that further infections can be prevented and the risk reduced. A recent survey by family doctors of children in their practices suggested that 11 of 23 children with renal scarring received suboptimal care, mainly failure to investigate UTI.[8]

The advent of new imaging techniques allows the implementation of alternative schemes for investigation which are less invasive or involve less irradiation than the established combination of intravenous urography (IVU) and micturating cysto-urethrography (MCU). These new techniques are undergoing further development, standardization and assessment. While follow-up studies are made and experience in their use and expertise in interpretation is being gained more generally, the clinician may be faced with greater uncertainty in planning management. Recent experience makes it clear that ultrasonography alone is not a technique which can exclude vesico-ureteric reflux or detect inflammatory change.

At the present time there is unfortunately no single comprehensive non-invasive method of investigation.

Imaging methods (Figures 14.1 and 14.2)

Radiology

Intravenous urography
This gives a well-defined structural assessment of the kidneys and urinary tract. Renal dimensions can be measured and retained for serial reassessment, including parenchymal thickness, renal pelvis and ureteric calibre. The bladder size and post-micturition residue can be judged and a loaded large bowel observed, often deforming the bladder or displacing the ureter in a constipated child. Spinal defects and stones can also be seen on the preliminary plain film. Four films usually suffice on an initial study and one for follow-up in a well-prepared child. Parents are able to see and understand their child's problem – a great help in obtaining compliance in treatment.

Disadvantages include the radiation dose, which can be cut down by preparing the child well, reducing the number of exposures and, on follow-up, limiting the area exposed to the kidneys. The gonadal radiation is higher in a full IVU than a DMSA scan, but the renal radiation dose is lower. Useful information can be gained from the infant IVU, but the renal outline is less well defined than later and bowel shadows can be troublesome. Another disadvantage is that acute inflammatory changes such as swelling or a reduced nephrogram may be overlooked and passed as normal unless careful measurements are made. Renal scars may not be apparent until scar tissue has contracted and the surrounding normal parenchyma has grown, several months after the process has been initiated.

Contrast micturating cysto-urethrography
The contrast cystogram gives an estimate of bladder capacity, structure, diverticula, function and residual urine, reliably demonstrates vesico-ureteric reflux and its severity, and may show intrarenal reflux. The urethra is also visualized, which is important in young boys to exclude urethral valves and show calibre variations. In older girls the wide bladder neck or spinning top urethra are typical, in association with an increased residue and constipation, of an unstable bladder.

Disadvantages are the catheterization and radiation involved. Experienced staff, the use of an image intensifier and follow-up with isotope cystography will minimize these.

Radionuclide imaging

^{99m}Tc-dimercaptosuccinic acid (DMSA) scan
The DMSA scan provides a functional assessment of the renal parenchyma based upon proximal tubular uptake of isotope, and also a measure of the percentage of total function provided by each kidney. Acute changes during

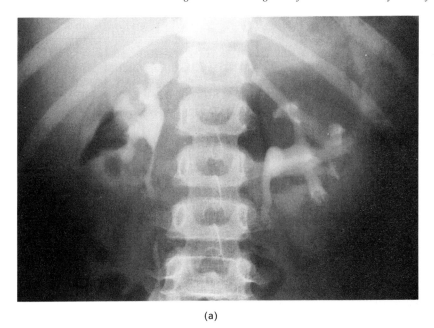

(a)

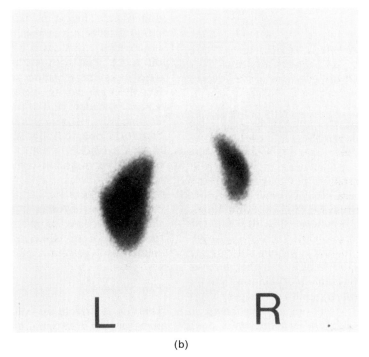

(b)

Figure 14.1 (a) IVU showing bilateral renal scarring. (b) DMSA scan, posterior view, with impaired function of right kidney and focal defects of left kidney (differential function: R. 25%, L. 75%)

or immediately after an infection tend to be diffuse and may disappear after 3–9 months, particularly if antibacterial treatment has been given rapidly.[9] The significance of these acute changes remains uncertain, but at the present time the early DMSA scan can be used as a screen for acute renal involvement and indicate those children needing further follow-up.

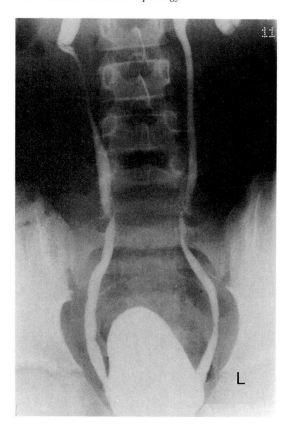

Figure 14.2 MCU showing bilateral VUR in an 8-year-old girl with history of recurrent symptomatic infections. Same patient as Figure 14.1 (a) and (b).

A variety of permanent changes in DMSA uptake are seen in children with established renal scarring. Here it provides a functional assessment, complementing structural changes seen on the IVU. [10–13]

Disadvantages include a 4-hour study, often inconvenient for the family, a higher level of renal, though lower gonadal, radiation than the IVU, and variation in quality of images. There may be technical variations and problems in interpretion, e.g. bilateral scarring with small smooth kidneys and symmetrical function, or duplex kidneys. Techniques are becoming standardized and equipment more widely available, and the significance of the acute changes is being explored. The interpretation of scans remains dependent on scan quality and observer.

[99m]Tc-diethylenetriaminepenta-acetic acid (DTPA) scan and MAG3 scan

These isotopes, with a shorter half-life than DMSA, give a measure of glomerular filtration and are used mainly in indirect cystography applicable only in older children or as a secondary investigation to locate and assess obstruction, and individual renal function.

Direct isotope cystography

This is a reliable means of diagnosing moderate to severe VUR and can be combined with urodynamic studies. The gonadal radiation dose is lower than in contrast cystography.

The disadvantages are that it involves catheterization and does not show the urethra or permit reflux grading.

Ultrasonography

This technique has the great attraction of being non-invasive and, as far as is known, is free from side effects. It detects changes in interface and thus defines solid and cystic structures and is of value in demonstrating renal cysts and dilatation. This is particularly useful in the infant in detecting persistent urinary tract dilatation which had been observed antenatally. In the older child who can co-operate, it can be used to estimate bladder capacity and residue. Renal length can be measured but this is observer dependent and not as yet reliably reproducible as a measure of renal growth. Ureteric dilatation due to VUR may also be detected but if the bladder is empty or the infant poorly hydrated, a negative result does not exclude reflux.

Disadvantages are therefore observer dependency, and unreliability in diagnosing VUR or scars and recognizing inflammation. In general, the nature of any abnormality found on ultrasound has to be confirmed by further imaging.

Plan of imaging

There is at present no consensus on a detailed plan for the investigation of infants and children with their presenting UTI.[14] A number of schemes have been put forward[15–17] but their feasibility and implementation depend upon availability of equipment and local expertise and interest. For instance, surgeons are concerned to exclude stones and obstruction; and physicians wish to identify not only those with established scars but those at risk of developing them, before they occur.

In the *infant* it is important to exclude obstruction and VUR and confirm that the kidneys are normal. This needs ultrasonography, cystography, and either a DMSA scan and plain abdominal film or a limited IVU.

Between *1 and 5 years* the author still considers a cystogram to be necessary following a proven symptomatic urinary infection. In the younger child there may be a chance to prevent or limit scarring; in the 4 or 5 year old it is unlikely to be the first infection and a cystogram would be indicated for a recurrence.

Over the age of 5 years the chances of new scarring taking place become progressively less likely. It is important to know whether the kidneys are normal, as this is the main determinant of prognosis, and a limited IVU or a DMSA is desirable. Some would consider ultrasonography adequate. Children in this age group may have problems with micturition control. Half of those with day wetting have UTI and many of them have some form of bladder instability which can be elucidated by contrast cystography, or urodynamics (and by a careful history).

There is general agreement that cystoscopy has no place in the primary investigation of childhood UTI.

Further management

This depends upon the response to treatment and on the results of investigation.

Obstruction and stones
In this small group in which infection may persist with the same or another organism or relapse early, ultrasound may reveal pelviureteric dilatation or an enlarged bladder; stones may also be detected by ultrasound or on a plain abdominal X-ray.

Surgical consultation is indicated

No obstruction
In the great majority, the presenting infection is quickly eradicated but, without prophylaxis, reinfection with a fresh organism can be expected in at least half of them, most commonly within the first three months and then with a decreasing risk over the next 12–18 months.[18]

- *If VUR is present* there is a need to prevent further infection, assess the renal status and continue to follow the child.
- *Diffuse or focal areas of impaired DMSA*

uptake within 3 months of UTI require further evaluation, continued prophylactic antibacterial treatment and follow-up. A suggested course would be to continue prophylaxis for 6–12 months and then repeat the DMSA scan. If the photon deficiency persists, a limited IVU will confirm the nature and significance of the abnormality. A cystogram is also indicated.

- *No reflux detected; no impairment of DMSA uptake; IVU normal after 12 months.* These children should have an excellent renal prognosis but may need symptomatic treatment or instruction in preventative measures. If acute pyelonephritic episodes recur, further investigation should be considered. Detrusor–sphincter dyssynergia or bladder instability must be suspected.

Prevention of further infection

Attention to detail and explanation to parents, preferably with visual aids, are essential.

Complete bladder emptying
Residual urine can be minimized by regular unhurried voiding, at least every 2 or 3 hours, with double micturition at bedtime (two or three voidings spaced 5 min apart). Enquiries should be made into the toilet facilities and their use and the availability of drinks at school, both often avoided by school children.

A normal *fluid intake* is recommended in infancy. In children, a drink at breakfast and at socially acceptable intervals is encouraged. Excessive drinking may become habit forming, reduce the efficacy of antibacterial therapy and is usually unnecessary.

In infancy as well as in childhood, *constipation* may need correction by attention to diet or by a regular small evening dose of a suitable laxative until records show a daily motion for at least a month, when the dose can be gradually reduced. Parents are often unaware of their children's bowel habits and either a diary or the appearance of a loaded bowel on abdominal film or IVU with a post-micturition residue may help to convince them of the presence and importance of constipation. Local irritation can be reduced by the application of barrier creams before swimming, by treating threadworms and by discouraging close-fitting trousers. The possibility of sexual abuse should be remembered.

Low-dose antibacterial prophylaxis

The purpose of prophylaxis is to protect the susceptible urinary tract from reinfection after the initial infection has been successfully treated, and not to suppress inadequately treated infection. (It is contraindicated in children who have persistent infection due to outflow obstruction.) Low-dose antibacterial prophylaxis can therefore be recommended: (a) during a bladder retraining programme; (b) while acute inflammation of the uroepithelium subsides; (c) while vesico-ureteric reflux is present. It is also recommended (d) during the actively growing stage of a scarred kidney, in order to allow optimal growth of any normal renal tissue, and (e) in the first year of life when the kidneys are more vulnerable, the symptoms of recurrence are less specific and the collection of a suitable sample of urine in emergency more difficult.

Suitable drugs. The qualities needed in a urinary prophylactic drug include efficacy against urinary pathogens, little induction of resistant organisms in the faecal flora, a high urinary excretion level, palatability and freedom from side effects. At the present time these requirements are best fulfilled by co-trimoxazole, trimethoprim and nitrofurantoin. They should be given in the lowest effective dose to keep the urine sterile (see Table 14.1). Recurrence with resistant organisms usually suggests that either too high a dose is being given, or there is some obstruction to outflow, detrusor–sphincter dyssynergia or an abnormality such as a bladder diverticulum.

Duration of prophylaxis This is empirical, but in a child with a structurally normal urinary tract and a history of recurrent infection, 6–12 months of prophylaxis will very considerably reduce the recurrence rate, when combined with bladder and bowel training.[18]

No controlled studies have been made of the appropriate duration of prophylaxis in children with vesico-ureteric reflux.[19] It has been suggested that prophylaxis is no longer necessary after the age of 7 and if the child is well, with sensible, well-motivated parents, discontinuing prophylaxis may be appropriate. If there are symptomatic recurrences, treatment can be started immediately, prophylaxis can be resumed and further investigation considered. The author has usually continued prophylaxis

until the reflux has disappeared or until puberty as part of a standard protocol. Most uncomplicated vesico-ureteric reflux will already have resolved spontaneously before this time. New scars have been reported after the age of 5 in both normal and scarred kidneys of children with VUR receiving intermittent treatment.

Follow-up control Regular supervision during prophylaxis is advisable to ensure compliance and check the urine if indicated. Children with previous recurrent symptomatic infections which have been prevented by prophylaxis are often reluctant to discontinue antibacterial treatment. If there is no vesico-ureteric reflux or evidence of renal involvement, it is appropriate to stop prophylaxis and culture the urine monthly for 3–6 months thereafter and if symptoms recur.

Side effects and toxicity No side effects have been observed or reported in children receiving long-term co-trimoxazole, trimethoprim or nitrofurantoin in a low dose (see Table 14.1).

Special situations

Newborn and infants

The detection, rapid treatment and investigation of young infants with UTI is critical. Presentation may be with any of the common symptoms of infancy such as diarrhoea and vomiting, feeding difficulty, 'colic', fever, convulsions, failure to gain weight and metabolic disorders. Initial investigation should include an ultrasound scan to exclude obstruction, and an MCU to detect reflux. A DMSA scan will demonstrate any impaired function without interference from bowel shadows, but an IVU is a very useful alternative. Tomography may be needed. It is the author's practice to keep all infants with proven UTI and no obstruction on prophylaxis during their first year. The symptoms of UTI are non-specific and since prophylaxis is effective, parental anxiety and the need for repeated urine collections are lessened.

Covert bacteriuria

Epidemiological studies of bacteriuria at school entry have shown a prevalence of 1–2% in girls and 0.08% in boys. Studies have therefore been largely confined to girls. Similar proportions of VUR and renal scarring have been found in schoolgirls with screening bacteriuria as in children with symptomatic infection. However, after the age of 5 continued untreated asymptomatic bacteriuria does not appear to be harmful even when VUR is present.[20,21] The late prognosis in these girls during pregnancy is related to the presence of renal scarring rather than VUR or persisting bacteriuria.[22] Compliance in any treatment regimen is difficult to achieve in asymptomatic schoolchildren. Kunin in the Charlottesville screening survey[23] and more recent studies suggest that antibacterial treatment of 'symptomless' bacteriuria in schoolgirls may distort the symbiosis between the host and organism so that a symptomatic infection with a different bacterial species may follow. This will depend also upon the antibacterial agent used. For example, nitrofurantoin has little effect upon the bowel flora resistance pattern, while amoxycillin treatment is rapidly followed by amoxycillin resistance in bowel and periurethral flora.

For these reasons the consensus of opinion is that truly asymptomatic bacteriuria in children of school age can be left untreated unless a symptomatic infection develops spontaneously.

Under the age of 5, population screening has been shown to be impractical in this country and not cost-effective. It is, however, advisable to collect a specimen of urine from any child presenting with fever or non-specific symptoms in this age group and treat and investigate appropriately. A busy mother may have overlooked, for example, delayed bladder control.

The child with a neuropathic bladder[24]

The same principles of management apply as outlined above:

- Any *symptomatic infection* when the child is feverish or unwell should be treated with full-dose antibacterial treatment.
- Urodynamic studies should be made to assess *bladder function* and whether there is low- or high-pressure voiding, the latter having more serious consequences for the kidneys, and to identify and grade any vesico-ureteric reflux. The renal status can be evaluated (a) by a DMSA scan and (b) by an IVU if there is recurrent urinary infection.

- Satisfactory *bladder emptying* should be established. This can be achieved by intermittent self-catheterization or drugs such as oxybutynin, and an adequate fluid intake. When these measures are unsuccessful, various surgical procedures may be considered.
- Provided that there is satisfactory bladder drainage, low-dose *antibacterial prophylaxis* can be used very effectively, and is particularly important if vesico-ureteric reflux is present. Prophylaxis is less likely to be successful when there is a large volume of residual urine. Frequent urine culture is unnecessary and may cause confusion; asymptomatic bacteriuria should not be treated, so that effective antibacterial treatment will be available for symptomatic urinary tract infection. Treatment should then be started as soon as a sample has been collected and some form of drainage introduced.
- *Follow-up.* Further assessments of bladder capacity, function and residual urine and of upper tract dilatation can be made by ultrasonography and of differential renal function on serial DMSAs. A limited IVU of the renal areas at intervals of several years will assess renal growth and parenchymal thickness and any progression of papillary damage from raised pelvicalyceal pressure.

Vesico-ureteric reflux

Significance

VUR or the backflow of urine from bladder to ureter through an incompetent ureteric valve is found in 30–40% of children with UTI. It allows infecting organisms and voiding pressure to be transmitted from bladder to renal pelvis, and on return to the bladder, refluxed urine increases the residual urine, encouraging reinfection. Any child with reflux is at potential risk of developing renal scarring if infection occurs. About 30% of children with UTI and reflux have reflux nephropathy, but almost all of those with renal scarring have, or have had, VUR. The severity of VUR varies (Figure 14.3) and this influences its effect and its outcome and management. There is a high resolution rate in children managed on a strict medical regimen of up to 90% of ureters with mild VUR, but only 30–40% or less of the more severe grades. The proportion of children with scarred kidneys also increases with severity of reflux, but scarring

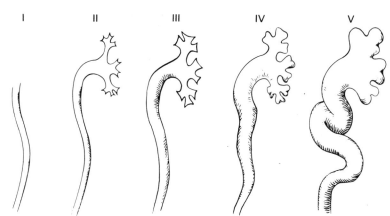

Figure 14.3 Grades of reflux (International Classification). I. Ureter only. II. Ureter, pelvis and calyces: no dilatation. Normal calyceal fornices. III. Mild or moderate dilatation and/or tortuosity of the ureter and mild or moderate dilatation of renal pelvis but no, or only slight, blunting of the fornices. IV. Moderate dilatation and/or tortuosity of ureter and moderate dilatation of renal pelvis and calyces; complete obliteration of sharp angle of fornices but maintenance of papillary impressions in majority of calyces. V. Gross dilatation and tortuosity of ureter: gross dilatation of renal pelvis and calyces: papillary impressions are no longer visible in majority of calyces. (From Ref. 25 with permission.)

can be found in association with mild VUR and insignificant symptoms.[7,25,26]

Objectives of management

The objectives in managing children with VUR and UTI infection are first to prevent urinary infection reaching the kidney, secondly to eliminate residual urine which will predispose to recurrence of infection, and thirdly to maintain, as far as possible, a low bladder pressure in order to ensure normal renal growth without parenchymal damage.

Prevention of urinary infection reaching the kidney
- *Rapid treatment and prevention of recurrence of urinary infection.* A medical regimen for the management of these children is based on the protocol already outlined, aimed at improved bladder and bowel function with uninterrupted low-dose prophylactic antibacterial cover. Attention to detail in each individual and ensuring the parents' or child's understanding in order to obtain compliance are important.

  With such a medical regimen, infection can be almost completely prevented, kidneys will grow with a minimal risk of scarring and reflux will tend to improve and stop spontaneously with time in over 80% of children.[27,28] The

prognosis is least good in those with persistent severe VUR and established scarring.
- *Anticipation of infection.* An early diagnosis of VUR can be made by investigating infants with urinary tract dilatation detected antenatally or by screening offspring and siblings of index patients for VUR by cystography. Up to a quarter of these may show VUR. Prophylactic measures can then be used to prevent infection developing until VUR either disappears or is corrected surgically.
- *Stop reflux.* This can be successfully achieved by *surgical procedures* in over 90% of patients in the hands of the best paediatric urologists, and particularly for the lesser grades of reflux. Where there are dilated atonic ureters, some tailoring of the lower end of the ureter may be necessary. More recently, O'Donnell and Puri have introduced the 'STING' technique (sub-endothelial teflon injection) which is carried out under direct visual control. The main attraction is that it can be performed as a day case and short-term results have been successful, although the procedure may have to be repeated. It is less satisfactory in patients with more severe grades of reflux where surgical reimplantation is more usual. There are as yet no long-term studies of the outcome regarding the permanence of the result, or the possibility of progressive narrowing of the vesico-ureteric junction.[29] There is also

concern about the reported migration of teflon to the lungs, meninges and other sensitive areas in experimental animals. Alternative materials are being explored.

All surgically treated children require follow-up (a) initially to confirm successful prevention of reflux and to exclude any obstruction at the vesico-ureteric junction; (b) over the first year to detect recurrence of infection; and (c) if there is any renal scarring, lifelong supervision of their blood pressure and renal function will be needed, the interval depending on the extent of the scarring.

Await natural disappearance
It has been indicated that there is a natural tendency for reflux to resolve spontaneously with time. This is less likely in children with marked dilatation of the ureter or renal pelvis persisting after the first few years. Nevertheless in the International Reflux Study, Reflux Grade III or IV (reaching the kidney with dilatation) improved or stopped during a 6 months pre-entry period in 25% of the children originally recruited. Some VUR persisted, however, in 83% of those who entered the study and were treated medically over a period of 5 years,[30] and in over half of those in the Birmingham Study.[31]

There is some evidence in children with VUR and an unstable bladder that oxybutynin may speed up the resolution of reflux. These children are also helped by training in regular, complete voiding, combined with double micturition at bedtime and by correction of constipation, during a period of antibacterial prophylaxis.

Reduce bladder pressure
Stones or posterior urethral valves, ureteroceles or neuropathic disorders impairing outflow should be searched for and corrected. Frequent voiding, preferably two-hourly and at intervals not greater than 3 hours, should be encouraged.

Follow-up

Children with normal kidneys
It is important to prevent renal damage. A limited IVU or a DMSA scan 1 year after the presenting urinary infection will indicate whether any permanent change is present. Subsequently, normal renal growth or unchanged

differential function on a DMSA scan is a more important guide than persistence of VUR.

Children with scarred kidneys
Further damage should also be limited or prevented in infants or children with or without VUR who have segmental scarring or parenchymal thinning on IVU or defects of DMSA uptake seen immediately after UTI and which persist 1 year later. Follow-up supervision includes monitoring the blood pressure, renal growth, function (plasma creatinine, GFR and differential function by isotope methods), urine culture and somatic growth.

Urine culture
Opinions differ about the value of regular urine culture and the intervals at which it should be carried out.

In infancy and early childhood, regular urine culture 3-monthly and if the child is unwell are particularly important. Growth and development and compliance in the prescribed regimen can also be checked. Antibacterial treatment of febrile illnesses should be preceded by collection of a satisfactory urine sample, preferably by suprapubic aspiration.

In the older child, regular supervision is needed to reinforce the therapeutic regimen, with further explanation of the objectives to parent and child. Some of the late developing new scars reported have followed a symptomatic UTI occurring a short time after interruption of prophylaxis. It is natural to doubt the need for prophylaxis in a well child if the status of the kidney and ureter are unknown. If a medical regimen is undertaken, it should be carefully adhered to if optimal results are to be obtained.

Medical or surgical treatment of children with VUR

Randomized prospective studies comparing the outcome of medical and surgical management of children with UTI and severe VUR have been conducted in Birmingham and in a multicentre international study. After 5 years there was no significant difference in either study between the treatment groups in renal growth and function, or in the development of further renal damage.

The Birmingham Study[31] of 104 children with either reflux corrected by one of two surgeons, or careful follow-up by paediatricians, showed equal numbers of children developing new scars in each group. They were all observed at the 2-year follow-up and no further new scars were seen between the 2- and 5-year follow-up.

Three hundred and four children with Grades III and IV VUR, 49% with scarred kidneys, entered the European limb of the IRSC, involving 8 centres. Nineteen of the 155 children treated medically, and 20 of the 151 children treated surgically, developed new scars; in 5 of the medical and 7 of the surgical groups, these developed in previously normal kidneys.[32]

In summary, the evidence so far emerging from controlled trials of medical and surgical management of severe reflux suggests that optimal medical or surgical treatment should be selected once reflux is diagnosed and the child carefully supervised while the kidneys are at risk. Even more important is the rapid diagnosis and treatment of the presenting infection. The choice of medical or surgical management for an individual child will depend upon social and geographical factors and upon local expertise as well as parental choice. The main indication for surgical correction is a social one, when there is poor compliance in a medical regimen with recurrent urinary infection, or if there is a paraureteric diverticulum when reflux is unlikely to resolve.

Urinary tract infection and renal scarring

The coarse irregular segmental scarring seen in chronic atrophic pyelonephritis or reflux nephropathy remains a major cause in this country of hypertension and of end-stage renal disease. It accounts for a lower proportion of young Swedish adults requiring dialysis and transplant, possibly because of greater interest in childhood UTI or a different health care system.

Experimental and clinical studies indicate that scars tend to be acquired in the young growing kidney, particularly in the first year or two of life when a refluxing urinary tract is infected,[5,33] although they can develop throughout childhood.[34] Delay in treatment is an important factor[2,3,5] and rapid treatment can prevent or limit the scarring process.[35,36] The distribution of scars is determined initially by the renal anatomy and the siting of compound papillae which allow the retrograde flow of urine (intra-

renal reflux) into the papillary collecting tubules.[33,37,38] Urine which may be infected or under pressure can flow from the bladder to the renal pelvis through an incompetent VU valve. Since 75% of normal human kidneys have at least one compound papilla, initial treatment should be planned on the assumption that the kidney is at risk. A refluxing unit repeatedly exposed to infection without developing scars may contain no compound papillae and remain intact.

Prevention of scarring

There is a possibility that scar development may be prevented by diagnosing VUR before infection occurs: (a) by screening the sibling and offspring of index patients with VUR and renal scarring; and (b) by following up infants with antenatal dilatation of the urinary tract.[39] In infants with VUR and previously normal scans, abnormal DMSA uptake has been found following UTI.[40] Infants presenting with VUR and UTI within 6 months of birth had twice as many abnormal DMSA studies as infants with VUR diagnosed postnatally and without known infection.[41] These findings emphasize the potential for preventing renal scarring in this age group. Further follow-up of such infants is needed.

The optimal management of children with bilateral renal scarring and severe reflux is uncertain. The duration of prophylaxis is empirical, but children with VUR and renal scarring are susceptible both to UTI and to the development of fresh scars in normal areas of scarred kidneys. For this reason the author usually continues low-dose prophylaxis until puberty and particularly if VUR persists.

Follow-up should include a regular check of blood pressure, renal function and for proteinuria.

Long-term effects of UTI, VUR and renal scarring

In early reports of childhood urinary infection, the prognosis was very poor but has improved since the advent of antibacterial agents.[42] The main sequelae are recurrent UTI in females and the consequences of renal scarring, namely hypertension and impaired renal function.

In a 10–17-year follow-up of 141 children with reflux treated by reimplantation, 12.8%

were hypertensive, 18% of those who had bilateral scarring preoperatively. All of those who developed hypertension had an abnormal IVU 6 months after surgery.[43] In a 30-year follow-up of 30 children treated in childhood for UTI associated with chronic pyelonephritic renal scarring, 7 (23%) were hypertensive, 2 had raised blood pressure during pregnancy and 3 had end-stage renal disease.[44] In a personal follow-up of 230 patients treated in childhood for UTI associated with VUR, 11% were hypertensive, 4% had a raised plasma creatinine, and 3, all of whom were hypertensive with impaired renal function in childhood, had received renal transplants. Further infection, mostly single episodes, had been reported in 30%, but very few had febrile symptomatic episodes.[45]

These follow-up studies represent, to some extent, an unnatural history of the condition, since in any patient the prognosis generally improves when they come under interested medical care. It has also been the practice to correct most severe vesico-ureteric reflux surgically. Studies comparing medical management and surgical correction of reflux persisting into adult life have not, however, shown any advantage of surgical treatment.[46] Adult complications have recently been reviewed.[34]

References

1. Smellie J.M., Edwards D., Hunter N., Normand I.C.S. and Prescod N. Vesicoureteric reflux and renal scarring. *Kidney Int.* 1975, **8S**, 65–72
2. Smellie J.M., Normand I.C.S., Ransley P.G. and Prescod N. The development of renal scars: a collaborative study. *Br. Med. J.* 1985, **290**, 1957–1960
3. Winter A.L., Hardy B.E., Alton D.J., Arbus G.S. and Churchill B.M. Acquired renal scars in children. *J. Urol.* 1983, **129**, 1190–1194
4. Berg U.B. and Johansson S.B. Age as a main determinant of renal functional damage in urinary tract infection. *Arch. Dis. Child.* 1983, **58**, 963–969
5. Winberg J., Bollgren I., Kallenius G., Mollby R. and Svensson S.B. Clinical pyelonephritis and focal renal scarring. *Pediatr. Clin. North Am.* 1982, **29**, 801–814
6. Smellie J.M., Hodson C.J., Edwards D. and Normand I.C.S. Clinical and radiological features of urinary infection in childhood. *Br. Med. J.* 1964, **2**, 1222–1226
7. Ozen H.A. and Whitaker R.H. Does the severity of presentation in children with vesico-ureteric reflux relate to the severity of the disease or the need for operation? *Br. J. Urol.* 1987, **60**, 110–112
8. South Bedfordshire Practitioners Group. Development of renal scars in children: missed opportunities in management. *Br. Med. J.* 1990, **301**, 1082–1084
9. Tappen D., Murphy A.V., Mocan H., Shaw R., Beattie T.J., McAllister T.A. and Mackenzie J.R. A prospective study of children with first acute symptomatic *E. coli* urinary tract infection. *Acta Paediatr. Scand.* 1989, **78**, 923–929
10. Goldraich NP, Ramos O.L. and Goldraich I.H. Urography versus DMSA scan in children with vesico-ureteric reflux. *Pediatr. Nephrol.* 1989, **3**, 1–5.
11. Smellie J.M., Shaw P.J., Prescod N.P. and Bantock H.M. ⁹⁹ᵐTc-dimercaptosuccinic acid (DMSA) scan in patients with established radiological renal scarring. *Arch. Dis. Child.* 1988, **63**, 1315–1319
12. Smellie J.M., Prescod N., Shaw P., Bantock H.M. and Normand I.C.S. Comparison of radiology and nuclear imaging in the assessment of patients with renal scarring. In: Host Parasite Interactions in Urinary Tract Infections. Kass E.H. and Svanborg Eden C. (eds) *Proceedings of 4th International Symposium on Pyelonephritis, 1986.* Chicago, University of Chicago Press, 1989: 280–284
13. McLorie G.A., Aliabadi H., Churchill B.M., Ash J.M. and Gilday D.L. ⁹⁹ᵐ-Technetium-dimercaptosuccinic acid renal scarring and excretion urography in diagnosis of renal scars in children. *J. Urol.* 1989, **142**, 790–792
14. Working Group of Research Unit, Royal College of Physicians. Guidelines for the management of acute urinary tract infection in childhood. *J. Roy. Coll. Phys.* 1991, **25**, 36–42
15. Haycock G.B. Investigation of urinary tract infection. *Arch. Dis. Child.* 1986, **61**, 1155–1158
16. Whyte K.M., Abbott G.D., Kennedy J.C. and Maling T.M.J. A protocol for the investigation of infants and children with urinary tract infection. *Clin. Radiol.* 1988, **39**, 278–280
17. Gordon I. Urinary tract infection in paediatrics: the role of diagnostic imaging. *Br. J. Radiol.* 1990, **63**, 507–511
18. Smellie J.M., Katz G. and Grüneberg R.N. Controlled trial of prophylactic treatment in childhood urinary tract infection. *Lancet* 1978, **2**, 175–178
19. Smellie J.M., Grüneberg R.N., Leakey A. and Atkin W.S. Long term low-dose co-trimoxazole in the prophylaxis of childhood urinary tract infection, clinical aspects. *Br. Med. J.* 1976, **2**, 203–206
20. Claesson I. and Lindberg U. Asymptomatic bacteriuria in schoolgirls. *Radiology* 1977, **124**, 179–183
21. Aggarwal V.K., Verrier-Jones K., Asscher A.W., Evans C. and Williams L.A. Covert bacteriuria: long term follow up. *Arch. Dis. Child.* 1991, **66**, 1284–1286
22. Sacks S.H., Roberts R., Verrier-Jones K., Asscher A.W., Ledingham J.G.G. Effect of symptomless bacteriuria in childhood on subsequent pregnancy. *Lancet* 1987, **2**, 991–994
23. Kunin C.M. A ten year study of bacteriuria in schoolgirls: final report of bacteriologic, urologic and epidemiologic findings. *J. Infect. Dis.* 1970, **122**, 382–393
24. Borzyskowski M. and Mundy A.R. (eds) *Neuropathic Bladder in Childhood.* Oxford, MacKeith Press, 1990

25. International Reflux Study Committee. Medical versus surgical treatment of primary vesico-ureteral reflux. *Pediatrics* 1981, **67**, 392–400

26. Smellie J.M., Normand I.C.S. and Katz G. Children with urinary infection: a comparison of those with and those without vesico-ureteric reflux. *Kidney Int.* 1981, **20**, 717–722

27. Edwards D., Normand I.C.S., Prescod N. and Smellie J.M. The disappearance of vesico-ureteric reflux during long term prophylaxis of urinary tract infection in children. *Br.Med.J.* 1977, **2**, 285–288

28. Smellie J.M., Edwards D., Normand I.C.S. and Prescod N. Effect of vesico-ureteric reflux on renal growth in children with urinary tract infection. *Arch.Dis.Child.* 1981, **56**, 593–600

29. Puri P. Endoscopic correction of primary vesico-ureteric reflux by sub-ureteric injection of polytetrafluoroethylene. *Lancet* 1990, **335**, 1320–1322

30. International Reflux Study in Children, European Branch. Cessation of vesico-ureteral reflux during 5 years in infants and children allocated to medical treatment. *J.Urol.* 1992, **148**, 1662–1666

31. Birmingham Reflux Study Group. Prospective trial of operative versus non-operative treatment of severe vesico-ureteric reflux in children: 5 years' observation. *Br.Med.J.* 1987, **295**, 237–241

32. International Reflux Study in Children: A five year study of medical or surgical treatment in children with severe reflux: radiological renal findings. *Pediatr.Nephrol.* 1992, **6**, 223–230

33. Ransley P.G. and Risdon R.A. Reflux and renal scarring. *Br.J.Radiol.* 1978, **51**, Suppl. 14, 1–35

34. Smellie J.M. and Daman-Willems C.E. Vesico-ureteric reflux: recent research and its effect on clinical practice. In: Catto G.R.D. (ed.) *Urinary Tract Infection.* Lancaster and Dordrecht, Kluwer Academic Publishers, 1989: 39–86

35. Ransley P.G. and Risdon R.A. Reflux nephropathy: effects of antimicrobial therapy on the evolution of the early pyelonephritic scar. *Kidney Int.* 1981, **20**, 733–742

36. Wikstad I., Hannerz L., Karlsson A., Eklöf A.-C., Olling S. and Aperia A. [99m]Technetium dimercaptosuccinic acid scintigraphy in the diagnosis of acute pyelonephritis in rats. *Pediatr.Nephrol.* 1990, **4**, 331–334

37. Rolleston T.L., Maling T.M.J. and Hodson C.J. Intrarenal reflux and the scarred kidney. *Arch.Dis.Child.* 1974, **49**, 531–539

38. Hannerz L., Wikstad I., Johansson L., Broberger O., and Aperia A. Distribution of renal scars and intrarenal reflux in children with a past history of urinary tract infection. *Acta Radiol.* 1987, **28**, 443–446

39. Najmaldin A., Burge D.M. and Atwell J.D. Fetal vesico-ureteric reflux. *Br.J.Urol.* 1990, **65**, 403–406

40. Gordon A.C., Thomas D.F.M., Arthur R.J., Irving H.C. and Smith S.E.W. Prenatally diagnosed reflux: a follow up study. *Br.J.Urol.* 1990, **65**, 407–412

41. Sheridan M., Jewkes F. and Gough D.C.S. Reflux nephropathy in the first year of life – the role of infection. *Pediatr.Surg.Int.* 1991, **6**, 214–216

42. Smellie J.M. and Normand I.C.S. Urinary infections in children, 1985. *Postgrad. Med. J.* 1985, **61**, 895–905

43. Wallace D.M.A., Rothwell D.L. and Williams D.I. The long-term follow up of surgically treated vesico-ureteric reflux. *Br.J.Urol.* 1978, **50**, 479–484

44. Jacobson S.H., Eklöf O., Eriksson C.G., Lins L.-E., Tidgren B. and Winberg J. Development of hypertension and uremia after pyelonephritis in childhood: 27 year follow-up. *Br.Med.J.* 1989, **299**, 703–705

45. Smellie J.M.. AUA Lecture: Reflections on 30 years of treating children with urinary tract infections. *J.Urol.* 1991, **146**, 665–668

46. Neves R.J., Torres V.E., Malek R.S. and Svensson J. Vesico-ureteral reflux in the adult IV. Medical versus surgical management. *J.Urol.* 1984, **132**, 882–885

15

Hypertension

M.J. Dillon

Introduction

In recent years there has been a growing interest in childhood hypertension. This is partly related to the accumulated evidence suggesting that adult essential hypertension has its origins in childhood and an increasing awareness that significantly raised blood pressure requiring treatment can and does occur in children, whereas in the past it was considered to be almost exclusively an adult disorder.

Severe untreated hypertension in childhood carries a high risk of morbidity and mortality.[1] In the majority of cases it is secondary to an underlying and often remediable cause and there are, therefore, considerable advantages to be gained by its detection and treatment. The benefits of recognizing mild to moderate degrees of hypertension are not so clear-cut and it is within this area that much controversy exists concerning investigation and management.

The increasing literature on childhood hypertension has tended to become polarized into two categories: that concerned with primary or essential hypertension dominated by epidemiologists and that concerned with secondary hypertension mainly contributed to by paediatric nephrologists, since 80–90% of secondary hypertension in children is due to renal disease. This chapter hopefully will go some way towards reconciling these areas of interest and put into perspective some of the important issues involved. Recommended further reading would include References 2–9.

Definition of hypertension

For hypertension to be identified it is important to know what constitutes normotension. Pickering[10] stated that, if secondary hypertension is excluded, blood pressure is a continuous variable which is not obviously bimodal and hence hypertension at any age represents an arterial pressure above an arbitrarily defined value. In children the problem is further complicated by the physiological increase in blood pressure with age and the various methodological problems encountered when attempting to measure blood pressure accurately, especially in young children.

A number of population studies have been published giving normal values of blood pressure from infancy to adolescence. Blood pressure measurements repeatedly exceeding a given percentile, for example the 95th, are thought to define hypertension rather than absolute values.[11] However, in view of the variability in both conditions and techniques of measurement, the available reference ranges are not directly comparable and this raises doubts about their validity when used to interpret blood pressure values in individual children. There is no problem when blood pressure is markedly increased; it becomes important the closer the value approximates to what is considered to be normal.

Blood pressure variance in childhood is dependent on a multitude of factors, both genetic and environmental. It is clear that blood pressure increases with age during the pre-adult

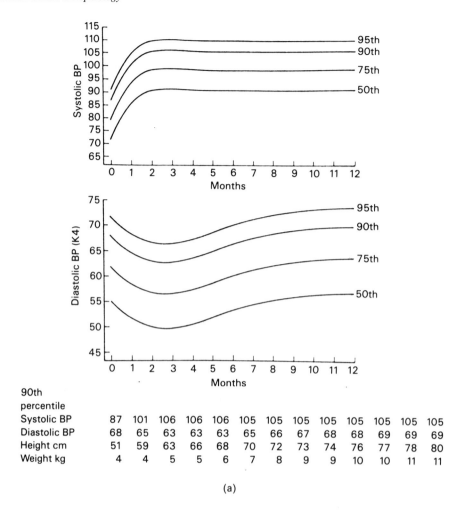

90th percentile													
Systolic BP	87	101	106	106	106	105	105	105	105	105	105	105	105
Diastolic BP	68	65	63	63	63	65	66	67	68	68	69	69	69
Height cm	51	59	63	66	68	70	72	73	74	76	77	78	80
Weight kg	4	4	5	5	6	7	8	9	9	10	10	11	11

(a)

years and this occurs in all populations studied, although the level and trend vary from population to population. Larger children (heavier and/or taller) have higher blood pressures than smaller children of the same age. It is therefore imperative that the level of a child's or adolescent's blood pressure is considered with respect to body size as well as to age.

Normative blood pressure data for children are available but have to be viewed with some circumspection since they may not reflect blood pressure norms for all racial groups and many omit to include some factorization for size, just relating blood pressure to age.

The National Heart, Lung and Blood Institute, Bethesda, USA has commissioned two reports of the Task Force on Blood Pressure Control in Children. The first report appeared in 1977 and enjoyed wide distribution, becoming a major reference for blood pressure stand-

ards in children.[12] The second report, published in 1987,[13] used data taken from nine different studies performed mainly in the USA, although there was one British source (the Brompton Study) included.[14,15] The initial report was criticized for several reasons: it was cross-sectional; only a white population was studied; only a single blood pressure measurement was made on each subject; and only chronological age was considered. The 1987 Task Force addressed some of these issues but some of the criticisms still apply.[8] The data included measurements on white, black and Mexican-American children, but it was still mainly cross-sectional in nature and used only one measurement per subject in the analysis. It changed from using the Korotkov phase IV (muffling) to phase V (disappearance) for diastolic blood pressure at the age of 13 years. An attempt was made, however, to take into account height and weight

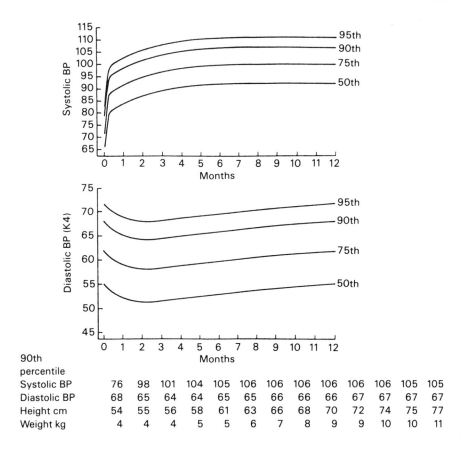

90th percentile												
Systolic BP	76	98	101	104	105	106	106	106	106	106	106	105	105
Diastolic BP	68	65	64	64	65	65	66	66	66	67	67	67	67
Height cm	54	55	56	58	61	63	66	68	70	72	74	75	77
Weight kg	4	4	4	5	5	6	7	8	9	9	10	10	11

Figure 15.1 Age-specific percentiles of blood pressure measurements in boys (a) and girls (b), from birth to 12 months of age (From Report of the Second Task Force on Blood Pressure Control in Children,[13] by permission)

by a cumbersome factorization technique (Figures 15.1–15.7).

Although the Task Force charts are extremely valuable, there are other reference values based on North West European studies that have been recently published[16] in which age, height and gender specific blood pressure centiles are presented (Figures 15.4–15.7). These are clearly of greater relevance to Europeans and define blood pressure as a function of height without the need for factorization. Alternatively there may be an argument for utilizing British (Brompton Study) age-related systolic blood pressure nomograms, at least for younger children.[17]

Methods of blood pressure measurement

The most convenient means of measuring blood pressure in children is the conventional sphygmomanometer. Of the various sources of error that are recognized with this technique, the most important is cuff size. A cuff that is too small produces an erroneously high blood pressure recording and can occasionally fail to occlude the underlying artery at all. A useful rule of thumb is to use the largest cuff, i.e. the widest cuff that still allows the vascular sounds to be heard easily with a stethoscope at the antecubital fossa. The length of the bladder should be at least two-thirds of the arm circumference and preferably longer. Four cuff sizes are recommended to cover most paediatric eventualities: suitable bladder measurements are 4 × 13 cm, 8 × 18 cm, 12 × 24 cm (adult cuff) and 14 × 33 cm (large adult cuff).[13,18]

The circumstances of measurement should be considered and ideally should minimize anxiety to avoid so-called 'white coat' hypertension well reported in adults. The child should be relaxed

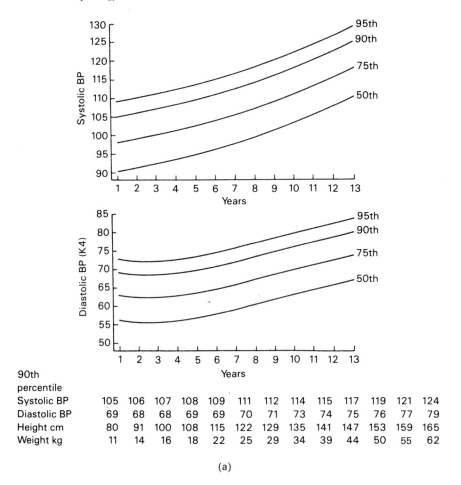

90th percentile													
Systolic BP	105	106	107	108	109	111	112	114	115	117	119	121	124
Diastolic BP	69	68	68	69	69	70	71	73	74	75	76	77	79
Height cm	80	91	100	108	115	122	129	135	141	147	153	159	165
Weight kg	11	14	16	18	22	25	29	34	39	44	50	55	62

(a)

and comfortable, sitting quietly (unless contraindicated) for 3 min in an acceptable ambient temperature. Ideally three recordings should be undertaken at 1-minute intervals with the arm supported at chest level. The average of the second and third readings should be utilized.[19]

The sytolic pressure is easier to define than diastolic. The fourth Korotkov sound, corresponding to the point of muffling rather than the disappearance of the sounds (fifth Korotkov sound), is the best estimate of the diastolic pressure, but this is of academic interest in the majority of clinical circumstances. However, in some circumstances (especially young children less than 1 year of age) the Korotkov sounds cannot be heard reliably, while in others they are detected continuously almost to zero with no identifiable muffle on auscultation. In these circumstances alternative methods may need to be used.

Instruments utilizing ultrasound based on the Doppler principle can record both systolic and diastolic pressures, but some doubt has been expressed about the accuracy of the diastolic estimate. In view of this, some have advocated Doppler systems that only measure systolic pressure and have the additional advantage of being relatively uncomplicated and inexpensive.[20] Alternative systems such as those that record low-frequency vibrations in arterial walls (infrasound) show unacceptable variability in measuring diastolic pressure in children, although they can measure systolic pressure accurately. However, oscillometric blood pressure recorders such as the Dinamap monitors have been validated by comparison with intra-arterial measurements in infants and young children, but do need to be calibrated regularly with reference to a mercury column, especially for epidemiological studies.

Other indirect methods of recording blood pressure, including palpation of the radial or brachial arteries as a sphygmomanometer cuff

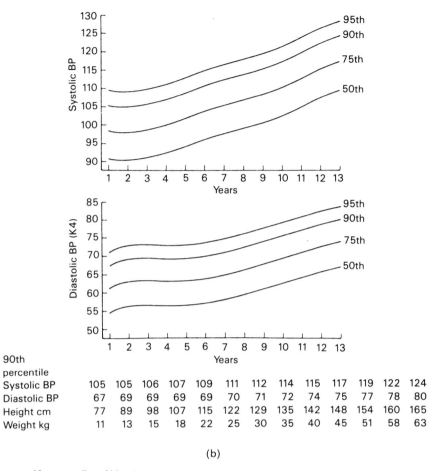

90th percentile													
Systolic BP	105	105	106	107	109	111	112	114	115	117	119	122	124
Diastolic BP	67	69	69	69	69	70	71	72	74	75	77	78	80
Height cm	77	89	98	107	115	122	129	135	142	148	154	160	165
Weight kg	11	13	15	18	22	25	30	35	40	45	51	58	63

(b)

Figure 15.2 Age-specific percentiles of blood pressure measurements in boys (a) and girls (b), 1–13 years of age (From Report of the Second Task Force on Blood Pressure Control in Children,[13] by permission)

is deflated, only give gross estimates of blood pressure and the so-called 'flush method' provides, at best, a mean blood pressure measurement.

Prevalence of hypertension

The prevalence of hypertension in childhood is not clearly defined and depends on the definition of hypertension chosen. Although considerable variation is reported in the literature, the true prevalence lies probably between 1% and 3%.[11] Studies reporting a much higher prevalence have often used a single blood pressure measurement, whereas in those in which multiple measurements have been undertaken the phenomenon of 'regression of blood pressure

toward the mean' is seen. The Muscatine Study[21] reported that 13% of their population were 'hypertensive' on initial measurements, but less than 1% had a persistently raised blood pressure.

The vast majority of children identified as having hypertension will have mild increases in blood pressure and presumably will come into the category of primary (essential) hypertension. However, a small number of children will have a much higher blood pressure (10% of those with hypertension; 0.1% of the population) and will, in the main, suffer from secondary hypertension and be the ones that will require treatment. In published series of hypertensive children, the proportion coming into the categories of primary and secondary depends very much on the nature of the referral pattern

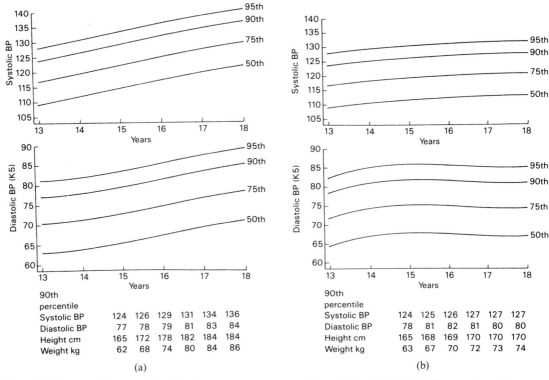

90th percentile						
Systolic BP	124	126	129	131	134	136
Diastolic BP	77	78	79	81	83	84
Height cm	165	172	178	182	184	184
Weight kg	62	68	74	80	84	86

(a)

90th percentile						
Systolic BP	124	125	126	127	127	127
Diastolic BP	78	81	82	81	80	80
Height cm	165	168	169	170	170	170
Weight kg	63	67	70	72	73	74

(b)

Figure 15.3 Age-specific percentiles of blood pressure measurements in boys (a) and girls (b), 13–18 years of age (From Report of the Second Task Force on Blood Pressure Control in Children,[13] by permission)

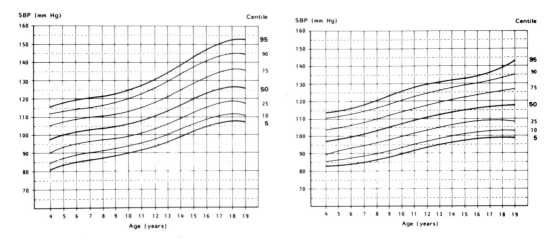

Figure 15.4 Age-specific percentiles of systolic blood pressure in boys (left) and girls (right) (From de Man *et al.*,[16] by permission)

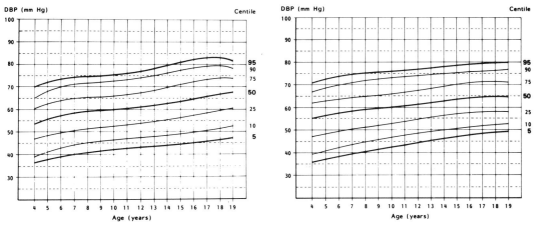

Figure 15.5 Age-specific percentiles of diastolic blood pressure in boys (left) and girls (right) (From de Man *et al.*, [16] by permission)

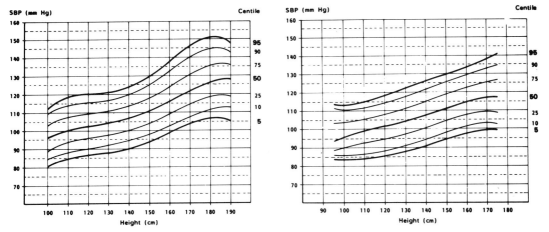

Figure 15.6 Height-specific percentiles of systolic blood pressure in boys (left) and girls (right) (From de Man *et al.*, [16] by permission)

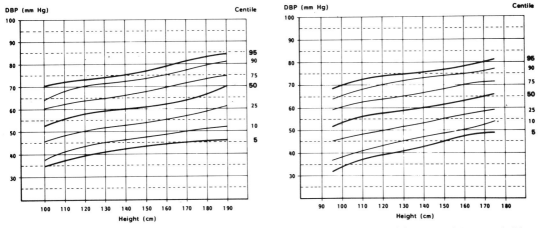

Figure 15.7 Height-specific percentiles of diastolic blood pressure in boys (left) and girls (right) (From de Man *et al.*, [16] by permission)

to the units concerned. Those dealing mainly with a relatively healthy population screened for hypertension as part of the routine clinical examination will identify a substantial proportion of mildly hypertensive children with primary hypertension. Tertiary referral hospitals to which are sent extremely sick children for treatment will proportionally have a much higher percentage of secondary hypertensive children within their hypertensive population.

Clinical features

Signs and symptoms of hypertension in childhood vary considerably and may be minimal even in the presence of markedly increased blood pressure. Unfortunately symptoms are often misinterpreted and children still present with features of malignant hypertension including loss of consciousness, convulsions and hemiplegia after a period of non-specific ill health during which the role of hypertension could only be detected by taking the blood pressure.

There are some differences in presenting features according to age. During infancy, congestive cardiac failure, respiratory distress, failure to thrive, vomiting and irritability are the most common features, whereas in older children headache, nausea, vomiting, polydipsia, polyuria, visual symptoms, tiredness, irritability, cardiac failure, facial weakness, epistaxis and growth retardation predominate.[11,22] Palpitations, sweating and pallor occur in catecholamine excess states but are not pathognomonic since they are also seen in other causes of hypertension such as renovascular disease.

Cardiomegaly or hypertensive retinopathy may be found on physical examination, but their absence does not exclude hypertension as a cause of symptoms and there may be other physical signs that might suggest an underlying cause for hypertension if detected or prompt the clinician to evaluate the blood pressure in an individual patient carefully. For example, delayed femoral pulses or a blood pressure difference between arms and legs may be found in coarctation of the aorta; a bruit in the abdomen or flank in renovascular disease; spinal, genital, perianal or abdominal wall abnormalities with neuropathic or obstructive bladder problems; abdominal masses with polycystic kidney disease, hydronephrosis, renal and adrenal tumours;

and clinical evidence of virilization or adrenocortical hyperfunction with adrenal enzymatic defects, adrenocortical malignancy or iatrogenic administration of steroids. A number of clinically recognizable syndromes are also associated with hypertension. Renovascular disease, for example, is seen in neurofibromatosis, Williams' syndrome, Marfan's syndrome, Klippel–Trenaunay–Weber syndrome, Feuerstein–Mims syndrome, and pseudoxanthoma elasticum; coarctation of aorta in Turner's syndrome and neurofibromatosis; phaeochromocytoma in von Hippel–Lindau disease, neurofibromatosis and multiple endocrine neoplasia syndromes types 1 and 2.

Complaints that are often not taken as seriously as they might but are particularly important include headache, facial palsy and visual impairment. It is mandatory to take the blood pressure in a child with a presenting feature of headache even though the history is suggestive of migraine or a refractive error. Similarly, a lower motor neuron facial palsy due to hypertensive damage to the facial nerve vasa nervorum is not an uncommon presenting feature of long-standing hypertension. The failure to take the blood pressure in a child with visual impairment may lead to permanent visual loss due to retinal damage, disc oedema, cortical pathway interruption, vitreous haemorrhage or ischaemic anterior optic neuropathy which are all serious manifestations of hypertensive end-organ damage. For further relevant reading, see References 3, 5 and 7.

Causes of hypertension

When considering the causes of hypertension in childhood there are advantages in differentiating between mild and severe hypertension, since the former is usually primary or essential in nature and the latter almost exclusively secondary. It is also helpful to distinguish between transient and sustained increases in blood pressure, although at presentation this may be impossible.

Transient hypertension

There are many conditions associated with short-lived increases in blood pressure that do not go on to develop sustained hypertension at a later stage. Within this group, although renal

Table 15.1   Causes of 'transient' hypertension in childhood

Acute glomerulonephritis
Henoch–Schoenlein nephritis
Haemolytic uraemic syndrome
Acute renal failure
Following urological surgery
Following renal transplantation

Acute hypovolaemia
- Nephrotic relapse
- Burns
- Renal, adrenal and gastrointestinal saline depletion

Central nervous system disease
- Tumour
- Infection
- Injury
- Fits

Guillain–Barré syndrome
Poliomyelitis
Familial dysautonomia
Hypercalcaemia
Lead poisoning

Drug therapy or overdose
- Corticosteroid
- Sympathomimetic
- Contraceptive pill

Excess administration of
- Blood
- Plasma
- Saline

Table 15.2   Causes of sustained hypertension in childhood

Coarctation hypertension
Saline-dependent hypertension
(advanced renal failure)
Renin–angiotensin hypertension
  Renovascular
  Parenchymal
  Tumours
Catecholamine hypertension
  Phaeochromocytoma
  Neuroblastoma
Corticosteroid hypertension
  Iatrogenic
  Congenital adrenal hyperplasia
  Conn's and Cushing's syndromes
Essential hypertension

disease predominates there are other causes that need to be considered, as listed in Table 15.1.

Sustained hypertension

In most cases, sustained hypertension, especially if severe, is likely to be due to renal disease. The major causes are given in Table 15.2.

The most important group numerically is that in which the hypertension is associated with activation of the renin–angiotensin system, although in the very young, coarctation of the aorta predominates. The proportion of children coming into the various categories as quoted in the literature depends, to an extent, on the clinical material referred to the centres involved and their particular expertise. Analysis of the experience at the Hospital for Sick Children, Great Ormond Street, London, of children admitted with severe sustained hypertension showed that 35.6% had coarse renal scarring, 23.3% glomerulonephritis, 9.5% renovascular disease, 5.5% renal polycystic disease, 4% previous haemolytic uraemic syndrome and 2.4% renal tumours. The remainder included 9.5% with coarctation of the aorta, 3.4% with essential hypertension, 2.8% with catecholamine excess and 4.6% who came into a miscellaneous group.[3,7,22]

Investigation

Strategy of investigation

How far investigation is justified depends on the severity and persistence of hypertension and the conditions under which it was detected. Mild hypertension found on routine examination in an asymptomatic child is a different situation to finding a markedly increased blood pressure in a symptomatic patient. If blood pressure is persistently increased, as opposed to a transient observation on an isolated occasion, investigation is indicated. The main question, however, is how far this should be taken and what is acceptable as an initial investigative protocol.

Borderline hypertension, namely systolic and/ or diastolic pressures within the upper range of normal but occasionally above, would require little more than a careful history and clinical examination with particular emphasis on family history of hypertension and the use of drugs, for example, the contraceptive pill in teenage girls. The most that might be indicated, in addition, would be a routine urine analysis, a check on renal function and perhaps an abdominal ultrasound.

Mild to moderate hypertension, namely blood pressure consistently exceeding the upper end of the normal range (for example the 95th percentile) without evidence of target organ involvement, will require more detailed evaluation. Apart from a full blood picture, routine plasma biochemistry including a plasma calcium

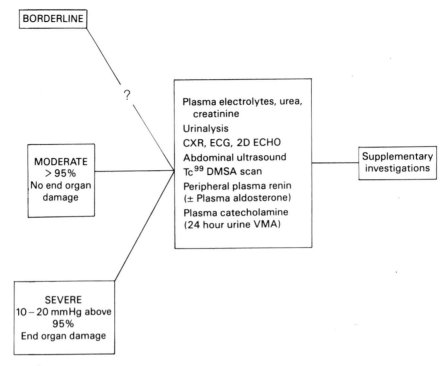

Figure 15.8 Evaluation strategy in childhood hypertension: initial investigations

measurement and urinalysis, slightly more detailed renal imaging should be undertaken such
as an abdominal ultrasound and a ^{99m}Tc-dimer-
captosuccinic acid (DMSA) scan. In addition, a
peripheral plasma renin activity, plus or minus
a plasma aldosterone concentration and some
measure of catecholamine production (24-hour
urine vanillyl mandelic acid excretion or a
plasma catecholamine measurement), would be
indicated. A measure of the end-organ effect of
the blood pressure on the heart might be judged
by a chest X-ray or electrocardiogram, but a
two-dimensional echocardiogram would be
more sensitive in detecting this.

Severe hypertension, namely blood pressure
consistently well above the upper end of the
normal range with or without target organ involvement, would require all the above investigations and, depending on the results, further
investigation as appropriate.

An attempt to illustrate the investigative steps
involved in evaluating hypertensive children of
varying severity is shown in Figures 15.8 and
15.9. References 3, 5, 7 and 23 will provide
additional detail for the subsequent sections on
specific aspects of investigation.

Renal imaging

For many years the intravenous urogram has
been the most appropriate means of demonstrating asymmetry of kidney size and function,
kidney displacement and the presence of structural abnormality including parenchymal loss.
Utilizing the rapid sequence technique, it has
been useful in demonstrating appearances suggestive of unilateral main renal artery stenosis (delayed nephrogram and dense prolonged pyelogram). However, its value in the investigation of
hypertension is now being questioned in view of
the availability of newer investigative modalities.

High-quality images obtained with ultrasound
have proved invaluable in assessing abdominal
masses, differentiating between solid and cystic
lesions, demonstrating gross degrees of scarring,
calculi and dilatation of the collecting systems.
However, it also has some limitations in terms
of hypertension investigation and can miss
upper renal pole pathology, is very much operator dependent and does not give information
regarding renal function. On the other hand, it
can provide non-invasively, information concerning renal blood flow using the so-called

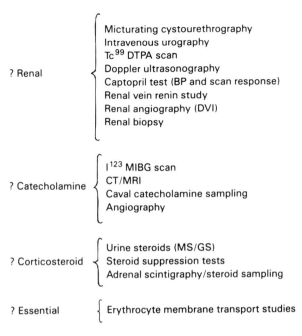

? Renal
- Micturating cystourethrography
- Intravenous urography
- Tc^{99} DTPA scan
- Doppler ultrasonography
- Captopril test (BP and scan response)
- Renal vein renin study
- Renal angiography (DVI)
- Renal biopsy

? Catecholamine
- I^{123} MIBG scan
- CT/MRI
- Caval catecholamine sampling
- Angiography

? Corticosteroid
- Urine steroids (MS/GS)
- Steroid suppression tests
- Adrenal scintigraphy/steroid sampling

? Essential
- Erythrocyte membrane transport studies

Figure 15.9 Evaluation strategy in childhood hypertension: supplementary investigations

'Doppler ultrasound' technique that can be helpful in renovascular disease evaluation.

Radionuclide imaging either by means of DMSA or ^{99m}Tc-diethylenetriaminepenta-acetic acid (DTPA) scanning has an important role in the investigation of childhood hypertension. DMSA is especially valuable in detecting pyelonephritic scarring and ischaemic areas due to renovascular disease as well as useful information concerning differential function. DTPA has not proved to be so helpful, although its value in obstructive uropathy and in providing information in terms of renal perfusion and glomerular function is acknowledged. Both scans, undertaken in conjunction with an oral dose of the ACE inhibitor captopril, may reveal evidence of renal ischaemia in renovascular disease not apparent in the non-captopril primed images. MAG3 scanning, recently introduced, may subsequently replace DMSA and DTPA since it appears to provide in one isotope study the information hitherto only available by undertaking both these longer established modalities of imaging.

Peripheral and renal vein renin measurements

In contrast with adult experience, peripheral plasma renin measurements are diagnostically valuable in children with secondary hypertension due to renovascular disease or renal scarring with values raised above the normal range in the majority of cases. Low values in a significantly hypertensive child point to a non-renin-dependent hypertensive state and if the values are extremely depressed suggest some form of mineralocorticoid excess.

Bilateral renal vein renin determinations have also been shown in childhood to be diagnostically valuable and to help in predicting surgical success in patients with renal lesions amenable to surgical treatment. In hypertensive children, a ratio of 1.5 or above between the renin values in the main renal veins points to asymmetrical release and, if the less affected kidney appears to have a suppressed renin release compared to the low IVC (< 1.3) and is otherwise normal, can be a predictor of success of surgery if this is indicated. A refinement of main renal vein renin sampling is to sample from segmental veins allowing local sources of renin release to be identified and eliminate false negative main vein ratios in situations where local scarring or segmental pathology exists.

Pharmacological blockade of renin–angiotensin system

The magnitude of the hypotensive response to an oral dose (0.7 mg/kg) of the ACE inhibitor captopril, has been shown to be of value in identifying children who have hypertension associated with hyperreninaemia.[24] The findings utilizing this technique do not help in terms of identifying the underlying pathology causing the hypertension nor in terms of predicting the outcome of surgical intervention, which is not surprising. Unfortunately some workers thought it might and inappropriately criticized the technique as a result. Administering captopril as a means of sensitizing DMSA and DTPA scans in suspected renovascular disease is another valuable extension of the above technique alluded to earlier in this chapter.

Angiography and digital vascular imaging

Angiographic investigation in childhood hypertension is most commonly indicated in renovascular disease to demonstrate abnormal main and intrarenal arterial anatomy. Other situations in which it has a role include coarctation of the aorta, renal tumours, phaeochromocytomas and adrenocortical tumours. Most studies nowadays are undertaken using the digital vascular imaging technique allowing very small quantities of contrast medium to be used, with obvious advantages in childhood. However, there is some loss of definition, especially in relation to small intrarenal vessels that can be a problem with very peripheral intrarenal vascular disease. This problem is very much more pronounced with intravenously administered contrast which is not recommended if arterial anatomy is to be examined. Cerebral angiography is at times required especially in relation to renovascular hypertension, since 50% of children with renovascular disease plus cerebral symptoms have arterial abnormalities in the intracranial vascular tree.[25]

Catecholamines and MIBG scanning

The measurement of urinary vanillyl mandelic acid (VMA) is the commonest screening test for phaeochromocytoma. However, a normal VMA excretion does not exclude the diagnosis of phaeochromocytoma and many units now utilize random plasma catecholamine measurements in addition. Plasma noradrenaline concentration is invariably increased in patients with phaeochromocytoma, irrespective of the level of the blood pressure and even betwen paroxysms.[26]

The localization of catecholamine-producing tumours involves, additionally, the utilization of radiolabelled (I^{123}) meta-iodobenzyl guanidine (MIBG) which concentrates in active sympathetic tissue[27] and vena caval plasma catecholamine sampling from the neck to the pelvis.[26,27]

Other investigative procedures

Urine steroid analysis may prove diagnostically helpful in the context of mineralocorticoid excess states such as 11β-hydroxylase deficiency, Conn's syndrome and cortisol 11β-hydroxysteroid dehydrogenase deficiency. In addition, a variety of stimulation and suppression tests are available for investigating Cushing's and Conn's syndromes and low renin hypertensive states. Computerized tomographic (CT) scanning and MRI scanning both have roles in identifying the presence of and the exact position of intra-abdominal masses such as phaeochromocytomas and other adrenal tumours. Measurement of erythrocyte intracellular sodium, the number of Na/K ATPase pump sites or Na/Li counter transport in red cells may provide clues to the propensity to develop essential hypertension, but so far are not reliably utilized to discriminate in individual cases.[28,29]

Treatment

This term encompasses the medical and surgical treatment of hypertension and can be considered under general management, antihypertensive drugs, medical management of the hypertensive emergency, medical management of moderate to severe hypertension, treatment of mild or borderline hypertension, and special situations including catecholamine excess, mineralocorticoid excess and surgical management. It is, however, important to appreciate that there is no clear-cut distinctions between various forms of treatment, and many hypertensive children require a combination of general measures, drug therapy and surgical intervention.

The difficult question to address is 'What are the indications for antihypertensive therapy?' There is usually no controversy about the need to treat severe hypertension in view of the known morbidity and mortality associated if treatment is not introduced. The problems arise when considering milder forms of hypertension. How much the blood pressure deviates from normal, its constancy, what is considered to be the cause and the presence of risk factors, such as a hypertensive family history, may all influence the decision to treat or not. A symptomatic child, a child with target organ involvement, a child with cardiomegaly or left ventricular hypertrophy or a child with an underlying cause that is known to be associated with an inevitable rise in blood pressure to unacceptable levels will require treatment. The balance that has to be achieved is one in which there is short- or long-term advantage to the child, bearing in mind the side effects and complications of the drugs or surgical procedures involved. This is not always easy to achieve and caution may be necessary at times, with a period of observation rather than therapy being the best course of action. A number of references are germane to the various aspects of treatment that follow and include References 3,5,7,23,30 and 31.

General management

The majority of hypertensive patients irrespective of whether they require drugs or surgical treatment will require general, non-specific advice concerning diet, exercise and life style. In circumstances of mild hypertension they may be the only therapeutic manoeuvres necessary.

Current evidence suggests that modest reduction in dietary sodium intake can have a blood pressure lowering effect in mildly hypertensive adults, although this is controversial. In children on treatment with antihypertensive drugs, sodium restriction is not mandatory but it is reasonable to restrict the addition of table salt or the use of salty processed foods. Popular 'junk foods' are heavily laden with sodium and it would seem appropriate that this particular type of food should be singled out for exclusion or limitation. Potassium supplementation may also have a hypotensive role and could be a useful adjunct in the management of essential hypertension but it is obviously contraindicated in the presence of renal impairment.

Weight loss would seem appropriate in view of the known association between blood pressure with body mass and there is evidence that it can lower blood pressure in hypertensive individuals.

Modest regular exercise, for example 'jogging', has been shown to reduce blood pressure in adults with essential hypertension. It would seem appropriate for exercise to be taken except in circumstances of poorly controlled hypertension.

Antihypertensive drugs

Experience with antihypertensive therapy is much more limited in children than in adults, so that subtleties differentiating individual drugs within particular groups have limited relevance. More important is the fact that a drug has been shown to be both safe and effective in clinical use, and this often means that drugs used in children are somewhat 'behind the times' by adult standards.

The main drugs available can be classified as (a) α- and β-adrenergic blockers, (b) diuretics, (c) vasodilators including calcium-channel blockers, and (d) renin–angiotensin inhibitors. The great majority of patients will be managed well by choosing from a very limited number of drugs. Dosages of the more commonly used agents are given in Table 15.3 and 15.4.

β-Adrenergic receptor blocking agents

These drugs act by competitive inhibition of catecholamines on β-receptor mediated effects on heart and kidney, at presynaptic β-receptors of postganglionic nerve endings, and in the central nervous system. Cardiac output falls, renin release is inhibited, noradrenaline release is impaired peripherally and there is also a centrally-mediated reduction in peripheral sympathetic activity.

Propranolol is the best-known example of this group and still remains one of the drugs of choice, in spite of potentially serious adverse effects, mainly on the heart and lungs. Side effects include the worsening of cardiac failure if present already, bradycardia, bronchospasm, hypoglycaemia, which is rare but can be a problem in diabetes, and some sodium and water retention. Others are Raynaud's phenomenon, nightmares and hallucinations, about which the family should be warned, nausea, diarrhoea and lethargy.

There is no convincing evidence that one beta-blocker is any more effective than any other in lowering the blood pressure if administered in appropriate dosage. More cardioselective drugs such as atenolol may have a place,

Table 15.3   Drug treatment of acute hypertension (From Houtman and Dillon,[31] by permission)

Drug	Dose	Action	Comment
Labetalol	1–3 mg kg^{-1} h^{-1} i.v.	Alpha- and beta-blocker	Drug of choice
Sodium nitroprusside	0.5–8.0 μg kg^{-1} min^{-1} i.v.	Direct vasodilator	Drug of choice
Nifedipine	0.25–0.5 mg/kg sublingually	Calcium channel inhibitor	Drug of choice
Hydralazine	0.1–0.2 mg/kg i.v.	Direct vasodilator	Second-line drug
Frusemide	0.5–2.0 mg/kg i.v.	Loop diuretic	Diuretic of choice
Diazoxide	2–10 mg/kg i.v.	Direct vasodilator	Second-line drug
Clonidine	2–6 μg/kg i.v.	Central adrenergic stimulant	Second-line drug

Table 15.4   Commoner oral drugs used in the treatment of hypertension (From Houtman and Dillon,[31] by permission)

Drug	Oral dose (mg kg^{-1} day^{-1}) Initial	Maximum	Action	Comment
Propranolol	1–2 mg	8–10 mg	Beta-blocker	A drug of choice
Atenolol	1 mg	2 mg	Cardioselective beta-blocker	Once daily
Phenoxybenzamine	1 mg	4 mg	Alpha-blocker	Drug of choice in phaeochromocytoma
Prazosin	0.05–0.1 mg	0.4 mg	Selective alpha-blocker	A drug of choice
Hydrochlorothiazide	1 mg	4 mg	Thiazide diuretic	A drug of choice
Frusemide	0.5–1 mg	15 mg	Loop diuretic	A drug of choice
Spironolactone	1 mg	3 mg	Aldosterone antagonist	Valuable in some mineralocorticoid excess states
Hydralazine	1–2 mg	8 mg	Direct vasodilator	A drug of choice
Nifedipine	0.25 mg	1–2 mg	Calcium channel inhibitor	A drug of choice
Captopril	0.3 mg	5 mg	Converting enzyme inhibitor	A drug of choice
Minoxidil	0.1–0.2 mg	1–2 mg	Vasodilator	Second-line drug

when a beta-blocker is considered essential, in the presence of an asthmatic history, but in moderate or severe asthma other antihypertensives should be used. Indeed there are some who would avoid the use of any beta-blocker, selective or not, in all patients with an asthmatic tendency. Atenolol is also attractive because of its long half-life and may be given once daily, although, as with many drugs, optimal oral dose and dosage frequency in children are not well defined.

α-Adrenergic receptor blockers

Phenoxybenzamine, which is a long-acting agent, has a special place in the management of phaeochromocytomas, both preoperatively and for prolonged treatment if the tumour is not amenable to surgery. A β-adrenergic antagonist is usually also employed in order to block the effects of catecholamines on the heart. The more general use of phenoxybenzamine is no longer recommended, in view of worries concerning carcinogenicity in animal experiments (Smith Kline Beecham, personal communication). The perioperative care of the patient may also include the use of phentolamine, a short-acting α-receptor blocking drug, effective within 30 s when given intravenously.

Prazosin, and more recently doxazosin, are two examples of drugs with high selectivity for $α_1$-adrenoceptors. Because of complex differential receptor structure at pre- and post-synaptic sites, these drugs preserve feedback control of noradrenaline release, consequently causing minimal reflex activation with its associated tachycardia and increased cardiac output, compared to the older classic α-adrenoceptor blockers, which were disappointing as antihypertensive agents used alone. Side effects are generally mild, with occasional postural dizziness, especially after the first dose, lethargy, fluid retention, blurred vision and dry mouth. Prazosin, often combined with a beta-blocker, is a popular agent in children, but it is debatable whether it has any advantage over a vasodilator such as hydralazine. This class of drugs is also of benefit for treating catecholamine-excess hypertension.

Labetalol

This is an agent with unique and complex pharmacological properties: it exhibits both selective α_1- and non-selective β-adrenergic blocking activity, although it is less active at α_1- than at β-adrenoceptors. It may be administered intravenously or orally, but has no clear advantage over alternative therapy for long-term use, in particular because of the inability to vary independently the relative degrees of alpha- and beta-blockade. Its main value in children is in the management of hypertensive emergencies (see below). Side effects and contraindications mainly relate to the β-blocking activity, but a toxic myopathy has been described.

Diuretics

The major action of the thiazide group of diuretics is to cause extracellular fluid volume depletion by inhibiting sodium transport in the early distal tubule, but they act in part by reducing peripheral vascular resistance. Most are readily absorbed from the gastrointestinal tract and cause a diuretic effect within an hour after administration. Clearance is primarily renal. Although the popular drugs in this group may be given 12 hourly to maintain maximal diuretic effect, they are usually given in the early morning so that diuresis does not interfere with sleep. The major unwanted effect is hypokalaemia, which may require either potassium supplementation or combination therapy with a potassium-sparing diuretic. Clinical toxicity is relatively rare, but sometimes results from unexpected hypersensitivity to the agents.

Unlike the thiazide diuretics with a relatively flat dose–response curve, the loop diuretics are capable of inducing a peak diuresis much greater than that with other agents. Their use is thus usually restricted to patients with significant fluid retention as part of their disease or as a result of the other hypotensive therapy being used. The main side effects are hypokalaemia, volume depletion and ototoxicity. The ototoxicity is related to high blood levels, and the risk is greatest in the presence of renal impairment. Frusemide is the recommended drug in this category for use in children.

Other diuretics have particular therapeutic use relating to hypertension. Spironolactone, a competitive antagonist of aldosterone, has a role in patients with aldosterone excess (adrenal hyperplasia or adenoma), and as an adjunct to a potassium-losing diuretic. Side effects include hyperkalaemia, gynaecomastia and menstrual irregularities. Amiloride and triamterene, also potassium-sparing drugs, are relatively weak diuretics used alone, but are often used in clinical states similar to those in which spironolactone is appropriate. They are particularly helpful in low-renin hypertension caused by 11β-hydroxysteroid dehydrogenase deficiency.

Vasodilators

These are a pharmacologically heterogeneous group of drugs which share vasodilatation as their major antihypertensive effect.

Although hydralazine was introduced into clinical practice well over 30 years ago, it fell into disfavour because of excessive side effects when it was given alone, or in combination with a ganglionic blocking agent. However it now enjoys new popularity, since many of its unwanted side effects are minimized when it is used in smaller doses concurrently with a diuretic and a β-adrenergic antagonist. Side effects include flushing, headache, tachycardia, palpitations, increased cardiac output, and salt and water retention. A lupus erythematosus-like reaction is dose-related and disappears when the drug is discontinued. The risk is greatest in slow acetylators who metabolize the drug more slowly, but in practice knowledge of acetylation status is not essential before commencing therapy.

Minoxidil is also a powerful vasodilator acting on systemic arterioles but its high incidence of side effects, including fluid retention and hypertrichosis, preclude it as a first-line hypotensive agent. However it is of value in relatively drug-resistant hypertensive states.

Sodium nitroprusside remains a drug of choice in the treatment of hypertensive crises (see below). Given intravenously it acts within seconds, and its effect lasts for a matter of minutes only. It requires considerable nursing care in order for its use to be considered safe, and a practical disadvantage is its inactivation by light. It is metabolized to cyanide and thiocyanate; in fact, cyanide toxicity is rare, but may occur when the patient receives an excessive dose or has liver impairment.

For many years diazoxide was the drug of choice for hypertensive emergencies. It is a non-diuretic thiazide with a direct vasodilator action. The effects of a single intravenous dose may last for up to 12 h, but there are serious risks of acute hypotension occurring shortly after the injection. Other side effects include salt and water retention, hyperglycaemia, hyperuricaemia, hypertrichosis, nausea, vomiting, and an unusual metallic taste in the mouth. It has been largely superseded by more easily titratable drugs, but it may still have a role if administered in small repeated bolus injections, or even perhaps in a carefully controlled infusate.

The calcium channel blockers have emerged as a new class of drug with great potential for manipulation of blood pressure. Their action interferes with the inward displacement of calcium ions through the slow channels of active cell membranes. However they differ in their predilection for the various possible sites of action, including myocardial cells, cells within the specialized conducting system of the heart, and those of vascular smooth muscle. Their therapeutic effects therefore differ, with much greater variation than that of beta-blockers. Nifedipine has now been used extensively, particularly in the management of acute hypertensive emergencies when given by the sublingual route (see below), but also in other hypertensive situations, including the successful medical management of a number of patients with phaeochromocytomas when used alone prior to surgery. Side effects include headache, flushing and tachycardia. Verapamil, used extensively in adults, has also been used in childhood, but it has a greater tendency to interact with other agents. It has a potential for major interaction with cyclosporin, resulting in reduced cyclosporin elimination, and should not normally be used in combination with a beta-blocker in view of the risk of hypotension and asystole, especially if there is coexisting cardiac impairment.

Angiotensin-converting enzyme (ACE) inhibitors

The introduction of the ACE inhibitors has been among the major pharmacological developments in recent years. These drugs are now assured of an important place in the current management of hypertension. They act by inhibiting the conversion of angiotensin I to angiotensin II resulting in lowered periperhal arteriolar resistance, although it is considered that the haemodynamic response is at least partially mediated by an effect on prostaglandins and the kallikrein–kinin system.

Captopril has now been used successfully in children for some years. It may be especially effective in hypertension associated with high peripheral renin. It is readily absorbed after oral dosage, and peak blood levels are reached in 30–90 min. Elimination is mainly by renal excretion, and although half-life is less than 2 h, the pharmacodynamic half-life is much longer, necessitating twice or three times daily dosage. Clearance is delayed in renal failure, so that dose frequency may require decreasing.

There are few side effects, but these include neutropenia and agranulocytosis, rashes and angioedema of the face, persistent cough, and a taste disturbance. The incidence of proteinuria associated with the drug, originally thought to be substantial, has diminished considerably more recently, concomitant with the use of relatively smaller doses. The most worrying feature of its use is in patients with reduced renal perfusion, as is the case in severe renovascular disease, especially critical main artery stenosis, in which there may be a serious deterioration in renal function, due to a deleterious effect on glomerular haemodynamics distal to the stenosis. These circumstances are a relative contraindication to the use of an ACE inhibitor, and certainly serum creatinine should be monitored regularly before and during treatment.

Enalapril is a newer drug in this group not used extensively in children, but has the potential advantage of once-daily administration, and overall treatment is cheaper.

Other agents

Clonidine lowers blood pressure primarily by stimulating α_2-adrenergic receptors in the brain, although the precise mechanism of action is still relatively obscure. It has the disadvantage of causing rebound hypertension on stopping the drug, a risk which is greater in children where adherence to therapy is often uncertain, but still has a role in multi-drug resistant hypertension. Methyldopa has a similar action to clonidine but is not now normally used because of its effect on mood and the risk of serious hypersensitivity reactions. Other drugs such as reserpine, guanethidine and hexamethonium are

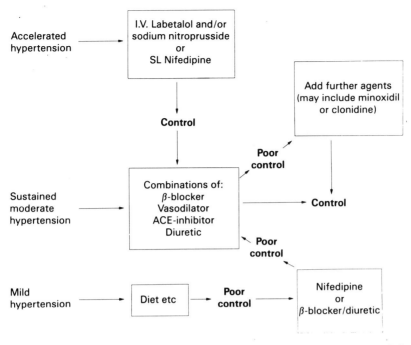

Figure 15.10 Flow chart of treatment in childhood hypertension (From Houtman and Dillon,[31] by permission)

not recommended, in view of their high incidence of troublesome side effects.

Management issues

How to go about managing hypertension, like so many things in medicine, is coloured by the experience of the clinician, the practice in the institution in which he or she works, the availability of hypotensive agents and the current climate relating to therapy both in adults and children. The outcome is a mixture of rational scientific medicine and clinical pragmatism based on experience. There are a number of 'right' ways to do it and rather more 'wrong' ways. In an attempt to illustrate the practice at the Hospital for Sick Children, Great Ormond Street, Figure 15.10 is a flow chart of suggested treatment of childhood hypertension, and the following sections will deal with several aspects in more detail.

Hypertensive emergencies

Emergency management is indicated when the level of blood pressure is a threat to life or to the function of vital organs. Drugs with a rapid action are necessary, but with no shortage of powerful antihypertensives available, the important issue is how to reduce the blood pressure safely to prevent sudden hypotension and the resulting failure to autoregulatory mechanisms. Thus, bolus injections of diazoxide are no longer recommended as first-line treatment, and drugs which can be infused to control blood pressure finely during the critical initial period are preferred. Sodium nitroprusside and labetalol are both effective; labetalol may be more appropriate for initial use as its method of administration is simpler. Intravenous therapy is indicated in non-co-operative patients, in the presence of encephalopathic symptoms, and when patients are vomiting. However, in recent years orally-administered drugs have been used in malignant hypertension, and in particular, sublingual nifedipine has gained favour as a first-line treatment of acute severe hypertension in childhood. Apart from its ease of administration and its absence of serious side effects, it may be that the risk of cerebral ischaemia is reduced as it tends to increase cerebral blood flow.

In order to reduce blood pressure sufficiently to avoid hypertensive complications, yet to maintain it at a level that permits autoregulatory mechanisms to function and ensure an adequate blood supply to the brain and other viscera, management goals need to be well defined. In this regard, it is important to be aware of the degree of chronicity of the hypertension. Thus, it may be sensible to decrease blood pressure in the first 6–12 h by not more than one-third of the total reduction planned, followed by a further third over the next 24 h and the final third over the next 2–4 days. Even slower approaches to the gradual reduction in blood pressure are often justified, especially if levels have been raised for a considerable period. An intravenous line should be accessible during the early period, so that plasma volume can be improved if the blood pressure drops unexpectedly. In difficult cases a central venous line is also valuable. It is safer to reserve the use of a diuretic until the acute phase is successfully managed, as many children with severe hypertension on presentation have extracellular fluid depletion. After the initial period of stabilization the transfer to suitable oral medication, if required, should be gradual, and the potential difficulties during this period should not be underestimated.

Moderate to severe chronic hypertension

In this situation, there is time to identify the cause of the hypertension and prescribe accordingly – a very different circumstance to that present when treating hypertensive emergencies. Special cases will clearly include those patients with coarctation of the aorta, catecholamine or corticosteroid excess hypertension, and renal failure, particularly those on dialysis or after renal transplantation.

Except for these special category patients, most chronically hypertensive children respond well to an approach which includes the combination of a vasodilator and a beta-blocker, with or without a diuretic. The International Committee of the Second International Symposium on Hypertension in Children and Adolescents[5] recommended a 'stepped-care' approach, starting with a low dose of either a diuretic or beta-blocker, building slowly to therapeutic levels. They caution against high-dose monotherapy because of side effects, and early combination of two or more drugs is recommended. Further approaches may include the use of an ACE inhibitor and another vasodilator, although it

is now controversial as to whether or not an ACE inhibitor should be among the first-line agents, especially as most children in this category will have some form of renin-dependent hypertension. The use of several drugs together should probably be supervised at a specialized centre and, as always, the principles of good prescribing apply in that it is best to keep to small numbers of drugs that are known well in the department caring for the child.

Mild hypertension

When a child is symptomatic or when there is evidence of proteinuria, cardiomegaly, or left ventricular hypertrophy, or if the cause is known to lead to progressive hypertension, treatment is clearly indicated. Mild hypertension poses a much greater problem in determining treatment. The non-pharmacological strategies mentioned above should be tried first if appropriate, but if blood pressure is still raised, there is a dilemma concerning the appropriateness of drug treatment. Unfortunately there are no follow-up studies of sufficient duration to allow accurate assessment of the effect of antihypertensives on morbidity and mortality when treatment is initiated in childhood or adolescence. In particular, there are worries concerning the adverse long-term effects of beta-blockers, and in particular, thiazide diuretics, on lipid metabolism,[24] so that, in the adult field at least, it may be that some of the newer agents acting on α-receptors are better drugs for first-line therapy of mild hypertension. Another concern is the possible effect on mental status and cognitive function of therapy, but there are few data concerning prolonged treatment. It is fair to say that there is as yet no unified agreement as to the best first-line agent for mild hypertension in childhood.

Special situations including surgical management

Treatment of hypertension of chronic renal failure

The treatment of the hypertension of chronic renal failure is essentially orientated towards salt and water depletion by dietary, diuretic or dialysis means. Standard hypotensive agents may also be required and, occasionally, bilateral native nephrectomy.

Renovascular disease

Renovascular disease may be managed surgically by nephrectomy, partial nephrectomy, revascularization by reconstructive vascular surgery, and autotransplantation. The development of interventional radiology has allowed intraluminal dilatation or angioplasty also to be undertaken. Decisions concerning surgical feasibility and likely outcome in terms of cure of hypertension require much care and the information provided by the refined investigative procedures already described.

The ideal lesion for revascularization surgery or intraluminal angioplasty is a unilateral, short-segment, main renal artery stenosis with no evidence of intrarenal or contralateral renal artery disease and clear lateralization of renin release to the affected side. To eliminate false positive or negative main renal vein renin ratios, segmental renal vein renin sampling is mandatory. Bilateral main renal artery stenosis and also intrarenal segmental artery stenoses are amenable to revascularization or angioplastic techniques, but preoperative anatomical and functional localization is essential before proceeding. For segmental lesions, heminephrectomy may prove to be the procedure of choice. Surgical techniques include saphenous vein bypass and autogenous arterial grafts, splenorenal, hepatorenal, internal iliac renal anastomoses, the use of Dacron grafts and autotransplantation.

Patients with renovascular disease may also have significant arterial abnormalities involving extrarenal arteries including the splenic, mesenteric, hepatic and cerebral vessels. Of these, cerebrovascular disease is the most important in view of the risks involved in controlling blood pressure with powerful hypotensive agents that might compromise the brain's blood supply. Revacularization of the brain by extra-intracranial arterial anastomosis has occasionally been necessary in these circumstances.[25]

Renal parenchymal disease

The mainstay of treatment in renal parenchymal disease is adequate medical management of blood pressure. However, in certain circumstances, there is a role for surgery. Cure of hypertension may be possible by removal of a small scarred kidney affected by reflux nephropathy, renal dysplasia or renal vein thrombosis, or even partial nephrectomy on occasions for polar scarring. Preoperative ^{99m}Tc-DMSA scanning and segmental renal vein renin sampling will allow identification of local areas of scarring amenable to selective surgery.

Phaeochromocytoma

Surgery is the treatment of choice in phaeochromocytoma once adequate sympathetic blockade has been achieved pharmacologically. The drug treatment of catecholamine excess hypertension is aimed at controlling the blood pressure by adequate α- and possible β-sympathetic blockade. Phenoxybenzamine and propranolol or prazosin and propranolol are useful combinations, but recently nifedipine has been shown to be of considerable value. Parenteral labetolol is at times necessary in accelerated hypertensive states, but the blood pressure can also be managed by agents such as sodium nitroprusside if alpha-blockers are seemingly only partly successful. Adequate localization of the catecholamine-producing lesion must be achieved preoperatively utilizing a combination of investigation procedures already outlined, including ultrasound, MIBG scanning, computerized tomography and caval catecholamine sampling. Surgery should be undertaken with arterial and venous lines *in situ* and adequate supplies of short-acting hypotensive agents available (phentolamine, labetalol, sodium nitroprusside) and supplies of plasma or blood to replete the vascular space if necessary. The type of anaesthesia needs careful selection to avoid utilizing an agent that elicits sympathetic activity. Halothane is the favoured agent. Handling the tumour can produce catastrophic increases in blood pressure and, on ligating the tumour veins, there can be a sudden expansion of the vascular compartment causing hypotension. The outlook surgically is good but occasionally malignant change is seen.

Corticosteroid excess hypertension

Hypertension due to 11β- and 17α-hydroxylase deficiency is treated with hydrocortisone, Conn's syndrome with spironolactone followed by surgery for adrenal adenoma or with spironolactone alone for hyperplasia. Cushing's syndrome hypertension may be controlled with spironolactone, but usually requires standard hypotensives as well, in addition to surgical intervention eventually. Cortisol 11β-hydroxysteroid dehydrogenase deficiency causing hypertension is treated with spironolactone and triamterene.

Blood pressure screening

Screening for asymptomatic elevation of blood pressure in children could be justified on two grounds.[19] First, it will allow the detection of secondary hypertension due to potentially serious underlying disorders such as coarctation of the aorta, renal or endocrine disease prior to symptoms becoming apparent. However, of the 1% or so of schoolchildren with a raised blood pressure, only 10% (0.1% of the population) will have such hypertension and the remainder will have mild hypertension that will turn out to be, if anything, primary or essential. There are certainly advantages in detecting these severely hypertensive children, but the number detected by screening programmes is likely to be very small (1 in 1000) for the effort that would be required.

The second ground for considering a screening programme would be that it would detect children with mild increases in blood pressure who have an increased risk of developing essential hypertension in adult life. Unfortunately the cost–benefit ratio in identifying those with primary hypertension remains unclear.[8] This conclusion is based on the analysis of tracking data in a number of studies in childhood. Although it is known that some children maintain their peer rank order of blood pressure as they mature, there are others who increase or decrease their rank order. The correlation coefficients between initial and follow-up blood pressure levels in a number of studies are relatively low and insufficiently consistent to allow predictions of future blood pressure levels from initial recordings, especially in young children. However, this may not apply in adolescence, where blood pressure recordings in the upper quintile of the normal range for age or size may have greater predictive value for future hypertension than in early childhood.

The British Hypertension Society Working Party on Blood Pressure Measurement and the Joint Working Party on Child Health Surveillance have both considered this issue and neither recommended that there should be mass screening for blood pressure at school medical examinations.[32]

In the USA the Task Force also takes this view by not recommending mass community screening programmes for children and adolescents.[13] It does, however, focus on surveillance of blood pressure of children under continuous care by primary physicians and recommends, in accordance with the guidelines of the American Academy of Pediatrics, annual determinations of blood pressure in children by their primary physicians. These somewhat ambiguous messages might cause confusion but are of no relevance in countries where primary physicians are predominantly concerned with treating the sick rather than undertaking health checks on well children.

References

1. Still J.L. and Cottom D. Severe hypertension in childhood. *Arch. Dis. Child.* 1967, **42**, 34–49
2. Giovannelli G., New M.I. and Gorini S. (eds) *Hypertension in Children and Adolescents.* New York, Raven Press, 1981
3. Inglefinger J.R. *Pediatric Hypertension.* Philadelphia, Saunders, 1982
4. Portman R.J. and Robson A.M. Controversies in pediatric hypertension. In: Tune B.M. and Mendoza S.A. (eds) *Pediatric Nephrology*, pp. 265–296 (in *Contemporary Issues in Nephrology*, Vol. 12. New York, Churchill Livingstone), 1984.
5. Proceedings of the Second International Symposium on Hypertension in Children and Adolescents. *Clinical and Experimental Hypertension*, 1986: 479–918
6. Hofman A., Grobbee D.E. and Schalekamp M.A.D.H. (eds) *The Early Pathogenesis of Primary Hypertension.* Amsterdam, Excerpta Medica, 1987
7. Ingelfinger J.R. and Dillon M.J. Evaluation of secondary hypertension. In: Holliday M.A., Barratt T.M. and Avner A.D. (eds) *Pediatric Nephrology*, 3rd edn. Baltimore, Williams and Wilkins, 1994: 1146–1164
8. Dillon M.J. Blood pressure. *Arch. Dis. Child.* 1988, **63**, 347–349
9. Adelman R.D. and Bullaboy C.A. Pediatric hypertension. *Curr. Opinion Pediatr.* 1991, **3**, 268–271
10. Pickering G.W. *High Blood Pressure.* London, Churchill, 1955
11. Leumann E.P. Blood pressure and hypertension in childhood and adolescence. *Ergebn. Inn. Med. Kinderheilk.* 1979, **43**, 109–183
12. Report of the Task Force on Blood Pressure Control in Children. *Pediatrics*, 1977, **59**, 797–820
13. Report of the Second Task Force on Blood Pressure Control in Children. *Pediatrics*, 1987, **79**, 1–25
14. de Swiet M., Fayers P. and Shinebourne E.A. Blood pressure survey in a population of newborn infants. *Br. Med. J.*, **2**, 9–11
15. de Swiet M., Fayers P. and Shinebourne E.A. Systolic blood pressure in a population of infants in the first year of life: the Brompton Study. *Pediatricss*, 1980, **65**, 1028–1035
16. de Man S.A., Andre J.-L., Bachmann H., Grobbee

D.E., Ibsen K.K., Laaser W., Lippert P. and Hofman A. Blood pressure in childhood: pooled findings in six European studies. *J. Hypertens.* 1991, **9**, 109–114.

17. de Swiet M., Fayers P.M. and Shinebourne E.A. Blood pressure in the first 10 years of life – the Brompton Study. *Br. Med. J.* 1992, **304**, 23–26

18. de Swiet M., Dillon M.J., Littler W., O'Brien E., Padfield P.L. and Petrie J.C. Measurement of blood pressure in children. Recommendations of a Working Party of the British Hypertension Society. *Br. Med. J.* 1989, **299**, 497

19. Houtman P. and Dillon M.J. Routine measurement of blood pressure in school children. *Arch. Dis. Child.* 1991, **66**, 567–568

20. Dillon M.J. Blood pressure measurement in childhood. In: O'Brien, E. and O'Malley K. (eds) *Handbook of Hypertension*, Vol. 14: Blood Pressure Measurement. Amsterdam, Elsevier 1991: 126–138

21. Rames L.K., Clarke W.R., Connor W.E., Reiter M.A. and Lauer R.M. Normal blood pressure and the evolution of sustained blood pressure elevation in childhood. The Muscatine Study. *Pediatrics*, 1978, **61**, 245–251

22. Gill D.G., Mendes da Costa B., Cameron J.S., Joseph M.C., Ogg C.S. and Chantler C. Analysis of 100 children with severe and persistent hypertension. *Arch. Dis. Child.* 1976, **51**, 951–956

23. Dillon M.J. Investigation and management of hypertension in children. A personal perspective. *Ped. Nephrol.* 1987, **1**, 59–68

24. Daman Willems C., Shah V., Uchiyama M. and Dillon M.J. Captopril as an aid to diagnosis in childhood hypertension. *Arch. Dis. Child.* 1989, **64**, 229–234

25. Daman Willems C.E., Salisbury D.M., Lumley J.S.P. and Dillon M.J. Brain revascularization in hypertension. *Arch. Dis. Child.* 1985, **60**, 1177–1179

26. Sever P.S., Roberts J.C. and Snell M.E. Phaeochromocytoma. *Clin. Endocrin. Metab.* 1980, **9**, 543–568

27. Deal J.E., Sever P.S., Barratt T.M. and Dillon M.J. Phaeochromocytoma – investigation and management of 10 cases. *Arch. Dis. Child.* 1990, **65**, 269–274

28. Uchiyama M., Shah V., Daman Willems C.E. and Dillon M.J. Sodium transport in erythrocytes: differences between normal children and children with primary and secondary hypertension. *Arch. Dis. Child.* 1989, **64**, 224–228

29. Deal J.E., Shah V., Goodenough G. and Dillon M.J. Red cell membrane sodium transport: possible genetic role and use in identifying patients at risk of essential hypertension. *Arch. Dis. Child.* 1990, **65**, 1154–1157

30. Dillon M.J. and Ingelfinger J.R. Pharmacological treatment of hypertension. In: Holliday M.A., Barratt T.M. and Avner A.D. (eds) *Pediatric Nephrology*, 3rd edn. Baltimore, Williams and Wilkins, 1994: 1165–1174

31. Houtman P. and Dillon M.J. The medical management of hypertension in childhood. *Child Nephrol. Urol.* 1992, **12**, 154–161

32. Hall D.M.B. *Health for All Children. A Programme for Child Health Surveillance.* Oxford, Oxford University Press, 1989

16

Classification and concepts of glomerular injury

A.J. Fish

Classification of glomerular injury

Various classifications of glomerulonephritis have been proposed based on pathogenetic mechanisms, histopathological features of the glomerular lesions, and disease aetiology. Some forms of glomerulonephritis are known to be immunologically mediated, but in many instances the pathogenetic mechanisms responsible for the glomerular injury are not known (Table 16.1). In the immunologically mediated forms of glomerulonephritis different mechanisms have been elucidated: (a) glomerular deposition of circulating immune complexes; and (b) reaction of circulating autoantibodies to glomerular basement membrane components. Glomerular injury by immune or non-immune mechanisms can be part of a systemic disorder or restricted to the kidney.

In children, immune complex glomerular injury is the most common form of glomerulonephritis and is encountered in the following order of relative frequency: post-infectious glomerulonephritis secondary to streptococcal infection, IgA nephropathy (Berger's disease), idiopathic membranous glomerulopathy, and types I and II mesangiocapillary glomerulonephritis. Anti-glomerular basement membrane autoantibody mediated glomerulonephritis with or without pulmonary haemorrhage occurs infrequently in the paediatric age group.

In the strict sense, nil lesion glomerulopathy is not a form of glomerulonephritis but is included in this classification since this disorder which is associated with heavy proteinuria and nephrotic syndrome closely mimics some of the clinical aspects of glomerulonephritis. Unlike the glomerulonephritides described above, there is no significant glomerular deposition of immunoproteins. The aetiology of this disorder,

Table 16.1 Classification of glomerular injury

Primary glomerulonephritis
Immune complex glomerulonephritis
    Post-infectious acute glomerulonephritis (streptococcal)
    Membranous glomerulopathy (idiopathic)
    Mesangiocapillary glomerulonephritis (types I and II)
    IgA nephropathy (Berger's disease)
Anti-GBM antibody mediated glomerulonephritis
Unknown aetiology
    Nil lesion nephrotic syndrome (nephrosis)
    Focal segmental glomerulosclerosis (steroid resistant)

Glomerulonephritis associated with systemic disorders
Immunologically mediated
    Systemic lupus erythematosus and other autoimmune 'collagen diseases' (scleroderma, mixed connective tissue disease)
    Anaphylactoid purpura
    Periarteritis nodosa, Wegener's granulomatosis, other vasculitides
    Mixed cryoglobulinaemia
    Systemic infectious (subacute bacterial endocarditis, shunt nephritis, syphilis, malaria, hepatitis)
    Sarcoidosis
Other aetiology
    Diabetes mellitus
    Amyloidosis
Hereditary disorders
    Nail-patella syndrome
    Familial nephritis (Alport's syndrome)
    Sickle cell anaemia

which is responsive to steroid therapy, and focal segmental glomerulosclerosis (steroid resistant) is unknown. There are a number of avenues of evidence which point to an abnormality in the cell-mediated immune system; however, none of these clues has been specifically conclusive (see Chapter 18).

In many systemic disorders with immunological abnormalities glomerular injury can be an important feature, but renal involvement is not necessarily always present in systemic lupus erythematosus, anaphylactoid purpura, periarteritis nodosa, cryoglobulinaemia, and sarcoidosis. Glomerular injury may also be associated with generalized disorders which are not immunologically mediated: diabetes mellitus, amyloidosis, familial nephritis, and nail-patella syndrome.

Clinical features of glomerulonephritis

The clinical features of glomerulonephritis may be manifest by an acute nephritic state or nephrotic syndrome; in milder forms of glomerulonephritis the patients may be asymptomatic and only have low-grade proteinuria or minimal urinary sediment abnormalities. These clinical presentations are not only found in primary forms of glomerulonephritis but may also be present in systemic disorders with associated glomerular involvement. Although there may be overlap of the clinical manifestations of glomerulonephritis, it is usually possible for the clinician to analyse the various signs and symptoms of glomerulonephritis.

The presence of proteinuria and/or haematuria may be encountered in children who present with few other signs of renal disease (normal renal function, normal blood pressure and no oedema). The proteinuria is usually minimal, occurs with or without haematuria, and is usually discovered on routine urinalysis. Proteinuria may be variable if related to posture (orthostatic proteinuria), which is a benign entity in most cases. However, persistent proteinuria is a sign of significant glomerular abnormality. Haematuria (more than 3–5 RBC per high power field) may be only microscopic. However, in other cases gross haematuria may occur. If haematuria is not accompanied by a systemic disorder or by an anatomical abnormality of the urinary tract, it may represent an early manifestation of glomerulonephritis.

Acute glomerulonephritis in children is most often preceded by streptococcal infection with a latent period of 10 days. Haematuria is regularly present, either microscopic or gross, the latter presenting as smoky or tea-coloured urine. Oliguria is common but total anuria is rarely encountered. Hypertension is a frequent manifestation of acute glomerulonephritis and is due to fluid overload. Oedema is often present in periorbital areas, being worse in the recumbent position. Hypervolaemia can produce dyspnoea, cardiomegaly, and pulmonary oedema due to fluid and sodium retention. Encephalopathy due to hypertension may present with headache, confusion, and less commonly seizures and papilloedema. Non-specific signs and symptoms such as fever, malaise and abdominal pain can also be present.

In childhood, nephrotic syndrome is rarely seen with acute glomerulonephritis, but more commonly with other forms of glomerulonephritis. Periorbital oedema, usually worse in the morning on rising, is frequently associated with ascites and pitting oedema of the lower extremities. The nephrotic syndrome can be complicated by poor appetite, gastrointestinal symptoms, tachypnoea, increased frequency of infection (peritonitis, cellulitis), and thromboembolic problems. The most common cause of nephrotic syndrome of childhood is nil lesion (minimal change) nephrotic syndrome, especially under the age of 6–7 years. In older children, other disorders such as membranous nephropathy, focal segmental glomerulosclerosis and mesangiocapillary glomerulonephritis should be considered, and a percutaneous kidney biopsy performed. Although conditions other than nil lesion may cause nephrotic syndrome in children less than 6 years of age, if the clinical and laboratory findings are compatible with this diagnosis, a trial of steroid therapy is recommended without performing a percutaneous needle biopsy of the kidney.

Pathophysiology

A clinical feature commonly observed in patients with glomerulonephritis is oedema. It is apparent to us that when practising physicians first encounter this physical finding it is mistakenly diagnosed as 'allergic oedema'. This, of course, is an incorrect diagnosis and a consequence of missing either the history of

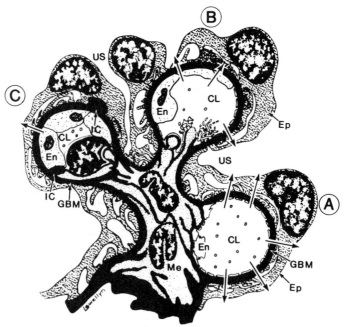

Figure 16.1 Graphic depiction of three capillary loops from a glomerular lobule. *Loop A* shows normal mesangial cells (Me), normal glomerular capillary lumen (CL), endothelium (En), with normal serum levels of albumin (open circles), no loss of albumin into the urinary space (US), and normal glomerular filtration (arrows). Glomerular epithelial cells (Ep) are normal with intact foot processes on the glomerular basement membrane (GBM). *Loop B* depicts the situation in nephrotic syndrome with normal glomerular filtration, low serum albumin and proteinuria and fused epithelial cell foot processes. In *Loop C* the acute nephritic state is associated with marked endothelial cell proliferation, immune complex (IC) deposition, capillary lumen narrowing, decreased glomerular filtration and oliguria (After Vernier *et al.*,[5] by permission)

oliguria or failing to detect the presence of proteinuria.

As emphasized above, the observation of proteinuria is the hallmark of glomerular injury and is a laboratory observation of specific significance which must be carefully investigated. Proteinuria is an important indicator of damage to the glomerular capillary filter mechanism. It is worth while to note that the sensitivity of the urinary dipstick method to detect proteinuria is directed toward screening for low levels of urinary protein. Consequently, a 4 + reading does not quantitate the true degree of proteinuria which can vary from 1 or 2 to 10 g in a young child. In some patients with glomerulonephritis, large urinary losses of protein result in depletion of serum albumin, lowering of plasma oncotic pressure, and the development of frank nephrotic syndrome (Figure 16.1, loop B). Since the latter is associated with hypoalbuminaemia and hypercholesterolaemia, these oedematous patients are difficult to clinically differentiate from children with idiopathic nephrotic syndrome or

'nil lesion' nephrosis. The presence of hypertension, loss of renal function, hypocomplementaemia, and formed elements in the urinary sediment are valuable clues that glomerulonephritis may be present.

Another form of oedema may be found in patients with glomerulonephritis which develops by a mechanism different from nephrotic syndrome. This type of oedema is due to fluid overload secondary to oliguria. Frequently, it is difficult to obtain a significant history of decreased urine output. Fluid homeostasis is normally kept under tight control with total intake and output normally balancing within a narrow range. In many instances the patient is not aware of a decreased urinary output; since oral intake of fluid continues, there is a progressive gain in weight and the development of oedema. The pathogenesis of oliguric oedema is a consequence of severely reduced glomerular filtration. In glomerulonephritis, there may be varying degrees of glomerular capillary endothelial cell proliferation, narrowing of the

Table 16.2 Laboratory investigations of glomerulonephritis

Blood
Haematology
　Haemoglobin, haematocrit
　Platelet count
　Sedimentation rate
　Coagulation parameters
Chemistry
　BUN, creatinine
　Electrolytes
　Total serum proteins and albumin
　Triglycerides, cholesterol
Serology
　Complement components: C3, C4, haemolytic
　　complement
　Circulating immune complexes, cryoglobulins
　Immunoglobulins
　Anti-streptolysin O titre, anti-DNAase B titre
　FANA, anti-DNA antibody, and other autoantibodies
　Anti-GBM antibody
　Anti-neutrophil cytoplasmic antibody

Urine
Urinalysis
24-hour urine collection for estimation of creatinine
　clearance and urinary protein

Renal biopsy

Other
Chest X-ray
Renal ultrasound
Cultures of urine, throat, blood

glomerular capillary lumina, and reduction in glomerular blood flow (Figure 16.1, loop C). These abnormalities may lead to an obvious decrement of glomerular filtration and oliguria. When the latter occurs, hypervolaemia, pulmonary oedema, cardiomegaly, and peripheral oedema ensue.

In summary, different pathophysiological mechanisms are active in the development of oedema when nephrotic syndrome is present versus oliguric fluid overload. It is important for the physician to determine which of these two states exists. The choice of strategies using treatment with fluid restriction or dialysis in the acute nephritic oliguric state, versus diuretics and possible colloid administration for nephrotic patients, rests upon a clear understanding of the nature and pathogenesis of oedema in each patient.

Laboratory investigation

Laboratory investigation of glomerular injury is guided by the clinical features, i.e. the presence of isolated urinary abnormalities or nephrotic syndrome or the nephritic state. Specific

Table 16.3 Serological findings in glomerulonephritis

	C3	C4	Immune complexes	Cryoglobulins
Primary glomerulonephritis				
Immune complex glomerulonephritis				
Acute post-streptococcal glomerulonephritis*	↓	N	+	+
Membranous glomerulopathy	N	N	Variable	−
Mesangiocapillary glomerulonephritis	↓	↓		
Type I			+	Variable
Type II	↓	N	+	−
IgA nephropathy	N	N	+	−
Anti-GBM nephritis†	N	N	N	−
Unknown aetiology				
Nil lesion nephrotic syndrome	N	N	−	−
Focal segmental glomerulosclerosis	N	N	−	−
Glomerulonephritis associated with systemic disorders				
Immunologically mediated				
SLE	↓	↓	+	+
Anaphylactoid purpura	N	N	Variable	−
Vasculitis/Wegener's‡	N	N	−	−
Cryoglobulinaemia	↓	↓	+	+
Systemic infection	N/↓	N/↓	+	+
Diabetes mellitus	N	N	N	N
Hereditary disorders	N	N	N	N

*Positive anti-streptolysin O titre.
†Positive anti-glomerular basement membrane antibody.
‡Positive anti-neutrophil cytoplasmic antibody.

laboratory investigation of glomerulonephritis is outlined in Table 16.2. Table 16.3 shows the results of the specific serological findings in glomerulonephritis and systemic disorders; depression of C3 levels is a significant indicator of immune mediated glomerulonephritis, especially in post-streptococcal glomerulonephritis, systemic lupus erythematosus, and membranoproliferative glomerulonephritis.

The majority of children with glomerulonephritis require a kidney biopsy for definitive diagnosis, although a biopsy is rarely indicated in nil lesion nephrotic syndrome or in post-streptococcal glomerulonephritis. The indications for biopsy in nephrotic syndrome are: age (less than 1 year and over 8 years), unresponsiveness to steroid therapy, gross haematuria, hypocomplementaemia and severe hypertension. Although the clinical diagnosis of post-streptococcal glomerulonephritis may tentatively be made, the presence of persistent nephrotic syndrome, prolonged oliguria, low C3, gross haematuria and heavy proteinuria suggests that a more serious form of glomerulonephritis is present and a renal biopsy is indicated. In systemic diseases with renal involvement, a renal biopsy will have two goals: (a) establish a definitive diagnosis of the disease (familial nephritis), or (b) document the severity of the renal involvement (systemic lupus erythematosus, diabetes mellitus), as it may influence the treatment of the disease.

References

1. Wilson C.B. and Dixon F.J. The renal response to immunological injury. In: Brenner B.M. and Rector F.C. Jr. (eds) *The Kidney*, 3rd edn. Philadelphia, W.B. Saunders, 1986: 800–889
2. Roy L.P., Fish A.J. and Michael A.F. Renal disorders. In: Stiehm E.R. and Fulginiti V.A. (eds) *Immunologic Disorders in Infants and Children*, 2nd edn. Philadelphia, W.B. Saunders, 1980: 561–579
3. Jennette J.C. and Falk R.J. Diagnosis and management of glomerulonephritis and vasculitis presenting as acute renal failure. *Med. Clin. North Am.* 1990, **74**, 893–908
4. Jayne D.R.W., Marshall P.D., Jones S.J. and Lockwood C.M. Autoantibodies to GBM and neutrophil cytoplasm in rapidly progressive glomerulonephritis. *Kidney Int.* 1990, **37**: 965–970.
5. Vernier R.L., Resnick J.S. and Mauer S.M. Recurrent haematuria and local glomerulonephritis. *Kidney Int.* 1975, **7**, 224–231

17

Acute nephritic syndrome

L.B. Travis, A. Kalia

This chapter will focus on the evaluation and management of the child who presents with the acute nephritic syndrome. The term 'nephritis', or more properly 'glomerulonephritis', refers to a specific renal disease in which inflammation and proliferation of cells within the glomerulus are the major abnormalities. The inflammatory changes are due primarily to immunological mechanisms. Acute glomerulonephritis is characterized by the sudden, often explosive, onset of symptoms of glomerular injury, which include haematuria, hypertension, oedema, and a varying degree of renal insufficiency. Although the disease may present at any age, the greatest prevalence is between 2 and 10 years of age. In children, the majority of cases of acute glomerulonephritis (AGN) will be post-infectious, most commonly following infection with group A β-haemolytic streptococci. It is on this particular disease entity, post-streptococcal acute glomerulonephritis (PSAGN) that the majority of this discussion will centre. In addition, there will be a brief review of other glomerulonephritides which may present in a similar manner and thus be confused with PSAGN.

Incidence, epidemiology and pathogenesis

Even though the prevalence of the disease has diminished in recent years, post-streptococcal acute glomerulonephritis (PSAGN) is still the most common non-suppurative renal lesion in children. The true incidence cannot be assessed with accuracy because of the wide range of clinical manifestations. Studies of relatives and sibling contacts of children with biopsy-proven PSAGN reveal that a high percentage of such family contacts have either abnormalities of urinary sediment or blood pressure elevations suggesting a mild form of the disease.[1,2] Recently, Lange and associates[3] have demonstrated that such patients have elevated titres of endostreptosin, a cytoplasmic protein of the group A streptococcus. Since such patients are unlikely to be brought to the attention of a physician, statistics may grossly underestimate the true incidence of this disease.

Studies designed to look at the incidence of glomerulonephritis following documented infection with group A β-haemolytic streptococci have revealed a variable 'attack rate' of as low as 1% to as high as 20%.[4-6] This variability appears to depend at least in part on the type of antecedent infection, with a higher incidence reported following skin infection in some studies.[7] PSAGN may occur following either nasopharyngeal or skin infection with streptococci, with a seasonal variability related to the prevalence of such infections. Pharyngitis-related PSAGN tends to peak in the winter and spring months, and pyoderma-related PSAGN is more prevalent in the summer and autumn, although this is by no means absolute. Roy and Stapleton[8] have shown that, in Memphis, Tennessee, pharyngitis-related PSAGN has become the more common, particularly in children over the age of 6 years. The single exception appears to

Table 17.1   Infectious agents associated with acute nephritis

Staphylococcus spp.
Pneumococcus spp.
Klebsiella spp.
Meningococcus spp.
Salmonella typhi
Mycoplasma pneumoniae
AIDS virus
Coxsackie virus
Echo virus
Epstein–Barr virus
Hepatitis B virus
Influenza virus
Mumps virus
Rubeola virus

be in black children where antecedent pyoderma is still most common.

PSAGN is most commonly seen in the younger school age child, but may occur at any age, even in the first few months of life. There is a male-to-female ratio 2:1 in most series, for reasons which are unclear. Some suggestions exist that there may be a genetic predilection towards development of PSAGN,[9,10] but the majority of studies do not seem to support this contention.

While group A β-haemolytic streptococcus is the most common infectious agent associated with acute nephritis, other bacterial and viral agents may be capable of producing a syndrome that is, often, clinically indistinguishable from PSAGN (Table 17.1). These infectious agents include *Pneumococcus* spp., *Staphylococcus* spp., typhoid fever, *Mycoplasma* spp., Coxsackie virus, mumps virus, echo virus, influenza virus, AIDS virus, and others. Since the long-term prognosis of non-streptococcal, post-infectious acute nephritis is less certain than that of PSAGN, attempts should be made to identify the causative agent whenever possible.

While there is little doubt about the temporal relationship between the streptococcal infection and the development of PSAGN, the exact mechanism by which renal injury is produced in this disease is not fully understood. Certain virulent properties of the organism may be important. Not all strains of group A streptococci are nephritogenic. In the USA, type 12 has been most frequently associated with pharyngitis-related AGN but types 1, 4, 6 and 25 have occasionally been identified. Type 49 is most often found in pyoderma-related AGN, although other strains (i.w.; 53, 55, 56, 57 and 58) have been implicated. As noted earlier, endostreptosin, a cytoplasmic protein antigen obtained from the nephritogenic streptococci, appears in the mesangium of patients with early PSAGN and suggests that immune complexes may be formed *in situ*.[11,12] Nephritic strain-associated protein (NSAP), a protein with an amino acid sequence identical to streptokinase, has been isolated from type 12 streptococci.[13,14] In addition, there appear to be features peculiar to the host that increase susceptibility to nephritis, as only a few of those infected with a nephritogenic strain of *Streptococcus* spp. develop nephritis. It has been suggested that an exuberant response of the host's immune system to the antigenic stimulus, with production of excess amounts of antibodies, may lead to the formation of the antigen–antibody complexes which traverse the glomerular basement membrane. There they activate the complement system, which leads to release of substances which attract neutrophils. Lysosomal enzymes released by the neutrophils are at least in part responsible for the damage to the glomerulus. Immunofluorescence microscopy of renal biopsy material in these patients will reveal deposition of IgG as well as the third component of complement, C3. On light microscopy, the glomeruli show an increase in cellularity with a swollen appearance and infiltration of neutrophils. Electron micrographs reveal electron-dense deposits which are felt to be aggregates of antigen–antibody complexes.

Clinical features

There is a wide range of variability in the presentation of patients with PSAGN. The 'typical' or classical case will present with a history of an upper respiratory tract infection with soreness of the throat approximately 2 weeks prior to the onset of swelling. This latent period may occasionally be as brief as 4–5 days, or as long as 3 weeks, with an average of about 10 days. In the case of pyoderma-related PSAGN, the interval between onset of infection and onset of nephritis may be difficult to determine. It is not uncommon for a child to have a chronic skin infection of several months' duration before experiencing the sudden onset of nephritis. The reason for this longer latent period is unknown. The child will usually have made an uneventful recovery from his respiratory illness by the onset of nephritis although, at times, fever and malaise may persist.

The first symptom of AGN noted will commonly be facial swelling. It will often be attributed to the child having 'slept too much', as it is prominent on awakening and disappears later in the day. Subsequently, however, the child or his parents will notice tightness of the child's shoes, or indentations left by socks and fullness of the abdomen may be present.

Either the onset of this oedema or the subsequent occurrence of gross haematuria will generally bring the child to the attention of the physician. Gross haematuria is present in 30–50% of hospitalized patients. Urine will usually be dark, mostly tea- or rust-coloured, sometimes smoky. The parent may note a decrease in the frequency of urination, although in older children the parent may be unaware of any alteration. In addition, a variety of non-specific symptoms may be present. Fever, malaise, abdominal pain, anorexia, headaches and weakness may be reported.

On physical examination, hypertension may be noted, and is present in the majority of hospitalized patients. The degree of hypertension is variable and not proportional to the degree of oedema. Occasionally the blood pressure may be markedly elevated, with systolic pressures in excess of 200 mmHg, and approximately 5% of hospitalized children may develop hypertensive encephalopathy, with headache, alteration of mental state, coma and convulsions.

Oedema may be mild, detectable only as minimal facial swelling or pretibial oedema, or may be severe, suggesting the picture of a nephrotic syndrome. As mentioned, the oedema is 'dependent' in nature, being more noticeable in the face upon arising, and gradually shifting to the lower extremities as the day progresses. Some ascitic fluid may be detected upon careful examination.

Many children appear pale, related in part to dilutional anaemia. However, oedema of the subcutaneous tissue also contributes to the appearance of pallor.

Circulatory congestion may be clinically evident. Tachypnoea and dyspnoea, due to pulmonary congestion and/or the presence of pleural effusion, are prominent features in some patients. Tachycardia, hepatic congestion and gallop rhythms can be noted when overt congestive heart failure is present. This is not commonly seen in children with previously normal cardiovascular systems.

Laboratory data

Urinalysis

Examination of the urine is of utmost importance in establishing the diagnosis of acute nephritis. The urine is often diminished in volume and with a dark or brownish hue. The colour is due to degradation of haemoglobin to acid haematin. Proteinuria is usually proportional to the degree of haematuria, and often in the range of trace to 2+ (up to 100 mg/dl). Protein excretion may, however, be greater and exceed 2 g/m² of body surface area per day.

Microscopic examination of the urine usually reveals numerous red and white blood cells. On careful inspection of the urine sediment under phase-contrast microscopy, the red blood cells appear crenated or distorted due to their passage through the glomerular basement membrane. The red blood cell (RBC) cast, considered as evidence of glomerular bleeding, may or may not be detected on routine urinalysis. It is often recommended that the urine be double or triple spun to look properly for such casts. This is done by centrifuging a specimen of urine and then discarding the supernatant. The pellet formed is resuspended in a second aliquot of urine and centrifuged again. This may be repeated a third time to obtain a very concentrated sample of urine sediment. The sediment may then be examined with or without a supravital stain. When performed in such a manner, RBC casts are reported to have been detected in greater than 80% of patients with acute nephritis.

Tests of renal function

A significant percentage of children admitted to the hospital with AGN will show elevations of blood urea nitrogen (BUN) and serum creatinine concentrations. In others, the BUN and serum creatinine may be normal, but the glomerular filtration rate is usually depressed. A few children will have severe azotaemia, with the development of metabolic acidosis and hyperkalaemia.

Haematological abnormalities

A mild normochromic, normocytic anaemia is present in many children. This is felt to be mainly dilutional in nature, since it parallels the degree of fluid retention and generally resolves as the oedema disappears.[15] There is also some evidence to suggest that alterations in the rate of red cell production or breakdown may contribute to the decrease in haematocrit.[16] The other blood components are usually normal, although there may be some elevation of the white blood cell count.

Bacteriological and serological examinations

Direct or indirect evidence of a preceding streptococcal infection should be sought in all children presenting with acute nephritis, regardless of history. If such proof is obtained it does not guarantee that the disease is PSAGN. Many chronic glomerulonephritides will exacerbate during an infection of any sort. Thus, evidence of an antecedent streptococcal infection supports, but does not prove, the diagnosis.

If the child has not received prior antibiotic therapy, and occasionally even if such therapy has been administered, group A β-haemolytic streptococci may be cultured from the nasopharynx or from skin lesions. Negative cultures may be seen if adequate antibiotic treatment has been received, or if the interval between initial infection and onset of clinical nephritis has been prolonged.

If direct cultural evidence of streptococcal infection is lacking, serological tests to demonstrate an immune response to streptococcal antigen should be pursued. Elevation of antibody titres to streptolysin-O (ASO) will be seen within 10–14 days following a streptococcal infection in most patients, and will remain elevated for several months. Unfortunately, the response of the ASO titre following skin infections with streptococci may be poor. This is felt to be due to the effect of skin lipids in interfering with the antigenicity of streptolysin-O. So, while this test is helpful, it may not be adequate when used alone. Other antibody titres, however, notably antihyaluronidase and antideoxyribonuclease B, will generally be elevated after a streptococcal infection, regardless of the site.[17] The 'streptozyme' test, employed in some laboratories, uses a mixture of extracellular products of the streptococcus, including the latter two mentioned.

Immunological tests

An important and very consistent finding in PSAGN is a lowering of the third complement

C3. C3 levels will be below normal at onset of symptoms in 80–90% of patients.[18,19] C3 activation can occur via two separate pathways. In the classic pathway, there will first be activation of C1, C4 and C2. This involves the properdin system, which includes properdin, C3 and several other factors.

While depression of C3 is common in PSAGN, C4 is less consistently lowered,[20] and if affected, tends to rise rapidly to normal. Properdin has been found to be low in the early stages of PSAGN[21] and has been demonstrated in biopsy specimens. This would support the notion that the alternative pathway of complement activation prevails in this disease.

Radiological studies

Chest roentgenograms may show findings considered by some to be pathognomonic of acute glomerulonephritis (Figure 17.1). The heart is generally of normal size and contour, although mild cardiomegaly may be seen. In contrast to the relatively normal cardiac silhouette, evidence of pulmonary fluid overload may be marked, with streaky densities radiating outward from the hilar areas in a 'sunburst' pattern. Unilateral or bilateral pleural effusions are not uncommon.[22] X-ray examination of the abdomen will usually show haziness suggestive of ascites.

Radiological and ultrasound evaluation of the kidneys will not reveal findings specific for AGN. The kidneys will be normal to increased in size. Small, contracted or scarred kidneys should prompt the physician to question the diagnosis and suspect an acute illness superimposed on chronic renal disease. The kidneys on ultrasound may have an increase in echogenicity compared to the liver parenchyma, which is non-specific and seen in a variety of renal disorders.

Differential diagnosis

The clinical course and long-term prognosis of PSAGN may be quite different from other forms of post-infectious nephritis. In addition, other renal diseases may present in a manner quite similar to PSAGN, but the implications for the patient with one of these diseases may be far greater. For this reason, it is important to distinguish between PSAGN and other conditions which may mimic it (see Table 17.2).

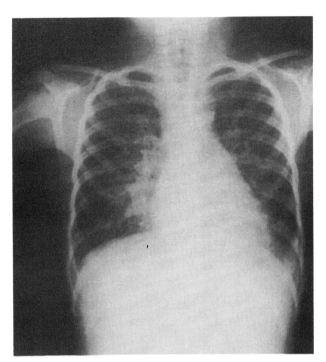

Figure 17.1 Chest X-ray of child with acute, post-streptococcal glomerulonephritis. There is moderate cardiomegaly with pulmonary oedema, particularly prominent in the hilar region. A right pleural effusion is present

The conditions which most commonly may be confused with PSAGN are: (a) any form of chronic glomerulonephritis, with an acute exacerbation, (b) Henoch–Schoenlein (anaphylactoid) purpura with renal involvement, (c) idiopathic haematuria (benign haematuria, recurrent haematuria, IgA nephropathy), (d) hereditary nephritis (Alport's syndrome) and, rarely, (e) systemic lupus erythematosus.

Acute exacerbation of chronic glomerulonephritis

As many as 10% of children hospitalized for acute nephritis may subsequently be found to have underlying chronic nephritis.[23] Since it is not uncommon for such conditions to be exacerbated by infections, bacteriological and serological tests for streptococcal disease may be present. Chronicity of the disease may be suggested by an abnormal growth pattern with short stature, or a history of pre-existing urinary abnormalities. Prior episodes of acute nephritis should arouse suspicion, as should haematuria which has its onset during 3–4 days following the onset of a respiratory infection.

Evidence of chronicity of disease may also be reflected by anaemia which is out of proportion to the degree of oedema and fluid retention. Additionally, a predominant picture of the nephrotic syndrome, while possible with PSAGN, is more suggestive of membranoproliferative glomerulonephritis. This is particularly so if the C3 remains depressed beyond 8 weeks.

Henoch–Schoenlein or anaphylactoid purpura with nephritis

This disease, in its more classic form, is unlikely to be confused with PSAGN. Patients with Henoch–Schoenlein purpura generally have a purpuric or petechial rash, significant abdominal pain and arthralgias. Occasionally, however, the renal manifestations will be the most prominent or may precede other findings.[23,24] This disease can usually be distinguished from PSAGN by the lack of evidence of antecedent streptococcal infection and the normal C3 value. In addition, the peripheral blood level of IgA is usually increased (see Chapter 1).

Table 17.2   Differential diagnosis of acute nephritis

Chronic glomerulonephritis
Abnormal growth pattern, short stature
Anaemia or azotaemia out of proportion to severity of
    illness
Past history of urinary abnormalities
Persistently depressed C3
Nephrotic syndrome

Henoch–Schoenlein purpura nephritis
Presence of purpuric and/or petechial rash
Severe abdominal pain, gastrointestinal bleeding,
    arthralgias
Normal C3
Elevated IgA levels in serum

Idiopathic haematuria
Recurrent bouts of haematuria
Absence of hypertension, oedema, renal insufficiency
Normal C3

Hereditary nephritis
Family history of renal disease
Hearing deficit in patient or family
Renal functional impairment out of proportion to severity
    of illness
Normal C3

Systemic lupus erythematosus
Systemic manifestations: rash, fever, arthralgias
Persistently depressed C3 and C4
Positive antinuclear antibody (ANA)

Idiopathic haematuria (benign haematuria, IgA nephropathy, Berger's disease, etc.)

Idiopathic haematuria is characterized by recurrent episodes of gross haematuria associated with respiratory infections. It is not generally complicated by hypertension or reduction in renal function.[25] Such patients will generally not have evidence of prior streptococcal infection and, again, C3 will be normal (see Chapter 1).

Membranoproliferative (mesangiocapillary) glomerulonephritis

MPGN may present with an almost identical picture as PSAGN and, in some instances, there may be evidence of a streptococcal illness. More often, these patients are nephrotic at onset and the degree of azotaemia greater. The C3 is decreased in well over 50% of cases and does not tend to return to normal after 6 weeks. In those instances where the C3 is not decreased, the failure of prompt resolution of the clinical features may alert to the need for renal biopsy.

Equally, when an initially depressed C3, fails to return to normal after 6 weeks, the probability of MPGN should be suspected.

Hereditary nephritis (Alport's syndrome)

This, like other forms of chronic glomerulonephritis, will tend to exacerbate with any infection, whether streptococcal or nonstreptococcal. There is, however, generally a history of renal disease in the family. Females have a much milder disease and are frequently asymptomatic; thus the family history may not always be positive. Many of these patients will have renal functional impairment greater than would be expected with PSAGN, and may have a history of hearing deficit (see Chapter 13).

Systemic lupus erythematosus

Systemic lupus erythematosus (SLE) may occasionally present with symptoms resembling PSAGN. This is a disease, along with membranoproliferative glomerulonephritis, in which C3 will be low. In SLE, however, the depression will generally persist beyond 8 weeks and will be accompanied by a decrease in C4 as well. Additionally, the patient with SLE will usually be older, and will have multi-system involvement. If doubt exists, determination of antinuclear antibody titres will generally distinguish the two diseases (see Chapter 20).

Management of the patient with acute nephritis

It is evident, given the wide range of severity of acute nephritis, that not all patients will need to be hospitalized during their illness. In the absence of hypertension or oliguria, many patients may be allowed to recover at home, provided that adequate follow-up can be obtained. We recommend hospitalization for those children with hypertension, significant oedema or oliguria.

Management of the child with acute nephritis centres on supportive and symptomatic care. There is little that can be done to alter the course of this disease once it becomes symptomatic. Many of the principles of therapy are those used to manage patients with acute renal failure of any cause, and the reader is referred to Chapter 21 for more in-depth discussion.

Often, the physician may find that the main task is reassuring anxious parents that conservative measures and watchful waiting are all that is required.

Hypertension

As noted, hypertension may be mild, or may be severe enough to lead to hypertensive encephalopathy with seizures. When the hypertension is mild (systolic pressure in the range of 130 mmHg and diastolic of 90 mmHg) and the patient asymptomatic, it is generally elected to observe the child without initiating treatment at first. Moderate hypertension (systolic pressure greater than 140–150 mmHg and diastolic greater than 100 mmHg) can be treated with intramuscular or oral hydralazine or with oral or sublingual nifedipine. This will generally result in lowering of the blood pressure within 30–40 min and can be repeated in 2–4 h if necessary.

It is our practice to treat the hypertension in this manner for the first day or two of hospitalization rather than to start the patient on chronic antihypertensive therapy. It is not uncommon for the hypertension to resolve rapidly, often after a single dose of an antihypertensive agent, and thus further medication may not be required.

Symptomatic or severe hypertension demands immediate action. Management is detailed in Chapter 15.

Oedema and circulatory congestion

Fluid retention in AGN is generally managed by fluid restriction. We allow our patients oral fluids in an amount equal to insensible water loss (400–500 ml/m^2 body surface area per day) plus one-half or less of their daily urine output. If weight loss does not result from such restriction, either further limitation of fluid or the use of an oral diuretic agent such as furosemide may be useful. As the patient's condition and renal function improve, fluid intake can gradually be liberalized.

Antibiotic therapy

The use of antibiotics has not been shown to alter the course of this disease once it is established.[26] In fact, documented PSAGN has occurred in patients who received appropriate antibiotic therapy shortly after onset of their streptococcal infection. Therapy should be instituted, however, in patients with positive cultures to eradicate the organism and prevent its spread to other individuals. An injection of benzathine penicillin 50 000 u/kg body weight intramuscularly or a 10-day course of erythromycin orally for the penicillin-allergic patients, will be effective in the majority of cases. Prolonged prophylactic therapy with penicillin does not appear to be indicated.

Bed rest

Bed rest was long advocated for the patient with acute nephritis. Studies have not shown that it is beneficial,[27] and may in fact have adverse social and psychological effects because of the limits it imposes on social interaction. In the absence of marked hypertension or significant oedema, bed rest does not appear to be indicated.

Persistent oliguria or anuria

Severe, persistent oliguria with azotaemia or total anuria is rare in PSAGN and its management will be that of acute renal failure from any cause. This is discussed in Chapter 21. With advances in techniques for the management of these patients, such as peritoneal and haemodialysis, mortality should be low.

Indications for renal biopsy

Renal biopsy should be considered if (a) renal function is severely impaired particularly if aetiology uncertain; (b) atypical presentation such as anuria, nephrotic syndrome; (c) delayed resolution with persistent hypertension, azotaemia, gross haematuria after 3 weeks, persistently low C3 levels at 6 weeks, persistent proteinuria after 6 months, persistent haematuria after 12 months.

Course of the illness

In general, the acute phase of illness in AGN with its most severe manifestations lasts 2–3 weeks (Figure 17.2). Thus, oliguria and azotaemia will generally resolve after 2 weeks, and blood pressure normalizes by 3–4 weeks.

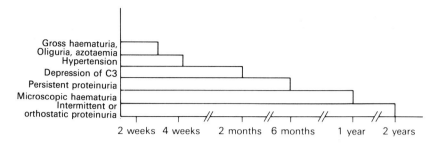

Figure 17.2   Time course of resolution for the usual clinical/chemical features of post-streptococcal glomerulonephritis

Urinary findings may take much longer to resolve. While gross haematuria is likely to clear by 3 weeks from onset of illness, microscopic haematuria may persist for up to 12 months, often accompanied by proteinuria for 6 months. Sometimes, proteinuria without haematuria may be the only demonstrable urinary abnormality.[28] C3 levels are expected to return to normal by 8 weeks, with the majority normalizing within 4 weeks.[29]

Follow-up

The frequency of need for follow-up examinations for patients with PSAGN will depend to a great extent on the individual patient and the severity of disease. We generally like to see patients at 4–6-week intervals for the first 6 months after onset of nephritis. Measurement of blood pressure and examination of urine for red cells and protein will be the best means to evaluate recovery. After 6 months, if haematuria and proteinuria have resolved, a yearly urinalysis and blood pressure determination should suffice.

Long-term prognosis

Controversy exists concerning the long-term prognosis in PSAGN. While it is generally agreed that the outcome is more favourable in children than in adults with this disease, follow-up studies report an incidence of impaired renal function that ranges from less than 1% to as high as 20–30%.[30-33] The difficulties in interpreting these studies stem from several factors. Often, the initial diagnosis of PSAGN was made solely on clinical grounds, without histological confirmation. Thus it is likely that some

of the patients had a pre-existing glomerulonephritis that was merely exacerbated by a streptococcal illness. Additionally, authors vary on their definition of what constitutes evidence of renal disease and chronic glomerulonephritis. Differences in severity of initial illness, possibly related to the strain of *Streptococcus* implicated, may affect ultimate outcome. On the whole, it can probably be said with a reasonable degree of assurance that greater than 90% of children with PSAGN should be expected to recover, without significant alteration in renal function.

Of children with post-streptococcal glomerulonephritis, a small minority of those hospitalized, 0.5–2.0% may have a rapid progression of their renal disease, reaching end-stage within weeks to months. Renal biopsy in these patients usually reveals extensive crescent formation.[34] Thus far, it is unclear whether early aggressive treatment of such patients with corticosteroids, cytotoxic agents and anticoagulants offers any advantage over supportive care alone in altering long-term prognosis.[35]

Finally, it should be recognized that second attacks of PSAGN can, and have, occurred. This is distinctly unusual, however, and a history of recurrent bouts of nephritis should raise the suspicion of an underlying chronic renal disease.

References

1. Dodge W.F., Spargo B.F. and Travis L.B. Occurrence of acute glomerulonephritis in sibling contacts of children with sporadic acute glomerulonephritis. *Pediatrics*, 1967, **40**, 1029–1030

2. Rodriquez-Iturbe B., Rubio L. and Garcia R. Attack rate of post-streptococcal nephritis in families. *Lancet* 1981, **i**, 401–403

3. Lange K., Azadegan A.A., Seligson G., Bovie R.C. and Majeed H. Asymptomatic post-streptococcal glomeru-

lonephritis in relatives of patients with symptomatic glomerulonephritis. Diagnostic value of endostreptosin. *Child. Neph. Urol.* 1988–89, **9**, 11–15

4. Hall W.D., Blumberg R.W. and Moody M.D. Studies in children with impetigo: bacteriology, serology and incidence of glomerulonephritis. *Am. J. Dis. Child.* 1973, **125**, 800–806

5. Anthony B.F., Perlman L.V. and Wannamaker L.W. Skin infections and acute nephritis in American Indian children. *Pediatrics* 1967, **39**, 263–279

6. Sagel I., Tresser G., Ty A. *et al.* Occurrence and nature of glomerular lesions after Group A streptococci infections in children. *Ann. Intern. Med.* 1973, **79**, 492–499

7. Anthony B.F., Kaplan E.L., Wannamaker L.W. *et al.* Attack rates of acute nephritis after Type 49 streptococcal infection of the skin and of the respiratory tract. *J. Clin. Invest.* 1969, **48**, 1697–1704

8. Roy S. III and Stapleton F.B. Changing perspectives in children hospitalized with poststreptococcal acute glomerulonephritis. *Pediatr Nephrol.* 1990, **4**, 585–588

9. Rodriguez-Iturbe B. and Garcia R. Isolated glomerular diseases: acute glomerulonephritis. In: Holliday M.D., Barratt T.M. and Vernier R.L. (eds) *Pediatric Nephrology*, 2nd edn. Baltimore, Williams and Wilkins, 1987: 407

10. Layrisse Z., Rodriguez-Iturbe B., Garcia R. *et al.* Family studies of the HLA system in poststreptococcal glomerulonephritis. *Hum. Immunol.* 1983, **7**, 177–183

11. Lange K., Seligson G. and Cronin W. Evidence for the *in situ* origin of poststreptococcal glomerulonephritis: glomerular localization of endostreptosin and the clinical significance of the subsequent antibody response. *Clin. Nephrol.* 1983, **19**, 3–10

12. Lange K., Cronin W. and Seligson G. Endostreptosin: its character and clinical significance. In: Holm S.E. and Christensen P. (eds) *Basic Concepts of Streptococci and Streptococcal Disease.* Windsor, Reedbooks, 1988: 260

13. Villareal H., Fischetti V.A., Van de Rijin I. and Zabriskie J.B. The occurrence of a protein in the extracellular products of streptococci isolated from patients with acute glomerulonephritis. *J. Exp. Med.* 1978, **149**, 459–472

14. Johnston K.H. and Zabriskie J.B. Purification and partial characterization of the nephritis strain-associated protein from *Streptococcus pyogenes. J. Exp. Med.* **163**, 697–712

15. Dodge, W.F., Travis L.B., Haggard M.E. *et al.* Studies of physiology during the early stages of acute glomerulonephritis in children. In: Metcoff J. (ed.) *Acute Glomerulonephritis.* Boston, Little, Brown, 1967: 319–331

16. Emerson C.P. The pathogenesis of anemia in acute glomerulonephritis: estimation of blood production and blood destruction in a case receiving massive transfusions. *Blood* 1948, **3**, 363–372

17. Wannamaker L.W. Differences between streptococcal infections of the throat and of the skin. *N. Engl. J. Med.* 1970, **282**, 78–85

18. Dodge W.F., Spargo B.H., Travis L.B. *et al.* Post-streptococcal glomerulonephritis. A prospective study in children. *N. Engl. J. Med.* 1972, **286**, 273–278

19. Derrick C.W., Reeves M.S. and Dillon H.C. Complement in overt and asymptomatic nephritis after skin infection. *J. Clin. Invest.* 1970, **49**, 1178–1187

20. Cameron J.S., Vick R.M., Ogg, C.S. *et al.* Plasma C3 and C4 concentrations in the management of glomerulonephritis. *Br. Med. J.* 1973, **3**, 668–672

21. West C.W., Ruley E.J., Forristal J. *et al.* Mechanisms of hypocomplementemia in glomerulonephritis. *Kidney Int.* 1973, **3**, 116–125

22. Kirkpatrick J.A. Jr. and Flersher D.S. The roentgen appearance of the chest in acute glomerulonephritis in children. *J. Pediatr.* 1964, **64**, 492–498

23. Edelmann C.M. Jr, Greifer I. and Barnett H.L. The nature of kidney disease in children who fail to recover from apparent acute glomerulonephritis. *J. Pediatr.* 1964, **64**, 879–887

24. Dodge W.F., Travis L.B. and Daeschner C.W. Anaphylactoid purpura, polyarteritis nodosa and purpura fulminans. *Pediatr. Clin. North. Am.* 1963, **10**, 879–897

25. Ayoub E.M. and Vernier R.L. Benign recurrent hematuria. *Am. J. Dis. Child.* 1967, **109**, 217–223

26. Freedman P., Meister H.P., Lee H.J. *et al.* The renal response to streptococcal infection. *Medicine* 1970, **49**, 433–463

27. McCrory W.W., Fleisher D.S. and Sohn W.B. Effects of early ambulation on the course of nephritis in children. *Pediatrics* 1959, **24**, 395–399

28. Travis L.B., Dodge W.F., Beathard G.A. *et al.* Acute glomerulonephritis in children. A review of the natural history with emphasis on prognosis. *Clin. Nephrol.* 1973, **1**, 169–181

29. Potter E.V., O'Keefe T.J., Svartman M. *et al.* Relationship of serum B₁C globulin to fibrinolysis in patients with post-streptococcal acute glomerulonephritis. *J. Lab. Clin. Med.* 1973, **82**, 776–783

30. Drachman R., Aladjem M. and Vardy P.A. Natural history of an acute glomerulonephritis epidemic in children. An 11- to 12-year follow up. *Isr. J. Med. Sci.* 1982, **18**, 603–607

31. Garcia R., Rubio L. and Rodriquez-Iturbe B. Long-term prognosis of epidemic post-streptococcal glomerulonephritis in Maracaibo: follow up studies 11–12 years after the acute episode. *Clin. Nephrol.* 1981, **15**, 291–298

32. Potter E.V., Lipshultz S.A., Abidh S. *et al.* Twelve to seventeen-year follow up of patients with post-streptococcal acute glomerulonephritis in Trinidad. *N. Engl. J. Med.* 1982, **307**, 725–729

33. Baldwin D.S., Gluck M.C., Schacht R.G. *et al.* The long term course of post-streptococcal glomerulonephritis. *Ann. Intern. Med.* 1974, **80**, 342–358

34. Gill D.G., Turner D.R., Chantler C. *et al.* The progression of acute proliferative post-streptococcal GN to severe epithelial crescent formation. *Clin. Nephrol.* 1977, **8**, 449–452

35. Roy S., Murphy W.M., Arant B.S. Jr Post-streptococcal crescentic glomerulonephritis in children: comparison of quintuple therapy versus supportive care. *J. Pediatr.* 1981, **98**, 403–410

18

Steroid responsive nephrotic syndrome

G. B. Haycock

Introduction

The nephrotic syndrome is defined as the combination of heavy proteinuria, hypoproteinaemia and oedema. Hyperlipidaemia, of variable degree, is invariably present but is not conventionally included as part of the diagnosis. The nephrotic syndrome is part of the clinical spectrum of proteinuric states and it is neither possible nor desirable to make a sharp distinction between nephrotic and non-nephrotic proteinuria. Two children may have the same disease according to histopathological criteria, one being clinically nephrotic and the other not. A third may have the nephrotic syndrome at some times and not others as a result of the interaction of various renal and non-renal factors: these include spontaneous changes in the amount of proteinuria, dietary energy and protein intake and the effects of drug and other treatment. In physiological terms, the nephrotic syndrome exists when the rate of urinary protein loss exceeds the rate at which the liver can replace it, leading to depletion of the extracellular albumin pool and a fall in the plasma albumin concentration below the normal range. Because of the influence of non-renal factors, the correlation between the magnitude of proteinuria and the severity of the resulting hypoalbuminaemia is rather weak, though present. Roughly speaking, proteinuria greater than about 50 mg kg^{-1} day^{-1} (approximately equivalent to 100 mg m^{-2} h^{-1}) for a few days or more is likely to cause hypoalbuminaemia. This corresponds to a value of about 3–5 g/day for an adult-sized patient and proportionally less for smaller individuals. The normal range for plasma albumin concentration in well-nourished children is 36–44 g/litre, but fluid retention and oedema are unusual until it has fallen below 25–30 g/litre, and in some children very much lower levels are seen. Depending on the nature of the underlying glomerular lesion, the urinary protein may be almost entirely albumin (selective proteinuria) or a mixture of albumin and higher molecular weight proteins (non-selective proteinuria). In either case the salt and water retention leading to nephrotic oedema is determined by the effect on the plasma albumin concentration, although losses of other proteins may be linked to some of the other events which may complicate the syndrome, such as infection and vascular thrombosis.

Causes of the nephrotic syndrome

As stated above, any disease that alters glomerular function so as to cause a large albumin leak from the plasma into Bowman's space may lead to the nephrotic syndrome. Causes include primary glomerulopathies, in which the disease is apparently confined to the glomeruli, and multisystem diseases with a renal component such as Henoch–Schoenlein purpura and systemic lupus erythematosus. A comprehensive list of causes, including the rarest entities and single case reports, is very long indeed but a relatively small number of diseases account for at least 99% of childhood cases and these are

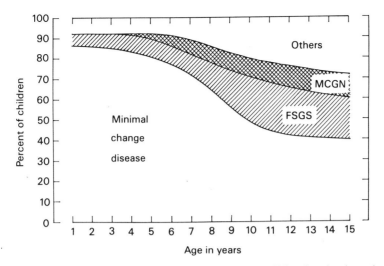

Figure 18.1 'Smoothed' representation of the distribution of major causes of childhood nephrotic syndrome by age (MCGN, mesangiocapillary (membranoproliferative) glomerulonephritis; FSGS, focal segmental glomerulosclerosis). Based on pooled data from the International Study of Kidney Disease in Childhood and patients investigated at Guy's Hospital, London (*n* = 566)

Table 18.1 Main causes of nephrotic syndrome in children aged 1–15 years

Primary glomerular disease
Minimal change disease (MCD)
  'Pure' MCD
  MCD with mesangial proliferation
Focal segmental glomerulosclerosis
Mesangiocapillary glomerulonephritis*
Membranous nephropathy

Multisystem diseases
Henoch–Schoenlein purpura
Systemic lupus erythematosus

* Mesangiocapillary glomerulonephritis is also known as membranoproliferative glomerulonephritis.

listed in Table 18.1. The mix of causes varies with age: the relative frequency of the commonest causes at different ages from 1 to 15 is shown in Figure 18.1. Note that infants are excluded from this analysis: the nephrotic syndrome in the first year of life, especially in the first 6 months, is dominated by congenital (usually hereditary) diseases with an almost uniformly bad prognosis (see Chapter 19). In adult populations the same primary and secondary diseases that affect children are seen but their relative importance is different, with membranous nephropathy being the commonest and minimal change disease being lower down the list. The remainder of this chapter will be confined to a discussion of the steroid sensitive nephrotic syndrome of childhood (SSNS), i.e. those cases in which proteinuria is abolished by high-dose corticosteroid therapy. In histopathological terms, this means minimal change disease and some cases of focal segmental glomerulosclerosis.

The mechanism of proteinuria in the nephrotic syndrome

The concepts of glomerular and tubular proteinuria have been discussed in Chapter 2. The proteinuria of the nephrotic syndrome is predominantly glomerular in type. In minimal change disease, and steroid sensitive patients generally, the proteinuria is usually purely glomerular, but in patients with nephrotic syndrome and progressive loss of renal function it is often mixed with tubular proteinuria superimposed on the underlying glomerular pattern. This is most typical of focal segmental glomerulosclerosis of steroid resistant, progressive type: even in this subgroup, however, the glomerular albuminuria is responsible for the hypoalbuminaemia and the other, contingent features of the nephrotic syndrome.

Glomerular filtrate is formed by *ultrafiltration* of plasma across the glomerular capillary wall. This structure has three layers: an inner, fenestrated *endothelium*, a *basement membrane*

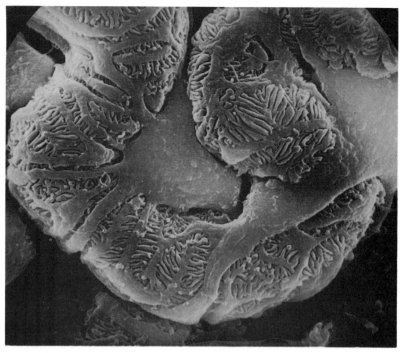

Figure 18.2   Scanning electron micrograph of a normal rat glomerular capillary loop, showing interdigitation of foot processes (pedicels) from adjacent epithelial cells (podocytes) (From Arakawa,[18] by permission; original print kindly supplied by Dr Arakawa)

consisting of a hydrated gel rich in proteoglycans, and an outer *epithelium* consisting of highly specialized cells called *podocytes*. Each podocyte possesses a cell body from which arise several octopus-like arms, each of which gives rise to numerous lateral *foot processes* which interdigitate with those of adjacent podocytes to invest the outer surface of the basement membrane like complex, jigsaw puzzle pieces (Figure 18.2). All three layers are negatively charged due to the presence of sialic acid residues on the 'glycocalyx' covering both epithelial and endothelial cells, and of sulphated glycosaminoglycans throughout the basement membrane. Plasma albumin is negatively charged at physiological pH, and there is evidence for both a *size-specific* barrier (a sieve) and a *charge-specific* barrier (an electric fence) to the passage of albumin molecules from capillary lumen to Bowman's space.

Most patients with SSNS have minimal changes on renal biopsy, with no structural changes to the glomerular capillary wall except an appearance usually described as 'fusion' of the epithelial foot processes. This is actually a misnomer: considered in three dimensions, the epithelial cells have altered their shape, with loss of foot processes, so that they now abut one another like simple squames or paving stones. This results in the appearance of a single thin epithelial sheet in the two dimensions of a thin section examined by electron microscopy, instead of the numerous little 'islands' of adjacent foot processes. The nature of the functional change in the properties of the glomeular filter has been the subject of intensive physiological study over two decades. The consensus view at present is that the albuminuria is due, mainly or entirely, to loss of the negative electrical charge on the basement membrane and perhaps the epithelium, impairing the charge-specific component of the filtration barrier. The evidence is complex and based on clinical and experimental physiological work as well as ultrastructural studies. It will not be reviewed here: the reader is referred to authoritative reviews on the subject.[1]

The proximate cause of the glomerular lesion

The central, unsolved problem concerning SSNS is: what causes the change in glomerular permeability to albumin that underlies the disease? It is widely assumed (though on circumstantial evidence only) that the condition has an immunological basis. Various observations support this hypothesis. All the drugs known to be effective (steroids, alkylating agents, cyclosporine, levamisole) have effects on the immune system. There is an increased incidence of atopy in affected children and their families. Children with nephrotic syndrome are notoriously susceptible to bacterial peritonitis and sepsis, especially due to *Streptococcus pneumoniae*. A form of minimal change nephrotic syndrome is associated with Hodgkin's disease and other lymphomas, themselves T-cell proliferative disorders. Certain infections (measles and malaria) that depress T-cell function are capable of inducing remissions of the disease. Serum IgG levels are low, and IgM levels frequently raised, in relapses of nephrotic syndrome and do not always normalize in remission. These and other considerations led Shalhoub[2] to propose that SSNS is the consequence of a primary, generalized disorder of T-cell function, a hypothesis that is still under investigation by several groups. The disease has been associated with various class 1 and class 2 HLA antigens in different populations: the known genetic linkage between the HLA system and the immune system makes this a promising area for research using the techniques of modern immunogenetics and molecular biology. The current state of knowledge of the immune system in SSNS was reviewed recently by Schnaper.[3]

Many workers have pursued the rather obvious possibility that the alteration in charge and permeability of the glomerular capillary wall might be due to the presence of a circulating factor. This is entirely compatible with the immunological hypothesis in that the factor(s) might be produced by cells of the immune system, either as the result of immunological reaction to antigen exposure or due to a primary abnormality of the immune system itself. Candidates for the role of the proposed factor include lymphokines such as *vascular permeability factor* and *soluble immune response suppressor*, and other circulating substances such as *platelet activating factor*, a kallikrein-like substance labelled *100-KF* and various crude, poorly characterized plasma fractions. This aspect of research is being actively followed in several laboratories at the time of writing: though promising, no one factor yet fulfils the equivalent of Koch's postulates as the cause of the disease. The current state of knowledge was recently summarized by Bakker and van Luijk.[4]

Pathophysiology of nephrotic oedema

Oedema is the cardinal clinical feature of the nephrotic syndrome. At least two hypotheses have been advanced in explanation of the renal salt and water retention involved: they are not entirely mutually exclusive. (The mechanisms of oedema formation in nephrotic syndrome have already been extensively discussed in Chapter 3.) The 'traditional' model based on alteration in Starling forces is questioned because there is evidence that the nephrotic patients are heterogeneous with respect to indices of plasma volume[5] or generally have a normal or increased plasma volume.[6] These and other observations indicate that, in at least some nephrotic subjects, the proximate cause of oedema may be a primary alteration in renal function leading to salt and water retention, circulating volume expansion and 'overflow' transudation into the interstitial space. This is the model usually proposed to account for the oedema of the *acute nephritic syndrome*. The subject is well reviewed by Tulassay *et. al.*[7] who conclude that the weight of evidence favours the hypovolaemic (underfilling) model in minimal change disease in children.

The question has practical implications as well as theoretical interest. Infusion of plasma or hyperoncotic albumin is logical therapy in a hypovolaemic child but may be dangerous in one who is volume replete. There is no doubt that some children present in acute nephrotic relapse with gross clinical evidence of hypovolaemia supported by laboratory evaluation: equally, others are clinically envolaemic. Volume must be carefully assessed and treatment tailored to his or her individual requirements, as described below under Clinical features and Laboratory findings.

Clinical features

Epidemiology

The disease occurs in both sexes, in all races

and at all ages but is commoner in males, in some races and at some ages rather than others. It is found in all parts of the world: geographical factors have not convincingly been implicated in its causation.

Sex

There is a consistent male predominance, the M:F risk ratio being in the range 1.5–2:1. The reasons for this are unknown.

Race

Steroid sensitive nephrotic syndrome is commoner in Arabs and the peoples of the Indian subcontinent than in white Europeans and their descendants in North America and Australasia: the per capita risk ratio is about 6:1 if Asian immigrants to the UK are compared with white children living in the same cities.[8] It is less common in Africans and Afro-Caribbeans than in whites. The incidence in oriental children is probably intermediate between that in Europeans and that in southern Asians. Beyond indicating a probable genetic predisposition to the disease in some populations, the significance of this distribution is not known.

Age

The disease is uncommon in the first year of life, and very rare under 6 months. The highest incidence is in the age range 2–5 years, with a smaller peak in later childhood. It becomes progressively less common with advancing age thereafter, both in absolute terms and as a proportion of all causes of the nephrotic syndrome, but occasional new cases present even into old age.

Genetic factors

Steroid sensitive nephrotic syndrome is clearly not inherited as a single gene disorder, but indirect evidence strongly implicates a genetic component in its causation. Several human leucocyte (HLA) antigens, singly and in combination, have been found to be over-represented in different populations of patients as compared with matched controls. HLA-DR7 is the single antigen most commonly identified, while the extended haplotype HLA-B8, -DR3, -DR7 predicted a relative risk of 21.5 in one recent

report.[9] The differing prevalence of the disease in different racial subgroups, referred to above, also favours the view that some individuals are genetically more predisposed to the disease than others. So does the slight but definite increased risk to siblings of affected children, especially within consanguineous marriages, and the association with atopy, itself a genetically determined trait. The molecular nature of this genetic predisposition is not understood, and it has no implications for practical management.

Symptoms and signs

The usual presenting feature is oedema. This is generalized and distributed by gravity: thus the face, particularly the periorbital regions, tends to be swollen in the morning and the ankles later in the day. Serous effusions (transudates) are commonly present and ascites without gross oedema is sometimes seen, particularly in very young children and infants, whose tissues are more resistant to the formation of interstitial oedema than those of older patients. Pleural effusions are often present, although rarely clinically significant. Children who are untreated or who fail to respond to treatment may progress to massive anasarca, and gross scrotal or vulval oedema can be particularly distressing. When oedema is severe, minor trauma may breach the continuity of the skin, leading to oozing of fluid from the exposed oedematous tissues.

Blood pressure is usually normal or low, but may be paradoxically raised in severely volume contracted patients, probably due to excessive secretion of renin, aldosterone and perhaps other vasoconstrictor hormones in response to hypovolaemia. Circulating volume should be carefully assessed before treatment is given (see below). The child is usually miserable but not acutely ill, unless a complication such as infection or severe hypovolaemia is present.

Clinical assessment of circulating volume

The purpose of the circulation is to supply the tissues with blood. In normal conditions this means that even the most peripheral parts of the body are well perfused, and therefore warm due to the transfer of heat from the centre of the body by the circulating blood. In a warm room, a person with a normal circulation is warm all over and the temperature of the great toe, under thermoneutral conditions, is an excellent indicator of this. If the patient is in bed with the feet covered, the toes should be warm to the touch: if the toe temperature is formally measured, it should be no more than 2°C less than the core temperature, i.e. not less than 35°C in an apyrexial patient. The palms, soles, finger and toe pulps should be pink with prompt capillary return after being blanched by pressure. Signs of functionally significant hypovolaemia therefore include cold periphery and diminished capillary return: venous pressure is reduced, although it is often difficult or impossible to assess the jugular venous pressure in an oedematous child. Abdominal pain is common in hypovolaemia, probably due to underperfusion of the splanchnic circulation: it may also be due to peritonitis, which must be excluded in any nephrotic patient presenting with this symptom.

Laboratory findings

Urine

Formed elements
Haematuria is usually absent, or present only intermittently, at the microscopic level in steroid sensitive disease. Continuous or macroscopic haematuria is a pointer to a more serious form of glomerulonephritis, as is the presence of cellular or granular *casts*.

Protein
The urine contains large amounts of *albumin*, typically > 50 mg kg^{-1} day^{-1} (100 mg m^{-2} h^{-1}) but sometimes much more, up to 20–30 g/day. The proteinuria is usually *selective*, that is to say mainly albumin with only small quantities of higher molecular weight proteins. This may be quantified by measuring the urine (U) and plasma (P) concentrations of two representative proteins such as transferrin (small) and IgG (large), from which the ratio of their renal clearances can be simply calculated ($U_{transferrin} : P_{IgG} / U_{IgG} : P_{transferrin}$): a value of < 0.1 is conventionally described as *highly selective*, > 0.2 as *poorly selective* or *non-selective* and 0.1–0.2 as *moderately selective*. The higher the degree of selectivity, the greater the probability that the patient has minimal change, steroid sensitive disease; conversely, poorly selective proteinuria predicts some other form of glomerulonephritis (see Table 18.1). However,

the correlation between selectivity and diagnosis, though significant, is weak. It is not helpful in the management of individual cases and most paediatric nephrologists have abandoned it as a clinically useful investigation.

Lipid
Lipiduria is also present, and fat globules and fat-laden macrophages ('oval fat bodies') may be seen on microscopy.

Electrolytes, urea and creatinine
Measurement of the urinary *sodium* concentration (U_{Na}) is valuable in the diagnosis of suspected hypovolaemia, which is a powerful stimulus to renal sodium retention. In the appropriate clinical setting, $U_{Na} < 10$ mmol/litre is diagnostic of reduction of effective circulating volume, while a value > 20 mmol/litre makes it unlikely. *This rule is invalidated if the patient has received a diuretic*, particularly a powerful loop diuretic such as furosemide. Urinary *potassium* excretion varies in response to dietary intake, as in normals, and measuring it yields no useful information. The urine is usually concentrated with respect to *urea* and *creatinine*, reflecting the reduced urine flow rate that underlies the fluid retention. Fractional sodium excretion (the fraction of filtered sodium excreted in the urine, calculated as $U_{creatinine} : P_{Na} / U_{Na} : P_{creatinine}$) is low ($< 0.01$) as in all salt-retaining states with normal or near-normal glomerular filtration rate. It will be very low indeed if hypovolaemia is present, but clinically this test is not more discriminating than simple measurement of U_{Na}.

Blood

Proteins
Hypoalbuminaemia is necessary for the diagnosis of nephrotic syndrome (plasma albumin concentration < 30 g/litre, often much lower). As would be expected, there is a rough inverse correlation between the plasma albumin and the severity of the clinical manifestations of the disease. *IgG* levels are also reduced but to a lesser extent than albumin: plasma *IgM* is usually raised. There are no consistent abnormalities of the plasma *complement* proteins C3 and C4, a point which helps to differentiate SSNS from that due to certain forms of glomerulonephritis in which the C3 may be reduced,

Table 18.2   Major complications of the steroid sensitive nephrotic syndrome

Infection
Hypovolaemia
Thrombosis
Acute renal failure
Hyperlipidaemia
Malnutrition
Side effects of treatment
    Corticosteroids
    Alkylating agents
    Cyclosporin A
    Levamisole

either transiently (acute post-streptococcal glomerulonephritis) or over a sustained period (mesangiocapillary or membranoproliferative glomerulonephritis, lupus and the nephritis of bacterial endocarditis or an infected ventriculo-atrial shunt). Of these, only mesangiocapillary glomerulonephritis is likely to be confused with the steroid sensitive disease.

Lipid
The plasma concentrations of total *cholesterol, low-density* and *very low density lipoproteins* are increased, often grossly, while those of *high-density lipoproteins* are usually normal. The plasma may be frankly lipaemic to the naked eye.

Urea, creatinine and electrolytes
Plasma *urea* and *creatinine* concentrations are usually normal but may be slightly to moderately raised in some cases due to hypovolaemia and renal underperfusion (*prerenal azotaemia*). Plasma *electrolyte* levels are normal in most cases, although *hyponatraemia* is occasionally seen. This is a complication of hypovolaemia: if plasma volume is contracted by more than a few per cent of normal, antidiuretic hormone (ADH) is secreted in response to baroreceptor stimulation even if plasma osmolality, the usual stimulus to ADH release, is normal. Since the normal diet contains proportionately more water than salt, the consequent impairment of water excretion leads to dilutional hyponatraemia. Hyponatraemia may be severe if a diuretic is used, inappropriately, in a hypovolaemic patient. A different form of hyponatraemia, often called *pseudohyponatraemia*, may be seen if the serum is lipaemic. This is because electrolytes are dissolved in the aqueous phase of plasma, and extreme hyperlipidaemia may reduce the

fraction of a given volume of serum or plasma which is water. This applies if sodium is measured by flame photometry: increasingly, cations in plasma are estimated using ion-selective electrodes, which measure *activity* rather than *concentration*, and activity is not affected by changes in plasma non-aqueous solids.

Calcium
The total plasma *calcium* concentration is reduced in parallel with the albumin, since it is partly albumin bound. The *ionized calcium* is normal, and it is not necessary to treat the low total concentration of the ion, which normalizes when the hypoalbuminaemia is corrected.

Haematology
The *haemoglobin* concentration and *haematocrit* are raised in proportion to reduction in plasma volume. The absolute values of these variables at presentation are, of course, influenced by other factors such as pre-existing anaemia, but *changes* in them are a reliable guide to changes in volume. There are no other specific or characteristic changes in the blood count.

Complications

The major complications of the nephrotic syndrome are listed in Table 18.2.

Infection

In modern (post-corticosteroid) times, the nephrotic syndrome has come to be regarded as a fairly benign condition, but before steroid therapy was available as many as 30% of affected children died of their illness, and before the introduction of antibiotics the proportion was even higher. As this historical note suggests, infection was the major cause of mortality, commonly with *Streptococcus pneumoniae* which was, and is, prone to cause fulminating peritonitis and septicaemia. This reflects the fact that nephrotic patients are immunocompromised in a number of ways involving not only humoral factors but also probably lymphocyte function (Table 18.3). In nephrotic children, as in the population generally, the proportion of individuals with preformed antipneumococcal antibody rises with age, which probably accounts for the decreased incidence of serious pneumococcal infection in older patients – it is rarely seen in

Table 18.3   Causes of susceptibility to infection in children with steroid sensitive nephrotic syndrome

Low plasma IgG
Low serum factor B (C3 proactivator)
Impaired opsonization
Impaired lymphocyte transformation
Drug-induced immunosuppression

Table 18.4   Factors predisposing to thrombosis in steroid sensitive nephrotic syndrome

Thrombocytosis
Increased platelet aggregability
Increased plasma concentrations of clotting factors
    Factor V
    Factor VII
    Factor VIII
    Factor X
    Fibrinogen
Accelerated thromboplastin generation
Reduced plasma concentration of antithrombin III
Hypovolaemia
    Circulatory sluggishness
    Increased blood viscosity
Corticosteroid therapy

adult nephrotics. Low levels of serum factor B (C3 proactivator), probably due to urinary loss, may be of particular importance in this respect since this substance is necessary for the efficient opsonization and killing of capsulated bacteria in the absence of specific antibody. The significance of the circulating inhibitor of lymphocyte transformation which has been found in the sera of nephrotic patients in relapse, but not in remission, is less certain. Infection remains a serious threat to nephrotic patients during relapse, and fever or other clinical evidence of infection should be treated as a medical emergency. It is important to remember that a significant proportion of serious infections in nephrotic children are caused by Gram-negative bacteria, and until an organism has been identified in a particular case a broad-spectrum antibiotic combination (including parenteral benzyl penicillin unless the patient is allergic to it) should be prescribed.

Thrombosis

Both arterial and venous thromboses are prone to occur in patients with the nephrotic syndrome; affected sites include the deep veins of the legs and pelvis, the renal veins, mesenteric veins, the pulmonary vasculature and the arterial supply to the lower limbs. Cerebral thrombosis has been described, fortunately rarely.

Renal vein thrombosis has been recognized as a feature of the nephrotic syndrome for many years; it is particularly associated with membranous nephropathy and use to be considered a *cause* of the syndrome, although it is now thought rather to be a *complication*. Membranous nephropathy is uncommon in childhood, which may account for the relative rarity of renal vein thrombosis in this age group.

The tendency to thrombosis is probably due to a combination of haemodynamic factors and hypercoagulability (Table 18.4). Hypovolaemia, when present, probably affects both: the former by causing circulatory sluggishness and the latter by producing haemoconcentration and hyperviscosity. The increased plasma concentrations of clotting factors may be the consequence of a general drive to increased protein synthesis secondary to hypoalbuminaemia: accelerated synthesis and turnover of fibrin have been directly demonstrated. The reduced plasma antithrombin III levels are probably due to increased urinary loss, as suggested by clearance studies and by the close correlation between the plasma concentrations of albumin and antithrombin III. The increased platelet aggregability may also be caused by the urinary loss of albumin, or some substance bound to albumin, since it has been shown to be reversible by the *in vitro* addition or the *in vivo* infusion of albumin, and by the addition of concentrated protein from nephrotic urine although, interestingly, not by aspirin.

Acute renal failure

Prerenal uraemia, usually of mild degree, is quite commonly seen in nephrotic patients in association with hypovolaemia, as discussed above. Much less commonly, acute renal failure unresponsive to volume replacement is seen. The cause of this is not completely understood. It is usually precipitated by hypovolaemia, especially if complicated by sepsis, and the histological appearances are those of acute tubular necrosis (ATN). However, most hypovolaemic episodes and infections do not lead to ATN, and why it should occur in a few cases remains a mystery. Very rarely, SSNS presents with ATN as the initial manifestation. Complete recovery is the rule, although dialysis may be necessary if the renal failure persists for more than a few days.

Hyperlipidaemia

The abnormality of plasma lipids characteristic of the nephrotic syndrome is elevation of total cholesterol, low-density and very low density lipoproteins with high-density lipoproteins remaining relatively normal. Despite several decades of research, the mechanism underlying these changes is poorly understood, but the cause seems to be directly related to hypoalbuminaemia. Whether the hyperlipidaemia of the nephrotic syndrome predisposes to atherosclerosis is an important but unanswered question: fortunately, few children are exposed to it for sustained periods due to the intermittent nature of the disease in most cases.

Malnutrition

Children with unremitting nephrotic syndrome for a long period may develop severe muscle wasting. This may be masked by oedema, and only becomes manifest when this is abolished. This is particularly likely to occur in small children with focal segmental glomerulosclerosis (FSGS), in whom urinary protein loss is often very heavy and sometimes refractory to all forms of treatment. Such patients are at high risk of sudden overwhelming sepsis and the prognosis is poor: fortunately this 'malignant' variety of FSGS is uncommon. In the much commoner SSNS, significant wasting can also occur if relapses are frequent, although in this case it is difficult to determine the respective contributions of frequent episodes of heavy proteinuria and prolonged corticosteroid therapy.

Management

The initial episode

The child should be admitted to hospital for initial assessment and treatment. Enforced bed rest is not necessary in a child who feels well enough to want to be active. If hypovolaemia is present according to the criteria discussed above, volume repletion should be undertaken with a colloid-containing solution such as plasma or salt-poor human albumin, in a dose

calculated to provide 1 g albumin/kg body weight. This is *not* a routine measure to be given to all nephrotic patients in relapse: plasma or albumin infusion may be dangerous in children who do not show clinical or laboratory signs of volume depletion (see above). If the patient is febrile or feels systemically unwell, antibiotics should be given. Penicillin alone is usually appropriate but an aminoglycoside may be added, or a broader spectrum agent such as a third-generation cephalosporin substituted, if signs of peritonitis or septicaemia are present, until information on antibiotic sensitivities is available. The urine sediment should be examined, and urine and blood specimens sent to the laboratory for basic biochemical estimations (see above). In the absence of indications for early renal biopsy (see below), oral prednis(ol)one should be started in a dose of 60 mg $m^{-2} day^{-1}$ (approximately 2 mg $kg^{-1} day^{-1}$) in two or three divided daily doses. (Prednisone is usually used in North America, prednisolone in Europe. The two are therapeutically equivalent.) Calculations should be based on 'ideal weight for height' rather than oedematous weight – this can be obtained from standard growth charts. Urinary protein should be monitored using dipsticks, particular attention being paid to the first specimen passed in the morning, which can be assumed to be free of orthostatic (postural) proteinuria. Treatment should be continued at this dosage until remission of the nephrotic syndrome has been induced, defined as loss of oedema and disappearance of proteinuria (urine protein negative or trace positive to dipstick testing on 3 consecutive days). By convention, the patient is a 'non-responder' if remission has not occurred after 4 weeks of continuous treatment and 4 weeks of intermittent treatment (see below). In this case biopsy should be performed: the management of the patient whose nephrotic syndrome is persistently unresponsive to steroids is beyond the scope of this chapter.

In the child who does respond, it is usual to reduce the dose of prednisolone and stop it over a period of a few weeks. There is no universally agreed scheme for doing this, but the following method, slightly modified from the protocol originally used by the International Study of Kidney Disease in Childhood, is used by the author and is probably as good as any other. On the fourth day following remission, the prednisolone dosage is reduced to 40 mg/m², *given as a single morning dose on alternate days only* for 4 weeks. At the end of this period, treatment is simply stopped. It is not necessary to taper the dose either over the transition from daily to alternate-day treatment, or at the end of the month of alternate-day therapy, provided that the total period of steroid treatment has not exceeded 8 weeks. Studies from Germany suggest that the relapse-free interval following treatment of the initial attack is lengthened if prednisolone is given at the full induction dose for 4 weeks irrespective of when response occurs.[10] However, it has not been clearly shown that this results in the patients receiving less steroid in the long run, and it carries an increased cost in short-term steroid toxicity during initial treatment. In some children (unfortunately, the minority) no relapse occurs and no further treatment is necessary. After a reasonable period of outpatient observation (3–6 months) the child can be discharged and told to return if relapse occurs at a later date. No restrictions of any kind should be imposed once treatment has stopped and the child has been released from hospital. The prognosis in this group is excellent in every respect.

In most children with SSNS, one or more relapses will occur following the initial episode. The management of these patients ranges from relatively straightforward to extremely difficult, depending mainly on three factors: (a) the frequency of relapses; (b) the dose and duration of steroid therapy necessary to induce remission on each occasion; and (c) the tolerance of the individual to long-term steroid treatment, which varies greatly from patient to patient.

Relapsing nephrotic syndrome

Following the example of the International Study of Kidney Disease in Childhood, it is useful to stratify children with SSNS according to the frequency of their relapses. Four grades of severity are conventionally recognized. They are defined according to precise criteria, and it is important to use the agreed terminology accurately in order that like may be compared with like when the results of therapeutic trials are evaluated.

Non-relapsing nephrotic syndrome
Children who do not relapse after the first episode of the disease. As indicated above, they need no treatment after the initial attack.

Infrequently relapsing nephrotic syndrome
Children who relapse after the first attack, but less than twice within the first 6 months and less than 4 times within any subsequent 12-month period.

Frequently relapsing nephrotic syndrome without steroid dependency
This is subsequently referred to simply as frequently relapsing nephrotic syndrome (FRNS). Children who relapse 2 or more times within the first 6 months after the first attack, or 4 or more times in any 12-month period.

Frequently relapsing nephrotic syndrome with steroid dependency
This is subsequently referred to as steroid dependent nephrotic syndrome (SDNS). Children fulfilling the criteria for FRNS in whom 2 consecutive relapses, or 2 of 4 relapses in any 6-month period, occurred while a (usually reducing) dose of steroid was still being given or within 14 days of discontinuing steroid therapy.

Children with infrequent relapses can be treated in the same way as those presenting for the first time. The median time to remission in more than one study is 11 days from starting high-dose steroid treatment. If response is followed by not more than 4 weeks of consolidation therapy, it can be seen that these children will be receiving steroids considerably less than half the time, allowing recovery from the acute side effects before the next relapse occurs. It is rarely, if ever, necessary to consider using drugs other than corticosteroids in children in this group. Long-term prognosis is good, with spontaneous resolution after a period of months to years being the rule. The remainder of this section concentrates on the management of children in the most difficult categories, those with FRNS and SDNS.

Maintenance steroid therapy

Patients with FRNS and SDNS are at risk of severe steroid toxicity, mainly because of the frequency with which they are exposed to continuous, high-dose prednisolone for induction of remission. The main indication for considering treatment, other than intermittent steroid therapy as described above, is the development of major side effects. The adverse effects of glucocorticoids are legion and too well known to need listing here, but particular attention should be paid to impairment of statural growth, disfigurement of facial appearance and bodily habitus, and behavioural changes. The last of these is more common than is appreciated by many physicians and may be severe and distressing to the parents. Because disturbance of mood and conduct is often attributed to the disease or to unrelated factors, rather than to the treatment, it may go unmentioned in the clinic unless specifically asked for by the doctor. An individual clinical judgement must be made in every case as to whether the child's side effects are acceptable or not (that is, acceptable to him, his family and his peers). However, many children in the FRNS and most of those in the SDNS categories are best given at least a trial of some treatment other than intermittent, high-dose prednisolone.

If prednisolone is given on alternate days, as a single morning dose, clinical side effects are milder than if the same total dose is given in single or multiple daily doses – for example, 30 mg every other day is better tolerated than 15 mg daily. Children with FRNS and significant side effects may therefore be given a trial of alternate-day prednisolone in the hope of preventing relapses and the consequent exposure to high, toxic doses. By definition, patients with FRNS have not relapsed while still taking steroids and the initial dose should be low, in the range 0.2–0.4 mg/kg (5–15 mg/m²) per dose. The dose should not be divided into two or more doses on treatment days, since the relative freedom from side effects hoped for from the regimen depends critically on an inter-dose interval of > 36 h, preferably 48 h. This has been formally documented to be the case with regard to suppression of the hypothalamopituitary-adrenal axis and to growth, and clinical impression strongly suggests that it is true of other side effects also. If successful in preventing relapse this protocol can be safely followed for months or years, and there is usually a gratifying improvement in the patient's appearance and well-being within a few weeks. It is reasonable to attempt gently to withdraw treatment every 6 months or so, to see whether it is still needed, but it is usually extremely well tolerated and the paediatrician should not hesitate to resume the same maintenance regimen if relapse occurs.

Patients with SDNS present a more difficult problem. By definition, they have relapsed while still receiving steroids or within 2 weeks of stopping them, and are likely to need a higher alternate-day prednisolone dose than those with FRNS. The history will reveal the dose at which relapse occurred during the previous few months, and maintenance therapy should be commenced at a level just above this. If this dose is held for 2–3 months it will become apparent whether or not it allows the side effects to regress to a tolerable level. If so, the dose can be 'fine tuned' by trial and error to establish the minimum amount that will achieve the desired effect: that is, freedom from relapse without unacceptable toxicity. If such a trial is not successful, the use of other drugs must be considered. Particular attention needs to be directed to growth at the time of the expected pubertal growth spurt. Children who have been growing well on alternate-day prednisolone may fall significantly behind in the mid-teens due to steroid-induced pubertal delay.[11]

Alkylating agents

Alkylating agents impair DNA transcription by attaching alkyl chains to purine bases. They are cytotoxic and immunosuppressive. Some members of the group, such as cyclophosphamide, have two alkyl groups and therefore also prevent cell division by crosslinking paired DNA helices. The parent drug, nitrogen mustard (mechlorethamine), was shown to be capable of inducing remission in the nephrotic syndrome in the 1940s. In the last three decades, two orally effective congeners of nitrogen mustard, chlorambucil and cyclophosphamide, have been more widely used. There is no doubt that they work, but their precise role in the management of minimal change disease remains controversial. There are two reasons for this: first, their toxicity, and secondly, the presence of widely conflicting claims in the literature as to their effectiveness in producing sustained remission and allowing the patient to stop taking corticosteroids.

Early reports tended to be optimistic in their conclusions, reporting long-term relapse-free survival in half or more of treated patients. However, many of these reports are sketchy as to the details of the patients, in particular whether they had FRNS, SDNS or a mixture of the two, and exactly how much drug was given over what duration. More recent studies have been more consistent, and it is now reason-

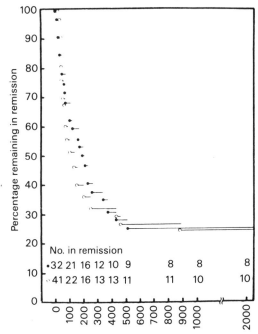

Figure 18.3 Time to relapse in children with steroid dependent nephrotic syndrome following cyclophosphamide in a dose of 2 mg kg^{-1} day^{-1} given for 56 days (●) or 84 days (○) (From Ueda *et al.*,[12] by permission)

ably clear that patients with FRNS respond well to alkylating agents, with 50–90% long-term remission, while those with SDNS are much more resistant to their action with only 20–30% long-term remission, as shown in Figure 18.3.[12]

Side effects of cyclophosphamide (much the most widely used of these drugs) can be divided into early, i.e. during or shortly after administration of the agent, and late or long-term. Early effects include bone marrow suppression, alopecia (always reversible), minor gastrointestinal upsets and haemorrhagic cystitis – the latter is rarely seen at the doses usually given in the nephrotic syndrome. Late effects include infertility, especially in males, and malignancy. Although both are obviously serious and worrying possibilities, they are undoubtedly dose related and a cumulative dose of cyclophosphamide of not more than 150–170 mg/kg has not been reported to cause either in a fairly extensive literature. Claims that nitrogen mustard and chlorambucil are more effective than cyclophos-

phamide have been made, but it is not clear whether the drugs were give in equivalent doses as regards both therapeutic and adverse effects. Most of the few malignancies that have been reported after alkylating agent therapy for nephrotic syndrome have followed the use of chlorambucil. However, the cumulative amount of chlorambucil used in these early trials was almost certainly equivalent to several times the amount of cyclophosphamide that is now conventionally given. It is therefore likely that the ability to cause secondary malignant disease is dose related rather than drug specific. At present there seems no compelling reason to prefer any other alkylating agent to cyclophosphamide, except perhaps for the occasional patient in whom compliance is so poor that four doses of nitrogen mustard, 0.1 mg kg^{-1} day^{-1} given intravenously in hospital, at least carries the assurance that the treatment has been given.[13]

The only indication for cyclophosphamide therapy is failure of intermittent or maintenance prednisolone therapy to achieve stable remission without poisoning the patient with the steroid. It should be given at a dose of 3 mg kg^{-1} day^{-1} for 8 weeks, the calculation being made on ideal weight for height rather than actual (i.e. oedematous or obese) weight. It is usual to start therapy with the patient in a steroid-induced remission but this is not essential: there is some evidence that proteinuria may remit faster if both drugs are given together in relapse than if prednisolone is given alone. Once in remission and on cyclophosphamide, prednisolone should be converted to an alternate-day regimen at 40 mg m^{-2} day^{-1} which is then tapered progressively to stop either just before or just after the cyclophosphamide.

Blood counts should be performed weekly during the first 4 weeks of treatment and 2-weekly during the second 4 weeks: occasionally treatment must be interrupted, usually because of neutropenia, but this is uncommon if the recommended dose is not exceeded. Patients should be advised to report any symptoms of intercurrent infection, or any exposure to infectious disease (especially chicken pox), during treatment so that necessary treatment or protection can be given.

Purine analogues

The purine analogues azathioprine, 6-mercaptopurine and 6-thioguanine have all been used sporadically in the nephrotic syndrome. However, the few controlled trials that have been performed have shown no evidence of a therapeutic effect.[14] These drugs have no place in the modern management of the disease.

Cyclosporin A

Cyclosporin A (CyA) is an immunosuppressive fungal metabolite which acts by modifying T-cell function. Specifically, the drug inhibits the release of interleukin 2 from activated T-helper cells and thus prevents the induction and proliferation of T-effector cells. The previously cited hypothesis of Shalhoub,[2] that steroid responsive nephrotic syndrome is a disorder of T-cell function, led several groups to assess the effect of CyA in the disease. Published reports are fairly consistent in that steroid responsive patients, including those with FRNS and SDNS, usually respond well to low-dose CyA and steroids can be withdrawn in most without relapse. The largest group of patients so far reported from a single centre is that of Niaudet *et al*.[15] who found that 17 of 20 steroid responsive patients were maintained in steroid-free remission for 2–8 months. However, *all* relapsed when treatment was withdrawn or shortly thereafter. This experience is confirmed in several other reports.

Side effects of CyA include tremor, hirsutism and gum hyperplasia. All of these are dose dependent and can be minimized or prevented by adjusting dosage according to blood levels of the drug. Unfortunately, CyA is also nephrotoxic and it is clear from the experience in transplant patients (especially those in whom the organ transplanted was not the kidney, e.g recipients of heart, liver and bone marrow grafts) that permanent kidney damage and even chronic renal failure can result if the drug is given at high dosage for long enough. The matter is made more difficult by the fact that there is also a reversible effect of CyA on renal function, probably due to inhibition of prostaglandin synthesis and consequent constriction of the renal microvasculature. Monitoring renal function by measurement of plasma creatinine or even formal GFR estimation is therefore inadequate to differentiate vasoconstriction from permanent damage.

At Guy's Hospital, we have adopted the following approach to CyA therapy in patients who have failed cyclophosphamide therapy and who remain severely affected by steroid side effects. First, the drug is introduced at a low dose, typically 4 mg kg^{-1} day^{-1} in two equal divided doses, and carefully adjusted to keep the measured trough blood level (measured 12–16 h after the last dose) below the upper limit of the target range for transplant patients. This value varies with the assay being used: in our laboratory, using a monoclonal antibody-based radio-

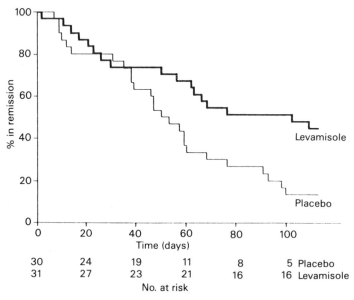

Figure 18.4   Percentage of children remaining in remission by time following levamisole therapy or placebo (From British Association for Paediatric Nephrology,[17] by permission)

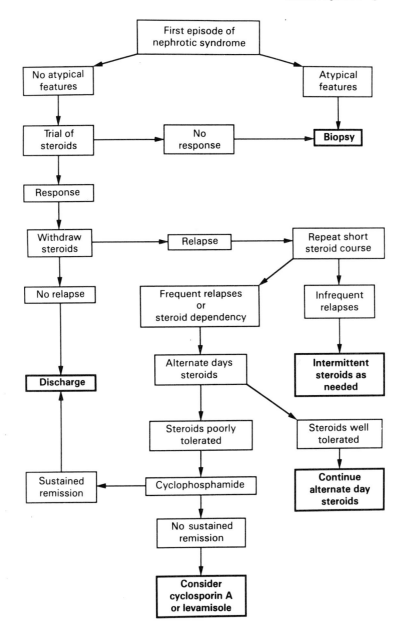

Figure 18.5 Suggested scheme for management of children with first and subsequent episodes of nephrotic syndrome

immunoassay, it is 150 ng/ml. The lower limit of the target range is defined as the smallest dose that keeps the patient in steroid-free remission. (This is different from the policy in transplant patients, in whom a predetermined lower limit is specified, in our laboratory 70 ng/ml.) Secondly, after 1 year of treatment a choice is made: either the drug is withdrawn, or a renal biopsy is performed. The latter alternative is selected if the patient expresses a strong desire to continue

taking CyA rather than risk further high-dose steroid exposure. If the biopsy shows no sign whatever of CyA toxicity the drug is continued for another year and the same choice then repeated. At the time of writing, 21 patients have been treated with CyA, of whom 17 have received it for more than 1 year and some are now in their fourth year of continuous therapy. So far, *no* patient has shown any sign of renal damage due to CyA, even in the 3-year biopsies. This is probably due to the fact that, in those patients who respond to CyA (17/21), the minimum effective dose is very low, often below the range usually considered effective in the prevention of graft rejection. These results have not yet been published in detail but encourage us to believe that CyA may have a future in the long-term management of children with FRNS and SDNS.

It must be emphasized that CyA is a potentially toxic drug. At present, it should probably only be used by, or in consultation with, a paediatric nephrologist with experience of its use in transplantation. Control of dosage by regular monitoring of the blood level is mandatory. It is very important to emphasize to the patient and parents that the likely effect of CyA is to substitute CyA dependence for steroid dependence, not to cure the disease.

Levamisole

The antihelminthic agent levamisole also alters T-cell function but, in contrast to the immunosuppressive agents discussed above, it stimulates rather than inhibits it. Sporadic reports in the early 1980s suggested that it might be effective in steroid responsive nephrotic syndrome. Two recent reports, one using children as their own controls[16] and the other a prospective, randomized, placebo-controlled study,[17] have now confirmed this effect. In the latter, 61 steroid-dependent patients, 38 of whom had relapsed following treatment with alkylating agents, were treated either with levamisole 2.5 mg/kg on alternate days or with placebo for 112 days. All patients were receiving maintenance alternate-day prednisolone therapy at the beginning of levamisole or placebo treatment: this was tapered and withdrawn over 56 days. At the end of the study, 14 of 31 levamisole-treated patients (45%) and only 4 of 30 placebo-treated patients (13%) were in remission (Figure 18.4): the difference was highly significant ($P = 0.008$). However, 4 of the 14 children in the levamisole group had relapsed within 3 months of stopping treatment. This agrees with the experience of Mongeau *et al.*[16] that, like CyA, levamisole can maintain a proportion of steroid-dependent patients in steroid-free remission as long as it is given, but is ineffective as a permanent cure of the disease. On the positive side, levamisole was well tolerated and no important side effects have been reported in either of the two studies cited or in other published accounts.

Other drugs

There is no evidence that any drugs other than those discussed above have any beneficial effect in the steroid sensitive nephrotic syndrome. Among those agents tried and found wanting are disodium cromoglycate, intravenous human gamma-globulin and high-dose, intravenous methylprednisolone.

It is evident from the foregoing that several options exist for the practical management of children with SSNS in whom steroid therapy alone is proving unsatisfactory. A suggested practical guide to treatment is given in Figure 18.5. Inevitably, given the 'soft' nature of most of the evidence for and against the various drugs now available, these proposals reflect the personal experience and prejudices of the author.

Members of a workshop convened by The British Association of Paediatric Nephrology and The Royal College of Physicians' Research Unit have produced a valuable consensus statement on management and audit potential for steriod responsive nephrotic syndrome and this is recommended reading.[19]

References

1. Carrie B.J., Salyer W.R. and Myers B.D. Minimal change nephropathy: an electrochemical disorder of the basement membrane. *Am. J. Med.* 1981, **70**, 262–268
2. Shalhoub R.J. Pathogenesis of lipoid nephrosis: a disorder of T-cell function. *Lancet* 1974, **ii**, 556–560
3. Schnaper H.W. The immune system in minimal change nephrotic syndrome. *Pediatr. Nephrol.* 1989, **3**, 101–110
4. Bakker W.W. and van Luijk W.H.J. Do circulating factors play a role in the pathogenesis of minimal change nephrotic syndrome? *Pediatr. Nephrol.* 1989, **3**, 341–349
5. Meltzer J.I., Keim H.J., Laragh J.H., Sealey J.E., Kung-Ming J., and Chien S. Nephrotic syndrome: vasoconstriction and hypervolemic types indicated by renin-sodium profiling. *Ann. Int. Med.* 1979, **91**, 688–696
6. Dorhout Mees E.J., Roos J.C., Boer P., Yoe O.H. and Simatupang T.A. Observations on edema formation in the nephrotic syndrome in adults with minimal lesions. *Am. J. Med.* 1979, **67**, 378–384
7. Tulassay T., Rascher W. and Schärer K. Intra- and extrarenal factors of oedema formation in the nephrotic syndrome. *Pediatr. Nephrol.* 1989, **3**, 92–100
8. Sharples P.M. Poulton J. and White R.H.R. Steroid responsive nephrotic syndrome is more common in Asians. *Arch. Dis. Child.* 1985, **60**, 1014–1017
9. Ruder H., Schärer K., Opelz G., Lenhard V., Waldherr R., Müller-Wiefel D.E., Wingen A.-M. and Dirrell J.

Human leucocyte antigens in idiopathic nephrotic syndrome in children. *Pediat. Nephrol.*, 1990, **4**, 478–481

10. Arbeitsgemeinschaft für Pädiatrische Nephrologie. Short versus standard prednisone treatment for initial treatment of idiopathic nephrotic syndrome in children. *Lancet* 1988, **i**, 380–383

11. Rees L., Greene S.A., Adlard P., Jones J., Haycock G.B., Rigden S.P.A., Preece M. and Chantler C. Growth and endocrine function in steroid sensitive nephrotic syndrome. *Arch. Dis. Child.* 1988, **63**, 484–490

12. Ueda N., Kuno K. and Ito S. Eight and 12 week courses of cyclophosphamide in nephrotic syndrome. *Arch. Dis. Child.* 1990, **65**, 1147–1150

13. Fine B.P. Munoz R.A. Uy C.S. and Ty A. Nitrogen mustard therapy in children with nephrotic syndrome unresponsive to corticosteroid therapy. *J. Pediatr.* 1976, **89**, 1014–1016

14. Abramowicz M., Arneil G.C. Barnett H.L. Barron B.A. Edelmann C.M. Jr, Gordillo P.G. Greifer I., Hallman N., Kobayashi O., and Tiddens H. Controlled trial of azathioprine in children with nephrotic syndrome. *Lancet* 1970, **i**, 959–961

15. Niaudet P., Habib R., Tete M.-J., Hinglais N. and Broyer M. Cyclosporin in the treatment of idiopathic nephrotic syndrome in children. *Pediatr. Nephrol.* 1987, **1**, 566–573

16. Mongeau J.-G., Robitaille P.O. and Roy F. Clinical efficacy of levamisole in the treatment of primary nephrosis in children. *Pediat. Nephrol.* **2**, 398–401

17. British Association for Paediatric Nephrology. Levamisole for corticosteroid-dependent nephrotic syndrome in childhood. *Lancet* 1991, **337**, 1555–1557

18. Arakawa M. Scanning electron microscopy of the glomerulus in normal and nephrotic rats. *Lab. Invert.* 1970, **23**, 480–496

19. Consensus statement on management and audit potential for steroid responsive nephrotic syndrome. *Arch. Dis. Child.* 1994, **70**, 151–157.

19

Steroid resistant nephrotic syndromes

R.S. Trompeter

The clinical and biochemical features which suggest steroid unresponsive nephrotic syndrome have been discussed in the previous chapter.

This chapter reviews the present understanding of some of the commoner types of steroid resistant nephrotic syndrome that occur in childhood. A general review of the morphological classification of nephrotic syndrome is provided by Grishman *et al.*[1] and the treatment of nephrotic syndrome in children by Trompeter and Barratt.[2]

Focal segmental glomerulosclerosis (FSGS)

FSGS is a pathological diagnosis that describes a distribution of glomerular scarring without reference to aetiology or pathogenesis. It is the morphological expression of many pathological processes, and it occurs in a primary form not associated with antecendent glomerular or systemic disease. When FSGS is seen in a patient with the nephrotic syndrome, it has important prognostic implications because it identifies a group of children or adults who will have a poor response to steroid therapy and an unfavourable prognosis.

Histopathology

Focal glomerular disease describes a process that involves only some glomeruli while leaving others seemingly normal. Segmental glomerular disease describes lesions involving some lobules of a glomerulus, while others remain unchanged. FSGS and hyalinosis describes a disease that presents both of these features on optical microscopy. Similar lesions may be seen in association with a wide variety of glomerular disease, but its principal presentation is in patients with nephrotic syndrome. This lesion is usually observed near to the corticomedullary junction and is to be differentiated from the presence of an occasional globally sclerosed glomerulus in the outer cortex, which may occur as the result of part of the normal development or aging process. It may also be seen in longstanding cases of minimal change nephrotic syndrome (MCNS) and in this situation does not appear to be associated with a poor response to corticosteroids.

Controversy exists concerning the possible relationship between FSGS and MCNS. Many investigators believe that FSGS represents a varient of MCNS, whereas others view the disease as a separate entity. Proponents of the former concept argue that the lesion of FSGS is frequently observed in the patient who has had a previous biopsy, but demonstrates only the lesion of minimal change disease, and that the clinical features of FSGS and MCNS are similar. Those who support the position that MCNS and FSGS are separate entities view that sclerotic glomeruli are present early in the disease, as are the presence of haematuria and poorly selective proteinuria, and that it is unusual to observe spontaneous or drug-induced remission of the nephrotic syndrome.

Light microscopy

The pathological process in FSGS primarily involves the mesangium and glomerular basement membrane and therefore lesions are much easier to appreciate using stains that emphasize these structures, i.e. periodic acid Schiff (PAS) or the Jane silver methenamine. The mildest change consists of segmental lesions within the glomerular capillary tufts, and may involve only a very small number of individual glomerular loops. There is collapse of the capillaries, increase of mesangial matrix and deposition of variable amounts of hyaline material in the mesangium or capillary lumina. In well-developed lesions, cells loaded with fat droplets and 'foam' cells may be seen. In more advanced lesions, adherence to Bowman's capsule develops, and the process becomes less cellular, more sclerosing and resembles a scar. The lesion may occur anywhere in the glomerulus, but has a predilection for the vascular pole.

Immunofluorescence and histochemistry

On immunufluorescence microscopy, the segmental hyaline lesions most frequently show deposition of the immune globulin IgM. Fine granular or short linear deposits of IgM may also be scattered through the tufts either in the mesangial region or along the periphery of capillary walls in glomeruli that appear normal by light microscopy. In approximately two-thirds of biopsy specimens, C3 complement deposits are localized in the hilar regions, in arteriolar walls, along Bowman's capsule and along tubular basement membrane. There is inconsistent deposition of the early acting complement components C1q and C4, IgG, IgA and fibrin.

Electron microscopy

The optically normal glomeruli uniformly reveal abnormalities on electron microscopy; therefore, sampling problems, although real, are not as severe as one would expect from the light microscopic appearance of the disease. Progression of FSGS is characterized by involvement of more glomeruli and larger segments of glomeruli, until the process becomes diffuse and is difficult to differentiate from chronic non-specific sclerosing glomerulonephritis. The tubules reflect the consequence of heavy proteinuria, including hyaline and lipid droplets and casts. In later stages there is tubular atrophy and interstitial fibrosis.

On electron microscopy, the segmental lesions reveal collapse of capillaries and wrinkling of basement membrane. There may be an increase of mesangial matrix, and electron-dense deposits may be found in mesangial and subendothelial areas. FSGS is therefore a diffuse glomerular disease segmental only on light microscopy.

Natural history

The first clinicopathological study of FSGS in children was published approximately 50 years ago and described 20 children with the nephrotic syndrome all of whom died within 5 years of the onset of oedema. The characteristic histopathological lesion was that of focal and segmental sclerosis of their glomeruli. The prevalence of FSGS in the clinical spectrum of nephrotic syndrome is approximately 4% in children aged less than 4 years, rising to 25% in teenagers. FSGS is the predominant glomerular lesion associated with idiopathic nephrotic syndrome, which progresses to chronic renal failure.

Controversy exists concerning the possible relationship between FSGS and MCNS. The presence of even a single glomerulus with segmental sclerosis in a renal biopsy otherwise chacteristic of MCNS obtained early in the course of the nephrotic syndrome, carries an unfavourable prognosis. The likelihood of a response to treatment with corticosteroids is reduced.

In the clinical setting, FSGS can be broadly divided into two major groups. The first group includes those in whom the histopathological legion is present at the onset of the nephrotic syndrome. The majority of patients will have a refractory nephrotic syndrome, poorly selective proteinuria, persistent microscopic haematuria, hypertension, progressive renal insufficiency and corticosteroid resistance. The second group includes patients in whom the initial histopathology is consistent with MCNS but who subsequently develop a histological picture more closely resembling FSGS. They rarely become hypertensive or have haematuria, usually remain steroid responsive and do not always progress to renal failure.

Actuarial analyses from series of children with biopsy-proven FSGS suggest that renal survival is probably between 45% and 65% at

Table 19.1   Response of steroid resistant nephrotic children with FSGS to treatment with immunosuppression

Author		*n*	*Responded*	*%*
Newman *et al.* (1976)[3]	Azathioprine and cyclophosphamide	6	1	17
Gubler *et al.* (1978)[4]	Chlorambucil and nitrogen mustard	23	2	9
ISKDC (1980)[5]	Cyclophosphamide	23	9	39
Mongeau *et al.* (1981)[6]	Cyclophosphamide	11	0	0
Trompeter (1987)[7]	Cyclophosphamide, vincristine and prednisolone	21	13	62
Mendoza *et al.* (1990)[8]	Cyclophosphamide or chlorambucil and pulse methyl prednisolone	23	18	78

15–20 years, respectively. These data are invariably retrospective and include children treated with corticosteroids and immunosuppressive drugs and the survival figures are influenced by referral artefact and differing policies concerning the timing of renal biopsy.

Treatment

FSGS that remits probably has a good prognosis and treatment directed to this aim is therefore justified to improve both patient survival as well as to minimize complications of the nephrotic state. Collected series suggest a response to corticosteroids, i.e. the induction of remission, of approximately 30%. It is therefore justified to treat any child with at least one standard course of prednisolone in the hope that remission may be induced.

The response of steroid resistant nephrotic syndrome with FSGS to treatment with cyclophosphamide alone is variable. Analyses of results of collective series suggest that approximately 20% of this group enter remission or maintain a plasma albumin concentration of greater than 25 g/litre in the presence of proteinuria.

From within any population of children with FSGS, a subgroup with 'malignancy FSGS' can invariably be identified. These are children identified by the presence of a refractory nephrotic syndrome and/or rapid progression to end-stage renal failure. The association of persistent nephrotic syndrome with a poor outcome for renal function may simply reflect more severe disease. However, it may also be a consequence of the protracted nephrotic state itself, the damage mediated by hyperfiltration due to a low plasma oncotic pressure together with platelet deposition as a consequence of the hyperaggreable state. Aggressive immunosuppression may have a therapeutic role in this small group of patients. This treatment has usually involved more than one course of cyclosphosphamide, sometimes in combination with intravenous pulse corticosteroids and/or vincristine. Lasting remission may be induced in a small number of cases prior to progression to end-stage disease (Table 19.1).[3–8]

The results of treatment of steroid resistant nephrotic syndrome secondary to biopsy proven FSGS with cyclosporin A are disappointing. Although remission or partial remission can occasionally be induced in a small minority, review of published data imply no clear benefit in steroid resistant patients, and that any effect in FSGS may be related to a history of steroid sensitivity rather than to histopathology.

Therapy with anti-platelet drugs such as dipyridamole used in combination with anticoagulation, or non-steroidal anti-inflammatory drugs such as indomethacin, has failed to produce consistent results and the usefulness of these forms of treatment is limited.

Angiotensin converting enzyme inhibitors have been shown to reduce proteinuria and preserve renal function in adult patients with chronic renal insufficiency. Recent published data demonstrated that short-term treatment with captopril reduced urinary protein excretion in children with the nephrotic syndrome of varying histopathology including FSGS.

Recurrence of both proteinuria and the lesions of FSGS is well documented in the transplanted kidney.[9] The incidence of recurrence is greater in children than in adults, with a figure of up to 50% in children aged less than 10 years at apparent onset of the nephrotic syndrome. There is a steady decline in incidence with increasing age. Although the risk of recurrence is substantial, biopsy-proven FSGS as a cause of the idiopathic nephrotic syndrome in childhood is not a contraindication to transplantation.

Mesangiocapillary glomerulonephritis (MCGN)

MCGN (also called membranoproliferative glomerulonephritis) is a well-defined histopathological entity considered separate from the large group of chronic glomerulonephritides, because of its characteristic clinical and pathologic features. Several subtypes of this disease have been recognized. Type I, the classic or subendothelial deposit variety and type III closely related and differing mainly in the localization of immune deposits; type II, or linear dense deposit disease, though clinically similar, is characterized by considerable morphological differences in which refractile, electron-dense material almost completely replaces the lamina densa of the glomerular capillary basement membrane.

Histopathology

Type I

Light microscopy
As the name implies, MCGN is characterized by changes of the mesangium and capillary wall. The glomeruli appear large due to proliferation of mesangial cells and increase of mesangial matrix. At the same time, the proliferating mesangium encircles the capillary loops and becomes interposed between the basement membrane and endothelial cells, leading to apparent duplication of basement membrane, i.e. 'double track' or 'contour'. In silver methanamine-stained preparations, protein deposits can be seen in the mesangium and along the capillary wall in the so-called subendothelial position, but actually within the interposed mesangium.

In MCGN, type III, the deposits disrupt the basement membrane and extend from the subendothelial to the subepithelial side, thus partially replacing the basement membrane.

Immunofluorescence
In type I disease there is consistent deposition of C3 complement in the periphery of glomerular lobules and in the mesangium. Deposition of all immunoglobulins is variable, as is that of early-acting complement components. In type III MCGN, complement deposition is similar but also extends along the capillary wall.

Electron microscopy
Granular electron-dense deposits are found within the mesangial matrix and subendothelially and the 'double contour' appearance in type I MCGN is due to simultaneous staining of the matrix and capillary basement membrane. In type II, the deposits are found within the disrupted basement membrane.

Type II (dense-deposit disease)

Light microscopy
A moderate increase in mesangial cells and matrix is observed, but less than in type I MCGN, and there is no mesangial interposition. The basement membrane is thickened and strongly stained with PAS.

Immunofluorescence
Dense-deposit disease is characterized by the predominance of C3 deposits in the mesangium and along the capillary walls. Deposits of early complement components and immunoglobulins are rare.

Electron microscopy
The diagnostic appearance is of electron-dense material present within the glomerular basement membrane. The transition between these dense deposits and normal basement membrane is striking. Subendothelial deposit are absent.

Clinical features

MCGN is a disease of older children, only rarely occurring in those under 5 years of age, and is more common in girls than boys. It accounts for approximately 5% of childhood nephrotic syndrome. There is considerable evidence that genetic factors play a role in the pathogenesis of MCGN. All types are extremely rare in Blacks and Orientals and the frequency in siblings is greater than would be predicted from its rarity. Familial type II has, however, not been reported. Haematuria is invariable and children present with either an acute nephritic syndrome or recurrent haematuria. Hypertension and reduced glomerular filtration rate are frequently present, although less so compared with adults. The hypertension is exacerbated by treatment with corticosteroids. Significantly more children than adults have MCGN type II and hypocomplementaemia is characteristic. Mean C3 complement levels are lower in type II than in type I. A higher proportion of patients with type II show the presence of C3 activating material (nephritic factor) and there is an increased incidence of partial facio-truncal lipodystrophy.

Natural history

In general, both types of MCGN are progressive with more than 50% of patients affected dead or requiring treatment for end-stage renal failure within 10 years of onset of the disease. Epidemiological studies reveal that after 20 years some 90% of patients will have renal failure and about 10% will show remission. In general, children with MCGN fare better than adults with regard to renal failure. Children do better for the first 10 years; however, thereafter progression occurs at the same rate as for adult onset disease.[10] Levels of complement and hypertension at onset correlate poorly with outcome, whereas the presence of nephrotic syndrome and reduction in glomerular filtration rate correlates significantly with poor prognosis.

Treatment

There are no specific proven treatments for MCGN. The nephrotic syndrome associated with MCGN does not respond to corticosteroids and indeed may be aggravated by this treatment with increased oedema, gastric erosions and severe acute exacerbation of hypertension. It has been suggested that prolonged alternate-day steroid therapy retards the progression of disease; however, controlled trials resulted in a high withdrawal rate from the treatment group because of side effects, so that the result was inconclusive.

Combined treatment with corticosteroids, cyclophosphamide, dipyridamole and anticoagulant has resulted in survival rates much higher than previously observed in adult nephrotic patients. A similar regimen used principally in children was associated with a beneficial short-term result in patients with the most severe disease, i.e. associated with crescent. However, longer term results were less encouraging and the potential risks of the treatment must be weighed carefully against possible benefits. Prospective studies using dipyridamole and aspirin were associated with significantly higher levels of GFR compared to untreated patients.[11]

Recurrence of both types I and II in the allografted kidney is an invariable feature and although renal transplants have been lost due to recurrence of disease, the frequency is not great enough to justify refusing transplantation.

Mesangial proliferative glomerulonephritis (MPGN)

Pure MPGN is an unusual histopathological finding in the childhood nephrotic syndrome, accounting for approximately 5% of cases. Histologically it is defined as showing uniform enlargement and increase in cellularity of the mesangial areas containing at least 4 cells each.

Histopathology

Light microscopy

MPGN is characterized by an increase in mesangial matrix, but the capillary lumina are patent and capillary walls thin. Later stages are associated with mesangial sclerosis and capsular adhesions.

Immunofluorescence

A preponderance of mesangial IgM deposits are found although other immune globulins, especially IgA and complement, may also be found.

Electron microscopy

Small, scattered electron-dense deposits may be found in the mesangium and occasionally in subepithelial areas. In children, the higher grades of mesangial cellularity are associated with electron-dense deposits.

Natural history

The relationship of diffuse MPGN to minimal change disease in FSGS remains a controversial issue in nephrology. Occasional children respond to corticosteroids but the majority are steroid resistant and tend to go spontaneously into remission without specific therapy. Some, however, remain persistently nephrotic and sequential renal biopsy may reveal lesions of FSGS. In some cases IgM is present in the mesangium and occasionally there is IgA deposi-

Table 19.2 Causes of secondary membranous nephropathy

Infections	*Antigen-mediated*
Hepatitis B	SLE
Syphilis	Sjögren's syndrome
Malaria	Sarcoidosis
Schistosomiasis	Renal tubular antigen
Leprosy	Renal transplantation
Drugs and toxins	*Other associations*
Mercury	Malignancy
Gold	Diabetes mellitus
Penicillamine	Renal venous thrombosis
Protenacid	Rheumatoid arthritis
Captopril	Sickle cell disease
Volatile hydrocarbons	Guillain–Barré syndrome

tion. These findings do not appear to influence prognosis.

Membranous glomerulonephritis[12]

The progressive lesion in membranous glomerulonephritis is observed in the glomerular capillary wall and is a histopathological diagnosis made principally on electron microscopy. In all series of biopsied patients, the proportion of cases in children is far less than that in adults. It has been variably reported as representing between 20% and 30% of nephrotic syndromes and between 2% and 5% of paediatric nephrotic syndromes of which 20% is hepatitis B disease associated. Approximately one-third of cases of membranous glomerulonephritis are caused by or associated with a variety of systemic diseases, drugs or toxic agents (Table 19.2)

Histopathology

Light microscopy

Membranous glomerulonephritis is characterized by diffuse thickening of the glomerular capillary walls with widely patent lumina and hypertrophy of the epithelial cells. Subepithelial electron-dense deposits are argyrophilic strands, 'spikes', and appear to arise from the lamina densa of the basement membrane.

Immunofluorescence

The glomerular basement membrane characteristically contains granular deposits of IgG and C3, and less commonly IgM, IgA or early components of complement.

Electron microscopy

New electron-dense deposits are formed continuously and studies have distinguished several patterns of deposition according to their extent and intensity of reaction of the basement membrane. The extent of the histological lesion allows for staging of the disease. Stage II, subendothelial deposits, corresponds to the classic and most common form of membranous glomerulonephritis.

Natural history

The disease can occur at any age, presenting uniformly with a nephrotic syndrome. There is a predominance of males in both adult and childhood series. Gross haematuria and evidence of complement activation are seen only in a minority of patients. The classic course is highly variable but rarely severe, with progression to renal failure in only a small number. Following drug-induced membranous glomerulonephritis, recovery is usual following discontinuation of treatment, and long-term clinical recovery may coexist even in the presence of hepatitis B surface antigenaemia. Although steroids have been shown to be beneficial in idiopathic membranous glomerulonephritis in adults, treatment in children is generally not warranted.

Congenital nephrotic syndrome[13]

Clinical features

Infants with clinical onset of the nephrotic syndrome in the first 3 months of life form a distinct subgroup and behave very differently from children who present with nephrotic syndrome later during the first year of life. The term congenital nephrotic syndrome should be reserved for those infants with early onset. There is frequently a history of a similarly affected family member and the disease invariably runs an intractable course, the majority of infants not benefiting from specific therapies and ultimately dying of complications of their disease.

The disorders associated with the nephrotic syndrome in the first months of life are best classified on the basis of both clinical and pathological features (Table 19.3). The majority of

Table 19.3   Classification of nephrotic syndrome in the first 3 months of life

Primary
Congenital nephrotic syndrome – Finnish type
Diffuse mesangial sclerosis
Minimal change nephrotic syndrome
Focal segmental glomerulosclerosis

Secondary
Congenital syphilis, toxoplasmosis, cytomegalovirus
XY gonadal dysgenesis and Wilms' tumour
Nephroblastoma
Hereditary onycho-osteodysplasia (nail-patella syndrome)
Oculocerebrorenal syndrome (Lowe's syndrome)
Membranous gloerulopathy
Mercury toxicity
Systemic lupus erythematosus (SLE)

infants with congenital onset have proteinuria at birth, although clinical signs may not appear for a few months. Many infants have been shown to have proteinuria *in utero*. The presence of inter-uterine proteinuria and elevated amniotic fluid levels of alpha-fetoprotein before 20 weeks' gestation enables in *utero* detection of this disorder.

The majority of reported cases have the congenital nephrotic syndrome of the Finnish type, which has a well-described autosomal recessive inheritance. The incidence of this disease has been estimated to be 12 cases per 100 000 births in Finland, but is much lower in other parts of the world, with occurrence in most racial groups. Nearly all infants are born prematurely, typically between 35 and 38 weeks, and are small for their gestational age. The placenta is usually much larger than normal, often weighing more than 25% of the infant's birth weight. The mean ratio of placenta to infant weight is 0.43 compared to 0.18 in normal infants. Breech presentation is relatively frequent and signs of fetal asphyxia are common. During the first weeks of life these infants often have non-specific feeding problems. Features such as widened cranial sutures, large fontanelles, pliable cartilagenous tissue and small nose with wide-set eyes and low-set ears have been frequently described. More than 50% present with oedema in the first week of life, and abdominal distension with ascites and umbilical hernia is common.

Early in the disease the typical laboratory findings of heavy proteinuria, > 50 mg kg body weight^{-1} 24 h^{-1}, hypoalbuminaemia and hyper-cholesterolaemia are evident. Renal function is always normal for age and haematuria and leucocyturia may also be present.

Failure to thrive and recurrent gastrointestinal symptoms such as vomiting and diarrhoea invariably complicate the persistent nephrotic state. Some infants may have gastro-oesophageal reflux and pyloric stenosis. Immune defects secondary to both malnutrition and excessive urinary losses of immunoglobulins and complement factors are characterized by severe bacterial infection. Severe oedema and ascites further predisposes to peritonitis and pneumonia. Excessive urinary losses of low molecular weight clotting factors and fibrinolytic proteins lead to a hypercoagulable state, with high incidence of arterial and venous thromboembolic complications. Specific deficiency states such as hypothyroidism due to urinary loss of T4 and thyroid-binding globulin, iron-deficiency anaemia due to loss of transferrin and vitamin D deficiency due to loss of vitamin-D-binding proteins and vitamin D are common. As a consequence, profound neurodevelopmental delay is apparent during the first year of life and seizure disorders secondary to hypocalcaemia or other metabolic disturbance may occur.

The rate of deterioration of renal function is variable, but end-stage renal disease is inevitable during the second and third years of life. As the glomerular filtration rate declines, the nephrotic state may become less clinically apparent, although proteinuria continues, and the physical and biochemical features of chronic renal failure dominate.

Histopathology

Finnish type

The morphology of Finnish-type nephrotic syndrome depends on the stage of the disease at which a renal biopsy is performed. The classic light microscopy finding of 'microcysts', i.e. diffuse cystic dilatation of the proximal tubule, may not be present in all biopsy samples obtained from infants in the first few months of life. Proteinuria of glomerular origin probably precedes 'microcyst' development; similar lesions are seen in biopsy specimens of older infants with steroid sensitive nephrotic syndrome and would suggest that this lesion is acquired. Immature fetal glomeruli, characterized by prominent epithelial cells around the periphery of the glomerular tuft, and an increase in mesangial matrix and cellularity, are early changes. There are no glomerular or mesangial immune deposits. As renal function declines there is glomerular capillary collapse and sclerosis, tubular atrophy and interstitial fibrosis.

Diffuse mesangial sclerosis

The rare and lethal lesion of diffuse mesangial sclerosis displays a distinct histopathological process in the early stages of the disease. Glomerular obliteration and mesangial sclerosis without hypercellularity dominates. With progression of the disease, i.e. deteriorating renal function, glomerular sclerosis and tubulointerstitial fibrosis are found.

Natural history

There is probably no place for the use of corticosteroids or other immunosuppressive drugs in the treatment of primary congenital nephrotic syndrome. Rare spontaneous remissions occur, but historically the majority of infants died of infection, neurological deterioration or renal failure. Many infants with secondary forms of congenital forms of nephrotic syndrome benefit from specific forms of treatment such as antibiotics for syphilis or toxoplasmosis and corticosteroids for SLE.

Every infant with congenital onset of nephrotic syndrome who remains proteinuric throughout the first 2 years of life will develop renal failure. The aim of medical treatment for such children is to promote linear growth with the ultimate objective of renal transplantation. Bilateral native nephrectomy, dialysis and high-calorie nasogastric or gastrostomy feeding ensures the dramatic weight gain necessary for successful transplantation. Patient and graft survival are excellent and are paralleled by improved psychomotor development.

Diffuse mesangial sclerosis is the typical histological finding in Drash syndrome.[14] It is unclear whether or not patients with diffuse mesangial sclerosis, without other features, are a forme fruste of this syndrome and are at risk of Wilms' tumour. In view of the association between pseudohermaphroditism and early onset nephropathy (typically in Drash syndrome), it is wise to check the karyotype of any female infant with early onset nephropathy.

General management of the chronically nephrotic child

Plasma volume expansion

Recognition of early signs of hypovolaemia and an awareness of circumstances predisposing to hypovolaemic crises are important in the management of the chronically nephrotic state. Abdominal pain is a particularly worrying symptom of hypovolaemia, the differential diagnosis including peritonitis and pancreatitis and peptic ulceration in the patient receiving corticosteroids. Plasma infusions must be carefully monitored by regular observation of pulse, blood pressure, jugular venous pressure, respiratory rate and peripheral/central temperature gradient. In health, the plasma volume is approximately 40 ml/kg body weight, so that plasma infusions of 20 ml/kg are appropriate. However, in order to avoid circulatory overload, the use of 20% albumin concentrate is preferable, infusing 1 g protein/kg body weight over a period of 2–3 h. This regimen may be repeated every 12 h until symptomatic improvement is achieved.

Control of oedema

The control of long-standing oedema is potentially a difficult problem. Restriction of dietary sodium intake while maintaining a generous oral protein intake of up to 5 g/kg body weight/24 h, combined with diuretic therapy, are appropriate measures. Frusemide, up to 5 mg kg^{-1} day^{-1}, alone or in combination with other loop diuretics or aldosterone antagonists, may be effective in producing a natriuresis.

Thromboembolic complications

Proteins involved in initiating both coagulation and fibrinolysis show altered synthesis, turnover and loss in the urine. As a consequence there is a small but significant incidence of both arterial thrombosis, approximately 0.7%, and about 1.1% venous thrombosis in nephrotic children. This complication is largely avoided by early recognition and treatment of the hypovolaemic state. Meticulous attention to venepuncture and intravenous infusion sites is mandatory. Femoral vein puncture must be avoided. In the hypercoagulable state, mobilization rather than bed rest is indicated. Major thrombotic episodes require anticoagulation.

Infection

Bacterial infection due to Gram-negative and Gram-positive organisms are common. Cellulitis, peritonitis, pneumonia and otitis are common and must be treated promptly and aggressively. Susceptibility to 'pneumococcus' is significant and penicillin prophylaxis is therefore recommended. Immunization with pneumococcal vaccine appears of limited value in the nephrotic patient.

References

1. Grishman E., Ehrenreich T. and Churg J. The morphologic spectrum of primary and secondary nephrotic syndrome in man. In: Cameron J.S. and Glassock R.J. (eds) *The Nephrotic Syndrome*. New York, Marcel Dekker, 1988: 285–372

2. Trompeter R.S. and Barratt T.M. Treatment and management of the nephrotic syndrome in children. In: Cameron J.S. and Glassock R.J. (eds) *The Nephrotic Syndrome*. New York, Marcel Dekker, 1988: 423–460

3. Newman W.J., Tisher C.C., McCoy R.C., Gunnells J.C., Krueger R.P., Clapp J.R. and Robinson R.R. Focal glomerular sclerosis: contrasting clinical patterns in children and adults. *Medicine (Baltimore)* 1976, **55**, 67

4. Gubler M.C., Waldherr R., Levy M., Broyer M. and Habib R. Idiopathic nephrotic syndrome with focal and segmental sclerosis and or hyalinosis: clinical course, response to therapy and long term outcome. In: Strauss (ed.) *Pediatric Nephrology*. Garland STMP Press, New York, 1978: 193–212

5. International Study of Kidney Disease in Children. Proceedings of the 5th International Paediatric Nephrology Symposium 1980 (Abstract *Ped. Res.* 1980, **14**, 1006)

6. Mongeau J.G., Corneille L., Robitaille P., O'Regan S. and Pelletier M. Primary nephrosis in childhood associated with focal glomerular sclerosis: is long term prognosis that severe? *Kidney Int.* 1981, **20**, 743

7. Trompeter R.S. Steroid resistant nephrotic syndrome: a review of the treatment of focal segmental glomerulosclerosis in children. In: Murakami K., Kitagawa T., Yubata K. and Sakai T. (eds) *Recent Advances in Pediatric Nephrology*. Amsterdam, Excerpta Medica, 1987: 363–371

8. Mendoza S.A., Reznik V.M., Griswold W.R., Krensky A.M., Yorgin P.D. and Tune B.M. Treatment of steroid-resistant focal segmental glomerulosclerosis with pulse methyl prednisolone and alkylating agents. *Pediatr. Nephrol.* 1990, **4**, 303–307

9. Senggutuvan P., Cameron J.S., Hartley R.B., Rigden S.P.A., Chantler C., Haycock G.B., Williams D.G., Ogg C.S. and Koffman G. Recurrence of focal segmental glomerulosclerosis in transplanted kidneys: analysis of incidence and risk factors in 59 allografts. *Pediatr. Nephrol.* 1990, **4**, 21–28

10. Cameron J.S., Turner D.R., Heaton J., Williams D.G., Ogg C.S., Chantler C., Haycock G.B. and Hicks J. Idiopathic mesangiocapillary glomerulonephritis. Comparison of Types I and II in children and adults and long-term prognosis. *Am. J. Med.* 1983, **74**, 175–192

11. Donadio J.V., Anderson C.F., Mitchell J.C., Holley K.E., Ilstrup D.M., Fuster V. and Chesbro J.H. Membranoproliferative glomerulonephritis. A prospective clinical trial of platelet-inhibitor therapy. *New Engl. J. Med.* 1984, **310**, 1421–1426

12. Kleinknecht C. and Habib R. Membranous glomerulonephritis. In: Holliday M.A., Barratt T.M. and Vernier R.L. (eds) *Pediatric Nephrology*, 2nd edn. Baltimore, Williams and Wilkins, 1987: 462–470

13. Sibley R.K., Mahan J., Mauer S.M. and Vernier R.L. A clinicopathological study of forty-eight infants with nephrotic syndrome. *Kidney Int.* 1985, **27**, 544–552

14. Manivel, J.C. *et.al.* Complete and incomplete Drash syndrome. *Human. Pathol.* 1987, **18**, no. 1

20

Renal manifestations of systemic disorders

A.J. Fish

Renal involvement is present in many systemic disorders of children. In some instances the prognosis of the disease will depend on the severity of the renal lesions (systemic lupus erythematosus, anaphylactoid purpura), and in other diseases renal involvement will be rare and will not significantly alter the prognosis (mixed connective tissue disease). In other disorders, such as diabetes mellitus, the renal lesions will usually not cause significant problems during childhood, but will be the cause of significant morbidity in later years. In this chapter, we discuss the renal manifestations of systemic diseases with renal involvement most commonly encountered in childhood.

Systemic lupus erythematosus

Systemic lupus erythematosus (SLE) is an immune complex mediated disorder which has an autoimmune basis. Multiple organ involve-

ment appears to be caused by vascular bed localization of circulating immune complexes. The biological properties of immune complexes, including complement activation and inflammatory cell chemotaxis, result in vascular injury and increased vascular permeability. When immune complexes localize to the glomerular capillary wall, lupus glomerulonephritis develops.

Systemic manifestations of SLE

The clinical manifestations of systemic injury in SLE are summarized in Table 20.1. The onset of SLE in the childhood population is observed between the ages of 11 and 15 years, although the disease may present earlier in life.[1,2] The presence of fever, skin rash and arthritis are most commonly encountered. The typical skin eruption is an erythematous rash over the bridge of the nose and malar areas, resulting in a butterfly distribution. The lesions may become vesicular and bullous, depending on the extent of vasculitic involvement, and ultimately focal areas of epidermal and dermal necrosis may develop. The rash is not limited to the face and may spread to involve the scalp with alopecia, neck, upper chest and arms. Periungal inflammation with secondarily infected paronychiae may be observed. The photosensitive nature of the skin lesions is typical, with worsening of the dermal manifestations associated with sun exposure. Mucous membranes of the nose and oral mucosa may be involved with painful ulcerations. Acute joint symptoms affect-

Table 20.1 Findings at the time of diagnosis of SLE

Symptoms and findings	%
Fever	60
Rash	80
Arthritis	60
Weight loss	30
Splenomegaly or lymphadenopathy	30
Cardiovascular	25
Central nervous system	20
Renal involvement	50

ing the small joints of the fingers and toes, wrists, ankles and knees result from synovitis and joint effusion. Destruction of joint surface cartilage, resulting in deforming arthritic disabilities, is seldom found.

Central nervous system involvement in SLE is difficult to assess. Based on vasculitic involvement of the brain, children often manifest personality changes, loss of intellectual capacity and subtle reduced academic achievement. More obvious neurological abnormalities manifest as seizures, cranial nerve lesions and chorea. Of interest, the latter may precede the other manifestations of SLE, and when combined with fever and joint symptoms, chorea may be mistakenly diagnosed as a component of rheumatic fever. This is further confounded by the recognized association of mitral (Libman–Sacks endocarditis) and aortic valvular inflammation.

Myocarditis, pericarditis and pericardial effusions may additionally occur. Secondary to vasculitic involvement of large vessels, arterial thrombosis, venous thromboses and pulmonary emboli have been observed in SLE. Bilateral or unilateral pleuritic chest pain due to pleural inflammation and effusions may develop.

Renal manifestations of SLE

A wide spectrum of clinical findings relating to renal involvement of SLE is observed. Regardless of the nature of the extrarenal involvement due to SLE, the overall incidence of renal disease in childhood SLE is 75%. One-quarter of the patients have normal renal function and no proteinuria. Severe renal disease with significant loss of renal function or heavy proteinuria is evident in 40% of patients. In the remaining patients, lesser degrees of proteinuria with or without mild impairment in renal function is observed. Depending upon the severity of glomerular injury, hypertension will be found. Without adequate therapy for SLE, progressive renal injury can be anticipated, leading to worsening nephrotic syndrome, uraemia and ultimately death due to renal insufficiency.

Renal histopathological findings

Studies of the natural history and overall prognosis of childhood and adult cases of SLE have been most closely correlated with the nature of pathological renal lesions. It is therefore recommended that SLE patients presenting with evidence of renal disease have a kidney biopsy to establish the severity of the histological changes. Because of the life-long duration of SLE and the chronic state of remission and exacerbations related to steroid therapy, a renal biopsy more accurately documents the nature and extent of the renal disease at the time of onset of SLE as well as long-term prognosis. Since complexities exist with respect to the various histopathological changes, the following basic classification of renal SLE has been adopted: normal, mesangial lupus nephritis, proliferative lupus nephritis (focal and diffuse), and membranous lupus nephritis.

In mesangial lupus nephritis there is mild mesangial cell proliferation, slight glomerular capillary endothelial reaction and minimal white cell infiltration; fibrinoid deposition, segmental glomerular necrosis and karyorrhexis are not present. By immunofluorescence, mesangial deposits of complement and immunoglobulins are observed which correspond to small deposits found in the mesangium by electron microscopy. Patients with these findings probably will have normal renal function, mild proteinuria and haematuria. In proliferative lupus nephritis, more severe endothelial cell proliferation is present with glomerular capillary lumen narrowing and significant polymorphonuclear leucocyte infiltration. Areas of glomerular necrosis, 'wire loop' lesions and epithelial cell crescents may be present. If the abnormalities are present in over 80% of glomeruli, the diffuse category is designated; the prognosis is somewhat worse in this situation compared to the focal form of proliferative lupus nephritis. By immunofluorescence and electron microscopy, extensive mesangial and subendothelial deposits are found. Scattered subepithelial deposits or 'humps' are also observed; however, the extensive subendothelial deposits which contain immunoglobulin and complement components make up the 'wire loop' lesion seen by light microscopy. These patients have the most severe clinical findings with hypertension, nephrotic syndrome and loss of renal function. During the course of steroid therapy there can be a remarkable improvement of these abnormalities; serial kidney biopsies have revealed regression of the inflammatory reaction and progressive decrease in the size and extent of immunoglobulin and complement deposition. The necrotic lesions and glomerular hyalinization will not respond to therapy, resulting in residual scarring or glomerular obsolescence. Extra-glomerular renal lesions such as interstitial fibrosis and extensive tubular and vascular lesions are not likely to respond to therapy. Therefore, the extent of glomerular scarring and interstitial fibrosis will determine the degree of residual impairment of renal function which is permanent and which will not recover with immunosuppressive therapy. Sequential kidney biopsies are of help in establishing these findings and guiding the clinical use of steroid therapy.

The fourth type of renal lesion found in SLE is membranous lupus nephritis. This lesion is quite different from the abnormalities described above, since usually only minimal glomerular endothelial proliferation is evident. Instead, extensive diffuse thickening of the glomerular basement membrane is seen. By immunofluorescence and electron microscopy, fine regular deposits of immunoglobulin are found in an epimembranous/subepithelial localization; the deposits are small, but regular and uniform in size and distribution. These lesions are indistinguishable from the findings in idiopathic membranous glomerulopathy in other patients who do not have SLE. Unlike the response to steroid therapy described above in proliferative lupus nephritis, the membranous lupus nephritis lesions do not respond well to this type of treatment. Clinically these patients have proteinuria with or without nephrotic syndrome, which waxes and wanes over many years. In some cases progressive glomerular scarring ensues, and ongoing renal failure cannot be prevented by immunosuppressive therapy.

Laboratory findings

As described above, SLE patients may have normal renal function with normal urinalyses. Those patients with proliferative lupus nephritis have low creatinine clearance and increased urinary protein excretion. When proteinuria is marked, nephrotic syndrome with hypoalbuminaemia and hypercholesterolaemia are found. SLE patients with active lupus nephritis usually have increased formed elements in the urine with red and white blood cells, cellular and granular casts.

Various serological and immunologic parameters are assessed in SLE patients. The fluorescent antinuclear antibody (FANA) test detects the presence of serum autoantibodies to nuclear antigens. The test is performed by overlaying SLE sera on a normal tissue target and examining the binding of patient IgG to nuclear constituents. The homogeneous pattern of nuclear staining indicates antibodies to deoxynucleoprotein and is not specific for SLE. Similarly, the speckled pattern of nuclear staining which is directed against several other nuclear antigens is found in SLE, as well as other connective tissue disorders. Peripheral nuclear staining or 'rim pattern', however, is almost virtually diagnostic of SLE; this pattern is associated with autoantibodies to native DNA. The activity of SLE with the risk of ongoing tissue injury is well correlated with the level of anti-DNA autoantibodies, and is well suppressed by steroid therapy. Anti-DNA antibody levels can also be measured by ELISA to more closely monitor disease activity and response to therapy.

Measurements of serum complement are also a useful guide to diagnosis and treatment of SLE. Levels of C3 or total haemolytic complement titres are low in the acute phases of SLE and usually return to normal with steroid therapy. Other serological tests are frequently abnormal in SLE but are not useful as guides in therapy; these include biologically false positive syphilis test, rheumatoid factor, circulating immune complexes, and cryoglobulins which may be present. Abnormalities in blood clotting tests include prolongation of the partial thromboplastin time; when the latter is due to autoantibodies to specific blood clotting factors such as factor VIII, a significant bleeding diathesis exists. Leucopenia, thrombocytopenia and Coombs' positive haemolytic anaemia are all caused by autoantibodies to these formed blood elements. Most of the latter abnormalities are corrected by steroid therapy and serve as indicators of SLE activity during the course of therapy.

Differential diagnosis of SLE

There are a number of diseases which are closely related to SLE and at times may be difficult to differentiate from SLE. On the other hand, true overlap syndromes exist where other collagen diseases such as scleroderma, dermatomyositis and mixed connective tissue disease are actually present in association with SLE.

Acute rheumatic fever is difficult clinically to separate from SLE because of the presence of arthritis, chorea, fever, and mitral or aortic valvular disease. These patients may have erythema marginatum and subcutaneous nodules which are characteristic of rheumatic fever, and the complement levels are normal and FANA antibodies are negative.

At onset, juvenile rheumatoid arthritis is associated with arthralgia, fever, weight loss, splenomegaly and elevated sedimentation rate; together these findings resemble SLE. Mixed connective tissue disease has a number of features typical of rheumatoid arthritis (arthritis), SLE (fever, lymphadenopathy, splenomegaly and cardiac findings), and scleroderma (oesophageal motility abnormalities and Raynaud's phenomenon). This disorder is diagnosed by very high FANA titre (speckled pattern) which is specific for ribonucleoprotein antigens; these patients have normal serum complement levels and lack anti-DNA antibodies.

Patients with a variety of vasculitic disorders such as periarteritis nodosa, anaphylactoid purpura and (drug-induced) serum sickness frequently develop renal disease and may resemble SLE. The individual characteristics of these and other disorders including thrombotic thrombocytopenic purpura and malignant hypertension usually permit easy differentiation from SLE.

Subacute bacterial endocarditis with glomerulonephritis may be remarkably difficult to differentiate from SLE; these patients have weight loss, fever, splenomegaly, valvular heart murmurs and cutaneous purpura. Low serum complement levels, positive rheumatoid factor, FANA titres and high sedimentation rates closely mimic SLE. This diagnosis must be carefully excluded by repeated blood cultures of severely ill patients with suspected SLE before starting steroid therapy.

Immunofluorescence of skin biopsies of normal or affected skin lesions in SLE reveals IgG deposition along the dermal–epidermal junction; this finding is present in approximately one-half of SLE patients, being more frequently observed when significant renal disease is evident. This test is relatively non-invasive and may be of help in differentiating other diseases from SLE.

Treatment of SLE[3–5]

Steroid therapy is used in the treatment of SLE; beneficial effects from this medication are quickly seen with early control of systemic manifestations of the disease. Malaise, fever, skin rash and arthritis are easily controlled, even with low doses of steroid. In the absence of significant renal disease, we recommend a 2–3-week course of prednisone 60 mg/m^2 in divided doses until the serum complement levels return to normal and anti-DNA antibody titres disappear. Thereafter prednisone can be reduced to 60 mg/m^2 every other day.

The management of SLE when major organ involvement exists with renal disease, central nervous system or cardiac complications, involves the addition of immunosuppressive therapy with azathioprine. As outlined below, the prognosis in SLE is related to recovery and healing of the severe renal lesions. Since relapse of active SLE frequently occurs, with falling serum complement levels and rise in anti-DNA titres when prednisone is tapered to an every other day regimen, this appears to be significantly less frequent when azathioprine is used along with prednisone. Although never critically evaluated by controlled clinical studies, the long-term survival in SLE has dramatically improved with this approach, and most investigators have adopted this concept. Along these lines, other investigators have used cyclophosphamide immunosuppressive therapy employing monthly intravenous bolus doses.

We recommend continuing alternate-day prednisone and azathioprine (1–2 mg kg^{-1} day^{-1}) over several years, to allow complete healing of the glomerular lesions of focal and diffuse lupus nephritis. Clinically there is return of normal renal function, disappearance of proteinuria, and repeat kidney biopsies show restoration of normal glomerular architecture. Although it was initially thought that normal or mild renal involvement at the outset of SLE had a good prognosis, it is now appreciated that, without continuous maintenance of serological suppression in SLE, there can be progressive renal injury. Unlike the approach given to proliferative lupus nephritis, the treatment of membranous lupus nephritis with low-dose steroids is recommended since this lesion does not respond to steroid therapy. Although the beneficial response to steroid therapy in SLE is well established, long-term administration of steroids may result in the following complications: hypertension, osteoporosis, infections, avascular necrosis, carbohydrate intolerance, lens cataracts, pseudotumour cerebri and psychosis. Considerable attention to these risks must be given as long-term administration of steroids to SLE patients is carried out. To this end, slow tapering of prednisone to 20–30 mg/m^2 on alternate days is tried, with close monitoring of blood serology and renal parameters.

Prognosis in SLE

The prognosis and survival in SLE has improved remarkably. From the pre-steroid era when the 5-year survival was less than 10%, today we are achieving 10-year survival figures of nearly 90%. The outlook in SLE correlates with the nature of the renal involvement, with the poorest survival being those patients with severe lupus nephritis. The improved outcome among the latter seems to be related to closely monitoring steroid and azathioprine dosage by following the serum complement and anti-DNA titres; the latter have been the most useful parameters of SLE activity. Although stricter and aggressive modes of steroid therapy have probably improved survival in SLE, one must allow that newer diagnostic techniques, improved dialysis, transplantation and more potent antimicrobial drugs have contributed to the better outcome in SLE.

The most serious complications in SLE remain related to infections of bacterial aetiology. Secondary infections are also due to opportunistic pathogens such as fungal (*Candida albicans*, aspergillus, cryptococcus), viral (cytomegalovirus), and parasitic (*Pneumocystis carinii*) agents. With increasing survival there is a changing pattern of complications leading to death, these relating to increased incidence of malignancy, myocardial infarction and arteriosclerotic thromboses.

In the majority of patients, renal SLE can be successfully treated with complete restoration of normal renal function. In a few patients active renal disease persists since adequate suppression of SLE cannot be achieved. Furthermore, some patients have irreversible renal involvement with glomerular scarring and interstitial fibrosis before adequate therapy can be started. Ultimate renal failure leads to dialysis and transplantation. The results with the latter have been excellent without evidence of significant recurrence of renal SLE in the grafted organ.

The key to the long-term success and favourable outcome in SLE appears related to a constant vigil with very close monitoring of SLE activity. The long-term suppression of autoimmunity, achieving a balance to avoid complications of therapy itself is the major objective in the care of patients with renal SLE.

Henoch-Schoenlein purpura

Anaphylactoid (Henoch-Schoenlein) purpura is one of the most common systemic diseases with renal involvement encountered in children. This disorder is more frequent in boys than in girls and occurs at any age, being more common between the ages of 2 and 8 years. It is often preceded by an upper respiratory tract infection and occasionally associated with streptococcal infection. This disorder has also occurred following immunization and exposure to drugs. Although the aetiology is unknown, it has been suggested that allergy may play a role in the pathogenesis of the disease; however, definite pathogenetic mechanism(s) are unknown. Affected organs show evidence of small vessel vasculitis, most frequently involving the capillaries but also the arterioles and venules. The affected vessels are surrounded by polymorphonuclear and round cell infiltrates, with varying amounts of nuclear debris, red cell extravasation and oedema.[6-9]

Systemic manifestations

Henoch-Schoenlein purpura is a multi-organ disease, affecting most frequently the skin, joints, gastrointestinal tract, kidneys and, less frequently, the central nervous system and testes. The onset of this disorder is variable, often accompanied by constitutional symptoms such as fever and malaise. Initially, multiple organ involvement may be evident, or the onset may be more gradual with appearance of different manifestations of the disease over the course of a few weeks.

Skin involvement is present in all patients and represents the hallmark of the disease. Characteristic cutaneous lesions involve the lower extremities and buttocks and less frequently the upper extremities, face and trunk. The lesions may initially appear urticarial, beginning as small wheals or erythematous papules and evolve into dark red purpuric macules that do not blanch on pressure. The purpura will usually fade but occasionally can develop into small vesicles and desquamate. The lesions appear in crops, and can be present in different stages at one time. The pathology of the skin lesion is a typical leucocytoclastic vasculitis, with deposition of IgA and fibrin in small dermal vessels of affected skin and occasionally in unaffected areas. A less common skin finding is angioedema of the scalp, face and extremities.

Gastrointestinal tract signs and symptoms are present in about 75% of patients, consisting of colicky abdominal pain, often accompanied by vomiting, melaena, ileus and haematemesis. Abdominal pain may precede the appearance of the purpuric rash by a week and make the diagnosis of anaphylactoid purpura difficult. Other gastrointestinal manifestations which are less common but much more severe are intussusception, massive gastrointestinal haemorrhage and intestinal perforation secondary to bowel wall necrosis. In 50% of patients, the stool will be positive for blood.

Joint manifestations are usually present in 60% of the patients, and usually involve large joints of the knees and ankles. Affected joints are swollen and painful on motion; often periarticular swelling and effusions have been observed. The joint symptoms are transient and do not lead to permanent deformity. Central nervous system manifestations are infrequent but can have serious sequelae, resulting from cerebral vasculitis or intracranial hemorrhage; the latter may be secondary to severe hypertension when renal involvement is present. The most common manifestations are seizures, coma and cerebrovascular accidents. Testicular swelling secondary to vasculitis has been reported in up to 10% of male patients. Other miscellaneous manifestations of anaphylactoid purpura have been reported infrequently: acute haemorrhagic pancreatitis, hepatomegaly, intramuscular haemorrhage, pulmonary haemorrhage, epistaxis, parotiditis, carditis and optic neuritis.

Renal manifestations

The renal involvement in Henoch–Schoenlein purpura is common, its frequency varying from 25% to 50% in different series, depending on the extent of renal assessment. The clinical manifestations of renal involvement are most often present within the first month of the disease, almost always present within 3 months after the initial rash, but occasionally noted to appear several months after the onset of disease.

The clinical manifestations are variable: microscopic haematuria, gross haematuria, proteinuria with or without nephrotic syndrome, acute nephritis and progressive renal failure can occur. All children with renal disease have

haematuria and proteinuria, approximately one-half have nephrotic syndrome or renal insufficiency early in the course of the disease, and 25% of the latter followed for more than 1 year develop end-stage renal failure.

Renal pathology

Glomerular involvement in anaphylactoid purpura is variable. The classification by Meadows and co-workers and by the International Study of Kidney Disease in Children is most frequently used: (I) minimal change, (II) mesangial proliferation, (IIIa) focal mesangial proliferation with less than 50% crescents, (IIIb) diffuse mesangial proliferation with less than 50% crescents, (IVa) focal mesangial proliferation with 50–75% crescents, (IVb) diffuse mesangial proliferation with 50–75% crescents, (Va) focal mesangial proliferation with greater than 75% crescents, (Vb) diffuse mesangial proliferation with greater than 75% crescents, (VI) membranoproliferative glomerulonephritis. The outcome of the renal disease seems to be related to the severity of the histological lesions. Groups I, II and III rarely progress to end-stage renal failure and usually have normal renal function with only mild haematuria and proteinuria. Most children who develop progressive renal failure have more than 50% of glomeruli involved with crescent formation.

By electron microscopy, dense deposits are observed in the mesangium in all patients, and less commonly in the subendothelial and subepithelial areas. Varying degrees of widening of the mesangium, segmental mesangial interposition, mesangial hypercellularity and polymorphonuclear leucocytes in glomerular capillary lumina may be present.

Immunofluorescent findings reveal in all cases the presence of mesangial IgA deposits. In contrast to the usually focal nature of lesions seen on light microscopy, IgA deposits are generalized and diffuse throughout the glomerular population. IgG, C3, fibrin and occasionally IgM can also be found in the mesangium. These deposits are usually mesangial but can also extend along the capillary walls as subendothelial deposits.

Laboratory investigation

There is no laboratory test which is diagnostic of Henoch–Schoenlein purpura. Moderate leucocytosis is present in 50% of patients with normal platelets, and occasionally low haemo-globin and haematocrit when there has been significant gastrointestinal haemorrhage. Anti-nuclear antibody and rheumatoid factor are negative. IgA levels are elevated in approxi-mately 50% of patients at the onset of disease, and C3 levels are normal. The stools are positive for blood in 50% of patients. Blood clotting tests are usually normal unless nephrotic syn-drome is present, and then coagulation abnor-malities will be those associated with nephrotic syndrome.

In patients with renal involvement, varying degrees of haematuria, proteinuria and decrease in glomerular filtration rate will be found. A renal biopsy will be helpful in establishing the severity of the renal involvement and the need for therapy. A biopsy is indicated when there is significant proteinuria, nephrotic syndrome or evidence of renal insufficiency.

Differential diagnosis

The classic triad of purpuric skin rash, gastro-intestinal symptoms and joint involvement is sug-gestive of anaphylactoid purpura. Since there is no definitive laboratory test for this dis-order, the diagnosis rests mostly on clinical assessment.

The differential diagnosis includes systemic lupus erythematosus, acute poststreptococcal glomerulonephritis, haemolytic-uraemic syn-drome, other vasculitides (Wegener's granulo-matosis, periarteritis nodosa, mucocutaneous lymph node syndrome) and other causes of purpura and glomerulonephritis. Systemic lupus erythematosus can present with a similar purpuric skin rash, joint involvement and renal manifestations; the presence of antinuclear anti-bodies, the decreased levels of complement C3 and C4, and the clinical and laboratory evi-dence of other manifestations of systemic lupus erythematosus, will establish the diagnosis. Acute poststreptococcal glomerulonephritis can occasionally present with a purpuric skin rash. The presence of low C3, and serological evidence of an antecedent streptococcal infec-tion, will rule out anaphylactoid purpura. Haemolytic-uraemic syndrome needs to be con-sidered since it also can present with a purpu-ric skin rash, abdominal manifestations and renal involvement; thrombocytopenia and a microangiopathic anaemia will establish the diagnosis.

Other causes of purpura, disseminated intra-vascular coagulation, and abnormalities of blood clotting must be excluded by laboratory testing. Other vasculitides such as Wegener's granulomatosis, periarteritis nodosa, can be difficult to differentiate. The clinical character-istics of these diseases and the findings of granulomas in Wegener's granulomatosis, an-eurysms in periarteritis nodosa, and positive antineutrophil cytoplasmic antibodies, will es-tablish these diagnoses. The renal disease of anaphylactoid purpura must be differentiated from the following glomerular disorders: IgA nephropathy, poststreptococcal glomerulone-phritis, systemic lupus erythematosus, mem-branoproliferative glomerulonephritis. With the exception of IgA nephropathy and SLE, which also have mesangial IgA deposits, the renal histopathology will differentiate these dif-ferent diseases.

Treatment

The prognosis of Henoch–Schoenlein nephritis is dependent upon the extent of glomerular lesions. Clinical evidence of renal insufficiency and/or nephrotic syndrome, histological find-ings of glomerular necrosis and sclerosis, or extensive crescent formation are indications of a poor prognosis.

In mild cases of Henoch–Schoenlein nephritis therapy consists mostly of conservative manage-ment and careful monitoring to detect the major serious complications of the disease. Steroid therapy is indicated when there is severe abdomi-nal pain and haemorrhage, which respond fa-vourably to this therapy. Steroid therapy is also of benefit to manage the neurological manifesta-tions, testicular swelling and pulmonary haem-orrhage; however, it is not useful to treat cuta-neous purpura.

The value of immunosuppressive therapy of the renal disease is uncertain since controlled studies have not been performed, and there is also variability in the natural course of Henoch–Schoenlein nephritis. It is generally agreed that patients with mild renal involve-ment do not require immunosuppressive therapy. We recommend that patients with severe renal involvement clinically and the exten-sive histological abnormalities discussed above be treated with immunosuppressive drugs to reduce the risk of developing progressive renal failure. Prednisone ($2\ mg\ kg^{-1}\ day^{-1}$) and azathioprine (2 mg kg^{-1} day^{-1}) are given initially. Renal transplantation has been performed successfuly in patients with end-stage renal failure and only occasional reports of recurrence have been described.

Scleroderma

Scleroderma, also known as 'progressive sclerosis', is a multisystem disease which frequently involves the kidney.[10,11] It is a rare disease in the paediatric population, although it has been described in children as young as 3 years of age. The aetiology remains unknown. Renal involvement is unusual at the onset of scleroderma, but occurs within 3 years of presentation and is characterized by the presence of proteinuria, hypertension and various degrees of azotaemia. The presence of azotaemia in patients with scleroderma is a poor prognostic

Table 20.2   Classification of vasculitic syndromes in childhood

Necrotizing vasculitis of small and medium size muscular arteries
    Polyarteritis nodosa
    Infantile polyerteritis nodosa – Kawasaki syndrome
    Allergic angiitis and granulomatosis
      (Churg–Strauss syndrome)
Vasculitis of small size vessels
    Henoch–Schoenlein purpura
    Cutaneous hypersensitivity vasculitis
    Hypocomplementaemia-urticarial vasculitis
    Serum sickness
Vasculitis of small size arteries and veins with granuloma
    Wegener's granulomatosis
Vasculitis of medium and large arteries with giant cells
    Systemic or temporal arteritis
    Takayasu's arteritis
Miscellaneous vasculitides

sign and, until recently, was uniformly fatal within 1 year of its appearance. Scleroderma renal crisis presents with an abrupt onset of malignant hypertension with oliguric renal failure and, if untreated, results in death.

Steroid treatment is of no benefit in the management of the renal manifestations of the disease. Calcium channel blockers have been reported to relieve symptoms of Raynaud's phenomenon.

Mixed connective tissue disease

Mixed connective tissue disease is characterized by overlapping features of systemic lupus erythematosus, rheumatoid arthritis and scleroderma.[12,13] Myositis, arthritis, lymphadenopathy, fever, anaemia and leucopenia are prominent clinical manifestations which will often improve with steroid therapy early in the course of the disease. Raynaud's phenomenon, sclerodactyly and oesophageal disorders have a less favourable response to therapy. There is a high titre of antibodies directed against a saline extractable nuclear antigen (ENA), termed anti-RNP (ribonucleoprotein) autoantibody. Renal involvement is uncommon and has been reported in 5–15% of patients. Membranous nephropathy or proliferative glomerulonephritis may be encountered; these abnormalities are usually non-progressive, and only in rare cases has progression to renal insufficiency occurred.

Vasculitis

Vasculitis is characterized by inflammation and necrosis of blood vessels. Clinical manifestations of vasculitis may result from primary blood vessel involvement or may accompany systemic disorders such as systemic lupus erythematosus or infections. The classification of primary vasculitides is difficult as these diseases are heterogeneous and have overlapping features.[14] A practical approach uses the size and nature of the vessels involved in the disease processes as outlined in Table 20.2. Many vasculitides have involvement of renal vessels with additional various clinical features which are detailed below.

Polyarteritis nodosa

Polyarteritis nodosa is a necrotizing vasculitis of small and medium size muscular arteries; the lesions are segmental and frequently located at bifurcation points along arteries. Many organ systems are involved in the disease process, the kidney being the most frequent, followed by the musculoskeletal system, gastrointestinal tract, liver, peripheral nerves, skin, heart and central nervous system. It is more commonly seen in males after the fourth decade, but this disorder occurs in children.[15–17]

The clinical presentation may be non-specific with constitutional symptoms of fever, malaise, weight loss and leucocytosis. Abnormal urinary sediment, decreased renal function and hypertension are the presenting signs of renal vascular involvement and underlying glomerulonephritis. Eighty per cent of patients with 'pauci immune' vasculitis have elevated antineutrophil cytoplasmic antibodies (P-ANCA).

The diagnosis of polyarteritis nodosa requires the demonstration of necrotizing vasculitis of small and medium size arteries. However, histopathological confirmation of the disease cannot usually be obtained since involved organs are inaccessible to biopsy. A characteristic angiographic feature of periarteritis nodosa is the presence of aneurysms in hepatic, abdominal and renal vessels; documentation of arterial aneurysms will help establish the diagnosis when histological analysis is unavailable. The prognosis of childhood periarteritis nodosa depends on the organ systems involved; without treatment, severe cases have a poor outlook. Extensive renal involvement with renal failure has a poor prognosis. Steroid therapy and, more recently, immunosuppressive therapy have considerably improved the prognosis. Prednisone 2 mg kg^{-1} day^{-1} in divided doses, combined with cyclophosphamide 2 mg kg^{-1} day^{-1} is the treatment of choice in severely affected individuals.

Kawasaki syndrome – infantile polyarteritis nodosa

Infantile polyarteritis nodosa and Kawasaki disease represent the same entity. Epidemics of Kawasaki disease have been described and have focused more attention on this entity.

Young children with infantile polyarteritis nodosa have different clinical features than older children and adults.[17–19] Infants usually less than 1 year of age, predominantly boys, have a clinical syndrome with the onset of prolonged fever accompanied by rash, conjunctivitis and respiratory symptoms. Some patients have hypertension and evidence of coronary artery thrombosis with myocardial infarction which often leads to death.

The pathological lesion is a necrotizing arteritis with predilection for the coronary vessels; renal vessels are involved but less frequently than the cardiac vessels. The prognosis of infantile polyarteritis nodosa with coronary artery involvement is poor. Death usually occurs,

within a few months after onset of the disease, from myocardial infarction. Therapy with steroids and immunosuppressive agents has been unsuccessful.

Kawasaki disease is a systemic vasculitis closely resembling infantile periarteritis nodosa which has been described in infants and children. The clinical manifestations are fever, rash, oral mucous membrane lesions, conjunctivitis, lymphadenopathy, arthritis, gastrointestinal dysfunction, cardiac disease and central nervous system signs. Haematuria and proteinuria are occasionally present, but progressive renal insufficiency is uncommon. The prognosis is dependent upon the severity of the cardiac lesions; treatment with salicylate therapy as an inhibitor of platelet function is the treatment of choice.

Allergic angiitis and granulomatosis

Allergic angiitis and allergic granulomatosis (Churg–Strauss syndrome)[20] is rare in children. The histopathological lesions and clinical manifestations are different from polyarteritis as there is a high incidence of eosinophilia with pulmonary vessel involvement, frequent granuloma formation, eosinophilic infiltrate (Loeffler's pneumonia) and high frequency of chronic asthma. Renal involvement is less frequent than in polyarteritis nodosa.

Vasculitis of small sized vessels

Anaphylactoid purpura has been described in detail elsewhere in this chapter. Hypocomplementaemic urticarial vasculitis is characterized by recurrent episodes of urticaria, secondary to necrotizing vasculitis, hypocomplementaemia, arthralgia, abdominal pain and renal disease. Proliferative glomerulonephritis which is not progressive may be encountered.

Vasculitis of medium and large arteries with giant cells

Giant cell arteritis usually does not involve the renal vessels. Takayasu's arteritis is a form of vasculitis affecting the aorta, its major branches and the pulmonary arteries. The disease has female predominance, and in the paediatric population there is a higher frequency in adolescence. Renal vessel involvement is uncommon, and hypertension is a frequent presenting sign when there is aortic involvement. The classical absence of pulses is accompanied by constitutional symptoms. Anti-inflammatory drugs have been used with moderate success.

Wegener's granulomatosis

Wegener's granulomatosis is characterized by necrotizing vasculitis with granuloma formation involving the upper and lower respiratory tract most frequently; many other organs may be involved including kidneys, joints, eyes, skin, central nervous system and heart.[21] This disorder has a male:female ratio of 2:1 and is more common in adults; however, children may be affected. Constitutional symptoms and respiratory tract manifestations are the most common presenting features. Rhinorrhoea, sinusitis, mucosal ulcerations and otitis media are encountered with upper respiratory tract involvement, while haemoptysis, cough and chest pain are evidence of lung disease. Elevated C-ANCA antibody titres are found in 90% of Wegener's patients, which is of diagnostic importance. Renal disease is common, ranging from mild urinary sediment abnormalities with no renal function impairment, to severe glomerulonephritis with acute renal insufficiency. The histopathology of the renal lesion varies from mild focal glomerulonephritis to severe necrotizing glomerulonephritis with crescent formation, renal granulomas are infrequently found, and immunofluorescent studies are negative. Renal involvement is usually preceded by other clinical manifestations of the disease. The most serious complications of Wegener's granulomatosis are uncontrollable pulmonary haemorrhage and the progression to chronic renal failure.[22-24] The current approach to treatment with steroids and immunosuppressive therapy has been effective in preventing these complications when therapy is instituted early in the course of the disease and continued for at least 1 year after remission is achieved. Prednisone and cyclophosphamide are the drugs of choice. Relapses may occur but remissions can be achieved by restarting therapy. Renal transplantation has been successful when progression to end-stage renal failure has occurred.

Diabetic nephropathy

Renal involvement secondary to the metabolic abnormalities of insulin deficiency is seen in juvenile onset (type I) diabetics.[25-31] Diabetes mellitus in childhood is normally not associated with significant clinical manifestations of renal disease; however, it has become apparent that the ultimately serious complications of this disorder have their origins shortly after the onset of the diabetic state.

Systemic manifestations

The clinical signs of insulin deficiency are well known; hyperglycaemia leads to polyuria, polydipsia and weight loss, with the eventual development of ketosis and coma. These features can be mistakenly diagnosed as signs of renal parenchymal disease; however, the presence of severe glycosuria readily establishes the diagnosis. These initial findings of the diabetic state are well controlled by replacement insulin therapy.

The more severe systemic manifestations of diabetic vascular disease are not seen in childhood. Older individuals will have progressively increasing difficulty with hypertension, retinopathy and neuropathy. Retinopathy in young patients is initially manifest by arteriolar wall thickening and exudative retinal lesions; the progression of retinal changes can be assessed by fluorescein angiography. A variety of neurological abnormalities in diabetes may be evident, but the earliest findings of diabetic neuropathy are detected by abnormalities of nerve conduction.

The aetiology of diabetes mellitus is unknown. A variety of factors have been implicated. While precipitating events such as viral infection have been observed, genetic predisposition to develop diabetes mellitus has been documented; there is a 50% concordance rate in identical twins with the onset of diabetes mellitus under the age of 40 years. There may be a multifactorial aetiology, since the development of renal disease varies considerably from one patient to another. Although the multisystem abnormalities of retinopathy, neuropathy and nephropathy are collectively felt to be due to diabetic vascular disease, there is considerable heterogeneity among individuals with respect to which of these organ systems will be involved.

Renal manifestations and laboratory findings

The earliest clinical evidence of diabetic nephropathy is the development of microalbuminuria. Unfortunately, this test does not accurately detect or predict the thickening of renal basement membranes described below, since the latter may develop without evidence of increased microalbuminuria. Underlying renal basement membrane abnormalities can be somewhat more accurately predicted by measuring microalbuminuria after stress or exercise. Early in the course of diabetes mellitus, supernormal levels of glomerular filtration rate (creatinine clearance) are observed as well as increased size of total renal mass by radiological analysis. Hypertension is not seen early in diabetic nephropathy, but elevated blood pressure appears later in the course of the disease associated with decreases in glomerular filtration rate and renal insufficiency. Diabetic patients have elevated plasma levels of haemoglobin A_{1C} which represents post-synthetic glycosylation of the haemoglobin molecule and correlates with the elevated blood glucose levels.

Renal histopathological findings

Specific studies have been carried out to elucidate the earliest evidence of renal histological changes in diabetes mellitus. Within a short time following onset of diabetes mellitus, increased volume measurements of total glomerular size, capillary loop area, mesangial volume and glomerular basement membrane width have been documented. With increasing time, overt glomerular basement membrane thickening, mesangial sclerosis with Kimmelstiel–Wilson nodules, capillary loop narrowing and fibrin cap formation may be found. These patients develop tubular basement membrane widening and more severe vascular wall thickening with characteristic arteriolar hyalinosis.

By immunofluorescent microscopy, diabetic glomerular and tubular basement membranes show progressively increasing linear staining for various plasma proteins such as albumin and IgG; the latter does not have an immunological basis, and in fact is also found in basement membranes of other organs such as skin, muscle and thyroid gland. It is, therefore, apparent that in diabetes mellitus generalized increased microvascular permeability exists, with apparent trapping of plasma proteins in thickened basement membranes. When examined by analytical methods, it has been revealed that collagenous components are increased while heparan sulphate proteoglycan, an important component of basement membranes, is reduced. It is of interest that the markedly expanded glomerular mesangial regions in diabetic kidneys contain significantly increased amounts of smooth muscle myosin, although the composition of Kimmelstiel–Wilson lesions which are part of the expanded mesangial matrix is unknown.

Treatment

While insulin therapy is used to control the gross metabolic abnormalities of diabetes mellitus such as hyperglycaemia and ketosis, attention is now being focused upon prevention of the long-term complications of basement membrane thickening. Tight glycaemic control using frequent doses of short-acting insulin may prevent the mild physiological derangements of increased glomerular filtration rate and microalbuminuria; established diabetic nephropathy with extensive basement membrane thickening cannot be reversed. Treatment strategies of this nature are further complicated by the lack of accurate predictability in individual patients of progressive diabetic nephropathy, since the latter is not closely correlated with other abnormalities in these patients such as retinopathy. Our current recommendation is that urinary microalbumin excretion be closely monitored, and when this parameter becomes elevated, further assessment of renal damage due to basement membrane thickening be made by percutaneous renal biopsy. Because of the variable clinical course in these patients, it may be possible to more accurately predict which patients will require or benefit from prophylaxis by tight glycaemic control during the childhood and adolescent years.

Prognosis

While end-stage renal failure due to diabetic nephropathy has been managed by renal transplantation, recurrence of histological evidence of this disorder in the transplanted kidney limits the long-term benefits from this approach. Transplantation of pancreatic tissue or isolated preparations of pancreatic islets is being approached on an experimental basis.

From the above it can be appreciated that increased knowledge and understanding of the initial pathogenetic events in the development of diabetic nephropathy have been acquired. Although specific recommendations regarding therapy cannot be given, it appears likely that close monitoring of individual patients will be predictive of those young patients at risk to develop progressive diabetic nephropathy. Further focus upon these patients during the childhood and adolescent years may prevent serious sequences of diabetes mellitus later in life.

References

1. Platt J.L., Burke B.A., Fish A.J., Kim Y. and Michael A.F. Systemic lupus erythematosus in the first two decades of life. *Am. J. Kid. Dis.* 1982, **2** (Suppl. 2), 212–222

2. Lehman T.J.A., McCurdy D.K., Bernstein B.H., King K.K. and Hanson V. Systemic lupus erythematosus in the first decade of life. *Pediatrics* 1989, **83**, 235–239

3. Austin H.A. III, Klippel J.H., Balow J.E., LeRiche N.G.H., Steinberg A.D., Plotz P.H. and Decker J.L. Therapy of lupus nephritis: controlled trial of prednisone and drugs. *N. Engl. J. Med.* 1986, **314**, 614–619

4. Lehman T.J.A., Sherry D.D., Wagner-Weiner L., McCurdy D.K., Emery H.M., Magilavy D.B. and Kovalesky A. Intermittent intravenous cyclophosphamide therapy for lupus nephritis. *J. Pediatr.* 1989, **114**, 1055–1060

5. Lehman, T.J.A. and Mouradian J.A. Systemic lupus erythematosus. In: Holliday M.A., Barratt T.M. and Avner E.D. (eds) *Pediatric Nephrology*, 3rd edn. Baltimore, Williams and Wilkins, 1994: 849–870

6. Levy M., Broyer M. and Arsah A. Anaphylactoid purpura nephritis in childhood, natural history and immunopathology. In: Hamburger J., Crosnier J. and Maxwell M.H. (eds) *Advances in Nephrology*, Vol. 6. Chicago, Year Book Medical Publishers, 1976: 183

7. Meadow S.R., Glasgow E.F., White R.H.R., Monrieff M.W., Cameron S. and Ogg C.S. Schonlein–Henoch nephritis. *Quart. J. Med.* 1972, **41**, 241–258

8. White R.H.R. and Yoshikawa N. Henuch–Schöntein nephritis. In: Holliday M.A., Barratt T.M. and Avner E.D. (eds), *Pediatric Nephrology*, 3rd edn. Williams and Wilkins, Baltimore, 1994: 729–738

9. Bunchman T.E., Mauer S.M., Sibley R.K. and Vernier R.L. Anaphylactoid purpura: characteristics of 16 patients who progressed to renal failure. *Pediatr. Nephrol.* 1988, **2**, 393–397

10. Steen V.D., Medsger T.A. Jr., Osial T.A. Jr., Ziegler G.L., Shapiro A.P. and Rodnan G.P. Factors predicting development of renal involvement in progressive systemic sclerosis. *Am. J. Med.* 1984, **76**, 779–786

11. Dabich L. Scleroderma. In: Cassidy S.T. (ed.) *Textbook of Pediatric Rheumatology*. London, John Wiley, 1982: 433

12. Singsen B.H., Swanson V.L., Bernstein B.H., Heuser E.T., Hanson V. and Landing B.H. A histologic evaluation of mixed connective tissue disease in childhood. *Am. J. Med.* 1980, **68**, 710

13. Nimelstein S.H., Brody S., McShane D. and Holman H.B. Mixed connective tissue disease: a subsequent evaluation of the original 25 patients. *Medicine* 1980, **59**: 239–248

14. Fauci A.S. The spectrum of vasculitis. Clinical, pathologic, immunologic, and therapeutic consideration. *Ann. Intern. Med.* 1978, **89** (Part 1), 660–676

15. Fink C.W. Polyarteritis and other diseases with necrotizing vasculitis in children. *Arthritis Rheum.* 1977, **20**, 378–384

16. Ettinger R.E., Nelson A.M., Burke E.C. and Lie J.T. Polyarteritis nodosa in childhood. A clinical pathologic study. *Arthritis Rheum.* 1979, **22**, 820–825

17. Cohen R.D., Conn D.L. and Ilstrup D.M. Clinical features, prognosis and response to treatment in polyarteritis. *Mayo Clin. Proc.* 1980, **55**, 146–155

18. Yanaglhara R. and Todd S.K. Acute febrile mucocutaneous lymph node syndrome. *Am. J. Dis. Child.* 1980, **134**, 603–614

19. Burns J.C., Wiggins J.W., Jr., Toews W.H., Newburger J.W., Leung D.Y.M., Wilson H. and Glode M.P. Clinical spectrum of Kawasaki disease in infants younger than 6 months of age. *J. Pediatr.* 1986, **109**, 759–763

20. Chumbley L.C., Harrison E.G. and De Remee R.A. Allergic granulomatosis and angitis (Churg–Strauss syndrome). Report and analysis of 30 cases. *Mayo Clin. Proc.* 1977, **52**, 477–484

21. Fauci A.S., Haynes B.F., Katz P. and Wolff S.M. Wegener's granulomatosis: prospective clinical and therapeutic experience with 85 patients for 21 years. *Ann. Intern. Med.* 1983, **98**, 76–85

22. Jennette J.C., Wilkman A.S. and Falk R.J. Anti-neutrophil cytoplasmic autoantibody-associated glomerulonephritis and vasculitis. *Am. J. Pathol.* 1989, **135**, 921–930

23. Jayne D.R.W., Marshall P.D., Jones S.J. and Lockwood C.M. Autoantibodies to GBM and neutrophil cytoplasm in rapidly progressive glomerulonephritis. *Kidney Int.* 1990, **37**, 965–970

24. Jennette J.C. and Falk R.J. Diagnosis and management of glomerulonephritis and vasculitis presenting as acute renal failure. *Med. Clin. North Am.* 1990, **74**, 893–908

25. Gundersen H.J., Mogensen C.E., Seyer-Kansen K., Osterby R. and Lundbach K. Early and late changes in the diabetic kidney. In: Hamburger J., Crosnier J., Grunfeld J.P. and Maxwell M.W. (eds) *Advances in Nephrology*, Vol.8. Chicago, Year Book Medical Publishers, 1979: 43–62

26. Brown D.M., Andres G.A., Hostetter T.H., Mauer S.M., Price R. and Venkatachalam M.A. Kidney complications. *Diabetes* 1982, **31** (Suppl. I), 71–81

27. Davies A.G., Price D.A. and Postlethwaite R.J. Renal function in diabetes mellitus. *Arch. Dis. Child.* 1985, **60**, 299–304

28. Hostetter T.M. Diabetic nephropathy. *N. Engl. J. Med.* 1985, **312**, 642–643

29. Silverstein J.M., Fennell R., Donnelly W. *et al.* Correlation of biopsy-studies nephropathy in young patients

with insulin dependent diabetes mellitus. *J. Pediatr.* 1985, **106**, 196–201

30. Viberti G. and Keen M. The patterns of proteinuria in diabetes mellitus: relevance to pathogenesis and prevention of diabetic nephropathy. *Diabetes* 1984, **33**, 686–692

31. Mogensen C.E., Mauer S.M. and Kjellstrand C.M. Diabetic nephropathy. In: Schrier R.W. and Gottschalk C.W. (eds) *Diseases of the Kidney*, Vol.3. Toronto, Little, Brown and Company, 1988: 2395–2437

21

Acute renal failure

G.S. Arbus, M. Farine, J.-P. Guignard

Acute renal failure (ARF) is a sudden decrease in renal function accompanied by the retention of nitrogenous wastes and a disturbance of water and electrolyte balance. It occurs much less commonly in children than in adults. ARF develops either secondary to a severe illness or as a result of acute renal disease. Because it is often associated with a major disease process, ARF is seen primarily in highly specialized centres, where patients with such conditions are referred for investigation and treatment.

In some cases, considerable clinical and investigative skill may be required to determine the aetiology of the kidney dysfunction. Optimum management necessitates careful monitoring and treatment of the patient's biochemical derangements.

Definitions applicable to acute renal failure

Oliguria

Oliguria is a reduction in urine output to less than 300 ml m^{-2} day^{-1}; this is the minimum amount necessary to excrete the daily solute output of approximately 500 mosmol/24 h in an adult. Assuming a maximum urinary concentrating ability of 1000 mosmol/litre, the minimum urine volume needed to excrete these wastes is 500 ml or about 300 ml m^{-2} day^{-1}. Definitions appropriate for neonates are given in Chapter 31.

It should be noted that an older patient urinat-ing less than 300 ml m^{-2} day^{-1} does not necessarily have ARF. A normal adult with limited access to fluids may be maximally conserving water. Although oliguria is considered a hallmark of ARF, the non-oliguric state may be seen in up to 50% of children.[1]

A normal or even increased urine output (a) commonly occurs in tubular dysfunction secondary to aminoglycoside toxicity, (b) may develop when acute tubular necrosis (ATN) is resolving, or (c) may be seen when there is intermittent or partial ureteral obstruction.

Anuria

Anuria technically means no urine, but because of so-called 'bladder sweat' it is defined as the excretion of less than 75 ml urine/day in an adult. In children, we define anuria as a urine output of less than 1 ml/kg body weight per day.

Azotaemia

Azotaemia is an abnormally high accumulation of nitrogenous wastes in the blood as indicated by the urea content. Although it is usually a reflection of acute or chronic renal dysfunction, non-renal causes should be considered. These include a high-protein diet, hormones (especially glucocorticoids), anti-anabolic drugs, e.g. tetracycline, and increased degradation of endogenous proteins as a result of inadequate caloric intake, surgery, trauma, infection, burns, fever or blood in the bowel.

Uraemia

Uraemia is the symptom complex reflecting organ dysfunction that occurs when the kidneys fail to regulate body composition.

Pathogenesis

The inability of kidneys in patients with ARF to excrete wastes effectively has been attributed to various causes, including alteration in glomerular permeability, renal tubular obstruction, filtrate backflow and vascular problems.[2] Animal studies have shown that, with gentamicin and heavy metal administration or renal ischaemia, there is a profound decrease in glomerular capillary permeability. Other studies, however, have demonstrated a high intratubular hydrostatic pressure secondary to obstruction by debris and casts which may be responsible for the decreased glomerular filtration rate (GFR) noted in ARF. The filtrate backflow theory suggests that, despite a normal amount of glomerular filtration, damage to the renal tubular epithelium allows the filtrate to leak back into the peritubular circulation, thereby accounting for a net imbalance of waste excretion. Despite the uncertainty of some of the proposed theories, there is agreement that decreased blood flow to the glomerulus is a major cause of altered kidney function in ARF. This may occur in several ways.[3]

Some studies have shown that there is a relatively greater decrease in renal blood flow to the cortex in patients with ARF and that renal function returns when cortical perfusion resumes.[3] Others have suggested that swelling of the capillary endothelial cells is responsible for the decreased renal blood flow.[4] In addition, Conger and Schrier discuss other vascular theories.[3] For example, the damage to the proximal tubule in ARF has been thought to allow extra salt to arrive at the macula densa, thereby stimulating an increase in intrarenal angiotensin II which, in turn, leads to arteriolar constriction and a decrease in the GFR. It has also been suggested that the GFR is reduced in ARF either because of high preglomerular (afferent) arterial resistance or because of low efferent resistance.

It is likely that there are different causes for both the initiation and maintenance phases of ARF. Recently the endothelial cell swelling theory as a cause for the decreased renal blood flow in the initiation phase of ischaemic ARF has regained support.[5] On the other hand, following reperfusion of an ischaemic kidney, there appears a surplus of damaging oxygen-free radicals which may be responsible for the maintenance phase of ARF.[6] Also, although the main clinical derangements in ARF are related to GFR, other renal dysfunctions may occur either as a result of damage to parts of the renal tubule or because of damage to the renal tubular cell. Thus with an ischaemic cause for ARF there tends to be damage primarily to the outer medullary area,[5,6] while with some nephrotoxic agents (aminoglycosides), the insult is mainly to the proximal tubular portion of the nephron. During the maintenance phase of ARF, the tubular cells of the kidney exhibit (a) a reduction of high energy phosphates, (b) a loss of cellular protein synthesis capacity, (c) an increased concentration of intracellular calcium, (d) intracellular acidosis, and (d) activation of membrane degradation processes.[6,7]

Aetiology and incidence

The cause of acute prerenal, renal, and postrenal failure are listed in Tables 21.1–21.3 and

Table 21.1 Causes of prerenal (functional) azotaemia in children

Hypovolaemia
Gastroenteritis (vomiting, diarrhoea)
Gastrointestinal drainage
Diabetic acidosis
Hypoproteinaemic states
Haemorrhage
Third spacing (peritonitis, ileus, burns)

Peripheral vasodilatation
Sepsis
Antihypertensive medication

Impaired cardiac output
Congestive heart failure, pericardial tamponade

Bilateral renal vessel occlusion
Artery
Vein

Drugs
Prostaglandin synthetase inhibitors
Angiotensin-converting enzyme inhibitors
Cyclosporin, diuretics

Others
Increased intra-abdominal pressure (from ascites)
Hepatorenal syndrome

Table 21.2   Causes of intrarenal (renal parenchymal) azotaemia in children

Circulatory insufficiency (see Table 21.1)

Nephrotoxins (antimicrobials, contrast media, anaesthetics, heavy metals, organic solvents, petroleum distillates, insecticides, cytotoxic agents, non-steroidal anti-inflammatory drugs)

Diseases of the kidney or vessels
Acute glomerulonephritis associated with lupus, post-streptococcal disease, rapidly progressive glomerulonephritis, Goodpasture's syndrome, IgA nephropathy
Bilateral acute pyelonephritis
Haemolytic uraemic syndrome
Acute interstitial nephritis resulting from drug hypersensitivity or infection
Cortical or medullary necrosis
Vasculitis, polyarteritis
Hypercalcaemia, hyperphosphataemia, hyperuricaemia
Acute disease in the presence of chronic renal disease

Myoglobinuria, haemoglobinuria

Tumour infiltrate

Intratubular obstruction (*sulphonamides, uric acid, methotrexate*)

Iatrogenic factors
Removal of a solitary kidney
Renal arteriogram
Cardiac pump oxygenation
Excessive sodium and water losses during nasogastric suction or surgical drainage

Table 21.3   Causes of postrenal (obstructive) azotaemia in children

Posterior urethral valves
Blocked bladder catheter
Neurogenic bladder
Surgical accident
Calculi*
Ureterocele*
Tumours*
Trauma*

* More likely in patients with a solitary kidney.

Table 21.4   Drug-induced acute renal failure

Vasomotor nephropathy
Cyclosporin, non-steroidal anti-inflammatory drugs, converting enzyme inhibitors

Acute tubular necrosis
Antimicrobials (aminoglycosides, cephaloridine, amphotericin B, colistin)
Heavy metals, organic solvents, contrast agents

Interstitial nephritis
Antimicrobials (penicillins, cephalosporins, cotrimoxazole)
Non-steroidal anti-inflammatory drugs, diuretics

Obstructive ARF
Cytolytic immunosuppressive drugs

Table 21.5   Possible causes of oliguria following cardiovascular surgery

Poor renal perfusion
Inadequate 'effective' vascular volume
Hypotension

Renal damage
Mismatched blood transfusion
Damage from cardiac bypass
Excess angiographic dye

Blocked bladder catheter

Table 21.6   Possible causes of azotaemia in leukaemia and tumours

Shock secondary to:
Sepsis
Haemorrhage

Kidney damage as a result of:
Acute hyperuricaemic nephropathy
Hyperphosphataemia

Tumour cell infiltrate of renal parenchyma

Drug toxicity, renal vessel or aortic compression from swollen lymph nodes

approaches to diagnosis and management in Figure 21.1. Frequently, ARF in children is secondary to prerenal failure associated with such conditions as gastroenteritis or sepsis. Although these causes of ARF are still prevalent in some parts of the world, with improved understanding of fluid and electrolyte imbalance in paediatrics and the introduction of many new drugs, including antimicrobials, they are decreasing. Today, dose-related nephrotoxic agents are a major factor in ARF in many units (Table 21.4).[8]

Other forms of therapy have also resulted in ARF. For example, postoperative oliguria occurs in some patients after certain complex surgical procedures (Table 21.5).[9] There may also be a relative decrease in urine output after surgery owing to excess secretion of antidiuretic hormone and/or aldosterone.[10] In addition, diseases such as leukaemia may cause azotaemia in diverse ways (Table 21.6).[11] In neonates, severe or prolonged hypoxaemia causes oliguria, secondary to renal hypoperfusion and decreased GFR. The renal vasoconstriction has been ascribed to the release of vasoactive factors such as angiotensin II, catecholamines or

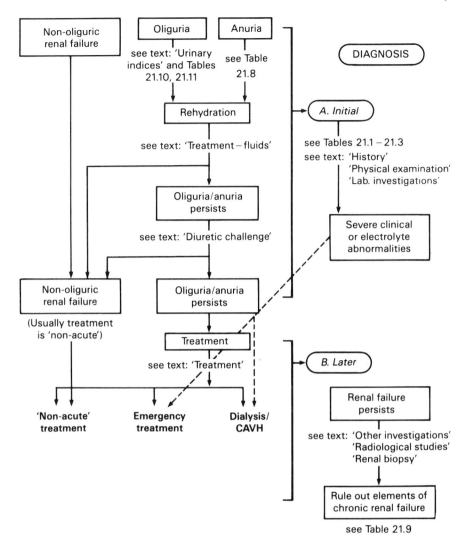

Figure 21.1 Outline for investigation and treatment of a child with acute renal failure

adenosine. Volume expansion can improve the state of renal hypoperfusion.[12]

Although these newer factors in ARF are important in major treatment centres, paediatricians will continue to see the more traditional causes, such as haemolytic uraemic syndrome and the various types of acute glomerulonephritis. Postrenal azotaemia is rare, especially in children. The specific causes of ARF in a large paediatric centre are shown in Table 21.7.[13]

Drug-induced renal failure (Table 21.4)

Vasomotor nephropathy

Some drugs such as cyclosporin, indomethacin and other non-steroidal anti-inflammatory drugs can increase renal vascular resistance and impair GFR. In young infants where the renin–angiotensin–aldosterone system is physiologically activated, the use of converting enzyme inhibitors may also induce vasomotor nephropathy.

Acute renal failure

A number of drugs, heavy metals and organic solvents can cause acute tubular necrosis. Hypertonic contrast agents carry the same risk, so that non-ionic agents should be preferred, especially in young infants whose renal concentrating ability is immature.

Table 21.7   Aetiology of acute renal failure in children as a function of age (After Loirat and Guesnu,[13] by permission)

Aetiology	Total no. children in each group		Age		
			1–12 months	1–4 years	> 4 years
Hypoperfusion	82	(38%)			
Acute dehydration	40		30	7	3
Septic shock	16		12	2	2
Major hyperthermia	14		8	5	1
Cardiogenic shock	8		4	1	3
Post-traumatic	4			1	3
Nephrotoxins	19	(9%)			
Endogenous toxins (myolysis, haemolysis, hyperuricaemia)	8		1	1	6
Exogenous toxins	11		3	4	4
Glomerulonephritis	34	(16%)		6	28
Haemolytic uraemic syndrome	65	(31%)	33	20	12
Obstructive uropathy	8	(4%)	1	4	3
Renal vein thrombosis	2	(1%)	2		
Others	3	(1%)	1		2
Total	213	(100%)	95 (45%)	51 (24%)	67 (31%)

Interstitial nephritis

Several drugs can induce idiosyncratic interstitial nephritis. This type of reaction is not related to the dose of drug administered: it is often associated with other signs of hypersensitivity including fever, rash and eosinophilia in a third of the patients. The condition improves upon drug withdrawal.

Obstructive ARF

Tubular lumen obstruction by uric acid crystals can occur after the use of cytolytic immunosuppressive agents such as methotrexate. The condition can be prevented by producing alkaline water diuresis and giving allopurinol, a xanthine oxidase inhibitor, before treatment.

Haemolytic uraemic syndrome

Haemolytic uraemic syndrome (HUS) is defined by the triad of microangiopathic haemolytic anaemia, thrombocytopenia and ARF. It is predominantly a disease of infants and young children, and is the commonest cause of ARF in otherwise healthy children living in temperate climates.

A few years ago we had shown that 30 of 40 paediatric patients with idiopathic HUS have evidence of infection by certain strains of *E. coli*.[14] These specific types of *E. coli* produce a cytotoxin, which has been called either verotoxin because it produces an irreversible cytopathic effect in vero cells (a line of African Green Monkey kidney cells) or Shiga-like toxin because of its close similarity in action and molecular structure to Shiga toxin from *Shigella dysenteriae* type 1.[15] Verotoxin is known to cause diarrhoea, haemorrhagic colitis, and our findings indicate a causal association with idiopathic HUS of childhood in North America. Recently such an association has been extended to other parts of the world, including South America, Europe and Japan.

Between 1980 and 1986 we had 86 children admitted to the Hospital for Sick Children, Toronto, with HUS. Of these, 91% had a classical, idiopathic presentation (that is, following a gastrointestinal upset) and 88% gave evidence of a verotoxin-producing *E. coli* infection. Of those with evidence of a verotoxin-producing infection, HUS was diagnosed a mean of 7.6 days after the onset of diarrhoea. Most cases were seen during the summer. Noteworthy presenting clinical features included anuria (44%), oliguria (27%), convulsions (24%), hypertension (13%), and coma (6.6%). Dialysis was performed in 60%. In our series, 82% made a complete recovery, 1 died, and 7 had a residual disability – 4 with some degree of renal failure (one with end-stage kidneys), and 3 with a neurological deficit. There was an association between the presence of convulsions on admission and an unfavourable outcome. Patients were hospitalized for a mean of 18.6 days, emphasizing that the condition is associated with considerable morbidity and places a significant burden on health care resources.

The mainstay of treatment is optimal supportive management of ARF. Patients with major neurological abnormalities need good supportive care including seizure control, avoidance of overhydration and early ventilatory support with frequent arterial blood gas monitoring.[16] There have been few trials of specific therapy and a number of vogues for various therapies. Few would now advocate the use of heparin, streptokinase or prostacyclin. Although in the past we have used fresh frozen plasma or plasmaphaeresis, we reserve the latter for children only when they appear to have a bad prognosis. Still to assess in the future would be the role of giving an antiverotoxin to patients when first admitted with HUS. Possibly the beneficial effects seen by some investigators with fresh frozen plasma or plasmaphaeresis was the giving of plasma with specific antibodies against the verotoxin. Thus far, the early giving of antimicrobials appears to have no effect on outcome and in HUS secondary to *Shigella dysenteriae* antimicrobials may actually worsen the outcome.[17]

Acute tubular necrosis

Any of the causes of prerenal azotaemia listed in Table 21.1, if uncorrected, will progress to acute tubular necrosis. In addition it can arise from the ingestion of nephrotoxins and has been described in acute pyelonephritis. The oliguric phase is often shorter in children than in adults and may even not be noticed at all. Mild proteinuria and microscopic haematuria are usually present.[18] The diagnosis is usually suspected from the clinical history and the absence of evidence of other forms of renal disease. Obstruction should be excluded by appropriate imaging.

Renal venous thrombosis

Seventy-five per cent of cases in childhood present in the first month of life. Unilateral or bilateral renal masses are usually palpable with proteinuria, haematuria and thrombocytopenia. The child of a diabetic mother, shock, twins, perinatal asphyxia and cyanotic heart disease are recognized associations, but some cases arise without any specific precipitating factor. Spontaneous recovery can occur even in bilateral cases. The role of heparin and surgical management is controversial and should probably only be considered in bilateral cases or in those cases that involve the inferior vena cava.

Myoglobinuria–haemoglobinuria

ARF may be associated with necrosis of skeletal muscle or massive intravascular haemolysis most likely due to a mismatched blood transfusion. The potential nephrotoxicity of myoglobin and haemoglobin is increased when renal ischaemia and/or systemic acidosis coexist. The sharp reduction in renal blood flow induced by myoglobinuria is best prevented by volume expansion. Intratubular obstruction certainly plays a role in myoglobinuria-induced ARF.

Cortical necrosis

This arises particularly in neonates, usually in association with acute tubular necrosis. Pure cortical necrosis occasionally occurs. Cortical necrosis can follow HUS. The prognosis is poor. Definitive diagnosis can only be made by examination of biopsy or autopsy specimens.

Investigation

Prompt assessment of the patient in ARF is essential to determine the aetiology of the renal failure, especially if a readily reversible cause is present, and to decide whether emergency treatment of fluid and electrolyte or metabolic disturbances is necessary.

History

Readily reversible causes of renal failure, which are usually prerenal or obstructive in nature, must be recognized and corrected to prevent ischaemic renal parenchymal damage. It is therefore necessary to enquire about events which could cause volume depletion since a decreased effective blood volume will lead to prerenal failure (Table 21.1). Gastrointestinal losses and

Table 21.8   Causes of anuria in childhood

Haemolytic uraemic syndrome
Bilateral renal arterial or venous occlusion
Cortical necrosis
Severe acute glomerulonephritis
Bilateral obstructive uropathy
Unilateral, ureteral obstruction (solitary kidney)
Acute tubular necrosis (infrequent)

Table 21.9   Factors suggestive of acute versus chronic renal failure

Acute	Chronic
Previously healthy	Poor growth
Gross haematuria	Family history of renal disease
Oedema	Chronically ill appearance
Large kidneys	Previous abnormal urine or hypertension
	Oedema (if terminal)
	Hypertensive retinopathy
	Anaemia
	Bone disease
	Small kidneys
	Broad waxy casts

dehydration are the most common causes of prerenal failure in non-hospitalized patients. A history of haemorrhage or third space losses, as with burns or pancreatitis, must be sought. Liver disease, cardiac disease, such as congestive heart failure, and peripheral vasodilatation secondary to shock predispose to prerenal failure. Obstructive causes of renal failure are not common (Table 21.3). However, it is important to enquire about the urinary stream if a bladder neck obstruction is suspected. A history of previous abdominal surgery or costovertebral angle pain suggests obstruction as the aetiology of the renal failure. Occasionally, intrarenal insults can cause readily reversible renal failure such as that resulting from nephrotoxins or hypercalcaemia.

Causes of ARF that cannot be easily reversed may become apparent from the history. HUS usually occurs after an episode of bloody diarrhoea. A history of antecedent sore throat 1–2 weeks before the onset of the present illness suggests post-infectious glomerulonephritis.

Anuria is found in only a few situations (Table 21.8). ATN causing anuria occurs infrequently.

When an otherwise healthy patient is first seen by a physician the differentiation of acute from chronic renal failure may be difficult, but it is necessary for management and prognostication (Table 21.9). Heights and weights, especially if known before the onset of ARF, are helpful in identifying a decrease in the rate of growth as is often seen with chronic renal failure. Evidence of bone disease and chronicity may be obtained by examining an X-ray of the fingers for signs of hyperparathyroidism or the knees and wrists for evidence of rickets. A high parathyroid hormone or alkaline phosphatase level may also indicate long-standing renal disease. Isosthenuria tends to occur in most patients with chronic renal failure but is also seen in those suffering from ARF due to ATN.

Physical examination

Vital signs

Hypertension usually indicates fluid (sodium) retention or a hyper-reninaemic state secondary to an intrarenal insult. Hypotension denotes a decrease in effective vascular volume and the possibility of prerenal failure. An increase in respiratory rate may suggest acidosis or pulmonary oedema. Tachycardia may be a sign of circulatory insufficiency, whereas a slow irregular pulse may indicate hyperkalaemia.

State of hydration

Decreased skin turgor, dry mucous membranes, sunken eyes and a sunken fontanelle indicate sodium and water depletion. Tachycardia, hypotension, coolness of extremities and a pasty-grey appearance are signs of shock necessitating immediate treatment. Overhydration may be seen when excess fluid has been given to an oliguric child and should be considered in the presence of hypertension, prominent neck veins (in the older child), râles on pulmonary examination and peripheral or periorbital oedema. It must be remembered that the nephrotic child may be intravascularly depleted and also oedematous. Accurate weights, especially when compared to these before ARF, are useful in assessing the state of hydration and monitoring ongoing fluid therapy.

Abdominal examination

A distended bladder, large palpable kidneys and costovertebral tenderness raise the possibility of obstruction or postrenal failure. A rectal examination may identify an obstructive mass.

Neurological examination

The state of mentation must be assessed. Confusion, nausea, vomiting and hiccups can be signs of uraemia. Carpopedal spasm, Chvostek's and Trousseau's signs, cramps, muscle twitching and convulsions suggest hypocalcaemia. An altered neurological state including irritability, seizures or coma may be seen in patients with HUS.

Other indicators

Features suggestive of underlying disease must be sought. For example, a maculopapular rash and fever may be seen in interstitial nephritis or viraemia. A purpuric rash and arthritis suggest Henoch–Schoenlein purpura. Haemoptysis may indicate that a patient has Goodpasture's syndrome, while multiple extrarenal signs and symptoms may be a manifestation of a collagen vascular disease such as lupus. The presence of rickets alerts one to the possibility of chronic renal failure.

Laboratory investigations

Various laboratory values are useful in determining the aetiology of ARF and in revealing homeostatic disturbances that may need correction.

Urinalysis

In patients with ARF, a marked discrepancy between the intensity of the haem test (large) and the number of red blood cells (few) on microscopic examination of a fresh urine sample suggests haemoglobinuria secondary to a mismatched transfusion or myoglobinuria as the aetiology for ARF. Pink-tinged serum is found in haemolytic states, whereas the serum is straw-coloured with myoglobinuria.

Mild proteinuria occurs in both prerenal failure and ATN, whereas extensive proteinuria suggests glomerular disease.

The urinary sediment may be helpful in differentiating prerenal oliguria from ATN. Hyaline and finely granular casts may be seen in prerenal failure, whereas in ATN, epithelial cells, degenerative cells and coarsely granular casts

are more likely. Red cell casts indicate glomerular disease, and white cell casts suggest pyelonephritis or interstitial nephritis. Eosinophiluria is found in drug-induced interstitial nephritis and can be demonstrated by Wright's stain. A telescoped urine is noted occasionally in an active vasculitis such as lupus and reflects the acute and chronic elements in kidney diseases. Thus, the acute phase is identified by red blood cells and cellular and granular casts, and the chronic phase primarily by waxy casts.

The specific gravity of the urine is helpful and is measured if only a few drops can be obtained; otherwise, the urine osmolality is preferred. In prerenal failure, urine is concentrated, whereas in ATN it closely resembles plasma in that its specific gravity is around 1.010 and its osmolality is approximately 300 mosmol/litre. Since proteinuria and glycosuria affect specific gravity, one should subtract approximately 0.003 from the specific gravity for each 10 g of protein or sugar per litre in the urine to obtain a more accurate indication of the concentrating ability of the kidney. Other substances, such as radio-opaque dye or mannitol, will also give a falsely high specific gravity when the urine is not truly concentrated.

Blood count and smear

Anaemia is present in chronic renal failure. It may also be seen following a bleed or when the haemoglobin is diluted by fluid accumulation, for example with nephritis. A microangiopathic haemolytic anaemia is found in HUS, with the blood smear showing fragmented cells and thrombocytopenia. Eosinophilia suggests an allergic interstitial nephritis such as from sulphonamides or the various penicillins.

Blood chemistry

In ATN with generally poor tubular function, the normal urea nitrogen/creatinine ratio of <100:1 is maintained. Acid-base, electrolyte, calcium, phosphorus and uric acid blood levels must all be determined and abnormalities corrected. In prerenal failure, the normal urea nitrogen/creatinine ratio of <100:1 (mmol/mmol) in the blood is increased because, with the low urine flow in the tubules, urea is reabsorbed but creatinine is not.

Table 21.10   Summary of urinary indices in oliguric renal failure*

	Prerenal	Oliguric ARF
Urine osmolality (mosmol/kg water)	> 500	< 350
Urine sodium (mmol/litre)	< 20	> 40
Urine/plasma urea nitrogen	> 8	< 3
Urine/plasma creatinine	> 40	< 20
Fractional excretion of filtered sodium (%)†	< 1	> 1

*After Miller *et al.*,[19] by permission.

†Fractional excretion of filtered sodium $= \dfrac{U_{Na} \times P_{Cr}}{U_{Cr} \times P_{Na}} \times 100.$

Table 21.11   Diagnostic indices in neonatal ARF*

	Prerenal	Intrinsic
Urinalysis	Normal	> 5 RBC/HPF
Urine osmolality (mosmol/kg water)	> 400	< 400
Urine sodium (mmol/litre)	31 ± 19	63 ± 35
Urine/plasma creatinine	29 ± 16	10 ± 4
Fractional excretion of filtered sodium (%)†	< 2.5 (mean 0.9)	> 2.5 (mean 4.3)

*After Anand,[20] by permission.
†See Table 21.10.

Urinary indices

An understanding of the pathophysiology of ARF is helpful, since physiological alterations form the basis of the laboratory tests used to differentiate prerenal azotaemia from oliguric ARF. In prerenal failure, the effective blood volume is decreased and the renal tubules retain a maximum amount of sodium and water in an attempt to increase the circulatory volume. As a result, the urine becomes concentrated with wastes, such as urea, being excreted in the small volume of water. In ATN, the damaged renal tubules are incapable of changing what was filtered and the composition of urine excreted tends to closely resemble that of plasma (Tables 21.10 and 21.11).[19,20]

The fractional excretion of filtered sodium is the most useful of these indices in identifying the aetiology of ARF. The fractional excretion of sodium has been shown to be greater than 1% in ATN, non-oliguric ATN and urinary tract obstruction and less than 1% in prerenal failure and acute glomerulonephritis.[19,21] Sodium excretion is based on both the glomerular filtration and the tubular sodium reabsorption. Fractional sodium excretion in the newborn is further discussed in Chapter 31. It should be recognized that these indices, in general, hold true but at times are not useful, for instance if the patient is a malnourished infant or has had a diuretic or mannitol in the hours before the urine sample is obtained.[20,22]

Other investigations

Further investigations depend on the suspected aetiology. For example, one might use the streptozyme test to confirm poststreptococcal glomerulonephritis, and antinuclear antibody if lupus nephritis is suspected and total serum complement, third and fourth components of complement in the presence of possible poststreptococcal glomerulonephritis or lupus nephritis.

Radiological studies

A chest X-ray may be useful when fluid overload is suspected. A plain abdominal film may show kidney size or calculi. Large kidneys suggest acute glomerulonephritis, tumour infiltrate, renal vein thrombosis (neonate), obstruction or infection, whereas small kidneys may indicate chronic renal disease. Ultrasound is useful in determining kidney size, showing renal cysts, demonstrating obstruction (evidenced by dilated pelvis and calyces) and assessing the patency of the renal arteries, veins and the inferior vena cava. The loss of corticomedullary differentiation on ultrasound suggests intrinsic renal disease. With Doppler ultrasound there is markedly diminished, absent or reversed diastolic flow during the oliguric/anuric phase of ARF,[23,24] and in the case of HUS it was shown that a diuresis occurred within 24–48 h of the diastolic flow returning to normal.[23] Radionuclear scans utilizing various isotopes help to differentiate the causes of ARF (Table 21.12).[1] An intravenous pyelogram may cause further deterioration of renal function and is usually not necessary. When obstruction is strongly suspected, a cystogram and/or cystoscopy may be done.

Diuretic challenge

A diuretic trial should be used only when lower tract obstruction has been ruled out and the

Table 21.12 Radionuclide studies in ARF (From Feld *et al.*,[1] by permission)

Cause of ARF	Study	Typical findings
Ischaemic or nephrotoxic renal failure	Tc-DTPA,* I-OIH†	Adequate perfusion, prompt parenchymal uptake, delayed excretion without collecting system dilatation
Hepatorenal syndrome	Tc-DTPA, I-OIH	Markedly diminished blood flow, faint or no parenchymal visualization
Acute pyelonephritis	Gallium	Unilateral or bilateral uptake
Acute interstitial nephritis	Gallium	Bilateral intense uptake
Renal artery embolism	Tc-DTPA	Absence of blood flow, diffuse or segmental absence of parenchymal uptake
Obstructive uropathy	Tc-DTPA, I-OIH	Delayed uptake, prolonged excretion, pelvic accumulation unchanged by diuretic
Renal lymphoma	Gallium	Bilateral uptake, often nodular

*[99m]Technetium-diethylenetriamine penta-acetic acid.
†[131]Iodine-orthoidohippurate.

patient is adequately hydrated (see below under 'Fluids'). It may be helpful in differentiating prerenal failure from ATN. Either frusemide 2 mg/kg body weight or mannitol 0.5–1 g/kg body weight can be used. A response to diuretics suggests that there is prerenal failure and that renal function will improve if the decreased vascular volume is corrected. A positive response may also indicate a conversion of oliguric ATN to non-oliguric renal failure in some patients. This conversion is considered of therapeutic benefit since not only is the patient easier to manage but there appears to be less morbidity and mortality associated with non-oliguric than with oliguric ATN.[25]

The diuretic challenge should generate more than 2–3 ml kg^{-1} h^{-1} (50 ml m^{-2} h^{-1}) in the subsequent few hours. If urine output is not augmented following an initial challenge, mannitol should not be repeated because it remains extracellularly and will draw water from the intracellular to the extracellular compartment if it has not been excreted. This may result in pulmonary oedema and factitious hyponatraemia.

Renal biopsy

Renal biopsies are not routinely performed in patients with ARF. A renal biopsy is done when there is serious doubt about the aetiology or prognosis of ARF or when it might affect the therapeutic course. Biopsy is also sometimes indicated in the recovery phase to predict if the problem is ultimately reversible or likely to be progressive in nature. The role of biopsy is further discussed in Chapter 12.

Treatment

Treatment for the various homeostatic derangements of ARF may have to be given before or during investigation of the causes of ARF. For example, dialysis may have to be started before any diagnostic investigation is undertaken. A suggested outline for sequential investigation and treatment of a child with ARF is shown in Figure 21.1.

Fluids

Emergency treatment

Children with signs of circulatory insufficiency or severe volume depletion need immediate treatment with lactated Ringer's or normal saline solution, 20 ml/kg body weight over 20–60 min. This treatment must be repeated until circulation is restored (see below) and the patient is urinating. If haemorrhage has occurred, blood will be the treatment of choice. In severe hypoalbuminaemic states an albumin infusion may be necessary to restore vascular volume. When a decreased circulatory volume is corrected early and is the sole reason for the oliguria, urination should increase within 2–4 h after normovolaemia is established. The bladder may need catheterization to exclude obstruction and to monitor urine output.

Central venous pressure monitoring is useful

if there are signs of shock and the urine output does not increase after a fluid challenge has been given. A low central venous pressure indicates that more fluid is necessary, whereas a high pressure suggests that if there is circulatory insufficiency, it may be due to cardiac failure. Volume overload is frequently a problem in ARF since it may lead to hypertension, congestive heart failure or pulmonary oedema.

At times a patient may mask the presence of volume depletion with a low normal systemic or central venous pressure. One should therefore always check the peripheral circulation for cold extremities (with a temperature probe) if one is suspicious of such a patient. A peripheral temperature probe can also prove useful in monitoring the adequacy of fluid replacement in volume depleted patients.

Non-acute treatment

Fluid management is difficult in the oliguric patient. Accurate and frequent weights must be obtained as a guide to treatment. A flow sheet on the patient's weight, intake and output, electrolytes, acid-base status, calcium and phosphorus is helpful in monitoring progress and planning further treatment. A patient who is not receiving adequate calories would be expected to lose about 0.2–1% body weight per day. Lack of weight loss in such a patient may indicate overhydration.

The calculation of maintenance water requirements in oligoanuria has already been discussed in Chapter 10. A 10% dextrose solution should be used in the anuric child, and serum electrolytes and acid-base status should be carefully monitored.

The patient who is non-oliguric requires frequent measurement of blood and urinary electrolytes and the use of appropriate replacement solutions. It is essential to guard against fluid overload and depletion at all times.

Maintaining fluid and electrolyte balance in the diuretic phase is a most difficult task. Diuresis often begins abruptly, increases progressively over several days and is accompanied by massive losses of sodium, chloride and potassium. It is believed to result primarily from the excretion of previously retained sodium, water and waste at a time that the kidneys are still not able to concentrate the urine. In the infant, who cannot regulate his oral intake, water and salt losses (urine plus insensible losses) should

be replaced quantitatively for the first few days until the kidneys would be expected to regain their concentrating ability. At that stage an attempt can be made to decrease the diuresis by withholding the replacement of insensible losses. We feel this approach is better than administering only a part of the urine replacement because that can lead to rapid, severe volume depletion if tubular function has not adequately recovered. Thereafter, one can prescribe a fixed amount of fluid (oral and i.v.) based on the previous few days of urine output and subsequently decrease this amount about 10% every day or two. In the older child, free access to salt and water may be a way to regulate fluid and electrolytes unless urinary losses are enormous. However, in addition to allowing older children free access to fluids, we tend to replace any significant loss compared to intake. Body weight and serum electrolytes must be monitored carefully in all patients.

Hyperkalaemia

Emergency treatment

Hyperkalaemia occurs when potassium elimination is reduced and tissue release continues. The clinical features and ECG changes in hyperkalaemia have been discussed in Chapter 10. ECG changes with hyperkalaemia constitute a medical emergency and therefore aggressive therapy should be started using any or all of the treatments outlined in Table 21.13. When 10% calcium gluconate is given (0.5–1.0 ml/kg body weight i.v. over 2–10 min), a cardiac monitor should be employed. Calcium gluconate provides the most rapid treatment for cardiac toxicity, but its action is brief. Although it directly antagonizes the cardiac toxicity of hyperkalaemia, it does not eliminate potassium from the body. Intravenous calcium gluconate should be used to treat hyperkalaemia only if there are ECG changes.

Sodium bicarbonate therapy (8.4% sodium bicarbonate, 2–3 mmol/kg body weight) should be used cautiously if the patient is hypocalcaemic, as correction of acidosis will decrease the amount of ionized calcium present and may precipitate tetany. Other side effects of bicarbonate therapy are hypertension and volume overload. Bicarbonate infusion has a short duration of action.

Hyperkalaemia can be corrected by giving

Table 21.13 **Treatment of hyperkalaemia**

Type	Dose	Onset	Mode of action
10% calcium gluconate	0.5–1.0 ml/kg body weight i.v. over 2–10 min	Immediate	Antagonizes the effect of potassium
8.4% NaHCO₃	2–3 ml/kg body weight i.v.	5 min	Shifts potassium into cells
20% glucose ± insulin	2.5–5 ml/kg body weight per hour i.v.	30 min	Shifts potassium into cells
Ion exchange resins	1 g Na or Ca polystyrene sulphonate/kg body weight orally or by enema	2 h when given orally 30 min when given per rectum	Removes potassium from body
Dialysis/haemofiltration	Haemodialysis	Rapid	Removes potassium from body
	Peritoneal dialysis	Gradual	Removes potassium from body
	Haemofiltration	Gradual	Removes potassium from body

20% glucose, 0.5–1.0 g/kg body weight per hour, until blood sugar is about 14 mmol/litre. Glucose facilitates the entry of potassium into cells. When this level is reached, an infusion of crystalline zinc insulin (0.2 u for each gram of glucose) may be given and adjusted according to blood sugar. A sodium–potassium exchange resin such as sodium polystyrene sulphonate (Kayexalate or Resonium A) or a calcium–potassium exchange resin such as calcium polystyrene sulphonate (Calcium Resonium), 1 g/kg body weight per dose orally or by enema, can be used and repeated every 4 h if necessary. The resins appear to be more effective as a high retention enema (retained for 30 min) than when given orally, since the colon is a major site for potassium–sodium exchange. It acts within 30 min when given rectally and within 2 h when given orally. The resin is diluted in a 70% sorbitol solution.

Salbutamol (a β₂-adrenergic agonist) is effective in lowering serum potassium. It can be administered intravenously (4 μg/kg in 10 ml of water over 10 minutes) or by nebuliser (2.5 mg weight < 25 kg, 5.0 mg weight > 25 kg). Nebulised salbutamol is probably the first choice emergency treatment of hyperkalaemia.[26]

It is important to stress that the emergency treatment of hyperkalaemia is rarely a definitive treatment. It is usually employed to stabilize the situation while dialysis is established.

Non-acute treatment

In a non-catabolic patient with ARF, the serum potassium level usually rises by less than 0.5 mmol/litre per day; above this rate, tissue catabolism and destruction are likely. Acidosis contributes to the hyperkalaemia by shifting potassium out of the cells. A mild elevation of serum potassium is treated by decreasing the amount of exogenous potassium, correcting acidosis and administering potassium exchange resins. The resins initially given up to every 4 hours can be reduced to 1 g/kg body weight per day when possible.

Hyponatraemia

Emergency treatment

Central nervous system (CNS) signs are not likely to be present unless the serum sodium is less than 120 mmol/litre or the hyponatraemia developed in less than 24 h. As hyponatraemia in ARF is usually due to fluid overload, treatment should be aimed at fluid removal. Administration of sodium is fraught with hazards such as volume overload, overcorrection and worsening of CNS signs. When CNS signs are present, sodium in the form of 3% sodium chloride (0.5 mmol/ml) may be administered cautiously. The theoretical amount of sodium to correct the hyponatraemia is given by the formula:

Na [mmol] = (Na level desired − Actual Na in mmol/l) × 0.6 × body weight in kg

Only half the calculated sodium should be replaced initially and if the patient does not improve, consideration should be given to commencing dialysis.

Non-acute treatment

In asymptomatic patients with hyponatraemia from fluid overload, a sodium infusion should be avoided and fluids should be restricted. By monitoring input and output carefully, it is possible to maintain a normal serum sodium in most patients.

Hypocalcaemia/hyperphosphataemia

Emergency treatment

Although hypocalcaemia is common in ARF, it seldom leads to symptoms. Alkali therapy decreases the amount of ionized calcium available and is the most common precipitator of symptoms. In symptomatic patients, 10% calcium gluconate must be given by continuous intravenous infusion. The starting dose is 0.1 mmol (0.5 ml) of a 10% calcium gluconate solution per kg body weight per hour. Initially the infusion is adjusted every 4 h as indicated by monitoring blood values. The rate is reduced slowly when terminating the infusion. Calcium, especially i.v., should be given cautiously while the phosphorus level remains high, as precipitation of calcium–phosphorus complexes can occur.

Non-acute treatment

A maintenance dose of calcium can be given intravenously using up to 120 ml of 10% calcium gluconate m^{-2} day^{-1} or orally using 50 mg of elemental calcium/kg body weight per day in the form of calcium carbonate or gluconate.[27] An oral phosphate binder (calcium carbonate or occasionally aluminium hydroxide) is given to help correct the hyperphosphataemia that occurs secondary to phosphate retention in ARF.

Metabolic acidosis

Emergency treatment

A sodium bicarbonate (8.4%) solution is used to treat metabolic acidosis when the serum pH falls below 7.25. The theoretical amount of bicarbonate necessary to correct the serum bicarbonate has been discussed previously (see Chapter 9). Additional bicarbonate infusion can be given as indicated until the pH is greater than 7.20 or the serum bicarbonate is greater than 12–13 mmol/litre. Frequent blood gas monitoring is necessary during this time, especially if there is a sudden change is the patient's status.

Bicarbonate therapy may cause sodium and fluid overload. Severe metabolic acidosis in the anuric child may be an indication for dialysis.

Non-acute treatment

Metabolic acidosis may develop in ARF as a result of the body's inability to excrete its daily endogenous production (1–3 mmol/kg body weight) of non-volatile acids. Measures to treat the metabolic acidosis include supplemental bicarbonate therapy (1–3 mmol/kg body weight per day), a low protein diet, correction of the catabolic state with adequate caloric intake and treatment of infection. Hyperalimentation may be necessary.

Hypertension

Emergency treatment

Severe symptomatic hypertension requires emergency treatment. Hypertension is usually due to fluid overload but the renin–angiotensin system may be contributory. Diuretic therapy, such as frusemide 2–3 mg/kg for patients with oliguria, and 5 mg/kg for anuria, given i.v. over 1–2 min, may be useful for patients with hypertension from fluid overload. Other treatment consists of restriction of sodium and fluid intake and antihypertensive medication as needed, or if the hypertension appears to be sustained, on a regular basis.

The emergency management of hypertension is discussed in Chapter 15.

Non-acute treatment

In addition to restricting sodium and fluid intake, an antihypertensive medication such as a beta-blocker is begun. Beta-blockers should be avoided in the presence of fluid overload. Usually propranolol is started orally at a dose of 1 mg/kg body weight per day or intravenously at a dose of 0.05–0.1 mg/kg body weight every 4–6 h. If additional antihypertensive medication is necessary, hydralazine can be given in a dose of 0.2 mg/kg body weight i.v. or i.m. every 4–6 h. Hydralazine starts to act within 10–15 min and remains effective for 2–6 h. Side effects include tachycardia, flushing and headache. Hydralazine is given orally when that becomes possible. We have been using a calcium channel blocker, nifedipine, either in place of the beta-blocker or instead of hydralazine.

Table 21.14   Indications for starting dialysis and/or CAVH

Signs of uraemia
Failure of fluid overload to respond to medical
   management
Symptomatic electrolyte problems
Certain nephrotoxins

Table 21.15   Selective indications for peritoneal dialysis, haemodialysis or CAVH

Peritoneal dialysis
Personnel not trained in haemodialysis
Very young patient
Very haemodynamically unstable patient
Gradual change in fluid or electrolyte problem sufficient
A nephrotoxin that can be removed by peritoneal dialysis

Haemodialysis
Personnel versatile in haemodialysis
Rapid change in fluid or electrolyte problem necessary
A nephrotoxin that is better removed by haemodialysis
Peritoneal dialysis not possible (e.g. abdominal surgery)
Peritoneal dialysis not working (e.g. repeat catheter
   blockage, not removing fluid or correcting an electrolyte
   problem)

CAVH
Dialysis not possible
Dialysis hazardous
Dialysis greater risk than CAVH
Certain nephrotoxins
Dialysis not necessary if CAVH successful

Nifedipine (0.25–0.5 mg/kg body weight/dose, maximum 20 mg) is available as a short-acting (every 4 h) or long-acting (every 8–12 h) preparation. The side effects are minimal compared to previous antihypertensive agents; nifedipine can only be given orally.

Convulsions

There are many possible causes for convulsions including hypertension, hypocalcaemia, uraemia and underlying kidney disease, such as HUS. Treatment should be geared to the prevention and elimination of possible precipitators. Intravenous or rectal diazepam 0.2 mg/kg body weight may be given slowly and repeated every 15 min as needed. Phenytoin may also be used. Because altered protein binding is possible in renal failure, phenytoin toxicity may be seen at lower than standard doses. Phenobarbital (6 mg/kg i.v.) is partially excreted through the kidneys and may therefore accumulate if given in standard doses to patients in renal failure. Consequently, careful drug monitoring is essential.

Dialysis and continuous arteriovenous haemofiltration (CAVH)

It is evident that the decision to undertake CAVH or dialysis is based on the patient's clinical condition and biochemical data and on the predicted course of the renal failure or nephrotoxin present. Frequently, patients who are non-oliguric and non-catabolic do not require CAVH or dialysis. For other patients, the use of CAVH may abort the subsequent need for dialysis, while at other times the anticipatory use of dialysis and/or CAVH therapy early in the course of ARF, before complications develop, usually alleviates the need to deal with repeated crises. Haemodialysis must be undertaken at an appropriate medical centre, but if the need arises peritoneal dialysis can usually be performed in a peripheral hospital.

Indications for starting dialysis or CAVH are as follows (Table 21.14): (a) signs of uraemia such as central nervous system disturbances, uraemic pericarditis or bleeding; (b) failure of fluid overload to respond to medical treatment, as in congestive heart failure or hypertension; (c) symptomatic electrolyte problems as seen, for example, with severe hyperkalaemia, hyponatraemia, metabolic acidosis, hyperphosphataemia or hypocalcaemia, and (d) the presence of a nephrotoxin that can be dialysed. A urea level above 50 mmol/litre is considered by some as an indication for dialysis.

The decision whether to use haemodialysis, peritoneal dialysis or CAVH is based on the relative risks and advantages of the three procedures (Table 21.15).

The advantage of peritoneal dialysis is that it can be done in any hospital not needing special machinery and trained personnel. Furthermore, it involves little risk of the dialysis disequilibrium syndrome because the return of homeostatic abnormalities towards normal occurs slowly. It is safer in the haemodynamically unstable patient because it avoids rapid changes in blood volume. In addition, it avoids the danger of hepatitis and bleeding associated with heparinization. In general, peritoneal dialysis is easier to perform in very small children. The risks of peritoneal dialysis include perforation of a viscus, haemorrhage on insertion of the catheter, peritonitis, septicaemia, hypoproteinaemia, catheter blockage, catheter leakage, pulmonary atelectasis, pleural effusion and hyperglycaemia.

Table 21.16　Some indications for the use of CAVH in controlling (diuretic-resistant) fluid/sodium retention

Hypervolaemia (with hypertension)
Interstitial pulmonary oedema
Inability to provide adequate nutrition because of severe fluid restriction
Inability to provide necessary medication because of severe fluid restriction

Table 21.17　Type of patient where CAVH may be preferable

Cardiovascular instability
Post-cardiac surgery
Post-abdominal surgery
Premature, newborn infant
Multiple organ system failure
Respiratory embarrassment from peritoneal dialysis
Pre-/post-liver transplantation
Removal of certain nephrotoxins
Generalized hypoperfusion/hypotension
To abort the need for dialysis
Patients on ECMO

Haemodialysis has the advantage of correcting biochemical derangements more quickly and efficiently than peritoneal dialysis. It is the treatment of choice in patients who have undergone abdominal surgery when peritoneal dialysis would not be advisable. CAVH is being used more and more as a possible alternative to dialysis. In paediatrics, it is done primarily in centres where there is expertise in haemodialysis, not so much because of the complexity of the procedure, but rather because of the critical nature of the patient requiring this treatment tends already to be in a highly specialized centre. CAVH uses blood lines to join the patient's artery and vein, with a filter inserted in the system. Substances with a molecular weight < 5000 are removed in a concentration similar to their plasma concentrations. The patient's arterial pressure drives blood through the system, with the filter removing fluid at a prescribed rate. With CAVH, a replacement fluid is added to the system. At times, CAVH is used in tandem with haemodialysis, i.e. CAVH haemodialysis. More recently, the technique of venovenous haemofiltration (CVVH) is being used. A double lumen catheter is inserted into a large vein (subclavian or jugular) and with the use of a blood pump the patient's blood is circulated through the filter. Thus, in this chapter, most instances of CVVH can substitute for CAVH.

Like peritoneal dialysis, CAVH is usually performed continuously over several days to weeks until the kidneys regain adequate function. The principal problems with CAVH include: (a) repeated clotting of the filter and lines, (b) ineffectiveness in controlling an electrolyte abnormality, and (c) complications with vascular access. Although CAVH can be employed either to correct many of the electrolyte imbalances seen in ARF or at times be used in lieu of dialysis to remove a nephrotoxin, its main use has been to maintain fluid balance (Table 21.16) in a very haemodynamically unstable patient (Table 21.17).

Most experience with CAVH, including ours, shows a high mortality rate. However, when one realizes that the type of patient needing CAVH is extremely ill and at high risk of dying even before starting this procedure, high mortality rates are not too unexpected.

Techniques for peritoneal dialysis

A knowledge of catheter insertion and peritoneal dialysis technique is necessary for performing peritoneal dialysis. If the patient has a bleeding disorder that is not amenable to correction, a surgeon should insert the catheter. A surgeon should also place a permanent type of catheter if one anticipates a rather prolonged period of peritoneal dialysis such as with HUS. We have the surgeon place a Tenchkoff catheter at the completion of cardiovascular surgery if there is a reasonably good chance dialysis will be necessary in the next few days. Disposable flexible peritoneal catheters are now available in all different sizes, including for prematures. With the help of a guidewire, the paediatrician can more readily introduce these catheters than the older stiffer one (described below). Strict aseptic technique is followed to prevent the development of peritonitis. An intravenous line should be running and blood should be available, since acute intra-abdominal bleeding occurs occasionally when the peritoneal catheter is inserted.

The patient should be sedated. At the authors' centre, CM_3 is used frequently for this purpose. A 1 ml mixture consists of chlorpromazine 6.25 mg, promethazine 6.25 mg and meperidine 25 mg. A dose of 0.1 ml/kg body weight (maximum dose 2 ml) is given i.m. 1 h before the procedure. In very young or semicomatose patients, the procedure can be performed without sedation.

The bladder should be emptied (by catheterization if necessary) to avoid perforation when the peritoneal catheter with stylet is being introduced. The patient is prepared and draped in a sterile manner. The skin and subcutaneous tissue are anaesthetized with 1% xylocaine without adrenaline at the site planned for the insertion of the peritoneal catheter. In most cases, a point in the midline of the abdomen, below the umbilicus and one-third of the distance between the symphysis pubis and umbilicus, is used. Other sites for insertion are just lateral to the rectus muscle at or above the level of the umbilicus or McBurney's point on the line connecting the umbilicus to the anterior superior iliac spine, two-thirds of the distance below the umbilicus. These sites are preferred in neonates and infants to minimize the risk of trauma to major vessels. To decrease the risk of perforating a viscus when the catheter is being inserted, dialysis fluid (20 ml/kg body weight) that has been warmed toward body temperature is introduced into the peritoneal cavity via a 16-gauge intravenous catheter inserted into the peritoneal cavity. The intravenous catheter is then removed. A small incision is made in the skin. The peritoneal catheter with the stylet in place is introduced into the peritoneal space. This is suggested by a 'pop' and decreased resistance to the introduction of the catheter and by efflux of fluid through the catheter. The stylet is removed and the catheter is advanced into the pelvic fossa. The dialysis fluid is run out by gravity to determine whether the system is working. Usually the catheter must be fixed in place using a purse-string suture and adhesive tape.

For each exchange, about 10–20 ml/kg body weight of warmed dialysis fluid is initially introduced into the peritoneal cavity. If no leaking occurs, and if the amount is well tolerated, the volume is gradually increased to 30–40 ml/kg body weight per exchange. Heparin (500 u/litre dialysis fluid) is used for the first few exchanges or until the dialysis fluid is clear to prevent the formation of fibrin clots. Normally, antibiotics are not added to the dialysis fluid. Dialysis solutions are available with different concentrations of glucose; usually 0.5, 1.5, 2.5 and 4.25% solutions are available. A decision on which solution to use is determined by the amount of excess fluid that must be removed. The standard dialysate solution is the 1.5% solution which contains 1.5 g sugar/100 ml of solution. A solution with higher glucose concentration is used when larger amounts of fluid must be removed. Potassium (3 mmol/litre) is added to the dialysis solution when the serum potassium is less than 4 mmol/litre. Normally the dialysis solution should not contain more than 4 mmol potassium/litre. If hypokalaemia persists, supplemental potassium can be given intravenously or orally.

The required amount of dialysate is usually run in over 5–10 min. The fluid is allowed to dwell in the peritoneal cavity for 30 min and is then run out over approximately 15 min. As the patient's condition improves, the dwell time can be gradually increased and in some stable patients the fluid exchanged only every 6 h, similar to continuous ambulatory peritoneal dialysis.

Weight, intake and output must be accurately recorded. The patient's intake is adjusted according to the amount of fluid removed through dialysis.

Some physicians feel that the acute peritoneal catheter should be changed every few days to prevent infection, while others leave the catheter in place, even for a few weeks.

Nutrition

Adequate nutrition prevents catabolism. Most of the calories should be provided in the form of carbohydrate or fat, since protein as a source of phosphate, sulphate and urea will contribute to metabolic acidosis and azotaemia. Daily energy intake should ideally be at least 1400 kcal m^{-2} body surface. For patients who are unable to take oral or enteral feeds, parenteral hyperalimentation must be started. In these cases, the amount of fluid may be a limiting factor and dialysis or CAVH may be required to allow for a fluid volume sufficient to provide for adequate calories. The provision of amino acids is controversial, especially since deleterious effects of amino acid hyperalimentation have been reported.[28]

Infection

Infection is one of the leading causes of death in patients with ARF. Invasive procedures should therefore be limited. One should try not to maintain a bladder catheter beyond a few days or beyond the polyuric phase of ARF. Prophylactic antibiotics are not recommended.

Table 21.18 Some factors affecting incidence and prognosis reporting of children with ARF

Definition of ARF
Rise in seum creatinine vs. oliguria vs. need for dialysis

Centre reporting
General hospital vs. referral centre

Type of problems
Warm vs. cold climate

Quality of basic care available
For example, routine fluid management

Centre expertise in preventing occurrence of ARF
Protocol for preventing tumour lysis, drug-monitoring programme

Type of patient included/excluded
Premature/newborn, oncological, transplant, surgical, terminal, multiple organ failure, chronic renal failure

Definition of outcome
Death vs. off dialysis

Drug therapy

Many drugs are excreted by the kidneys and will require adjustments of dosages in renal failure. Nephrotoxic drugs may be important in the causation of renal failure and should be avoided in established renal failure. Before commencing any drug in renal failure, it is essential to check specifically on its handling in renal failure. Information can usually be obtained from review articles,[29–31] local or national formularies,[32] and in case of doubt directly from the drug manufacturers.

Prognosis

The reporting of prognosis for patients with ARF depends on many factors (Table 21.18), especially the type of patient included in any series. Niaudet *et al.* remarked that they had only a 10% mortality in their children with ARF, which neither included any surgical or neonatal hypoxaemic patients, compared to other reports where the mortality was 60% and included these two types of patients.[33] Certainly, as tertiary hospitals continue to treat high-risk patients such as cardiac, surgical, transplantation, immune deficiencies, prematures, etc., the mortality rate for ARF will remain high.

References

1. Feld L.G., Springate J.E and Fildes R.D. Acute renal failure. I. Pathophysiology and diagnosis. *J. Pediatr.* 1986, **109**, 401–408

2. Siegel N.J., van Why S.K., Boydstun I.I. *et al.* Acute renal failure. In: *Pediatric Nephrology*, Holliday M.A., Barratt T.M. and Avner E.D. (eds). Baltimore, Williams and Wilkins, 3rd edn, 1994: 1176–1186

3. Conger J.D. and Schrier R.W. Renal hemodynamics in acute renal failure. *Ann. Rev. Physiol.* 1980, **42**, 603–614

4. Flores J., DiBona D.R., Beck C.H. and Leaf A. The role of cell swelling in ischemic renal damage and the protective effect of hypertonic solute. *J. Clin. Investi.* 1972, **51**, 118–126

5. Mason J. The pathophysiology of ischaemic acute renal failure. *Renal Physiol.* 1986, **9**, 129–147

6. Canavese C., Stratta P. and Vercellone A. The case of oxygen free radicals in the pathogenesis of ischemic acute renal failure. *Nephron* 1988, **49**, 9–15

7. Gaudio K.M. and Siegel N.J. Pathogenesis and treatment of acute renal failure. *Pediatr. Clin. N. Am.*, 1987, **34**, 771–787

8. Ellis D., Fried W.A., Yunis E.J. and Blau E.B. Acute interstitial nephritis in children: a report of 13 cases and review of the literature. *Pediatrics* 1981, **67**, 862–870

9. Chesney R.W., Kaplan B.S., Freedom R.M., Haller J.A. and Drummond K.N. Acute renal failure: an important complication of cardiac surgery in infants. *J. Pediatr.* 1975, **87**, 381–388

10. Geha A.S. Acute renal failure in cardiovascular and other surgical patients. *Surg. Clin. N. Am.* 1980, **60**, 1151–1156

11. Kaplan B.S., Herbert D. and Morrell R.E. Acute renal failure induced by hyperphosphatemia in acute lymphoblastic leukemia. *Can. Med. Ass. J.* 1981, **124**, 429–431

12. Guignard J.-P. and John E.G. Renal function in the tiny premature infant. *Clin. Perinatol.* 1986, **13**, 377–401

13. Loirat C. and Guesnu M. Insuffisance rénale aiguë. In: Royer P., Habib R., Broyer M. and Mathieu H. (eds) *Néphrologie Pédiatrique.* Paris, Flammarion Médecine-Sciences, 1983: 415–424

14. Karmali M.A., Petric M., Lim C., Fleming P.C., Arbus G.S. and Lior H. The association between idiopathic hemolytic-uremic syndrome and infection by verotoxin producing *Escherichia coli. J. Infect. Dis.* 1985, **151**, 775–782

15. Karmali M.A. Infection by verocytotoxin-producing *Escherichia coli. Clin. Microbiol. Rev.* 1989, **2**, 15–38

16. Steele B.T., Murphy N., Chuang S., McGreal D. and Arbus G.S. Recovery from prolonged coma in the hemolytic-uremic syndrome. *J. Pediatr.* 1983, **102**, 402–404

17. Butler T., Islam M.R., Azad M.A.K. and Jones P.K. Risk factors for development of hemolytic uremic syndrome during shigellosis. *J. Pediatr.* 1987, **110**, 894–897

18. Chantler C. Renal failure in childhood. In: *Renal Disease*, Black D. and Jones N.F. (eds). Oxford, Blackwell, 1979: 825–868

19. Miller T.R., Anderson R.J., Linas S.L., Henrich W.L, Berns A.S., Gabow P.A. and Schrier R.W. Urinary diagnostic indices in acute renal failure: a prospective study. *Ann. Intern. Med.* 1978, **89**, 47–50

20. Anand S.K. Acute renal failure in the neonate. *Pediat. Clin. N. Am.* 1982, **29**, 791–800

21. Espinel C.H. and Gregory A.W. Differential diagnosis of acute renal failure. *Clin. Nephrol.* 1980, **13**, 73–77

22. Mathew O.P., Jones A.S., James E., Bland H. and Groshong T. Neonatal renal failure: usefulness of diagnostic indices. *Pediatrics*, 1980, **65**, 57–60

23. Patriquin H.B., O'Regan S., Robitaille P. and Paltiel H. Hemolyticuremic syndrome: intrarenal arterial Doppler patterns as a useful guide to therapy. *Radiology* 1989, **172**, 625–628

24. Wong S.N., Lo R.N. and Yu E.C. Renal blood flow pattern by noninvasive Doppler ultrasound in normal children and acute renal failure patients. *J. Ultrasound Med.* 1989, **8**, 135–141

25. Brenner B.M. and Stein J.H. *Acute Renal Failure*, Vol. 6. *Contemporary Issues in Nephrology*. New York, Churchill Livingstone, 1980

26. McClure R.J., Prasad V.K. and Brocklebank J.T. Treatment of hyperkalaemia using intravenous and nebulised salbutamol. *Arch. Dis. Child.* 1994, **70**, 126–128

27. Wiggelinkhuizen J. and Pokroy M.V. Acute renal failure in infancy and childhood. *S. Afr. Med. J.* 1954, **48**, 2129–2136

28. Zager R.A. Amino acid hyperlimentation in acute renal failure: a potential therapeutic paradox. *Kidney Int.* 1987, **32**, S72–75

29. Wong A.F., Bolinger A.M. and Gambertoglio. Pharmacokinetics and drug dosing in children with decreased renal function. In: *Pediatric Nephrology*, 3rd edn, Holliday M.A., Barratt T.M. and Avner E.D. (eds), Baltimore, Williams and Wilkins 1994: 1305–1313

30. Bennett W.M. *et al.* Drug therapy in renal failure: dosage guidelines for adults. *Ann. Intern. Med.* 1980, **93**, 62–89 and 286–325

31. Trompeter R.S. A review of drug prescribing in children with end-stage renal failure. *Pediatr. Nephrol.* 1987, **1**, 183–194

32. British Medical Association Prescribing in Renal Impairment. *British National Formulary* 1984: 11–16

33. Niaudet P, Maher H.-I., Gagnadoux M.-F. and Broyer M. Outcome of children with acute renal failure. *Kidney Int.* 1985, **28**, S148–151

22

Chronic renal failure

S.P.A. Rigden

Renal failure is a continuum (Table 22.1), but for the purposes of this chapter, chronic renal failure (CRF) is defined by a GFR of < 50 ml min^{-1} 1.73 m^{-2} SA, i.e. to include chronic renal insufficiency (CRI), because below this level of renal function, growth impairment and metabolic abnormalities such as secondary hyperparathyroidism begin to become apparent and further progressive loss of function is likely to occur. Renal replacement therapy (RRT), either by dialysis or transplantation, does not usually become necessary until the GFR falls below 10 ml min^{-1} 1.73 m^{-2} SA. The initiation of RRT defines the onset of end-stage renal failure (ESRF), and pre-terminal renal failure (pre-TRF) defines those patients with CRF before RRT becomes necessary.

Incidence and prevalence

The incidence of ESRF in children is, fortunately, low; in 1987 the acceptance rate for new patients aged less than 15 years in the five European countries with the most active treatment programmes for children was 3.7–6.6 per million child population (pmcp).[1] In the UK, this translates to approximately 60–70 children commencing RRT each year. These children should be treated in specialized paediatric centres, where facilities can be concentrated and expertise developed. Data from the European Dialysis and Transplant Registry have shown better patient survival[2] and a higher chance of having a functioning transplant for children treated in specialized centres.[3]

The prevalence of pre-TRF is less well defined, but studies in Switzerland[4] and more recently in Sweden give figures of 18.5 and 26.1 pmcp, respectively. These children require careful conservative management in order to optimize their growth and to preserve their renal function for as long as possible which, for some, will be into adult life. They should be under the

Table 22.1 Stages of renal failure

	GFR (ml min^{-1} 1.73 m^{-2} SA)	
Impaired renal function	80–50	Asymptomatic
Chronic renal insufficiency	50–30	Metabolic abnormalities
Chronic renal failure	30–10	Impaired growth Progressive renal failure
End-stage renal failure	< 10	Renal replacement therapy required

Table 22.2 Causes of CRF

	EDTA[6] (%)	NAPRTCS[7] (%)	Sweden[5] (%) (pre-TRF + ESRF)
Glomerulonephritis	*25.8*	*21.3*	*9.6*
Focal segmental glomerulosclerosis	6.8	12.0	4.1
Other glomerulonephritis	19.0	9.3	5.5
Pyelonephritis/interstitial nephritis	*24.2*	*23.0*	*24.9*
Obstructive uropathy	10.8	16.0	17.8
Vesico-ureteric reflux	7.8	4.1	5.0
Other causes	5.6	2.9	2.1
Hereditary/familial nephropathy	*15.6*	*15.2*	*27.5*
Polycystic kidney disease	1.6	1.8	7.5
Medullary cystic disease, including nephronophthisis	6.3	2.9	11.0
Hereditary nephritis with nerve deafness	1.6	–	0.7
Other hereditary nephritis	0.6	3.0	3.4
Cystinosis	3.2	2.6	1.4
Primary oxalosis	0.9	1.0	–
Congenital nephrotic syndrome	–	3.9	1.4
Other causes	1.4	–	2.1
Congenital hypoplasia/dysplasia	*13.5*	*21.7*	*23.1*
Aplasia/hypoplasia/dysplasia	10.9	18.1	21.0
Prune-belly syndrome	0.8	3.6	2.1
Other causes	1.8		
Multisystem disease	*10.2*	*8.6*	*8.3*
Lupus erythematosus	0.8	–	2.1
Henoch–Schoenlein purpura	2.4	–	2.1
Haemolytic uraemic syndrome	4.8	3.9	2.7
Systemic immunological disease	–	4.7	–
Other multisystem disease	2.2	–	1.4
Renal vascular disease	*1.6*	*2.2*	*3.5*
Miscellaneous	*3.5*	*4.8*	*2.8*
Kidney tumour	0.7	0.7	0.7
Drash syndrome	–	0.6	1.4
Others	2.8	3.5	0.7
Chronic renal failure Unknown cause	*5.7*	*3.3*	*0.7*

supervision of a specialized paediatric centre, but often their care can be shared with their local paediatrician.

Causes of CRF

The causes of CRF, derived from three sources,[5–7] are summarized in Table 22.2. The primary renal diseases of 2372 children commencing RRT in Europe between 1981 and 1985 are shown in column 1,[6] and those of 725 children transplanted in North America between January 1987 and February 1989 in column 2;[7] in column 3,[5] the causes of CRF

(GFR < 30 ml min^{-1} 1.73 m^{-2} SA) in 146 Swedish children, 77 of whom required RRT during the period 1978–85, are given.

The proportional distribution of primary renal diseases has changed over time, mainly as a result of the increasing number of younger children now being treated. The age of 230 children receiving first renal transplants at Guy's Hospital in four consecutive 5-year periods is shown in Figure 22.1: between 1968 and 1972 only 2 of 8 children transplanted were less than 10 years old, whereas in the 5-year period 1983–87, 29% of the 116 children transplanted were aged 5–10 years and 18% less than 5 years.

The primary renal diseases of these children

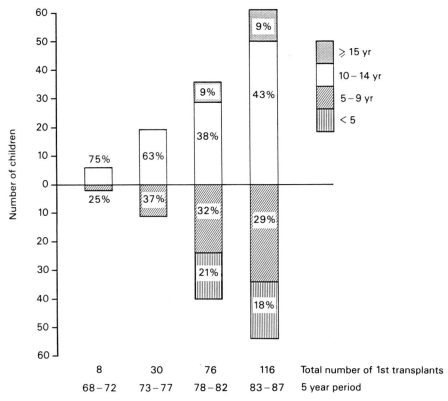

Figure 22.1 Age of children receiving first renal transplants in four consecutive 5-year periods at Guy's Hospital, London

are presented in a similar format in Figure 22.2. The increase in the proportion of children with congenital abnormalities from 33% to 52% is clearly seen. In this classification, vesico-ureteric reflux is considered a congenital abnormality. Inherited conditions form the second largest group of causes of ESRF. Now approximately 75% of children requiring RRT have a prenatal cause, which has important implications for genetic counselling, antenatal diagnosis and future research. It is also interesting to note that glomerulonephritis as a cause of ESRF is, in this series, relatively less common than in other larger series.[6,7]

Presentation of the child with CRF

Children with CRF present to their paediatricians in a wide variety of ways. The onset of CRF may be silent and its progression insidious, with symptoms only developing late in its course.

Antenatal ultrasound

The advent of routine antenatal ultrasound scanning has resulted in the increased detection of fetal renal tract abnormalities,[8] some of which are causes of CRF, e.g. obstructive uropathy due to posterior urethral valve, infantile polycystic kidney disease. Such an *in utero* diagnosis requires close co-operation between the obstetrician, local paediatrician and paediatric nephrologist to ensure the appropriate management of the fetus pre- and post-delivery and that the parents are given accurate information.

Abdominal mass – see Chapter 7

The discovery of a renal mass or a palpable bladder may be the first clue to underlying CRF. The scheme for investigation outlined in Chapter 7, together with an assessment of renal function, will lead to the correct diagnosis.

Failure to thrive

Chronic uraemia frequently results in vomiting

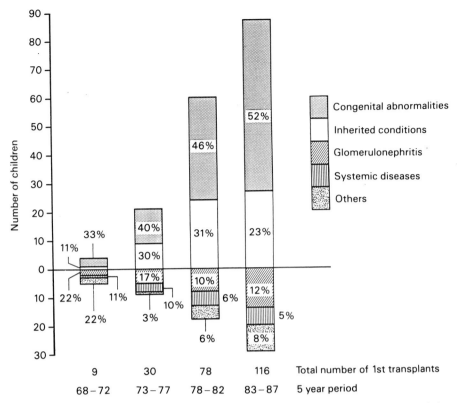

Figure 22.2 Primary renal disease of children receiving first renal transplants in four consecutive 5-year periods at Guy's Hospital, London

and failure to thrive, particularly in infants and young children, making an assessment of renal function mandatory in such children. Failure to thrive with dehydration and electrolyte disturbances is a common mode of presentation in children with renal tubular disorders (see Chapter 24), which are either associated with CRF, e.g. obstructive uropathy, or which will progress to CRF, e.g. Fanconi's syndrome due to cystinosis.

Short stature

Poor growth velocity, short stature and pubertal delay may all be caused by and presenting symptoms of CRF.

Lethargy, pallor

Pallor, due to the normochromic–normocytic anaemia which results from chronic uraemia, and lethargy are classic symptoms of CRF, but they may not develop until late in its course.

Occasionally a child with even less specific symptoms of ill health is found to have CRF.

Urinary tract infection

The investigation of a child with a urinary tract infection (see Chapters 13 and 14) may reveal a serious underlying renal tract abnormality or pyelonephritic scarring sufficient to result in CRF.

Enuresis

The large majority of children with enuresis will have no organic cause found (Chapter 6), but CRF may present in this way in a small number of children. Useful clues are the presence of daytime wetting, the onset of secondary enuresis, a history of urinary tract infection and a history of polydipsia and polyuria. An early morning urine osmolality is a very useful screening test and will often avoid the need for renal tract imaging studies.

Hypertension

Hypertension, usually symptomatic, is not infrequently the presenting feature of coarse renal scarring due, for example, to reflux nephropathy, which may also result in CRF. It follows therefore that all children with hypertension must have their renal function assessed (Chapter 15). Non-renin-dependent hypertension due to salt and water retention also occurs in children with CRF, but is less likely to be a presenting feature, unless it results in cardiac failure (see below).

Congestive cardiac failure

Congestive cardiac failure, resulting from untreated hypertension and/or salt and water overload, may be the first sign of underlying CRF in some children and requires urgent treatment with diuretics or, if necessary, dialysis and occasionally ventilation.

Haematuria

The causes and investigation of haematuria are discussed in Chapter 1. Rarely haematuria, usually macroscopic, is the first symptom of a condition which will ultimately cause renal failure, e.g. Alport's syndrome, adult-type polycystic kidney disease.

Nephrotic syndrome

The outcome for children with minimal-change nephrotic syndrome is generally excellent, but for those with steroid resistant disease the outlook is less favourable, with a proportion progressing to chronic and ESRF (Chapter 19). Infants with congenital nephrotic syndrome also have a poor prognosis, either succumbing to infection or eventually developing CRF.

Failure of resolution of acute renal failure

Occasionally a child with acute renal failure will make no or an incomplete recovery and be left in chronic or ESRF, e.g. in rapidly progressive glomerulonephritis, or there may be a very slow but inexorable decline in renal function, usually heralded by hypertension and/or proteinuria, in children in whom there had apparently been a good recovery from acute renal failure, e.g. haemolytic uraemic syndrome.[9]

Asymptomatic – detected by screening

Very rarely an asymptomatic child is found to have proteinuria or microscopic haematuria on routine urinalysis, which on investigation is found to be due to serious underlying renal disease.

It is important to screen even the apparently healthy siblings of children with genetically determined CRF, e.g. juvenile nephronophthisis, Alport's syndrome, reflux nephropathy, while realizing the potentially devastating effect on the family of finding a second affected child.

Investigation of the child with CRF

It may not be clear at presentation whether a child has acute, and therefore potentially reversible, or chronic renal failure (see also Chapter 21). A scheme for the assessment of such children is given in Table 22.3. In others, history and examination suggest chronic disease and appropriate investigations elucidate the underlying cause (Table 22.4). The investigations listed in Table 22.5 should be performed to assess the degree of CRF and the severity of any secondary metabolic derangements.

Conservative management of pre-terminal renal failure

The aims of conservative management are, from the child's viewpoint, to

- feel *normal*, i.e. not to have uraemic symptoms such as nausea or vomiting
- be *normal*, i.e. to be like your friends and have sufficient energy to take a full part in all school and extracurricular activities or, for the pre-school child, to achieve normal motor, social and intellectual development
- maintain *normal* growth

while

- preserving *normal* family functioning
- slowing progression to ESRF
- preparing the child and family for the treatment of ESRF.

For the child with moderate to severe CRF (GFR < 30 ml min^{-1} 1.73 m^{-2} SA), these objectives are best met by a team approach in

Table 22.3 Assessment of the child with renal failure of unknown cause

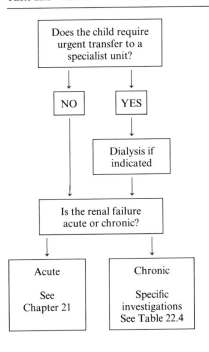

Indications for transfer
- anuria/oliguria
- symptomatic electrolyte abnormalities
  hyperkalaemia – K^+ > 6 mmol/litre
  hypernatraemia, hyponatraemia,
  metabolic acidosis
  hyperphosphataemia, hypocalcaemia
- severe hypertension
- pulmonary oedema

Features suggestive of:

acute renal failure

- normal or slightly
  enlarged kidneys
  on ultrasound

- micro-angiopathic
  haemolytic anaemia,
  thrombocytopenia

chronic renal failure

- small/asymmetrical
  kidneys
- cystic kidneys
- abnormal collecting
  systems/ureters/bladder
  on ultrasound
- normochromic,
  normocytic anaemia
- end-organ effects of
  hypertension,
  e.g. retinopathy
- poor growth
- radiological evidence of
  rickets or secondary
  hyperparathyroidism
- family history

Table 22.4 Specific investigations to elucidate the underlying cause of CRF

Renal tract ultrasound
Micturating cysto-urethrogram
Radioisotope scans – DMSA, DTPA
Antegrade pressure flow studies
IVU
Urinalysis
Urine microscopy and culture
C3, C4, ANF, DNA binding, ANCA
Renal biopsy
Purine excretion
Oxalate excretion
White cell cystine level

Table 22.5 Investigations to assess the severity of CRF

Full blood count	
Biochemistry:	blood electrolytes, urea, creatinine, calcium, phosphate, alkaline phosphatase, total protein, albumin, urate, blood pH and bicarbonate – using blood gas analysis
	urine creatinine, phosphate, protein, albumin
GFR:	of less value in severe CRF
PTH:	using an intact molecule assay
Left hand and wrist X-ray:	for bone age and evidence of renal osteodystrophy
Chest X-ray	
ECG or echocardiogram	

the setting of a dedicated clinic, where ample time can be spent with each patient and the family.[10]

Ideally the team should comprise or have access to: a paediatric nephrologist, a children's trained renal nurse, a paediatric renal dietitian, a teacher, a social worker, a child psychologist and/or a child psychiatrist, in addition to the most important team members, the child and family. For some children with less severe degrees of CRF, it may be appropriate for their care to be shared with their local paediatrician, but it is important that they are under the supervision of a specialist paediatric centre, particularly for the prevention, detection and treatment of secondary hyperparathyroidism and in order to promote maximal growth.

Management points

Management points to be considered at each outpatient visit include those in the following sections.

Growth

The assessment of growth and the multifactorial nature of growth impairment in CRF are reviewed in detail in Chapter 4 and elsewhere.[11,12] In our experience, and that of other large centres, the major loss of height has often already occurred prior to our seeing the child, emphasizing the need for early referral. With careful attention to and reversal of all possible growth-retarding factors, it is usually possible to restore normal growth velocity and sometimes to induce catch-up growth, particularly in young children.[13]

If a child with CRF has a height velocity below the normal range for age, it is mandatory to seek the reason why, with a view to correcting it, rather than simply ascribing the poor growth to 'CRF'. However there remains a group of children with CRF, who, despite optimal management, continue to grow poorly and

who may benefit from an alternative approach, such as transplantation before ESRF is reached, or treatment with recombinant human growth hormone in supraphysiological doses.[14]

Nutrition

A paediatric dietitian is an essential member of the team because nutritional therapy forms the backbone of conservative management in CRF.[15] The recommended intake of nutrients for children with CRF are given in Table 22.6, but certain points need to be emphasized:

(a) The intake of nutrients should be monitored by prospective 3-day dietary assessments performed at 1–3-month intervals.

(b) Children with CRF tend to be anorexic with spontaneous energy intakes frequently below the estimated average requirement (EAR) for age. The most important aim of dietetic therapy is to increase the energy intake to at least EAR for age, which usually requires the use of glucose polymers or fat emulsions as calorie supplements and sometimes the use of nasogastric or gastrostomy tube feeding, particularly in infants and young children.[13]

(c) In order to prevent or treat secondary hyperparathyroidism, plasma phosphate must be maintained between the mean and -2 SD for age,[17] by restriction of dietary phosphate and the use of calcium carbonate as a phosphate binder (see below and Chapter 5). As the major dietary sources of phosphate are dairy products, adequate phosphate restriction can be achieved by limiting the intake of cow's milk to less than half a

Table 22.6   Recommended nutrient intakes for children with CRF (From Department of Health[16])*

Age	Weight (kg)	Energy (kcal)	Protein (g)	Calcium (mg)	Phosphorus (mg)
0–3 m	5.9	115/kg	2.1/kg	525	400
4–6 m	7.7	100/kg	1.6/kg	525	400
7–9 m	8.8	95/kg	1.6/kg	525	400
10–12 m	9.7	95/kg	1.5/kg	525	400
1–3 y	12.5	1230	14.5	350	270
4–6 y	17.8	1715	19.7	450	350
7–10 y	28.3	1970	28.3	550	450
11–14 y M	43.0	2220	42.1	1000	775
F	43.8	1845	41.2	800	625
15–18 y M	64.5	2755	55.2	1000	775
F	55.5	2110	45.4	800	625

*Energy is expressed as estimated average requirement (EAR) in kcal kg^{-1} day^{-1} for infants and kcal/day for children over 1 year of age. Protein, calcium and phosphorus are expressed as reference nutrient intakes defined as EAR + 2 SD.

pint a day and by avoiding cheese and yoghurt.

(d) Further protein restriction is seldom necessary so long as energy intake is ensured to promote anabolism and dairy proteins are reduced. If, despite these measures, a child's blood urea remains above 20 mmol/litre, we introduce gentle step-wise protein restriction using the child's 3-day dietary assessments as the basis for advice, until the blood urea is less than 20 mmol/litre. We do not restrict protein to less than 6% of EAR for calories and carefully monitor not only height and weight, but also plasma albumin as a measure of the adequacy of protein nutrition. We never ask parents to weigh a child's diet nor to use special low-protein products which are often unpalatable and expensive. Several centres have investigated the use of low-protein diets supplemented with essential amino acids or a mixture of essential amino acids and their keto-acid analogues, with encouraging results in terms of patient well-being, growth and preservation of renal function,[18] but they are complex, unpalatable and not proven in controlled trials to be better than less complicated diets.

Fluid and electrolyte balance

Clinical assessment of hydration by skin turgor, mucous membrane moisture, blood pressure, jugular venous pressure and weight should be performed at each clinic visit. Children with obstructive uropathy or renal dysplasia are particularly likely to become salt depleted, which is detrimental to growth.[19] Sodium chloride supplements should be gradually increased until an improvement in growth is seen, without producing oedema, hypertension or hypernatraemia. Water is determined by the child to satisfy thirst. Children with primary renal disease resulting in hypertension may benefit from a modest reduction in sodium intake, but it is seldom necessary to restrict fluid until ESRF supervenes.

Most children with CRF are able to maintain potassium homeostasis satisfactorily despite fluctuations in intake.[19] If hyperkalaemia develops it is important to exclude catabolism and metabolic acidosis (see below) as correctable causes, before giving individually tailored advice based on the child's dietary assessments.

Metabolic acidosis

Maintenance of acid-base equilibrium is particularly important in infants and children. Persistent metabolic acidosis is frequently associated with failure to thrive in infancy and also contributes to bone demineralization and hyperkalaemia. We therefore aim to correct metabolic acidosis using sodium bicarbonate supplements in a starting dose of 2 mmol kg^{-1} day^{-1}. We then titrate the dose to each child's requirements using venous blood gas determinations of pH and bicarbonate concentration.

Renal osteodystrophy

The management of renal bone disease is discussed in detail in Chapter 5. We have shown in our clinic that it is possible to prevent and reverse established secondary hyperparathyroidism over long periods of time using a regimen of mild dietary phosphate restriction as outlined above, calcium carbonate given with meals as a phosphate binder and 1α-hydroxycholecalciferol (one-alpha HCC) or 1,25-dihydroxycholecalciferol (1,25-DHCC).[20] The dose of calcium carbonate is increased until the plasma phosphate falls between the mean and -2 SD for age, when if the PTH level is still high, one-alpha-HCC or 1,25-DHCC is introduced and increased until the plasma calcium is at the upper end of the normal range. Plasma calcium, phosphate and alkaline phosphatase are measured at each clinic visit: PTH levels, using an intact molecule assay, are checked monthly and therapy adjusted accordingly. If the biochemical parameters are normal and the child asymptomatic, it is only necessary to perform an annual X-ray of the left hand and wrist to assess bone age.

Hypertension

Satisfactory blood pressure control is not only important to prevent the morbidity and mortality associated with hypertension, but may also be important in retarding the progression of CRF (see below). The management of hypertension is discussed in detail in Chapter 15.

Infection

A urine sample should be cultured at each clinic visit to exclude infection. Those children prone to recurrent urinary infections, e.g. those with persisting vesico-ureteric reflux, should be maintained on low-dose prophylactic antibiotics, remembering that nitrofurantoin becomes less effective with declining renal function and the general measures to prevent reinfection, as outlined in Chapter 14, stressed.

Anaemia

CRF is associated with a normochromic, normocytic anaemia of variable severity. The pathophysiology of this anaemia is complex and may include shortened red cell survival, inhibition of erythropoiesis by uraemic toxins, particularly PTH, aluminium toxicity, and iron and folate deficiency, together with the most important factor, the inadequate production of erythropoietin. Recombinant human erythropoietin (rHuEPO) is now available and has been used successfully to treat the anaemia of children with ESRF maintained by dialysis (see below).[21,22] However, the majority of children with pre-TRF can maintain satisfactory haemoglobin levels without endogenous rHuEPO therapy, provided that careful attention is paid to nutrition, iron and folate supplements are given if indicated and secondary hyperparathyroidism is suppressed without the use of aluminium-containing phosphate binders.

Preservation of renal function

In the majority of patients with CRF, renal function continues to decline, irrespective of the primary renal disease and whether or not it is still active. Animal studies have resulted in several hypotheses to explain this non-specific progression of renal failure, but none has been definitely established in man.[23] Studies in animals suggest that various hypotensive agents and dietary restriction of protein and phosphorus may slow the rate of progression, but there is, as yet, little convincing data from well-designed clinical trials that similar benefits are derived by patients.[24,25]

Our present policy, therefore, is to control blood pressure to well within the normal limits for age and to prevent secondary hyperparathyroidism, but not to restrict protein intake beyond the limits set out above. We have in fact observed extremely slow rates of decline in renal function over long periods of time, in association with the control of secondary hyperparathyroidism.[20]

Education and preparation

The conservative phase of CRF management is an ideal time for an ongoing programme of education for the child and family. It is very important that everyone understands the rationale of conservative management and that ultimately RRT will be necessary. It is usually possible to predict with reasonable accuracy, when ESRF will supervene, from a plot of the reciprocal of the plasma creatinine or the calculated GFR. Using this prediction, there should, at an appropriate time, be full discussion of the various RTT options available (see below). It is very helpful for the child and family to meet other children on the various forms of dialysis and who have been transplanted. They should also meet the various staff involved, including the transplant surgeon, and visit the dialysis unit, so that by the time RTT becomes necessary, they are thoroughly acquainted with the various therapeutic options.

In addition to education there are also physical aspects of preparation for ESRF management to be considered:

- It is very important to ensure that a child approaching ESRF is fully immunized including, if indicated, BCG.
- In children whose CRF is associated with bladder dysfunction, e.g. neuropathic bladder, posterior urethral valve, it is essential to be sure that the bladder is 'safe' prior to transplantation. This will involve investigation with urodynamic studies and perhaps bladder surgery to increase the capacity and/or reduce the pressure within the bladder and/or management with clean intermittent catheterization (see Chapter 26).
- Children who are likely to require dialysis prior to transplantation, but who are not suitable for peritoneal dialysis, should have an arteriovenous fistula created to provide vascular access for haemodialysis.

Social and psychological support

Chronic life-threatening disease inevitably results in stress for the child and family. CRF and its treatment may be disruptive to a child's schooling, social life and family life: siblings may feel excluded and the parents' relationship put under stress; there may be financial difficulties as a result of a parent having to give up

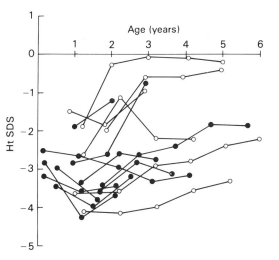

Figure 22.3 Growth of 16 children with pre-TRF presenting before 2 years of age. ●, Male; ○, female

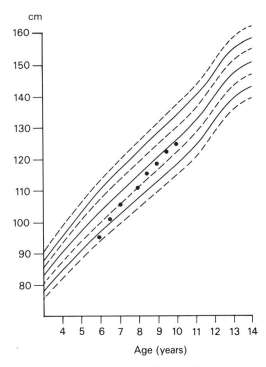

Figure 22.4 Growth chart of a girl presenting at age 6 with a calculated GFR of approximately 10 ml min^{-1} 1.73 m^{-2} SA. During 4 years of conservative therapy she has gained 1.39 SD in height and her GFR has fallen to approximately 7 ml min^{-1} 1.73 m^{-2} SA

work and the expense of travelling, sometimes long distances, to the specialist centre.

Good medical management will minimize illness and good patient and family education the fear of the unknown. It is important that the child attends a normal school, develops normal peer group relationships and takes part in out-of-school activities: liaison with the hospital-based teacher can be useful in this respect. The problems of denial and non-compliance with treatment may be helped by encouraging school friends, as well as siblings, to visit the hospital and to become part of the extended team. All families should have easy access to a social worker for help with practical and financial difficulties, as well as for psychological support. Many families derive support from each other, either informally or through a parents' support group. More difficult problems such as behavioural disorders, feeding problems and poor family functioning ideally require skilled intervention by a child psychologist or psychiatrist, who should be seen as part of the team.

Using these principles it is possible to improve the well-being, activity and growth of children with pre-TRF and possibly prolong the time until RTT is required.[13] Figure 22.3 depicts the growth of 16 children with pre-TRF who presented to our clinic before 2 years of age: 12 of the children were significantly short at presentation and 10 required nasogastric tube feeding. After 2 years in the clinic, 11 children had improved their rate of growth, with a mean

increase in height SDS of 0.9. GFR remained stable throughout, being 17 ml min^{-1} 1.73 m^{-2} SA at entry (range 7–37), 18 ml min^{-1} 1.73 m^{-2} SA (range 8–33) at 2 years and 22 ml min^{-1} 1.73 m^{-2} SA (range 7–40) at 4 years.

Catch-up growth is less common in older children with pre-TRF, but is possible as exemplified by the child whose growth chart is shown in Figure 22.4. She was referred for dialysis, at almost 6 years of age, with a plasma potassium of 7.0 mmol/litre, a urea of 31.6 mmol/litre and creatinine of 365 μmol/litre. After 4 years of conservative management, her height SDS has improved from −1.59 to −0.2, her potassium is 4.3 mmol/litre, her urea 23.6 mmol/litre and her creatinine 800 μmol/litre.

Moving on

Even with meticulous management, most children with pre-TRF eventually progress to ESRF: other children present in ESRF. The first decision to be made is whether it is indeed appropriate to treat a particular child. It is becoming increasingly rare not to treat, but ESRF management can be arduous and, after full discussion with the family, this may be the best decision for, for example, a child with multiple handicaps or a small infant. However, the majority of children are suitable for treatment which ideally is by renal transplantation, with dialysis only being used as a means to that end.

The treatment of ESRF is much better considered as a 'roundabout' (Figure 22.5) as opposed to a straight line, namely:

Pre-TRF $\longrightarrow$ Dialysis $\longrightarrow$
                Transplantation $\begin{array}{l} \longrightarrow \text{Success} \\ \longrightarrow \text{Failure} \end{array}$

We prefer to transplant children just before they become symptomatic from their renal failure and require dialysis.[12] This policy requires careful timing and sometimes more rapid progression of CRF than anticipated, or a lull in the supply of kidneys means that a child enters the 'roundabout' for a period of dialysis prior to transplantation, as will the child presenting in ESRF. The ideal exit is with normal renal function, but if this is not achieved and further treatment is appropriate, the child simply remains on the roundabout and returns to dialysis if necessary, with a view to another transplant.

Indications for initiating renal replacement therapy

For children with progressive pre-TRF, our usual policy is to place them 'on-call' for a cadaveric renal transplant when their calculated GFR has fallen below 10 ml min^{-1} 1.73 m^{-2} SA, with the aim of transplantation before dialysis becomes necessary.[26] Dialysis is indicated if the child develops:

- uraemic symptoms such as lethargy, anorexia or vomiting, which interfere with daily life
- dangerous biochemistry, e.g. hyperkalaemia, despite the measures outlined above
- evidence of circulatory overload
- impaired growth velocity unresponsive to optimal conservative management; ocasionally poor growth constitutes an indication for earlier initiation of RTT, preferably by transplantation.

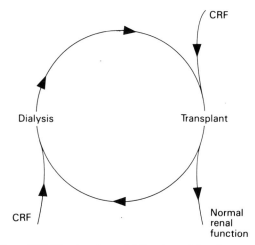

Figure 22.5 The chronic renal failure 'roundabout'

For children presenting in ESRF, the indications for dialysis are as in acute renal failure (see Chapter 21).

Dialysis options

The basic choice is between haemodialysis and peritoneal dialysis: both have advantages and disadvantages.

Haemodialysis

Haemodialysis requires access to the circulation: this is best provided by an arteriovenous fistula created from radial or brachial vessels of the non-dominant arm.[27] In young children surgically placed, double lumen central venous catheters may be preferable to avoid the trauma of placing dialysis needles in the fistula, although since the introduction of effective local anaesthetic cream (EMLA) this is less of a problem. Moreover central venous catheters are an infection risk and may result in stenosis or occlusion of large central veins, making further access difficult.

Haemodialysis is now mainly undertaken in specialist centres, since children and families who are suitable for home dialysis usually opt for peritoneal dialysis. In the UK on 31 December 1992, of 570 children receiving ESRF treatment, only 2 (0.4%) were maintained on home haemodialysis, while 54 (9.5%) received hospital-based haemodialysis and 120 (21%) were treated by continuous ambulatory peritoneal dialysis (CAPD) or continuous cycling peritoneal dialysis (CCPD) at home: 394 (69%) children had functioning transplants (data provided by the British Association for Paediatric Nephrology survey, 1993). As haemodialysis usually has to be performed three times a week for 3–5 h per session, depending on the patient's size, centre haemodialysis can be very disruptive to a child's education and social life. It does, however, relieve the family of the stresses and responsibility of performing dialysis. The educational disruption can be reduced by a teacher attached to the dialysis unit, who can liaise with the children's schools and maintain continuity of work.

Peritoneal dialysis

Peritoneal dialysis is a simple and effective technique that has gained in popularity since the advent of soft permanent peritoneal catheters and more recently automated cycling machines. It is particularly useful for treating small children, while it allows older children greater freedom from the hospital, little or no disruption to schooling and the chance to go away on holidays. The major disadvantage is peritonitis.[28] Peritoneal dialysis may be performed either intermittently, usually overnight using an automated cycling machine, or continuously by CAPD or by CCPD (see above). CAPD utilizes the peritoneum 24 h per day, with the child or carer performing four exchanges of dialysate during the day with a long overnight dwell. CCPD combines five or six overnight exchanges delivered by an automated cycling machine with a long daytime dwell. CCPD obviates the need for daytime exchanges and reduces the number of system disconnections to two per day: it may also reduce parent fatigue or CAPD 'burn-out', but it is expensive and, because it is machine dependent, allows less freedom than CAPD.

CAPD and CCPD usually result in better biochemical control with a less severe degree of anaemia than thrice weekly haemodialysis. However, peritoneal dialysis may prove impossible in children with intra-abdominal adhesions resulting from intra-abdominal surgery or peritonitis.

Limitations of dialysis

Both haemodialysis and peritoneal dialysis are safe and efficient modes of renal replacement but there are physical and psychosocial limitations.[29] Children treated by dialysis require regular review of all of the points listed under 'Conservative management of pre-terminal renal failure' (see above) and in addition will require an individually adjusted fluid restriction depending on their residual urine output, if any, and their mode of dialysis. Insensible fluid losses should be calculated as 300 ml/m^2 body SA per day. Several points deserve special mention:

- *Growth* – it is in general more difficult to achieve normal growth in children on dialysis,[12] although CAPD/CCPD may prove superior in this respect.[30]
- *Nutrition* – the nutritional strategy for children on dialysis is very similar to that discussed for the child with pre-TRF. An adequate energy intake is of paramount importance. Children on peritoneal dialysis may require an increase in protein intake to compensate for losses on dialysis.[15]
- *Anaemia* – with the advent of rHuEPO therapy, children on haemodialysis need no longer be profoundly anaemic and transfusion dependent[21] and although, in general, children on CAPD/CCPD are better able to maintain haemoglobin levels, some undoubtedly need and benefit from rHuEPO therapy (see below).[22]
- *Social and psychological support* become even more necessary during periods of dialysis, which increase stress for the child and family.[29]

Transplantation

Transplantation is the preferred treatment for children with ESRF, because this offers the potential for full rehabilitation to a near normal life style. Transplantation is performed using a cadaveric kidney or a kidney from a live relative over the age of consent, which for a child usually means a parent. With improved immunosuppression and cadaveric graft survival, the indications for live donor transplantation are diminishing, even in young children.[31] Overall in Europe, in the period 1984–88, 20% of children transplanted received a living related graft, although there was wide inter-country variation:[3] in North America, live donor sources accounted for 42% of grafts performed in children between January 1987 and February 1989.[7]

Immunosuppression

Immunosuppressive regimens at present in use vary widely,[7] from monotherapy using cyclosporin alone,[32] to quadruple therapy using a polyclonal antibody, steroids, azathioprine and cyclosporin A.[31] Some general points can be made:

- the intensity of immunosuppression required is in general inversely related to the degree of HLA matching achieved between the donor and recipient
- immunosuppression needs to be continued indefinitely, a fact not always appreciated by patients, particularly non-compliant teenagers
- cyclosporin A is nephrotoxic and therefore blood levels must be monitored to ensure an adequate immunosuppressive effect, while avoiding nephrotoxicity
- alternate-day steroid regimens are associated with better growth post-transplant than those utilizing daily steroids.[33]
- the increasing use of anti-lymphocyte antibodies, particularly if monoclonal antibodies, e.g. OKT3, are also given, is associated with an increased incidence of post-transplant malignancy.

Graft survival

The most recent EDTA data for patients transplanted before the age of 15 years in the period 1983–88 show a 1-year graft survival for living donor grafts of 87%, falling to 68% at 5 years and, for cadaveric grafts, a 1-year survival of 72%, falling to 50% by 5 years.[3] Similar 1-year graft survival figures of 88% for live donor grafts and 72% for cadaveric grafts have been reported by the North American Pediatric Renal Transplant Co-operative Study.[7]

Long-term graft survival data from two major paediatric centres are summarized in Table 22.7.[34] It is clear that even with good graft survival a child is likely to require two or three transplants for a normal life span.

Following transplantation there may be problems related to graft function, hypertension, infection and immunosuppressive therapy. Three particular problems deserve mention:

- *Recurrence of primary disease.* The only metabolic disease with recurrence is type I hyperoxaluria, but many forms of nephritis show histological recurrence, although fortunately in many patients this is only accompanied by mild or no clinical disease. Recurrence or *de novo* diseases account for only 5% of graft losses.[35]
- *Malignancy.* Wilms' tumour may recur post-transplant, particularly if the interval between primary treatment and immunosuppression for transplantation is less than 1 year.[36] Perhaps more worrying is the apparent increase in lymphoproliferative disorders, which may be associated with the increasing use of polyclonal and monoclonal antibodies.[7]
- *Growth.* In general, prepubertal children with successful transplants grow at an accelerated rate, but the growth of older children has been less satisfactory.[12] Steroid therapy, even when administered on alternate days, is probably an important factor, through its depressant effect on the hypothalamopituitary pulsatile secretion of growth hormone.[37] Some

Table 22.7   Long-term graft survival after living donor and first cadaver transplant

Centre (time period)	Transplants		Graft survival (years)		
			5	10	13
Hanover 1972–83	Total	106	–	–	61%
	Live donor	32			
	Cadaver	74			
Guy's Hospital 1968–87	Total	248	60%	54%	50%
	Live donor	73	80%	72%	–
	Cadaver	175	50%	45%	–
	< 5 years*	37	54%	–	–

*Recipients < 5 years old at time of transplant.

short transplanted children have now been treated with recombinant human growth hormone (see below).

Patient survival and rehabilitation

The survival of children with ESRF continues to improve: 88% of the 3436 children commencing RRT in Europe between 1983 and 1988 were alive 3 years later, compared to 84% of the 2422 children commencing treatment between 1977 and 1982.[3] Long-term survival is also good, with a 14-year actuarial survival of 81% for the 113 children treated in Hanover[34] and a very comparable figure of 79% at 15 years for the 248 children transplanted at Guy's Hospital. The 5-year actuarial survival for children transplanted at Guy's since 1983 has improved to 96%. The survival of young children is also improving: the overall 4-year actuarial survival rate for 44 cadaver transplants in children under 6 years old in Minnesota was 69%, but has improved since the introduction of cyclosporin A to approximately 90%.[31] Similarly at Guy's the 5-year actuarial survival for 37 children aged less than 5 years at transplant, 34 of whom received cadaveric grafts, was 80% but all 6 deaths occurred before the introduction of cyclosporin A in 1983.

Rehabilitation following a successful renal transplant during childhood is in general very good.[38] However, there are young adults, particularly young men, who commenced RRT during childhood who still have problems;[39] they were concerned about their physical appearance, particularly their height and the effect that this had on their social life and on forming lasting relationships with the opposite sex. The challenge now is to try and ensure that the present generation of children with ESRF achieve more complete rehabilitation in adult life.

Recent advances in the management of children with CRF

Recombinant DNA technology has resulted in two important and exciting new therapies for children with CRF.

Recombinant human erythropoietin

rHuEPO has now been used successfully in adults and children with ESRF to correct anae-

mia.[21,22] With rHuEPO therapy, children on chronic dialysis no longer require regular blood transfusions and the risk of blood-borne infection, iron overload and sensitization to HLA histocompatibility antigens are correspondingly reduced. Already established iron overload improves with rHuEPO therapy, while children with low or normal iron stores require iron supplementation to maintain haemopoiesis. HLA antibodies decreased in sensitized children, such that they are able to be retransplanted.[21] Several studies have now reported improved cardiovascular performance and exercise tolerance following correction of anaemia and, although difficult to document objectively, there is little doubt that the quality of life for these children has improved enormously. Fortunately, complications of rHuEPO therapy in children have, with careful monitoring, been relatively few, with a lower incidence of serious hypertension and cerebral events than observed in adults.

Recombinant human growth hormone

Poor growth remains a major problem for some children with CRF, despite optimal conservative management or successful transplantation to restore normal function. Recombinant human growth hormone (rHGH), given in supraphysiological doses, has now been studied in such children with, at least in prepubertal children, encouraging results.[14]

Growth velocity improved significantly in all groups, with the most impressive change in the prepubertal children with pre-TRF: these results have since been confirmed in a controlled trial. Treatment with rHGH also improved the rate of growth in prepubertal children with transplants, although the changes were less dramatic, which is likely to be due to steroid therapy.[37] The results for the pubertal patients are less easy to interpret and least encouraging: again, the central depressant effects of steroid therapy on hypothalamic-pituitary function are probably the cause.[37] The potential side effects of rHGH include possible increase in rate of progression of renal failure due to glomerular hyperfiltration, an increased rate of transplant rejection and effects on carbohydrate metabolism. These are under further investigation. In the meantime, it seems reasonable to offer rHGH therapy to prepubertal children with pre-TRF who are growing poorly, despite optimal conservative management: for children with transplants, particularly those approaching puberty, it is probably as important to reduce the dose of steroids to a minimum and to only prescribe rHGH after very careful consideration of the possible deleterious effects on transplant function.

Conclusions

The prognosis for children with CRF has changed immeasurably over the past 25 years, from almost certain death to, now, a good prospect of long-term survival and rehabilitation. Technical advances have made it possible to offer dialysis and transplantation to almost all children with ESRF, including the very young. However, problems persist particularly in the areas of growth and transplant rejection.

The future must lie with research into means of preventing the congenital and genetically determined causes of CRF; into methods of early detection of CRF in order to prevent growth retardation and perhaps the progression to ESRF; and into more specific methods of immunosuppression.

References

1. Rizzoni G., Ehrich J.H.H., Brunner F.P., Brynger H., Dykes S.R., Geerlings W., Fassbinder W., Tufveson G., Selwood N.H. and Wing A.J. Combined report on Regular Dialysis and Transplantation of Children in Europe, 1988. *Nephrol. Dial. Transplant.* 1989, **4** (Suppl. 4), 31–40
2. Rizzoni G., Broyer M. and Brunner F.P. Combined report on dialysis and transplantation of children in Europe, XIII, 1983. *Proc. EDTA-ERA* 1984, **21**, 69–95
3. Ehrich J.H.H., Rizzoni G., Brunner F.P., Brynger H., Geerlings W., Fassbinder W., Raine A.E.G., Selwood N.H. and Tufveson G. Combined report on Regular Dialysis and Transplantation of Children in Europe, 1989. *Nephrol. Dial. Transplant. 1991*, **6** (Suppl. 1), 37–47
4. Leumann E.P., Die chronische niereninsuffizienz im Kindersalter. *Schweiz. Med. Wschr.* 1976, **106**, 244–250
5. Esbjorner E., Aronson S., Berg U., Fodal U. and Linne T. Children with chronic renal failure in Sweden 1978–1985. *Pediatr. Nephrol.* 1990, **4**, 249–252
6. Brunner F.P., Broyer M., Brynger H., Dykes S.R., Fassbinder W., Geerlings W., Rizzoni G., Selwood N.H., Tufveson G. and Wing A.J. Demography of Dialysis and Transplantation in Children in Europe, 1985. *Nephrol. Dial. Transplant.* 1988, **3**, 235–243
7. Alexander S.R., Arbus G.S., Butt K.M.H., Conley S.,
8. Fine R.N., Greifer I., Gruskin A.B., Harmon W.E., McEnery P.T., Nevins T.E., Nogueira N., Salvatierro O. Jr and Tejani A. The 1989 Report of the North American Pediatric Renal Transplant Cooperative Study. *Pediatr. Nephrol.* 1990, **4**, 542–553
9. Smith D., Egginton J.A., Brookfield D.S.K. Detection of abnormality of fetal urinary tract as a predictor of renal tract disease. *Br. Med. J.* 1987, **294**, 27–28
10. Fitzpatrick M.M., Shah V., Trompeter R.S., Dillon M.J. and Barratt T.M. Long term renal outcome of childhood haemolytic uraemic syndrome *Br. Med. J.* 1991, **303**, 489–492
11. Rees L., Rigden S.P.A., Chantler C., Haycock G.B. Growth and methods of improving growth in chronic renal failure managed conservatively. In: Scharer K. (ed.) *Growth and Endocrine Changes in Children and Adolescents with Chronic Renal Failure. Pediatric and Adolescent Endocrinolology*, Vol. 20. Basel, Karger, 1989: 15–26
12. Barratt T.M., Broyer M., Chantler C., Gilli G., Guest G., Marti-Henneberg C., Preece M.A. and Rigden S.P.A. Assessment of renal function. *Am. J. Kidney Dis.* 1986, **7**, 340–346
13. Rigden S.P.A., Rees L. and Chantler C. Growth and endocrine function in children with chronic renal failure. *Acta Paediatr. Scand.* (Suppl.) 1990, **370**, 20–26
14. Rees L., Rigden S.P.A. and Ward G.M. Chronic renal failure and growth. *Arch. Dis. Child.* 1989, **64**, 573–577
15. Rees L., Rigden S.P.A., Ward G. and Preece M.A. Treatment of short stature in renal disease with recombinant human growth hormone. *Arch. Dis. Child.* 1990, **65**, 856–860
16. Rigden S.P.A., Start K.M. and Rees L. Nutritional management of infants and toddlers with chronic renal failure. *Nutrit. Health* 1987, **51**, 163–174
17. Department of Health. Dietary reference values for food energy and nutrients for the United Kingdom. *Report on Health and Social Subjects 41.* London, H.M. Stationery Office, 1991
18. Clayton B.E., Jenkins P. and Round J.M. *Paediatric Chemical Pathology.* Oxford, Blackwell Scientific, 1980
19. Jureidini K.F., Hogg R.J., van Renen M.J., Southwood T.R., Henning P.H., Cobiac L., Daniels L. and Harris S. Evaluation of long-term aggressive dietary management of chronic renal failure in children. *Pediatr. Nephrol.* 1990, **4**, 1–10
20. Rodriguez-Soriano J., Arant B.S., Brodehl J. and Norman M.E. Fluid and electrolyte imbalances in children with chronic renal failure. *Am. J. Kidney Dis.* 1986, **7**, 268–274
21. Tamanaha K., Mak R.H.K., Rigden S.P.A., Turner C., Start K.M., Haycock G.B. and Chantler C. Long term suppression of hyperparathyroidism by phosphate binders in uremic children. *Pediatr. Nephrol.* 1987, **1**, 145–149.
22. Rigden S.P.A., Montini G., Morris M., Clark K.G.A., Haycock G.B., Chantler C. and Hill R.C. Recombinant human erythropoietin therapy in children maintained by haemodialysis. *Pediatr. Nephrol.* 1990, **4**, 618–622
23. Offner G., Hoyer P.F., Latta K., Winkler L., Brodehl J.

and Scigalla P. One year's experience with recombinant erythropoietin in children undergoing continuous ambulatory or cycling peritoneal dialysis. *Pediatr. Nephrol.* 1990, **4**, 498–500

23. Klahr S., Schreiner G. and Ichikawa I. The progression of renal disease. *N. Engl. J. Med.* 1988, **318**, 1657–1666

24. Rosman J.B., Langer K., Brandl M., Piers-Becht T.Ph.M., van der Hem G.K., ter Wee P.M. and Donker Ab.J.M. Protein-restricted diets in chronic renal failure: a four year follow-up shows limited indications. *Kidney Int.* 1989, **36** (Suppl. 27), S96–S102

25. Wingen A.M., Fabian-Bach C. and Mehls O. for the European Study Group for Nutritional Treatment of Chronic Renal Failure in Childhood. Low-protein diet in children with chronic renal failure – 1-year results. *Pediatr. Nephrol.* 1991, **5**, 496–500

26. Nevin T.E. and Danielson G. Prior dialysis does not affect the outcome of pediatric renal transplantation. *Pediatr. Nephrol.* 1991, **5**, 211–214

27. Bourquelot P., Cussenot O., Corbi P., Pillion G., Gagnadoux M.F., Bensman A., Loirat C. and Broyer M. Microsurgical creation and follow-up of arterio-venous fistulae for chronic haemodialysis in children. *Pediatr. Nephrol.* 1990, **4**, 156–159

28. Neiberger R., Aboushaar M.H., Tawan M., Fennell R., Iravani A. and Richard G. Peritonitis in children on chronic peritoneal dialysis: analysis at 10 years. *Adv. Periton. Dial.* 1991, **7**, 272–274

29. Brownbridge G. and Fielding D.M. Psychosocial adjustment to end-stage renal failure: comparing haemodialysis, continuous ambulatory peritoneal dialysis and transplantation. *Pediatr.Nephrol.* 1991, **51**, 612–616

30. von Lilien T., Gilli G. and Salusky I.B. Growth in children undergoing continuous ambulatory or cycling peritoneal dialysis. In: Scharer K. (ed.) *Growth and Endocrine Changes in Children and Adolescents with Chronic Renal Failure. Pediatric and Adolescent Endocrinology*, Vol. 20. Basel, Karger, 1989: 27–35

31. So S.K.S., Gillingham K., Cook M., Mauer S.M., Matas A., Nevins T.E., Chavers B.M. and Najarian J.S. The use of cadaver kidneys for transplantation in young children. *Transplant.* 1990, **50**, 979–983

32. Salaman J.R. Renal transplantation without steroids. *Paediatr. Nephrol.* 1991, **5**, 105–107

33. Broyer M. and Guest G. Growth after kidney transplantation: a single centre experience. In: Scharer, K. (ed.) *Growth and Endocrine Changes in Children and Adolescents with Chronic Renal Failure. Paediatric and Adolescent Endocrinology*, Vol. 20. Basel, Karger, 1989: 36–45

34. Offner G., Aschendorff C., Hoyer P.F. *et al.* End stage renal failure: 14 years experience of dialysis and renal transplantation. *Arch. Dis. Child.* 1988, **63**, 120–126

35. Cameron J.S. Recurrent primary disease and de novo nephritis following renal transplantation. *Paediatr. Nephrol.* 1991, **5**, 412–421

36. Penn, I. Renal transplantation for Wilms' tumour: report of 20 cases *J. Urol.* 1979, **12**, 793–794

37. Rees L., Greene S.A., Adlard P., Jones J., Haycock G.B. *et al.* Growth and endocrine function after renal transplantation. *Arch. Dis. Child.* 1988, **63**, 1326–1332

38. Reynolds J.M., Garralda M.E., Postlethwaite R.J. and Goh D. Changes in psychosocial adjustment after renal transplantation. *Arch. Dis. Child.* 1991, **66**, 508–513

39. Henning P., Tomlinson L., Rigden S.P.A., Haycock G.B. and Chantler C. Long term outcome of treatment of end stage renal failure. *Arch. Dis. Child.* 1988, **63**, 35–40

23

Inherited kidney disease and genetic counselling

R.J. Postlethwaite, M. Super

Inherited kidney disease

Inherited kidney disease may come to attention in a number of ways. It may present like any other renal disease with various combinations of haematuria, proteinuria, urinary infection, hypertension, oedema and renal failure. Sometimes it is possible to detect it because a suspicion arises that disease in another member of the family may be inherited and study of the family reveals other cases. Sometimes it is found because the individual has a recognizable syndrome, one part of which is a renal abnormality.

It is important not to rely solely on a family history, however careful. The disease may have a varying expressivity, clinically obvious in some members of the family and occult in others. Clinical examination of family members, particularly blood pressure measurement and urinalysis, are important and ultrasound examination of the kidneys of relatives is often useful. One should be aware that the age of onset of the condition (as well as its severity) may be variable and absence of detectable disease in a child may not exclude its appearance later. Finally, just as 'all that glisters is not gold' neither is every reported instance of renal disease in a family bound to be relevant. Renal calculi in one member of the family, may or may not have relevance to the renal failure in another; detailed information of the type of renal disease in other family members must be obtained before assuming its relevance. Moreover, clinically or pathologically similar conditions may exhibit different modes of inheritance and each family may need to be individually studied before genetic counselling is possible.

Advances in molecular biology are at last beginning to shed light on the location of some of the genes associated with inherited kidney disease. This and the ultimate identification of the genes themselves should enormously increase our understanding of this important group of conditions.

Genetic counselling

The philosophy of genetic counselling in renal disease differs in no way from other system disorders, but the successful management of end-stage renal failure by dialysis and transplantation now allows for treatment possibilities to be discussed in greater detail, influencing resulting decisions. However, too few families do receive genetic counselling, perhaps because of the emphasis devoted to treatment. In counselling a family with renal disease, the diagnosis, severity, variability of expression, therapeutic options and possible availability of prenatal diagnosis need to be discussed, with the risk of recurrence.

Registers of families in which renal disease is segregating have important functions: (a) to allow surveillance, prevention, early diagnosis and treatment of renal damage, and (b) to ensure that genetic counselling can indeed occur.

Registers also facilitate the application of new molecular genetic techniques. Dominant polycystic kidney disease is a good example of this and is discussed in detail below.

Prenatal diagnosis

Due to the fact that very few of the gene loci associated with kidney disease have been accurately plotted, prenatal diagnosis is mostly limited at present to those conditions detectable either by prenatal ultrasound or by an increased concentration of alpha-fetoprotein (the fetal precursor of albumin) in maternal serum or amniotic fluid. During ultrasound screening in pregnancy as one is examining the kidneys, it is important to note the presence and size of the bladder. The presence of urine allows one to exclude bilateral renal agenesis and a large bladder may suggest a diagnosis of urethral obstruction.

As gene loci are discovered, prenatal diagnosis by DNA will become feasible, including much earlier testing in pregnancy, e.g. by chorionic villus biopsy.

Take-up of prenatal diagnosis with the option of termination is directly proportional to the severity of the burden imposed by the disease, the magnitude of the recurrence risk and the staging of tests in pregnancy.[1] When intragenic or closely linked extragenic probes exist, then diagnosis in DNA extracted from chorionic villi taken at 9 weeks of pregnancy becomes feasible. Introduction of techniques such as polymerase chain reaction allow rapid analysis, with results available after a few days. The rapid progress in the development of tests in Duchenne and Becker's[2] muscular dystrophy and cystic fibrosis,[3,4] shows just how quickly such advances can become part of clinical practice.

Progress in inherited kidney disease

The powerful tool of positional cloning (formally termed reverse genetics) by studying families with more than one affected individual can identify genetic markers which allow for chromosomal localization of the specific disorders. What one searches for is a polymorphic marker which gives consistent results within a family.[5] First one discovers the location of the gene before its product. This approach has been used most extensively in dominant polycystic kidney disease in which it localized the gene to the short arm of chromosome 16, very near the alpha-globin locus. In the study of large families with many affected individuals, linkage to chromosome 16 markers can be established and odds of 97% or 3% of having the gene can be given, depending on whether the polymorphism travelling with the gene has been inherited or not. The figures of 97% and 3% reflect the distance of hypervariable DNA markers (from within the alpha-globin locus) from the DPKD locus and reflect the chances of a meiotic crossover. The gene itself has not yet been identified. Some families do not show linkage with the alpha-globin locus[6] and in some of these it has been shown that the gene is probably on chromosome 2.

Tuberous sclerosis (TS) has suffered a similar fate, with linkage to both ABO groups and the oncogene Vi-abel on chromosome 9,[7] shown in some families, but with others showing chromosome 11 linkage,[8] with yet others showing linkage to neither. Very recently a locus for tuberous sclerosis has been found on chromosome 16 very near the DPKD locus.[9] This is very interesting, for sometimes children with TS have been born with clinical features of DPKD.

In nephrogenic diabetes insipidus, in an elegant series of studies it has been shown that (a) the condition is a generalized disorder of v2 receptors, (b) the gene for v2 receptors co-localizes with the nephrogenic diabetes insipidus gene, and (c) both these genes are located between the markers DXS52 and factor VIII close to the end of the long arm of the X chromosome.[10] These studies show that the region within which the NDI gene is located is at most four megabase pairs long making it amenable to reverse positional cloning, which should eventually result in the gene itself being cloned.

The gene for hypophosphataemic rickets has been localized to Xp22.[11]

Gene linkage allows for presymptomatic even antenatal diagnosis in informative families. It is of no use in the isolated case. Depending on the closeness of the flanking markers, there is an inevitable error in the accuracy of prediction (in both ways). It is also quite clear that different genetic defects may give the same or similar phenotypic disease.

One of the earlier accurate localisations was of the gene for nail-patella syndrome to the long arm of chromosome 9 about 10 centimorgans from the ABO blood group locus. This can be used within a family to make a preclinical even prenatal diagnosis (Figure 23.1). This diagnosis would have an error of 10% in both directions because of the distance between the

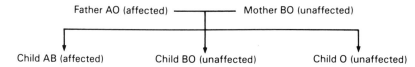

Figure 23.1 ABO blood group linkage in nail-patella syndrome

ABO and nail-patella gene. Nail-patella syndrome occurs both with and without chronic renal failure and is phenotypically consistent in any one family. When the actual gene is eventually localized it might very well show a different mutation in those families with and without renal disease.

The potential for pre-symptomatic diagnosis has created a dilemma best exemplified by DPKD. How soon in childhood does one need to know if the gene for DPKD which usually presents in adulthood has been inherited? Some people take the view that as no therapy is available the diagnosis should be delayed until the individual is considering having a family. It is also felt that the stigmatization of having a condition would adversely affect the child. Intuitively we have always felt that an accurate early diagnosis is helpful for the family; the parents are relieved to know with some degree of certainty that some of the children are not affected. Recent surveys have supported this view, with the majority of families favouring pre-symptomatic diagnosis while feeling it would not alter their management.[12] This is an important problem, with financial and humanitarian consequences. It needs careful study to confirm the correct approach.

With the identification of the gene, even more possibilities open up. In Alport's syndrome, where the gene is located to the X chromosome (Xq21.2 - q22.2),[13] it is hypothesized that the basic genetic defect lies in the gene for the $\alpha5$ chain of type IV collagen and as a consequence of this defect $\alpha3$ and $\alpha4$ chains of type IV collagen are not incorporated in the basement membrane. The gene is a large one and already at least 36 mutations have been described, ranging from single base substitution through to deletion of the whole gene. This should allow for more accurate diagnosis, diagnosis in families without a family history, understanding of the basic defect and explanation of phenotypic variations. This might have therapeutic implications. For example, a small number of patients with Alport's syndrome develop Goodpasture's syndrome after renal transplantation. This is because the Goodpasture antigen is absent in the kidney of a patient with Alport's syndrome. It might be that patients with a major deletion of the gene as opposed to less severe alterations such as point mutations are the ones likely to have this problem.

Thus far the gene for autosomal recessive polycystic kidney disease has not been localized, but 70% of the genome including chromosome 16 has been excluded.

Isolated renal malformations and renal involvement in malformation syndromes

Cystic dysplasia is usually sporadic and often associated with urinary tract obstruction. It may also be part of an inherited syndrome. Familial cases have additionally been observed. The empirical recurrence risks for close relatives of an isolated case with bilateral involvement is about 5%. It is extremely low in relatives of unilateral cases.

Isolated renal malformations

Bilateral renal agenesis is commonly a sporadic condition (possibly a lethal new dominant mutation), but occasional reports of autosomal dominant inheritance have been reported in which one parent had unilateral renal aplasia or hypoplasia. Renal hypoplasia, dysplasia, ectopia and fusion have occasionally been reported as familial and are not uncommon in association with various malformation syndromes; when present as an isolated abnormality, however, they are usually sporadic. Hydronephrosis is occasionally familial.

The most important inherited isolated malformation is vesico-ureteric reflux, although even here the majority of cases are not inherited. The incidence of vesico-ureteric reflux among siblings (symptomatic and/or asymptomatic) of children with vesico-ureteric reflux has been reported to be 8–52%.[14,15] The mode of inheritance is not agreed, but the most commonly

Table 23.1 Renal malformations in conditions lethal in the fetus or newborn

Syndrome	Renal malformation	Comment
Trisomy 13 or 18	Cystic kidneys	
Triploidy	Cystic dysplasia	
45 XO Turner's	Horseshoe	
Meckel–Grueber	Cystic dysplasia	Autosomal recessive
Chondrodysplasia punctata (rhizomelic type)	'Micromulticystic'	Autosomal recessive
Asphyxiating thoracodystrophy (not invariably lethal)	Mesangial thickening + sclerosis glomeruli	Autosomal recessive
Majewski short rib polydactyly	Cystic dysplasia	Autosomal recessive
Roberts	Horseshoe and cystic	Autosomal recessive
Saldino–Noonan short rib	Cystic dysplasia	Autosomal recessive
Thanatophoric dysplasia	Hydronephrosis	Sporadic (occ. autosomal recessive)

Table 23.2 Major renal abnormalities in Possum Database

Abnormality	No. of syndromes
Agenesis/hypoplasia	105
Normal large kidneys	3
Dysplastic/cystic dysplastic kidneys	80
Polycystic kidneys	25
Ureteric abnormalities (reflux/hydronephrosis)	66
Horseshoe/fused/ectopic kidney	50
Renal tubular defects	21
Renal failure/nephritis	67
Bladder abnormalities	35
Urethral abnormalities	22
Renal stones	10
Other urinary tract defects	43

accepted view is that it is an autosomal dominant gene with incomplete penetrance. Detection of asymptomatic individuals should allow for prevention of renal damage. Thus screening is recommended, but there is no agreement as to whether radionucleide cystography, direct or indirect, ultrasound or DMSA scan is the preferred investigations. We currently offer ultrasound and cystography to children under the age of 2 years and DMSA and ultrasound in older children. It is particularly important to screen newborn babies born into families with either a parent or sibling with a reflux.

In all these isolated malformations, ultrasound scan (and possibly other investigations) of the parents is recommended.

Renal involvement in malformation syndromes

In many of the chromosomal trisomy and deletion syndromes, renal malformations are an occasional feature; horseshoe kidneys, hydronephrosis reduplication and hypoplasia are some of the commoner findings. Renal lesions are especially common in Turner's syndrome and duplication of the short arm of chromosome 10. Also of special interest is the interstitial deletion of the short arm of chromosome 11 which leads to the aniridia–Wilms' tumour complex. In a number of conditions (Table 23.1), renal malformations are associated with chromosomal or genetic aberrations which are lethal in intrauterine or early neonatal life. These have been grouped together in a table because identification of the condition will often depend on accurate examination of the fetus or infant; while this has no relevance to the affected individual, it may be a most important step in the identification of a syndrome with vital connotations for the family.

An increasingly bewildering array of syndromes are described with renal involvement. These syndromes may or may not be inherited. Classification and identification of the syndromes is enormously helped by the use of a computer database such as the Possum Database. This lists over 300 syndromes in which renal involvement may occur, listed under 12 main headings (Table 23.2). This classification is pragmatic and necessarily eclectic and over-inclusive. In consequence there is much overlap between the different categories and imprecise terminology is accepted. There is, for example, much overlap between agenesis/hypoplasia, dysplastic/cystic dysplastic kidneys and polycystic kidneys and the latter term which should be confined to two specific entities (see Chapter 25) is used to encompass virtually any multiple cystic lesion of the kidney. Interrogation of the database also reveals considerable overlap between reflux/hydronephrosis, and hypoplasia/

agenesis, possibly hinting at shared mechanisms. Reflux excludes isolated familial reflux.

This or similar databases can be used in a variety of ways:

- In the presence of a recognized syndrome it can be established if a renal component is likely and appropriate investigation and/or monitoring organized.
- Given a set cluster of signs including renal abnormality, the possibility of a previously described syndrome can be explored.
- Presented with an isolated renal anomaly, the possibility that this might be a feature of an otherwise silent syndrome can be investigated.

A number of physical signs are associated with an increased risk of abnormalities and should prompt appropriate investigation for renal association usually by way of ultrasound, but again the appropriate investigations could be directed by interrogation of the database for likely associations. These associations have been discussed extensively in Chapter 7.

Fetal exposure to troxidone, thalidomide and phenytoin are occasionally associated with renal malformations; doubtless other maternally-ingested drugs will also be implicated in time.

Alport's syndrome and familial nephritis

Alport's syndrome and familial nephritis are not synonymous, indeed Alport's syndrome is one type, albeit the pre-eminent type, of familial nephritis. Further confusion arises because many patients do not meet all the criteria. Much light should be shed on this by the new genetic advances.

Alport's syndrome

Alport's syndrome is an hereditary disease characterized by haematuria, progressive renal failure, deafness, ocular malformations and typical ultrastructural abnormalities of the glomerular basement membrane. The gene for Alport's syndrome has been localized to the short arm of the X chromosome (see above).

Diagnostic criteria

The diagnosis of Alport's syndrome should be restricted to families fulfilling three of the following four criteria:[16,17]

1 *Positive family history of haematuria, with or without progressive renal failure.* The development of renal failure is less common in females.
2 *Electron microscopic evidence on renal biopsy of Alport's syndrome.* On light microscopy the findings include fetal-looking glomeruli, attenuation of glomerular basement membrane, reduction in size of capillary loops, infiltration with lymphocytes and plasma cells with clusters of foam cells, glomerular segmental sclerosis and obsolescence, tubular atrophy and interstitial fibrosis. These changes are non-specific, but some (e.g. foam cells) are suggestive of Alport's syndrome. Immunofluorescence is unhelpful.

   The characteristic changes are found on electron microscopy. The lamina densa of the basement membrane is seen to vary considerably in thickness; in some areas it is very thin and in others it is broadened and laminated, often showing a latticework appearance which has been likened to a 'basket weave' (Figure 23.2). In the interstices of this lattice may be found electron-lucent areas sometimes containing specks of denser material. These changes are almost pathognomonic of Alport's syndrome.[18]
3 *Progressive high tone sensorineural* – this usually becomes apparent around the end of the first decade; it is often progressive during childhood but tends to be stable in adulthood. Audiometry may be necessary to demonstrate clinically inapparent hearing loss.[19]
4 *Characteristic eye changes* – bilateral anterior lenticonus is the commonest lesion and is thought to be diagnostic.[20] Posterior lenticonus is seen less commonly. Various lens abnormalities have been described, none of which is specific to Alport's syndrome. Macular flecks and peripheral flecks are characteristic of Alport's syndrome but these are rarely seen in childhood clinical features.

In childhood, the disease characteristically runs a silent course. Microscopic haematuria and proteinuria are usually found in affected family members within a few years of birth – but not necessarily in the first one or two. There is progressive renal sclerosis in the males but in the female, although urinary abnormalities are usually detectable, the disease often does not progress to renal failure; inter-family variations are very important in this respect

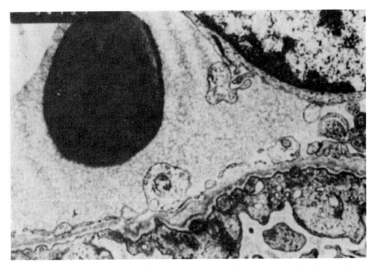

Figure 23.2 Electron micrograph of basement membrane in Alport's syndrome showing latticework appearance which has been likened to a 'basket weave'

however. In the male, by the late teens or twenties as the sclerosis proceeds, proteinuria becomes heavier, and hypertension and renal failure appear. Sometimes the proteinuria becomes so heavy as to cause hypoalbuminaemia and a nephrotic syndrome (which may rarely be the presenting feature), but in any event the male patients gradually progress to end-stage renal failure.

The deafness may ultimately be quite profound, again especially in the males. Ocular abnormalities may need attention, but bulk less obviously among the patient's problems. It is wise carefully to assess the hearing of all children with any type of inherited nephritis; it is often a more important problem in childhood than their renal disease.

Renal transplantation and dialysis are ultimately possible for most patients but no means of halting, or even delaying, the progress to renal failure are known. Of course, there are a number of effective supportive measures available for treating chronic renal failure and its complications, so regular supervision of pre-symptomatic patients is needed to ensure that they are started promptly. The rare occurrence of Goodpasture's syndrome after renal transplantation has already been discussed.

Thin glomerular basement membrane disease

In children with recurrent haematuria syndrome, the only finding on renal biopsy might be the diffuse attenuation of the basement membrane.[21] There are a number of possible explanations for this:

- A biopsy done early in the course of classical Alport's syndrome may only show this abnormality. Others members of the family should show typical changes.
- Some families with a pedigree of haematuria/ progressive renal failure with or without deafness only show this abnormality.[22] They should be considered to have a variant of Alport's syndrome rather than a typical Alport's syndrome.
- Some families show numerous members with haematuria, but no evidence of renal failure.[23] This is the condition of familial benign haematuria.
- In the absence of a family history it is not possible to assign any individual child to any of the above (or other) categories.

Other forms of familial nephritis

In addition to X-linked inheritance in classical Alport's syndrome, autosomal dominant and more rarely recessive variants may occur and in these variants families may be severely affected.

A number of other conditions have been associated with the familial nephritis, but without sufficient definition of the renal lesion to know whether it exhibits the basement membrane changes now believed to be a hallmark of (even if not exclusive to) Alport's syndrome.

Macrothrombocytopenia

This condition, in which platelets are few but about the same size as red blood cells, has been reported in a handful of families associated with sensorineural deafness and a progressive familial nephritis leading to end-stage renal failure.[24] Thrombocytopenia has usually produced only minor difficulties with haemorrhagic problems. The disease seems to be transmitted in a dominant fashion, although there are insufficient cases to decide if it is X-linkage or autosomal dominant.

Hyperprolinaemia

This has been one of the more common associations with clinically typical Alport's syndrome. However, it is possible that the two conditions are inherited separately and there are conflicting reports about the character of the histological changes; at least one case reported to show the typical renal changes of Alport's syndrome, but was reported not to exhibit the basement membrane abnormalities.

A small number of other associations have been reported, but there is no clear evidence that renal disease is, or is not, the same as Alport's syndrome; they include ichthyosis polyneuropathy and Charcot–Marie–Tooth disease among other.[25] Nail-patella syndrome used to be included in this category, but it is now quite clear that this is a genetically and morphologically distinct condition syndrome; one suspects at least some of the other Alport's 'variants' may in time follow the same path but this is currently speculative.

Isolated basement membrane nephropathy

One-third of children biopsied for recurrent haematuria syndrome show Alport-like changes or, less commonly, thin basement membrane disease. It is not clear if these represent new mutations estimated to cause 18% of cases, or some totally unrelated renal disease. The fact that some of these develop deafness, and progression to renal failure occurs both without but more commonly with deafness, reinforces the idea that these children have Alport's syndrome. Almost inevitably, however, the group

is going to turn out to be heterogeneous and it is likely that the problem will be more rapidly elucidated by gene probes than long-term clinical studies.

References

1. Thornton J.G. Decision analysis in prenatal diagnosis. In: Lilford R.J. (ed.) *Measuring Patients' Values in Prenatal Diagnosis*. London, Butterworths, 1990
2. Roberts R.G., Bentley D.R., Barby T.F.M. *et al.* Direct diagnosis of Duchenne and Becker muscular dystrophy by amplification of lymphocyte RNA. *Lancet* 1990, **336**, 1523–1526
3. White R., Woodward S., Lepport M. *et al.* A closely linked marker for cystic fibrosis. *Nature* 1985, **318**, 382–384
4. Super M., Ivinson A., Schwarz M.J. *et al.* Clinical experience: prenatal diagnosis of cystic fibrosis. *Lancet* 1987, **ii**, 782–784
5. Knepelman B., Antignac C., Subler M.C., Grünfeld J.P. A molecular approach to inherited kidney disorders. *Kid. Inf.* 1993, **44**, 1205–1216
6. Romeo G., Devoto M., Costa G. *et al.* A second genetic locus for autosomal dominant polycystic kidney disease. *Lancet* 1988, **ii**, 8–11
7. Fryer A.E., Connor J.M., Povey J. *et al.* Evidence that the gene for tuberous sclerosis is on chromosome 9. *Lancet* 1987, **i**, 659–661
8. Smith M.S., Smalley R., Cantor M. *et al.* Mapping of a gene determining tuberous sclerosis to human chromosome 11q 22–23. *Genemics* 1990, **6**, 105–114
9. The European chromosome 16 tuberous sclerosis consortium. Identification of the tuberous sclerosis gene. *Cell* 1993, **75**, 1305–1315
10. Omueland A.M.W., Dreesen T.C.F., Verdyte M. *et al.* Mutations in the vasopressin type 2 receptor gene ($AVPR_2$) associated with nephrogenic diabetes insipidus. *Nature Genet.* 1992, **2**, 99–102
11. Kainer G., Spence J.E. and Chan J.C.M. X-linked hypophosphataemia, progress in characterisation of genetic and metabolic defects. *Nephron* 1989, **51**, 449–453
12. Gabow P.A. Genetic counselling in ESRD patients with polycystic kidney disease. *Semi Dialysis* 1991, **4**, 2–9
13. Tryggvason K., Zhou J., Hostikka, S.C. and Shows T.B. Molecular genetics of Alport Syndrome. *Kid. Int.* 1993, **43**, 38–44
14. Van der Abbelle A.D., Treves S.T., Lebowitz R.L. *et al.* Vesicoureteral reflux in asymptomatic siblings of patients with known reflux. Radionuclide cystography. *Pediatrics* 1987, **79**, 147–152
15. Aggarwal V.K. and Verrier-Jones K. Vesicoureteric reflux: screening of the first degree relatives. *Arch. Dis. Child.* 1989, **64**, 1538–1541
16. Schroder C.H., Brunner H. and Monnens L.A.H. Genetic features of Alport's syndrome. *Contrib. Nephrol.* 1990, **80**, 3–8

17. Flinter F.A., Bobrow M. and Chantler C. Alport's syndrome or hereditary nephritis. *Pediatr. Nephrol.* 1987, **1**, 438–440

18. Rumplet H.J. Alport's syndrome: specificity and pathogenesis of glomerular basement membrane alterations. *Pediatr. Nephrol.* 1987, **1**, 422–427

19. Grunfeld J.P. The clinical spectrum of hereditary nephritis. *Kidney Int.* 1985, **27**, 83–92

20. Govan J.A.A. Ocular manifestations of Alport's syndrome: a hereditary disorder of basement membrane. *Br. J. Opthalmol.* 1983, **67**, 493–503

21. Gubler M.C., Beaufils H., Noel L.H. and Habib R. Significance of thin glomerular basement membranes in hematuric children. *Contrib. Nephrol.* 1990, **80**, 147–156

22. Habib R., Gubler M.C., Hinglais N. *et al.* Alport's syndrome. Experience at Hôpital Necker. *Kidney Int.* 1982, **21**, 520–528

23. Gauthier B., Trachtmon H., Frank R. and Valderrama E. Familial thin basement membrane nephropathy in children with asymptomatic microhematuria. *Nephron* 1989, **51**, 502–508

24. Parsa K.P., Lee D.B.N., Zamboni L. and Glassock R.J. Hereditary nephritis, deafness and abnormal thrombopoiesis. *Am. J. Med.* 1976, **60**, 665–668

25. Bernstein J. Hereditary renal disease. In: Churg J. *et al.* (eds) *Kidney Disease Present Status.* IAP Monograph No. 20. Baltimore, William and Wilkins, 1979: 295–315

24

Renal tubular disorders

J. Brodehl

Introduction

Electrolytes, inorganic and organic substances are reabsorbed from or secreted into the primary urine by tubular cells. These tubular functions are specific, mostly active and genetically controlled transport mechanisms. Disturbances of a single function are mostly congenital and inherited and, therefore, called 'primary tubulopathies'. Complex tubular disturbances involving more than one tubular system arise from generalized tubulopathies or extrarenal metabolic disorders. These can be congenital or acquired and are called 'secondary or symptomatic tubulopathies'.

Tubular dysfunction can lead to three different kinds of pathophysiological disturbances: (a) a derangement of the internal homeostasis by loss of an essential substance such as phosphate, bicarbonate or water, (2) pathological composition of the urine leading to supersaturation, as in cystinuria or hypercalciuria, and (c) alteration of renal parenchyma, as in nephrocalcinosis. Many tubulopathies, however, are non-diseases because neither homeostasis nor urinary composition nor renal parenchyma are pathologically affected. They, then, serve only biochemical, physiological, molecular biological and genetic interests.

Clinical signs of tubulopathies will only appear as long as glomerular filtration rate is high enough, to produce a quantitative net loss of a substance. In the case of global renal insufficiency which is often accompanied by tubular disturbances, signs of tubular dysfunction become clinically irrelevant. A list of the most frequent primary and secondary tubulopathies and their treatment approaches are shown in Tables 24.1 and 24.2, respectively.

Disturbances of tubular phosphate reabsorption

The renal handling of phosphate is best described by the maximum tubular phosphate reabsorption corrected by glomerular filtration rate (TmP/GFR). Direct measurement of this by phosphate loading and simultaneous GFR measurement is too cumbersome for routine practice in children. It can be estimated by the determination of phosphate and creatinine in a fasting blood sample and simultaneously obtained urine sample using the formula:[1]

$$TmP/GFR = PlPO_4 - \frac{[UPO_4 \times [PlCr]}{[UCr]}$$

where $PlPO_4$ = plasma phosphate, UPO_4 = urinary phosphate, $PlCr$ = plasma creatinine, and UCr = urinary creatinine.

The nomogram by Walton and Bijvoet,[2] which is widely used, overestimates the values in non-phosphate-loaded children and is, therefore, not recommended.

Table 24.1   Primary tubulopathies and their therapeutic approach

Phosphate reabsorption
    Familial hypophosphataemic rickets (C)
    Pseudohypoparathyroidism, types I and II (C)
Glucose reabsorption
    Renal glucosuria, types A, B, O (A)
    Renal glucosuria in congenital glucose-galactose
      malabsorption (B)
Amino acid reabsorption
    Hyperglycinuria (A)
    Hyperhistidinuria (A)
    Hypercystinuria (A)
    Iminoglycinuria (A)
    Hyperdibasicaminoaciduria (A)
    Classical cystinuria (C)
    Hyperdicarboxylaminoaciduria (A)
    Hartnup disease (C)
Bicarbonate reabsorption
    Proximal tubular acidosis (C)
Uric acid reabsorption and secretion
    Renal hypouricaemia (A)
    Renal hyperuricaemia (B)
H-ion secretion
    Distal tubular acidosis (C)
Electrolyte reabsorption and secretion
    Pseudohypoaldosteronism (C)
    Renal hypomagnesaemia (B)
    Bartter's syndrome (C)
    Idiopathic hypercalciuria (B)
    Hyperkalaemia with acidosis (B)
Water reabsorption
    Nephrogenic diabetes insipidus (C)
Endocrine tubulofunction
    Vitamin-D-dependent rickets (B)
Complex tubulofunction
    Glucophosphate diabetes (B)
    Glucoglycinuria (A)
    Glucoglycin-phosphate diabetes (B)
    Idiopathic renal Fanconi's syndrome (C)

(A), no treatment necessary; (B), symptomatic treatment;
(C), treatment as described in the text.

Table 24.2   Secondary (complex) tubulopathies and their therapeutic approach

In inborn errors of metabolism
Galactosaemia (G-1-P-uridyltransferase def.) (A)
Fructose intolerance (F-1-P aldolase B def.) (A)
Tyrosinaemia, type I (fumaryl-acetoacetate-hydrolase def.) (B)
Cystinosis (C)
Lowe's syndrome (B)
Wilson's disease (A)
Glycogenosis with Fanconi's syndrome (B)

In acquired diseases
Nephrotic syndrome (A)
Multiple myeloma (A)
Vitamin D deficiency (A)
Hypercalcaemia (A)
Hypokalaemia (A)

In intoxications
Heavy metals (A)
Drugs (A)
Vitamin D (A)

A, treatment of underlying disease; B, symptomatic treatment; C, treatment as described in the text.

increased urinary ethanolamine) and other forms of rickets.

Treatment of hypophosphataemic rickets aims to increase the extracellular phosphate concentration continuously, by which bone mineralization should be improved and growth retardation prevented or ameliorated. Children, therefore, should receive as early as possible neutral phosphates (Phosphate Sandoz) in a daily dose of 50–100 mg/kg body weight, given in 5 divided doses every 4–6 h during day and night time. In addition, cholecalciferol (Rocaltrol) is given in a starting dose of 25–50 ng kg^{-1} day^{-1} in order to increase the intestinal calcium and phosphate resorption and by this to prevent secondary hyperparathyroidism which should appear after phosphate loading. This treatment is able to heal rickety bone disease and to improve growth rates.[3] It must be monitored strictly in order to prevent side effects such as hypercalciuria, hypercalcaemia, hyperoxaluria (as the consequence of intestinal hyperresorption of oxalic acids[4]) and nephrocalcinosis. Urinary calcium excretion should not exceed 0.1 mmol kg^{-1} day^{-1} or calcium:creatinine ratio (mmol:mmol) 0.6; serum calcium should not surpass 2.75 mmol/litre and urinary oxalic acid excretion 0.6 mmol 1.73 m^{-2} day^{-1} or oxalic acid:creatinine ratio (mmol/mol) 268.

Hypophosphataemic vitamin-D-resistant rickets

The initial evaluation of hypophosphataemic rickets has been discussed in Chapter 5. For differential diagnosis, other forms of vitamin-D-resistant rickets have to be excluded as vitamin D dependency type I (low calcium and phosphorus, hyperparathyroidism and hyperaminoaciduria), vitamin D dependency type II (receptor resistance with signs as type I plus alopecia), renal osteodystrophy (elevated phosphorus, low calcium, hyperparathyroidism), hypophosphatasia (normal calcium and phosphorus, low alkaline phosphatase,

Pseudohypoparathyroidism

Pseudohypoparathyroidism describes a group of disturbances characterized by an end-organ resistance to the action of parathyroid hormone.[5] Resistance to parathormone could be identified at different levels of hormone–effector interaction[6] and is not only expressed in the renal tubules, but variably in the skeletal system and many other organs also. This explains the wide variations of clinical expressions of the diseases described as pseudohypoparathyroidism, pseudo-pseudohypoparathyroidism and Albright's osteodystrophy. Besides disturbances in calcium and phosphate metabolism, there are constitutional changes such as round facies, stunted growth, obesity, brachymetacarpaly, cataracts, soft-tissue and basal ganglia calcification and mental retardation. Diseases are mostly familial with different modes of genetic transmission (autosomal dominant, X-linked or recessive).

Diagnosis is confirmed by characteristic laboratory findings, i.e. low serum calcium, high serum phosphate and parathormone, normal renal function with high values of TmP/GFR, and renal resistance to the phosphaturic effect of exogenous parathormone. By determination of urinary cyclic AMP, two types can be differentiated: no increase of cAMP excretion after PTH application is type I, while normal increase of cAMP without phosphaturia is characteristic of type II. Determination of G protein in erythrocyte membranes allows a further differentiation of the disease entity in types Ia and Ib. G-protein is present in all cells. The G-protein signalling unit mediates the response of other hormones and this probably explains associated problems such as hypothyroidism and hypogonadism.

Treatment of pseudohypoparathyroidism is in general similar to the treatment of hypoparathyroidism. The serum calcium should be maintained in the low normal range, which is achieved with vitamin D or cholecalciferol. Starting dose is 10 000 iu vitamin D or 0.25 μg cholecalciferol, with an increase as required to achieve low normal serum Ca. By this, serum phosphorus is usually lowered to the normal range. Only rarely is it necessary to use additionally phosphate binders such as calcium carbonate. Therapy must be monitored carefully in order to avoid under- or overtreatment.

Renal glucosuria

Normally urine contains a slight amount of glucose which is less than 0.8 mmol/l. This amount is called *basal* glucosuria[7] and cannot be detected by strip tests, which require a concentration of more than 2.2 mmol/l, but only by enzymatic methods. The normal urinary excretion rates of glucose are 3.6–16.7 mmol 1.73 m^{-2} day^{-1}, with relatively higher amounts in newborns and premature infants.

Frank glucosuria (or hyperglucosuria) is defined as an excretion of glucose in amounts that exceed the upper limit of basal glucosuria. This is caused by a disturbance of active tubular glucose reabsorption. The diagnosis of primary renal glucosuria excludes glucosurias associated with other tubular defects such as Fanconi's syndrome, or renal insufficiency. Clinically there are two types of primary glucosuria: one is the pure renal type (so-called benign familial glucosuria), and the other is associated with an intestinal defect of glucose–galactose absorption (so-called congenital glucose–galactose malabsorption).

Benign renal glucosuria is a familial condition not associated with an intestinal defect or other tubular disturbances. It is inherited as an autosomal dominant or recessive trait. The daily urinary excretion rates are in the range 0.01–0.17 mmol, but occasionally may approach 0.56 mol. There are usually no signs of hypoglycaemia, ketosis, polyuria or polydipsia and, therefore, no therapy is required. The condition, however, must be diagnosed properly, in order to avoid iatrogenic mismanagement for assumed diabetes mellitus.

Renal function studies are generally not required, unless there is special interest in the pathophysiology and genetics. These include glucose titration studies with simultaneous measurement of glomerular filtration rate. By this, different types of renal glucosuria can be detected:[7] type A, with a low glucose threshold (T_G/GFR) and low maximal glucose reabsorption (Tm_G); type B, with a low threshold but a normal maximal reabsorption; and type O in which tubular glucose reabsorption is completely absent, i.e. threshold and maximal glucose reabsorption are not measurable.[8] In congenital glucose–galactose malabsorption, the renal defect is only mild and characterized by an exaggerated splay.[9]

Table 24.3 Types of hyperaminoacidurias

Prerenal hyperaminoaciduria
(due to extrarenal metabolic defect)
    Pure overflow h. (e.g. phenylketonuria)
    Competitive h. (e.g. hyperargininaemia)
    Non-threshold h. (e.g. cystathioninuria)
Renal hyperaminoaciduria
(due to tubular defect)
    Specific h.
        Individual-specific transport system
        involved (e.g. hypercystinuria)
        Group-specific transport system involved
        (e.g. classical cystinuria)
    Generalized h. (due to metabolic cell injury)
    (e.g. renal Fanconi's syndrome)

Hyperaminoacidurias

Amino acids are filtered freely through the glomerular basement membrane and subsequently reabsorbed by active processes. Tubular reabsorption is so effective that 98–99%, of the filtered amino acids are retrieved with a urinary loss of only 1–2%, which is called the physiological aminoaciduria. Any aminoaciduria larger than this amount is labelled hyperaminoaciduria.

Every amino acid detected in the blood is found in the urine; however, the pattern of amino acids is quite different in the two fluids. This is due to the fact that individual amino acids are handled specifically by the tubular cells, independent of their plasma concentration. The degree of reabsorption ranges from $92.8 \pm 1.8\%$ (for histidine) to $99.8 \pm 0.1\%$ (for valine) in healthy children and adults, with lower values in early infancy.[10]

The first step in the evaluation of the renal handling of amino acids is the measurement of free amino acids by screening or semi-quantitative methods such as thin-layer chromatography. If hyperaminoaciduria is suspected, urine should be examined by more accurate methods such as column-chromatography or gas-chromatography. The most sensitive parameter of tubular amino acid handling is the percentage tubular amino acid reabsorption, since it is almost independent of the tubular load. It can be estimated by measuring creatinine and amino acids in a spontaneously voided urine and simultaneously drawn blood specimen and by using the formula

$$\% \, TAA = 100 \left(1 - \frac{UAA \times PCr}{UCre \times PAA} \right)$$

where UAA and PAA are the amino acid concentration in urine and plasma, and UCre and PCre are creatinine concentrations in urine and plasma.

Types of hyperaminoacidurias

Hyperaminoaciduria is caused either by an increment of filtered load due to an overproduction or defective catabolism in the organism (= *prerenal* hyperaminoaciduria), or by a defective tubular reabsorption while filtered amounts of amino acids are normal (= *renal* hyperaminoaciduria) (Table 24.3). In the first type the defect is located outside the kidney, reflecting a systemic metabolic derangement. Recognition of prerenal hyperaminoaciduria with corresponding increased blood level establishes the metabolic diagnosis and will not be further considered here. It should only be realized that prerenal hyperaminoaciduria is expressed in three different categories depending on the mechanism of tubular transport of the involved amino acid:[11] (a) a pure 'overflow' hyperaminoaciduria without any additional tubular competition for resorptive sides (as in phenylketonuria with phenylalanine); (b) an overflow hyperaminoaciduria with additional competition in the resorption of related amino acids ('competitive' hyperaminoaciduria, as in hyperargininaemia with cystine-lysine-ornithine-argininuria); (c) a 'non-threshold' hyperaminoaciduria of amino acids with poor or no tubular resorption and absence of elevated plasma levels (as in cystathioninuria).

The renal hyperaminoaciduria reflects a tubular defect in the kidney which can involve either a specific tubular transport system at the tubular membranes, or a general tubular cell injury leading to defective cell metabolism. The defects in specific hyperaminoaciduria may involve either an individual-specific transport carrier or a group-specific transport system (see Table 24.1). The specific tubular hyperaminoaciduria is characterized by a constant and distinct pattern of amino acids in the urine, which in most cases renders the diagnosis easy. The excretion of other amino acids not involved in the specific defects remains completely normal. The blood concentration of the involved amino acids is normal or slightly lowered, and the tubular resorption rate is diminished.

The second group of renal hyperaminoaciduria is caused by systemic metabolic disturbances, intoxications, or deficiencies that secondarily affect tubular cell metabolism and lead to multiple non-specific tubular defects including the resorption of all amino acids and of other substances such as glucose, phosphate and bicarbonate (see Table 24.2). The hyperaminoaciduria is of generalized type. In its full expression it is described as the renal Fanconi's syndrome.

From the specific hyperaminoacidurias listed in Table 24.1, only two have clinical relevance, i.e. classical cystinuria and Hartnup disease. All the others are not associated with consistent clinical symptoms and, therefore, need no specific treatment. Patients should be diagnosed competently in order to exclude more severe and treatable diseases and receive adequate genetic counselling. The generalized hyperaminoaciduria will be discussed under the heading of Fanconi's syndrome.

Classic cystinuria

Cystinuria refers to a group of genetic disorders caused by defective intestinal and tubular transepithelial transport of cystine and of the dibasic amino acids arginine, lysine and ornithine. Due to poor solubility, cystine crystallizes in the urine, leading to the development of calculi in the urinary tract with the potential for obstruction, infection and ultimately renal insufficiency. The urinary loss of dibasic amino acids and the intestinal defect are of no clinical significance. Cystinuria is inherited as an autosomal recessive trait with at least three different alleles and variable expressions in the heterozygotes.[12] It is labelled classic cystinuria in order to distinguish it from isolated hypercystinuria and other types of cystine-lysinuria.[11]

The diagnosis of cystinuria should be suspected in any child with urinary calculi. It can be tested easily by microscopic examination of the urinary sediment, preferably of a morning specimen, which should be acidified with a few drops of acetic acid. In homozygous untreated patients the typical hexagonal, flat, birefringent crystals should appear in polarized light. As screening methods the cyanide nitroprusside test for disulphides should be used, the lower limit of sensitivity being 0.25 mmol/l or 38 mmol/mol creatinine, or thin-layer chromatography which easily detects cystine and the dibasic amino acids.[12] Quantitative analysis with column chromatography reveals excessive amounts of cystine and lysine, and high amounts of arginine and ornithine. Calculation of percentage tubular reabsorption results in negative values for cystine, i.e. a net secretion in homozygous carriers.

Treatment is directed toward prevention of urinary tract calculi and dissolution of stones that have already been formed. All homozygous carriers of cystinuria should be treated whether stones are already formed or not, while heterozygous carriers do not require prophylactic procedures, since their urinary cystine content remains below 1.0 mmol/l or 95 mmol/l of creatinine, respectively. Treatment consists of fluids, alkalinization of the urine and pharmacological reduction of cystine excretion. Since crystallization of cystine depends mainly on its concentration in the urine, the most important aspect of treatment is the maintenance of a high urinary output by a large fluid intake. This is especially important during night time, when the urine tends to be concentrated and acid. The urinary volume should be continuously not less than 2 ml min^{-1} 1.73 m^{-2}. Continuous fluid therapy is rewarded by prevention of stone formation and dissolution of stones already formed.[13] Cystine solubility can be enhanced by providing an alkaline urine with a pH value of at least 7.5. This can be achieved by administration of bicarbonate or citrate in large amounts, especially for the night time. For monitoring, urinary pH should be checked in the morning specimen.

In patients with recurrent urinary calculi often requiring lithotripsy or surgery, treatment with D-penicillamine or its analogues has offered great advantages. D-penicillamine is a dimethylcysteine that reacts with cysteine to form a soluble mixed disulphide and lowers the blood concentration of cystine. Its application reduces cystine excretion, thus preventing the formation of stones and promoting the dissolution of calculi. It is given daily in divided dosage of 30 mg/kg. Under this regimen the urinary cystine concentration should be kept below 0.63 mmol/l. Analogues such as N-acetyl-D-penicillamine and α-mercaptopropionylglycine seem to be as effective as D-penicillamine. Unfortunately, all have many undesirable side effects. Their use, therefore, should be restricted to those patients in whom the fluid and alkali therapy has failed.

Hartnup disease

Hartnup disease is a rare autosomal recessively transmitted complex disturbance in the epithelial transport of neutral amino acids.[14] It is characterized by a tubular and intestinal defect in the reabsorption and absorption of monocarboxylic-monoamino acids (cyclic and neutral amino acids), leading to a characteristic hyperaminoaciduria and to intestinal malabsorption with secondary decomposition of amino acids in the stool. The malabsorption, especially the defective tryptophan absorption, is responsible for the clinical signs, including pellagra-like photosensitive rash, attacks of cerebellar ataxia, and other central nervous symptoms.

Diagnosis is established by demonstration of specific hyperaminoaciduria, which is usually massive and remarkably constant. The urinary pattern of amino acids is unique and includes all cyclic and neutral amino acids, while the imino acids, glycine, dicarboxylic and dibasic amino acids are excluded. All other tubular functions are well retained. The urine contains increased quantities of indoles also, but this is secondary to the intestinal defect.

The hyperaminoaciduria of Hartnup disease, although massive, is of little clinical importance and has not been shown to result in any nutritional disturbance. Substitution of amino acids, therefore, is not necessary. Treatment is only directed to deficiency of endogenous nicotinamide formation, which is due to reduced tryptophan absorption and considered to be the cause of skin rash and ataxia. Nicotinamide is administered in a dose of 40–200 mg/day, which is usually followed by marked improvement of dermatitis and neurological picture, although such improvements could also occur spontaneously.

Renal tubular acidosis

Renal tubular acidosis (RTA) describes a group of transport defects of bicarbonate reabsorption, excretion of hydrogen ions, or both.[15] It leads to a metabolic acidosis associated with hyperchloraemia and a normal plasma anion gap. By definition, glomerular filtration rate is not primarily impaired, in contrast to uraemic acidosis, in which glomerular insufficiency is accompanied by normal or low serum chloride and increased anion gap.

The renal mechanism for acid-base homeostasis is achieved primarily by two processes: (a) the reabsorption of filtered bicarbonate (HCO_3^-), which occurs in the proximal tubules, and (b) the excretion of hydrogen ions (H^+), which takes place in the distal tubules. Filtered bicarbonate is reabsorbed to 80–90% in the proximal tubules by an active cellular transport mechanism and to a lesser extent by passive back-diffusion along the paracellular pathway. Distal urinary acidification is achieved by three related processes: (a) reabsorption of the small fraction of bicarbonate, which escapes the proximal reabsorption (10–20%), (b) secretion of H^+ to titrate the basic divalent phosphate (HPO_4^{2-}) to monovalent acid form ($H_2PO_4^-$) or titrable acid, and (c) accumulation of ammonium intraluminally which buffers H^+ to form non-diffusible ammonium (NH_4^+). H^+ secretion and titration of non-HCO_3^- urinary buffers can produce a urinary pH as low as 4.5 under conditions of acid loading.

From the pathophysiological and clinical point of view, three main types of RTA should be distinguished, as outlined in Table 24.4.[15] It is noteworthy that type 3 RTA, originally described as an own entity, has to be regarded as a transient phenomenon in infants and young children with primary RTA, in whom a tubular wasting of bicarbonate can occur.

Proximal renal tubular acidosis

The proximal RTA (type 2) is caused by an impairment of HCO_3^- reabsorption in the proximal tubules and characterized by a decreased HCO_3^- threshold. It results in urinary bicarbonate wasting and metabolic acidosis (blood pH 7.20–7.35) with low HCO_3^- (12–15 mmol/litre) and hyperchloraemia. Distal tubular acidification is intact; thus when plasma HCO_3^- is reduced below the bicarbonate threshold, the urinary pH can be lowered to less than 5.5 and adequate amounts of NH_4^+ can be excreted. Except for periods of dehydration, serum electrolytes, especially potassium, calcium and phosphorus, remain in normal ranges.

Proximal RTA is either an isolated tubular defect (very rare) or is associated with other tubular disturbances, as in Fanconi's syndrome (see below). The most prominent clinical features are failure to thrive, vomiting and stunted growth.[16] Rickets and osteomalacia are only found if the defect is combined with complex

Table 24.4   Pathophysiology and clinical classification of renal tubular acidosis (RTA) (After Rodriguez-Soriano and Vallo[15])

Type	Pathophysiology	Hereditary	Treatment
Proximal RTA (type 2)	Impaired proximal HCO_3^- reabsorption		Large doses of alkali $(10–15 \text{ mmol kg}^{-1} \text{ day}^{-1}$
Isolated	Isolated defect	Most sporadic, rarely familial	sodium bicarbonate)
Associated with other tubular defects	Multiple tubular defects (Fanconi's s.)	a.d., a.r., sporadic	plus phosphate, potassium, vit. D and fluids
Distal RTA (type 1)	Impaired distal H^+ secretion		$1–3 \text{ mmol kg}^{-1} \text{ day}^{-1}$
Secretory defect ('classic')	H^+ pump failure	a.d.	sodium and potassium,
Gradient defects	Increased back-leak		bicarbonate or citrate
Voltage-dependent defect	Reduced luminal negativity		
Hyperkalaemic RTA (type 4)	Impaired Na transport (aldosterone deficiency, pseudohypoaldosteronism), reduced ammoniagenesis	Sporadic	Hormonal substitution, high amounts of Na

a.d., autosomal dominant; a.r., autosomal recessive.

tubulopathies. In isolated RTA type 2 there is neither hypercalciuria nor nephrocalcinosis. Most cases are in the paediatric age group, and there is a tendency to improve with increasing age. Treatment requires large amounts of alkali, i.e. 10–15 mmol kg^{-1} day^{-1} of sodium citrate or sodium lactate, which has to be administered frequently in divided doses in order to maintain normal bicarbonate levels throughout the day and night time. By this, accelerated growth and normal thriving can be achieved.

Distal tubular acidosis

The distal RTA (type 1) is caused by an impairment of distal acidification and is characterized by the inability to lower urine pH maximally below 6.0 under acid load. The reduced excretion of titrable acid and ammonium is a consequence of the primary defect. In general, HCO_3^- reabsorption is normal, but because of the elevated urine pH a certain fraction of bicarbonate escapes reabsorption (< 5% of filtered load).

The pathomechanism of distal RTA includes the inability to secrete H^+ adequately ('secretory' defect or 'classic' distal RTA), to maintain a steep lumen-to-cell H^+ gradient due to increased back-leak of secreted H^+ ('gradient' defect) or to generate or maintain a distal lumen-negative transepithelial difference ('voltage-dependent' defect).[15] In children, distal RTA is mainly caused by a genetic defect of the H^+ pump, i.e. a primary disturbance. In

adults, it is generally an acquired disease, often seen in the course of an autoimmune-mediated interstitial nephritis.

Clinical features of distal RTA are characterized by failure to thrive, vomiting, polyuria, rickets, growth retardation, nephrolithiasis and nephrocalcinosis. Laboratory tests reveal a metabolic hyperchloraemic acidosis, with inability of the kidney to lower the urine pH below 6.0. Incomplete forms of distal RTA may exhibit these changes only after acid loading. Treatment of distal RTA requires alkali in the amount of a daily net acid production, i.e. 1–2 mmol kg^{-1} day^{-1} of sodium and potassium bicarbonate or citrate. However, since bicarbonate wasting is often found in children with distal RTA, higher amounts of alkali are sometimes required to correct completely the metabolic acidosis. Treatment then leads to normal thriving, healing of rickets and growth.

Hyperkalaemic renal tubular acidosis

The hyperkalaemic type of renal acidosis is often referred to as type 4 RTA,[17] although it rather should be named for its known primary defect, i.e. aldosterone deficiency or aldosterone unresponsiveness (pseudohypoaldosteronism). Acidosis in these patients is only a piece of the whole spectrum of metabolic derangement evoked by the impaired aldosterone effect. Hyperkalaemia due to aldosterone deficiency is associated with diminished H^+ secretion and reduced production of ammonium. After an

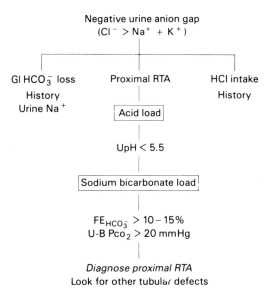

Figure 24.1 Diagnostic algorithm for a patient with hyperchloraemic acidosis and a negative urine anion gap (GI, gastrointestinal; RTA, renal tubular acidosis; UpH, urine pH; $FE_{HCO_3^-}$, fractional excretion of bicarbonate; U-B PCO_2, urine to blood PCO_2 gradient) (From Rodriguez-Soriano and Vallo[15] by permission)

acid load the urine can be acidified normally, but the net acid excretion remains subnormal due to low rates of NH_4 excretion. Renal HCO_3^- reabsorption is reduced at normal plasma levels, but there is no HCO_3^- wasting.

Hyperkalaemic RTA is most frequently observed in children with hypo- or pseudohypoaldosteronism, either isolated or associated with chronic renal parenchymal damage.[18] Nephrocalcinosis and nephrolithiasis are not part of this disease, and bone lesions appear only in uraemic acidosis.

Diagnostic procedures in metabolic acidosis

Metabolic acidosis is caused by a variety of diseases, the most common of them listed in Chapter 9. The first step in the evaluation of a patient with acidosis is to calculate the *plasma* anion gap ($Na^+ - (Cl^- + HCO_3^-)$) which normally is in the range of 8–16 mmol/litre. Acidosis with a normal anion gap reflects the loss of HCO_3^- either from the gastrointestinal tract or the kidney. Thus, RTA should be suspected when the metabolic acidosis is accompanied by hyperchloraemia and a normal plasma anion gap.

The next step should be the calculation of the *urine* anion gap, i.e. $Na^+ + K^+ - Cl^-$. The urine anion gap has been proposed as an indirect index of urinary NH_4^+ excretion. Its usefulness in the evaluation of tubular acidosis has been confirmed for children by Rodriguez-Soriano and Vallo.[15] When a urine sample of a patient with hyperchloraemic acidosis has a negative urine anion gap ($Cl^- > Na^+ + K^+$), a gastrointestinal or renal loss of HCO_3^- or a previous intake of an acid salt are the probable causes (Figure 24.1). The suspected diagnosis of proximal RTA then is established when the other disorders can be excluded. Definite diagnosis of proximal RTA is achieved by bicarbonate titration with calculation of HCO_3^- threshold and acid loading test with NH_4Cl (0.1 mg/kg) which should produce a urine pH below 5.4 when serum HCO_3^- drops below the renal threshold.

When a urine sample from a patient with hyperchloraemic acidosis has a positive urine anion gap ($Cl^- < Na^+ + K^+$), a defect in distal tubular acidification should be suspected (Figure 24.2). If plasma potassium is normal or low, the demonstration of an inability to lower urine pH below 5.5 either after NH_4Cl loading or frusemide (1 mg/kg orally) establishes the diagnosis of distal RTA. The fractional excretion of HCO_3^- at normal plasma HCO_3^- concentrations should not exceed 5% of the filtered load in these cases, unless in an infant below the age of 1 year. Diagnostic work-up should further include the search for nephrocalcinosis by ultrasonography and the measurement of urinary calcium.

When plasma potassium is increased, the search for distal abnormality in Na transport is mandatory. The diagnostic work-up should include an acid loading with measurement of minimal urine pH, the determination of plasma renin and aldosterone and investigation of a possible underlying chronic nephropathy.

Renal pseudo-endocrinopathies

Pseudohypoaldosteronism

This condition represents a rare sporadic or familial disorder of tubular unresponsiveness to mineralocorticoids mimicking the salt-losing syndrome of hypoaldosteronism. It is caused

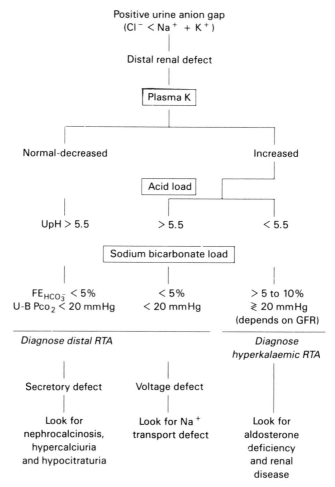

Figure 24.2 Diagnostic algorithm for a patient with hyperchloraemic metabolic acidosis and a positive urine anion gap (for abbreviations see Figure 24.1) (From Rodriguez-Soriano and Vallo[15] by permission)

by a receptor defect which could not only be expressed in the distal tubular cells, but also in other Na transporting cell membranes of saliva and sweat glands and colon mucosa. Sodium loss in early infancy is very severe and leads to hyponatraemia, hyperkalaemia and dehydration. In contrast to adrenocortical insufficiency or adrenogenital syndrome, plasma aldosterone and renin are adequately stimulated, but remain ineffective due to receptor resistance. There is an overlap between pseudohypoaldosteronism and renal tubular acidosis type 4, as described above, and it seems likely that pseudohypoaldosteronism and early childhood type 4 RTA are similar disorders with different degrees of salt wasting.[19]

Laboratory diagnosis is established by simultaneous measurement of blood and urine sodium, potassium, aldosterone and renin activity. In addition, the overall kidney function should be evaluated, in order to exclude chronic renal insufficiency, which could be associated with sodium loss. Rarely it is necessary to test the responsiveness of the kidney to the application of exogenous fluocortisone or aldosterone. Recent investigations demonstrated that the aldosterone receptor is also expressed in mononuclear leucocytes, which therefore could be studied especially in familial cases.[20]

Bartter's syndrome

This syndrome is characterized by persistent hypokalaemia, hypochloraemia, alkalosis, hyperreninaemia, and hyperaldosteronism in the presence of normal blood pressure, and elevated urinary K and Cl excretion in the absence of other conditions that might cause similar features.[19] In addition there are other clinical and biochemical findings, as hypercalcaemia, hypercalciuria, magnesium deficiency, excessive renal prostaglandin production and hypertrophy of juxtaglomerular apparatus in renal biopsy, which are not obligatorily found in all cases but could help to distinguish between the 'classic' syndrome, a 'Bartter-like' syndrome and the 'neonatal variant' of Bartter's syndrome.

The basic defect in Bartter's syndrome seems to be a disturbed tubular chloride reabsorption, which could be due to a defective chloride transporter (so-called Na-2 Cl-K-cotransporter) in the ascending limb of Henle's loop, which is also inhibited by frusemide. By this, sodium is delivered in excessive amounts to the distal tubules and reabsorbed there by exchange with potassium, which leads to potassium wasting.

The patient presents early in life with failure to thrive, vomiting and constipation, all signs of persistent hypokalaemia. There may be a history of polyhydramnios during pregnancy. The patient suffers often from polydipsia, polyuria, fatigue, muscle cramps and growth retardation. The blood pressure remains low in spite of hyperreninaemia. The familial cases demonstrate an autosomal recessive transmission.

The laboratory diagnosis can be established by the following findings: chronic hypokalaemia (2–3 mmol/litre), hypochloraemia (80–85 mmol/litre), metabolic alkalosis with bicarbonate 28–35 mmol/litre, low serum sodium, increased plasma renin and aldosterone, increased urinary prostaglandins, and normal blood pressure. Usually it is not necessary to test the (blunted) response of blood pressure to angiotensin or to perform a renal biopsy for the search of juxtaglomerular hypertrophy. The differential diagnosis includes incomplete distal RTA, use of loop diuretics, laxative abuse, chloride-deficient diet, congenital chloride diarrhoea, cystic fibrosis, mineralocorticoid excess, primary magnesium-losing kidney and the renal Fanconi's syndrome.

Treatment aims to normalize hypokalaemia in order to reverse the secondary hypokalaemic symptoms. Supplementation with KCl and NaCl is usually ineffective to normalize K blood levels persistently. This applies also for the use of spironolactone and potassium-sparing diuretics (triamterene). The best approach today is treatment with prostaglandin synthetase inhibitors such as indomethacin, which lead to a rapid correction of hypokalaemia with improvement in weight, appetite and growth. The starting dose of indomethacin is $1–2$ mg^{-1} kg^{-1} day^{-1} in 2–3 divided doses. Patients have to be checked regularly, since indomethacin could affect glomerular filtration rate, especially in those who had a reduced GFR at the onset of treatment.

Nephrogenic diabetes insipidus

The renal type of diabetes insipidus is characterized by a resistance of the kidney to the antidiuretic effect of vasopressin. By this, the kidney loses its ability to concentrate the urine, which leads to polyuria, polydipsia, chronic dehydration and, mainly in infants, to fever, obstipation, failure to thrive and mental retardation. It can occur as a congenital disorder, then mostly inherited as an X-linked recessive trait, or as an acquired disturbance caused by intoxications, systemic disease or obstructive uropathy.

In normal children the plasma osmolality is maintained very constant in the range of 275–285 mosmol/kg H_2O, despite wide variations in water and solute intake. This is very strictly regulated by vasopressin (adiuretin), an octapeptide of the posterior hypophyseal lobe. By increase of the extracellular osmolality of 1–2%, vasopressin release is stimulated via osmoreceptors, or by decrease of circulating volume of 10% via the baroceptors, respectively.[21] In the kidney, vasopressin binds to the contraluminal receptors both in cells of the medullary thick ascending limp of Henle and in the collecting tubules. It activates adenylate cyclase which releases cAMP from ATP. By this, in the thick ascending limb the absorption of NaCl is stimulated, which increases the hypertonicity of the renal medulla, and in the collecting ducts the apical water channels are increased which leads to a rise of water permeability. Thus, with circulating vasopressin normal individuals elaborate a urine hypertonic to plasma.

In the congenital form of nephrogenic diabetes insipidus, either the binding of vasopressin to the receptor or the activation of adenylate cyclase or a post-cAMP step may be disturbed.[21] The molecular mechanism has not been elucidated in humans so far, as could be investigated in mice. Probably the human disease is heterogeneous and produced by a variety of molecular defects. The gene locus for the X-linked recessive type could be assigned to the subtelomeric region of the long arm of the X-chromosome.[22]

The congenital type presents shortly after birth with irritability, poor feeding, vomiting, 'unexplained' fever, and failure to thrive. The infant is constantly dehydrated, and despite a reduced skin turgor the nappies remain wet and the urine diluted. In untreated patients the psychomotor development is retarded due to hypernatraemic brain damage. Later in life, dilatation of urinary tract occurs as a consequence of large urinary volumes retained voluntarily.

The laboratory examination reveals hypernatraemia (up to 180 mmol/litre), hyperchloraemia and hyperosmolality. In severe dehydration, retention of urea and creatinine and metabolic acidosis may be present. The diagnosis is established by determination of plasma vasopressin and performance of vasopressin test. Plasma vasopressin is inadequately high compared to urinary osmolality.[23] The vasopressin test is performed with lysine-vasopressin (2 mU/kg as i.v. bolus) or deamino-D-arginine vasopressin (DDAVP) which is administered as an intranasal spray in a dosage of 10–20 μg.[24] Urine is collected in timed intervals before and after vasopressin, and osmolality measured simultaneously in plasma and urine. By this, response to exogeneous vasopressin can be evaluated by changes in osmolality and calculation of the free-water clearance:

Osmolar clearance

$$C_{osm} = U_{osm} \times V/P_{osm}$$

Free-water clearance

$$C_{H_2O} = V - C_{osm}$$

In normals, the urinary osmolality increases to values well above the isotonicity, and the free-water clearance becomes significantly negative. In patients with nephrogenic diabetes insipidus, urine osmolality remains below isotonicity and free-water clearance remains positive.

It has been proposed to measure cAMP after vasopressin in order to differentiate between nephrogenic diabetes insipidus type 1 (no response) and type 2 (with increase). However, the response of urinary cAMP to vasopressin, in contrast to PTH, is only weak, even in normals; therefore it is doubtful whether one could use it for clinical diagnosis.

The differential diagnosis of polyuric states includes a variety of renal and non-renal diseases and should be considered in each case. A list of causes is shown in Chapter 7.

The treatment aims to prevent dehydration and hyperelectrolytaemia and, at the same time, to reduce the daily fluid intake to amounts which are tolerable for the patients and do not interfere with their daily activities and nightly sleep. Fluids have to be offered freely as soon as thirst regulates the need. In infants, a nasogastric tube allows a continuous drip of solute-free fluid, especially at night. A diet low in salt and protein keeps the obligatory fluid loss low and is therefore recommended. In addition to dietary treatment, drugs can be used to reduce the daily urinary volumes. The most effective drugs are hydrochlorothiazide (2 mg kg^{-1} day^{-1}) and indomethacin (1–2 mg kg^{-1} day^{-1}), which should be combined for optimal treatment.[25] The mechanism of these drugs is not fully understood. Hydrochlorothiazide induces natriuresis and contraction of extracellular fluid volume. By this, the sodium delivery to the distal tubules are reduced which could lead to a reduction of final urine. Prostaglandin synthetase inhibitors reduce the elevated levels of prostaglandins found in cases with nephrogenic diabetes insipidus, and by this could modulate the water handling of the renal tubules. Since the use of hydrochlorothiazide is associated with a potassium loss, one should substitute potassium chloride orally.

Fanconi's syndrome

The renal Fanconi's syndrome (de Toni–Debré–Fanconi syndrome) is characterized by generalized disturbance of tubular function, while glomerular filtration is not primarily affected. It leads to excessive urinary losses of amino acids, glucose, phosphate, bicarbonate, and other organic and inorganic substrates handled by the proximal and distal tubules. The metabolic consequences are acidosis, hypophosphataemia, hypokalaemia, dehydration, rickets, osteoporosis and growth retardation. The syndrome appears to be the final expression of many different injuries to the renal tubule, especially the proximal segment. It may either be congenital or acquired, primary or secondary, complete or incomplete. (For a recent review

Table 24.5   Aetiological classification of Fanconi's syndrome

Primary (idiopathic) Fanconi's syndrome
　Common type
　　Hereditary (autosomal dominant, autosomal recessive (?), X-linked recessive (?))
　　Sporadic
　Brush-border type
Secondary (symptomatic) Fanconi's syndrome
　In inborn errors of metabolism
　　Cystinosis (autosomal recessive)
　　Tyrosinaemia, type I (autosomal recessive)
　　Glycogenosis (autosomal recessive)
　　Galactosaemia (uridyl transferase deficiency) (autosomal recessive)
　　Hereditary fructose intolerance (autosomal (recessive)
　　Lowe's syndrome (X-linked recessive)
　　Wilson's disease (autosomal recessive)
　　Cytochrome-c-oxidase deficiency (autosomal recessive)
　In acquired diseases
　　Multiple myeloma
　　Nephrotic syndrome
　　Transplanted kidney
　　Tumour
　In intoxications
　　Heavy metals (mercury, uranium, lead, cadmium)
　　Maleic acid, lysol, toluene
　　Outdated tetracycline, methyl-3-chromone
　　Cisplatin, ifosfamide

see References 26 and 27). An aetiological classification of Fanconi's syndrome is given in Table 24.5.

The cardinal features of Fanconi's syndrome are hyperaminoaciduria, glucosuria and phosphate wasting. *Hyperaminoaciduria* is generalized, i.e. all free amino acids are involved, but to various extents. By quantitative determination of the percentage tubular amino acid reabsorption, as outlined above, it becomes obvious that the degree of disturbed reabsorption corresponds with the degree of normal reabsorption. Thus, the generalized hyperaminoaciduria is characterized by an exaggeration of the normal pattern. The severity of hyperaminoaciduria is variable and depends on the stage and cause of the disease, glomerular filtration rate, and additional factors such as vitamin D status or hyperparathyroidism.

Glucosuria is of renal origin and therefore usually accompanied by normal blood glucose levels. The tubular defect is characterized by a low threshold and a low maximal glucose reabsorption at saturation blood glucose levels.

Glucosuria is variable, usually moderate. The only exception is the glycogenosis with Fanconi's syndrome, in which glucosuria is massive, up to 1 mol/day.

The *phosphate wasting* (phosphate diabetes) is caused by reduced tubular reabsorption of inorganic phosphate, which leads to sustained hypophosphataemia. The fractional phosphate reabsorption Tmp/GFR which is easily determined by using spontaneous urine and plasma samples (as outlined above) is significantly reduced, and loading with phosphate does not increase the phosphate reabsorption. Persistent hypophosphataemia is associated with disturbed bone mineralization and is the main cause of rickets in Fanconi's syndrome.

Other tubular symptoms are encountered in most cases of Fanconi's syndrome, but to various extents. These include bicarbonate wasting which corresponds to type 2 RTA (see above) and leads to severe metabolic acidosis. Further signs are uric acid wasting associated with hypouricaemia, hypokalaemia which could lead to muscle weakness and cardiac dysrhythmias, low carnitine levels affecting muscle metabolism, hypercalciuria, polyuria and tubular proteinuria. Tubular secretion of p-aminohippurate (PAH) may be impaired in some types of Fanconi's syndrome out of proportion to the degree of glomerular filtration rate, leading to increase of filtration fraction. This is especially seen in cystinosis, multiple myeloma and some kinds of intoxication.

The diagnosis of a renal Fanconi's syndrome is not complete as long as its aetiology is not revealed. Therefore, in each case the search for the cause is mandatory, since many underlying diseases can well be treated, either by eliminating the cause or symptomatically. Most cases are secondary types caused by metabolic diseases, intoxications or other disturbance (see Table 24.5).

Idiopathic Fanconi's syndrome

This syndrome is rare. It occurs either sporadic or familial, with different modes of inheritance. The diagnosis of an idiopathic type is made by exclusion of all known causes leading to the complex tubular defect. One has to realize that the term idiopathic is only a preliminary one which can be used as long as the underlying metabolic derangement remains unknown. The idiopathic Fanconi's syndrome may develop at any age and last over a long life-span.

The tubular dysfunctions could appear successively over years, as in the so-called Luder–Sheldon syndrome which later progresses into an idiopathic Fanconi's syndrome.[28] These cases have an uncertain prognosis concerning renal function, since they may develop chronic renal insufficiency over a period of 10–30 years.

Cystinosis

The most common type of Fanconi's syndrome is that caused by cystinosis (cystine storage disease). This is an autosomal recessively inherited disorder of lysosomal cystine transport resulting in excessive intracellular accumulation of free cystine in many organs, including the kidney.[29] There are three different types of cystinosis, depending on the degree of involvement of certain organ systems: infantile (nephropathic) cystinosis is the most severe type, leading to progressive tubular and later glomerular insufficiency early in life; the adolescent (intermediate) type is characterized by a milder nephropathy presenting clinical signs not before the second decade of life; the adult (benign) type has no renal involvement but only cystine crystals located in the cornea, bone marrow and leucocytes.

The clinical signs of nephropathic cystinosis do not appear before the age of 3–6 months when affected infants start with episodes of unexplained fever, vomiting, anorexia and polydipsia. They show signs of dehydration, failure to thrive, rickets and growth retardation. The tubular signs develop at an age at which glomerular filtration is still normal or only slightly impaired. Therefore, severe glomerulotubular imbalance arises which could provoke life-threatening 'electrolyte crisis'. Beyond the age of 5–6 years the glomerular filtration rate falls progressively and serum creatinine increases accordingly. The median time for 'renal death' is 9.2 years.[30] Extrarenal signs of cystinosis are numerous.[31,32] High intracellular cystine is found in various organs, leading to photophobia and retinopathy, hypothyroidism, diabetes mellitus and exocrine pancreatic insufficiency, hepatopathy and cerebral involvement.

Diagnosis of cystinosis is established by determination of cystine content in leucocytes, rectal mucosa, conjunctiva or fibroblasts. In these cells the cystine content is elevated up to 100 times normal. Therefore, one does not wait for the appearance of clinical signs as crystals in the cornea, pigment degeneration of the retina, or crystals in rectal mucosa or bone marrow, which used to be the hallmark for diagnosis in former times. In renal biopsy, the early diagnosis of crystals can be achieved only by electron microscopy. The signs of Fanconi's syndrome are usually severe and distinguished by an early and severe defect in tubular PAH transport, leading to gross elevation of filtration fraction (C_{IN}/C_{PAH}).

Treatment of cystinosis should be symptomatic, as in other types of Fanconi's syndrome (see below). In addition, a specific treatment has been introduced,[33] with the aim of reducing the intracellular concentration of cystine and to prevent further cystine accumulation. Continuous treatment with cysteamine or phosphocysteamine has been shown to lower the cystine content of leucocytes to near normal levels. The long-term clinical results, especially in regard to preservation of renal function, however, await final proof. Therefore, this treatment must be considered to be still investigational and should be done only in controlled trials.

Renal replacement therapy is necessary when terminal renal failure is reached. In most children, continuous peritoneal dialysis such as CAPD or CCPD is preferred, which however has the disadvantage of delivering high amounts of glucose to the patient who already is prone to develop diabetes mellitus. The ultimate aim is kidney transplantation, which has been successfully performed since the late 1960s. In most reports the graft survival was the same or even superior to that in other causes of end-stage renal disease.[34,35] Rehabilitation of the patient is good; however, the long-term sequelae and complications of the disease make the final prognosis uncertain.

Treatment of Fanconi's syndromes

Treatment of Fanconi's syndrome is either specific or symptomatic. Specific treatment is possible in secondary types where the underlying metabolic defect should be eliminated (as in galactosaemia, fructose intolerance or drug intoxications). In those cases a return to normal can usually be obtained.

The symptomatic treatment for all other types is equally important as it may almost completely compensate for the deranged tubular function. It may not only prolong survival, but also provide in most cases full rehabilitation with normal activity and well-being.

Acidosis due to bicarbonate losses (type 2

RTA) requires large amounts of alkali (2–10 mmol kg^{-1} day^{-1} of sodium bicarbonate, citrate or lactate). Potassium depletion should be substituted with potassium (2–4 mmol kg^{-1} day^{-1}) as bicarbonate, citrate or phosphate, depending on the levels of these anions. Hypophosphataemia can be compensated partly by oral supplementation of 1–3 g neutral phosphate per day. In some cases, phosphate supplementation may produce or aggravate hypocalcaemia and stimulate hyperparathyroidism. Administration of additional oral calcium and vitamin D may prevent hypocalcaemia. Treatment with vitamin D (starting dose 5000 IU/day) or 1,25-diOH-Vit D (0.25–0.5 μg/day) is indicated in rickets. Careful monitoring of vitamin D treatment is necessary to avoid toxic side effects, especially nephrocalcinosis. Polyuria necessitates sufficient fluid intakes, in order to avoid dehydration. In practice, a fixed amount of fluid for the whole day is prepared with the required salts dissolved. Additional fluids may be ingested *ad libitum*. Finally, in a few patients who progress to renal insufficiency, dialysis and transplantation may be indicated (see cystinosis).

References

1. Brodehl J., Krause A. and Hoyer P. F. Assessment of maximal tubular phosphate reabsorption: comparison of direct measurement with the nomogram of Bijvoet. *Pediatr. Nephrol.* 1988, **2**, 183–189

2. Walton R.J. and Bijvoet O.L.M. Nomogram for derivation of renal threshold phosphate concentration. *Lancet* 1975, **II**, 309–310

3. Reusz G.S., Hoyer P.F., Lucas M., Ehrich J.H.H. and Brodehl J. X-linked hypophosphataemia: treatment, height gain and nephrocalcinosis. *Arch. Dis. Child.* 1990, **65**, 1125–1128

4. Reusz G.S., Latta K., Hoyer P.F., Byrd D.J., Ehrich J.H.H. and Brodehl J. Evidence suggesting hyperoxaluria as a cause of nephrocalcinosis in phosphate-treated hypophosphataemic rickets. *Lancet* 1990, **I**, 1240–1243

5. Spiegel A.M. Pseudohypoparathyroidism. In: Scriver C.R, Beaudet A.L., Sly W.S. and Valle D. (eds) *The Metabolic Basis of Inherited Disease*, 6th edn. New York, McGraw-Hill, 1989: 2013–2027

6. Radecke H.H., Auf'mKolk B., Jüppner H., Krohn H.-P., Keck E. and Hesch R.-D. Multiple pre- and postreceptor defects in pseudohypoparathyroidism (a multicenter study with twenty four patients). *J. Clin. Endocrinol. Metab.* 1986, **62**, 393–402

7. Brodehl J., Oemar B.S. and Hoyer P.F. Renal glucosuria. *Pediatr. Nephrol.* 1987, **1**, 502–508

8. Oemar B.S., Byrd D.J. and Brodehl J. Complete absence of tubular glucose reabsorption: a new type of renal glucosuria (type O). *Clin. Nephrol.* 1987, **27**, 156–160

9. Elsas L.J., Hillman R.E., Patterson J.H. and Rosenberg L.E. Renal and intestinal hexose transport in familial glucose-galactose malabsorption. *J. Clin. Invest.* 1970, **49**, 576–585

10. Brodehl J. and Gellissen K. Endogenous renal transport of free amino acids in infancy and childhood. *Pediatrics* 1968, **42**, 395–404

11. Bordehl J. Renal hyperaminoacidurias. In: Edelmann C.M. (ed.) *Pediatric Kidney Disease*. 2nd edn. Boston, Little, Brown, 1992, 1811–1840.

12. Byrd D.J., Lind M. and Brodehl J. Diagnostic and genetic studies in 43 patients with classic cystinuria. *Clin. Chem.* 1991, **37**, 68–73

13. Dent C.E., Friedman M., Green H. and Watson L.C.A. Treatment of cystinuria. *Br. Med. J.* 1965, **I**, 403–408

14. Levy H.L. Hartnup disorder. In: Scriver C.R., Beaudet A.L., Sly, W.S. and Valle D. (eds) *The Metabolic Basis of Inherited Disease*, 6th edn. New York, McGraw-Hill, 1989: 2515–2527

15. Rodriguez-Soriano J. and Vallo A. Renal tubular acidosis. *Pediatr. Nephrol.* 1990, **4**, 268–275

16. Edelmann C.M. Isolated proximal (type 2) renal tubular acidosis. In Gonick H.C. and Bukalew V.M. (eds) *Renal Tubular Disorders*. New York, Marcel Dekker, 1985: 261–279

17. Sebastian A., Schambelan M., Hulter H.N., Maher T., Kurtz I., Biglieri E.G. *et al.* Hyperkalemic renal tubular acidosis. In: Gonick H.C. and Bukalew V.M. (eds) *Renal Tubular Disorders*. New York, Marcel Dekker, 1985: 307–356

18. Rodriguez-Soriano J. and Vallo A. Renal tubular hyperkalemia in childhood. *Pediatr. Nephrol.* 1988, **2**, 498–509

19. Rodriguez-Sorigno J. Tubular disorders of electrolyte regulation. In: Holliday M.A., Barratt T.M. and Avner E.D. (eds) *Pediatric Nephrology*, 3rd edn. Baltimore, Williams and Wilkins, 1994: 624–639

20. Armanini D., Kuhnle W., Strasser T., Dorr H., Butenandt I., Weber P.C. *et al.* Aldosterone-receptor deficiency in pseudohypoaldosteronism. *New Engl. J. Med.* 1985, **313**, 1178–1181

21. Reeves W.B. and Andreoli T.E. Nephrogenic diabetes insipidus. In: Scriver C.R., Beaudet A.L., Sly W.S. and Valle D. (eds) *The Metabolic Basis of Inherited Disease*, 6th edn, Vol.II. New York, McGraw-Hill, 1989: 1985–2011

22. Knoers N., Heyden v.d.H., Oost v.B.A., Monnens L., Willems J. and Ropers H.H. Three point linkage analysis using multiple DNA polymorphic markers in families with X-linked nephrogenic diabetes insipidus. *Genomics* 1989, **4**, 434–437

23. Robertson G.L. Thirst and vasopressin function in normal and disordered states of water balance. *J. Lab. Clin. Med.* 1983, **101**, 351–371

24. Brodehl J. Nephrogenic diabetes insipidus. In: Belton N.R. and Toothill C. (eds) *Transport and Inherited Disease*, Lancaster, MTP Press, 1981: 207–230

25. Kaulitz R. and Brodehl J. Langfristige Verläufe von 6 Jungen mit kongenitalem nephrogenen Diabetes insipidus. *Klin. Pädiatr.* 1989, **201**, 425–430

26. Foreman J.A. Fanconi syndrome and cystinosis. In: Holliday M.A., Barratt T.M. and Avner E.D. (eds), *Pediatric Nephrology*, 3rd edn. Baltimore, Williams and Wilkins, 1994: 537–556

27. Brodehl J. Fanconi syndrome. In: Cameron J.S., Davison A.M., Grünfeld J.-P., Kerr N.S. and Ritz E. (eds) *Oxford Textbook of Clinical Nephrology*. Oxford, Oxford University Press, 1991, 723–740

28. Patrick A., Cameron J.S. and Ogg C.S. A family with a dominant form of idiopathic Fanconi syndrome leading to renal failure in adult life. *Clin. Nephrol.* 1981, **16**, 289–292

29. Adamson M.D., Anderson H.C. and Gahl W.A. Cystinosis. *Sem. Nephrol.* 1989, **9**, 147–161

30. Gretz N., Manz F., Augustin R., Barrat T.M., Bender-Götze C., Brandis M. *et al.* Survival time in cystinosis. A collaborative study. *Proc. Europ. Dialysis Transplant. Ass.* 1982, **19**, 582–588

31. Broyer M., Tete M.-J. and Gubler M.C. Late symptoms in infantile cystinosis. *Pediatr. Nephrol.* 1987, **1**, 519–524

32. Brodehl J. Cystinosis. In: Cameron J.S., Davison A.M., Grünfeld J.P., Kerr D.N.S. and Ritz E. (eds) *Oxford Textbook of Clinical Nephrology*. Oxford, Oxford University Press, 1991, 2220–2226

33. Gahl W., Reed G.F., Thoene J.G., Schulman J.D., Rizzo W.B., Jonas A.J. *et al.* Cysteamine therapy for children with nephropathic cystinosis. *New Engl. J. Med.* 1987, **316**, 971–977

34. Broyer M., Donckerwolcke R.A., Brunner F.D., Bryuger H., Jacobs C., Kramer P. *et al.* Combined report on regular dialysis and transplantation of children in Europe 1980. *Proc. Europ. Dialysis Transplant. Ass.* 1981, **18**, 60–87

35. Ehrich J.H.H., Brodehl J., Byrd D.J., Hossfeld S., Hoyer P.F., Leipert K.-P. *et al.* Renal transplantation in 22 children with nephropathic cystinosis. *Pediatr. Nephrol.* 1991, **5** 708–714

25

Cystic disorders of the kidney

M. Lendon, R.J. Postlethwaite

Introduction

Cystic diseases of the kidney are relatively common and at first sight seem to include a bewildering array of disorders. It is possible, taking into account epidemiology, demography, genetics, and clinical and morphological features, to produce classifications which are brief, acceptable both to clinicians and pathologists and have predictive features.[1] Despite this, many problems seem to remain which are at least partly explained by the differing experience of cystic disorders of, among others, radiologists, obstetricians, neonatologists, paediatric surgeons, paediatricians, geneticists, pathologists and adult physicians. This in turn gives rise to a confusion in terminology. In particular, there is a tendency to apply the term 'polycystic kidney(s)' to any lesion in which one or both kidneys show multiple cysts. The term 'polycystic kidney disease' should be reserved for two hereditary cystic diseases, recessive polycystic kidney disease (RPKD) and dominant polycystic kidney disease (DPKD) which are clearly distinct both by their modes of inheritance and by their pathological characteristics.[2] Similarly, 'cystic dysplasia' and 'multicystic kidney' have strict diagnostic criteria. In the initial assessment of multiple cysts in the kidney, particularly on imaging, it is better to use a non-specific descriptive term such as 'multiple renal cysts' until the condition has been more accurately defined following consideration of all its other attributes.

A recent review of renal cysts in children by Kissane,[1] provides an elegant and practical classification. It is reproduced in modified form in Table 25.1.

Renal cystic dysplasia

This is the commonest form of renal cystic disease in children and is essentially a histological diagnosis. It depends on the demonstration of cortical and medullary cysts with structural disorganization of the kidney and includes primitive ducts surrounded by fibromuscular collars. Islands of metaplastic cartilage are seen in approximately 40% of dysplastic kidneys. This embryological maldevelopment may affect

Table 25.1 Classification of renal cysts (After Kissane[1])

Renal cystic dysplasia
Multicystic dysplasia
Obstructive dysplasia
  bilateral
  unilateral
Cystic dysplasia in hereditary syndromes

Polycystic disease
Autosomal recessive polycystic disease
Autosomal dominant polycystic disease

Glomerulocystic renal disease

Medullary renal lesions
Juvenile nephronophthisis/medullary cystic disease
Medullary sponge kidney

Simple renal cysts

Acquired renal cysts

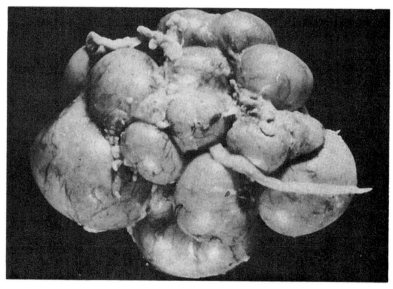

Figure 25.1 Multicystic dysplastic kidney – numerous thin-walled cysts of varying size with atresia of the distal end of the attached ureter

Table 25.2   Recent experience of multicystic dysplastic kidney at Royal Manchester Children's Hospital (Personal communication, Mr D.C.S. Gough)

Normal renal function – contralateral kidney normal		28 (74%)
Normal renal function – contralateral kidney abnormal		
Idiopathic hydronephrosis*	3	
Vesico-ureteric reflux	3	8 (21%)
Duplex	2	
Renal impairment		2 (5%)
Total		38

*Resolved on follow-up.

the whole kidney, a major segment or only be detected on microscopic examination. Clinically it is normally a presumptive diagnosis but there is rarely any indication for renal biopsy and indeed this may be a fruitless exercise as dysplastic foci may be segmental or widely dispersed. Cystic dysplasia occurs in three major situations: as a multicystic renal mass, in association with obstructive lesions of the lower urinary tract, and in association with various hereditary syndromes.

Multicystic kidney

The multicystic kidney consists of numerous thin-walled cysts surrounding a residual core of dysplastic tissue. Normally differentiated nephrons are rarely seen. The draining ureter is always atretic (Figure 25.1). It can be viewed as the extreme of the cystic dysplastic spectrum. Previously the commonest presentation was as an abdominal mass and a diagnosis was usually established at laparotomy. Thus nephrectomy was the usual treatment. Although the contralateral kidney was grossly normal, in 30–50% of patients there was impaired renal function.[3] Increasingly this lesion is identified antenatally. Of 302 patients assessed in this institution for antenatal urological problems, 38 (12.5%) had multicystic kidney (Table 25.2). In 28 (74%) the contralateral kidney was normal as was the renal function. In a further 8 (21%), though the contralateral kidney showed a structural anomaly, the renal function was normal. Thus in only 5% was the renal function abnormal. In these two patients the contralateral kidney showed pelvi-ureteric junction obstruction and acute renal failure was precipitated by infection.

This changing spectrum of presentation presumably represents a shift from symptomatic presentation to identification of pre-symptomatic cases. It does, however, create a dilemma. In the short term no morbidity or mortality arises from the multicystic dysplastic kidney (MDK),[4] but in the long term there is a small risk of hypertension, sepsis and a remotely possi-

Table 25.3   Renal cysts associated with hereditary syndromes (From Kissane,[1] by permission)

Cystic dysplasia associated with autosomal recessive syndromes
  Meckel–Gruber syndrome and variants
  Zellweger's cerebrohepatorenal syndrome
  Jeune's asphyxiating thoracic dystrophy
  Miscellaneous:
  Short-limb polydactyly syndromes
  Orofacial digital syndromes, type I, etc.

Cysts (and other renal lesions) associated with autosomal dominant disorders
  Tuberose sclerosis
  von Hippel–Lindau
  von Recklinghausen's neurofibromatosis

Cystic lesions associated with aneuploids
  Trisomy 13 and trisomy 18
  Turner's syndrome

ble risk of malignancy.[5] The lesion usually has a characteristic appearance on imaging (see below).[6] This has led some to recommend a conservative approach,[7] whereas others have advocated nephrectomy.[5] We have followed this latter advice, offering the parents a choice at 1 year between nephrectomy and continuing observation. Following nephrectomy, in view of the normality of the contralateral kidney follow-up can be discontinued in the majority. We feel this approach is preferable to repeated life-long investigation and blood pressure measurement which must otherwise be advised because of the risks of hypertension and malignancy. Regression of the cysts occurs in a minority over the first year.[4] Exploration of the renal area in patients who have shown regression usually identifies renal remnants (see Chapter 30). As the risk of malignancy and/or hypertension presumably relates to persistence of tissue rather than cysts, the significance of this regression is not clear.

Obstructive dysplasia

In some series, 90% of cases of cystic dysplasia have been associated with urinary tract obstruction, although the association has been less frequent in others.[8,9]

Bilateral dysplasia

Any anatomical or functional obstruction of the urinary tract during development may be associated with dysplasia. It is bilateral in urethral atresia, the 'prune-belly' syndrome, urethral valves, anterior urethral diverticulum or in spina bifida where there is intra-uterine bladder dysfunction. Bilateral dysplasia may have a widely varying expression, from being clinically silent to presenting with severe renal failure with Potter's sequence and massively enlarged kidneys (see Chapter 7).

Unilateral dysplasia

This is usually associated with ipsilateral obstruction, e.g. ectopic ureterocele. The severity of unilateral obstruction is correlated with the severity of cyst formation. Treatment is surgical excision (see Chapter 27).

Cystic dysplasia in hereditary syndromes and aneuploides

A variety of hereditary syndromes with multiple malformations in other organ systems are associated with cystic dysplastic changes in the kidneys. Both autosomal recessive and autosomal dominant disorders are involved and the more common syndromes are listed in Table 25.3. Aneuploides such as trisomy 13 or 18 and Turner's syndrome may be associated with renal cysts, but in Turner's syndrome structural lesions such as horseshoe kidney (the commonest), duplication, rotational abnormalities and hydronephrosis are much more important clinically, occurring in 60–80% of patients.

Imaging in cystic dysplasia

The appearance of a cystic dysplastic kidney on imaging depends on two factors: (a) the size and distribution of the cysts, and (b) the degree of renal function in intervening areas of renal tissue.

Multiple large cysts are easily seen on ultrasonography, but are usually associated with poor renal function so that IVP or radioisotope imaging is unsuccessful. This is seen at its most extreme in MDK where, on ultrasonography,[6] the kidney is replaced by a collection of macrocysts of varying sizes which do not communicate. Dysplastic echogenic septa are interspersed among the cysts and there is no demonstrable peripheral renal parenchyma. There is absence of function in the ipsilateral kidney on radioisotope scanning, both dynamic and static.

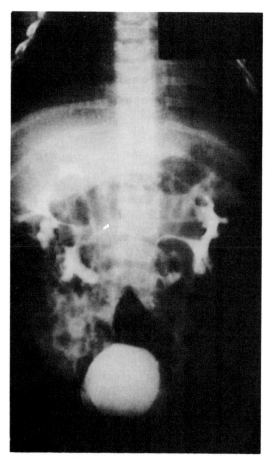

Figure 25.2 Multiple macrocysts with normal intervening renal tissue produce typical pericalyceal deformity on IVP and cold areas in DMSA scans. These appearances occur in DPKD in the second and third decade. In children, the appearances are commonly due to some other pathology such as tuberous sclerosis, as in this case

Occasionally it may be difficult to distinguish between severe hydronephrosis and MDK and puncture of the cysts with contrast examination may be necessary to make this distinction. The contralateral kidney should always be examined in MDK to exclude any lesion, including ureteric reflux.

The exception to this rule is tuberous sclerosis where, despite large cysts, the surviving renal tissue usually gives good renal function so that the large cysts can be visualized on IVP (Figure 25.2) and DMSA scan (Figure 25.3). The resemblance of this imaging appearance (not the clinical circumstances) to DPKD has often led to confusion.[10]

As the cysts become smaller they become more difficult to detect on ultrasound as discrete cysts and eventually the lesion is only appreciated as altered echogenicity of the kidney and/or loss of corticomedullary differentiation. Generally in these circumstances renal function is better preserved, so that visualization is obtained on other imaging techniques. Despite this, the cysts are not visualized because they are too small. Thus in most cases of obstructive dysplasia the kidneys are of varying sizes but rarely demonstrate discrete cysts on imaging.

The same principles apply to the findings in hereditary syndromes.

Genetics of cystic dysplasia

Cystic dysplasia in the hereditary syndromes is usually inherited in a Mendelian pattern. Obstructive cystic dysplasia is almost always sporadic, but family studies have shown an empirical recurrence risk of 2.1%.[11] Isolated cystic dysplasia, i.e without obstruction and without a defined syndrome, may be sporadic but there are increasing reports of familial cystic dysplasia.[12]

Polycystic disease

As mentioned earlier, polycystic kidney disease refers specifically to two conditions: autosomal recessive polycystic kidney disease (RPKD) and autosomal dominant polycystic kidney disease (DPKD).[2,13] These two diseases have distinct genetic, clinical, radiographic and morphological features, but in each group there is some clinical and pathological heterogeneity and at the extremes some overlapping of clinical presentation.[14]

An interesting feature of polycystic kidney disease is the evolving clinical, pathological and imaging pattern. Thus in DPKD, cysts generally develop in the second decade in what were previously normal kidneys. Evolution of the disease pattern is seen not only in RPKD and DPKD but also in the inherited medullary cystic diseases (see below) and in congenital nephrotic syndrome (Finnish-type congenital nephrotic syndrome pathologically could be considered a cystic kidney lesion). In obstructive dysplasia the pattern of cysts is fixed, and the renal function, although impaired, is

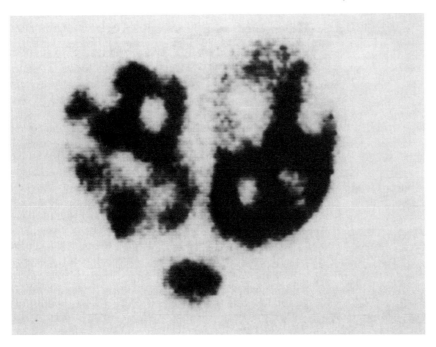

Figure 25.3 DMSA scan in multiple macrocysts – scan from same patient as Figure 25.2 (note that in DMSA scanning the images are reversed so that the right kidney is on the right of the picture)

Table 25.4   Age of presentation of RPKD (From data in Kaariainen et al.[15] and Kaplan et al.[16])

	$n = (73)^{15}$	$n = (55)^{16}$
Neonatal	93%	45%
6 months–1 year	1.5%	45%
> 1 year	5.5%	10%

frequently stable once the obstruction has been relieved.

Autosomal recessive polycystic kidney disease

RPKD is a rare condition. Its incidence is not known precisely, but recent estimates suggest an incidence of 1:40 000.[2]

Two recent large studies allow for a much more complete picture of the clinical presentation. The first study identified all the children who had been treated or investigated for polycystic kidney disease in Finland between 1974 and 1983.[15] The second is a report from a major paediatric nephrology centre.[16] Looking at the age distribution in the two series, there is a striking excess of neonatal cases in the Finnish series (Table 25.4). In this series 93% (66) pre-sented in the neonatal period. Of these, 56 did not survive the neonatal period and 52 of these 56 deaths were from respiratory failure. Clearly many of these neonates were not previously referred to paediatric nephrology centres. It is also important to note that only 4 of the 56 neonatal deaths were due to renal failure. Severe oliguria, often with hyponatraemia, is fre-quently present in the newborn period in the presence of well-preserved renal function. The mechanism is not clear, but it usually responds to frusemide and salt and water restrictions. This oliguria can be wrongly interpreted as a sign of severe renal failure. Some of the pitfalls in assessment and the possible improving out-look for these neonates with severe respiratory problems is illustrated by the case histories of the last three neonates referred to our depart-ment. All three required ventilation from days to months. One patient was dependent on dialy-sis from birth and required prolonged mechani-cal ventilation. At the age of 9 months he remains well on dialysis with no respiratory support. In the other two patients, a decision to stop ventilatory support had been considered in the referring units because of severe oliguria in ventilatory-dependent patients. Both are now

Table 25.5   Mode of presentation of RPKD (From data in Kaariainen *et al.*[15] and Kaplan *et al.*[16])

	%
Respiratory failure	44
Enlarged kidneys	34
Enlarged liver	10
Renal failure	2.5
Urinary tract infection	2.5
Vomiting	2.5
Failure to thrive	2.5
Proteinuria	1
Miscellaneous	1

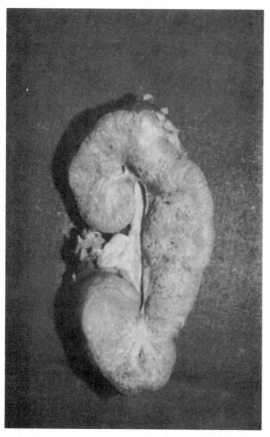

Figure 25.4 Infantile polycystic kidney in the neonate – radially arranged cysts extending from cortex to medulla, producing a characteristic spongy appearance to the cut surface of the kidney

over the age of 1 year with no respiratory problems and only moderate renal impairment. Thus RPKD presenting with respiratory failure in the neonate with or without renal failure is not the uniformly fatal condition it used to be.

Large kidneys predominate in patients presenting outside the neonatal period. The distribution of this and other presenting signs compiled from these two series[15,16] is demonstrated in Table 25.5. Hypertension is a frequent and often severe problem in infancy. This sometimes manifests itself as congestive cardiac failure. It is surprising that none of the 128 patients in these two series presented with hypertension or congestive cardiac failure and certainly RPKD should be considered in the differential diagnosis of these problems in infancy.

Most deaths occur in the neonatal period. A further 10–20% of patients die before the age of 1 year. The outlook is surprisingly good in patients surviving to 1 year, with no deaths in one series (aged 2–23 years)[15] and 85% 10 years and 79% 15 years life-table survival in patients alive after the first year in the other series.[16]

With improving survival, liver disease becomes more important. Though hepatocellular failure occurs rarely if ever, approximately 50% of patients surviving beyond 3 months of age develop splenomegaly and at least a quarter of these patients eventually require portocaval shunts for portal hypertension. In patients presenting outside the first year of life, liver involvement may predominate – a condition sometimes referred to as congenital hepatic fibrosis.[2,13]

Pathology[2,14–16]

At autopsy the kidneys are considerably enlarged and appear to fill the abdominal cavity. They have a smooth surface with exaggerated fetal lobulation. The cut surface shows a radial arrangement of cysts extending from the subcapsular cortex. Larger cysts are seen in the medulla (Figure 25.4). The pelvis and ureters are normal. Histology, microdissection studies and lectin binding show the cysts to be derived from collecting ducts and lined mainly by flattened cuboidal epithelium or occasionally by hyperplastic columnar epithelium with polyp formation.

The liver may also be enlarged and show macroscopic cysts, but more usually there are only the histological lesions, termed 'ductal plate malformation', consisting of dilated and tortuous bile ducts in enlarged and fibrous portal tracts.

The kidneys in the older child may show

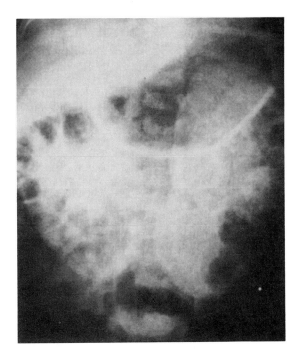

Figure 25.5 Infantile polycystic kidney disease – IVP appearance. Enlarged kidneys and diffuse mottled nephrogram. Other features not well shown

reduced numbers of cysts irregularly scattered throughout cortex and medulla. Blyth and Ockenden[17] have described a diminution in the percentage of tubules affected by cystic change with increasing age. Histologically there may be glomerular sclerosis, tubular atrophy and interstitial fibrosis to account for functional impairment. The liver shows increasing portal fibrosis with distortion of bile ducts – the histological picture of 'congenital hepatic fibrosis'. This may progress to portal hypertension.

Imaging in RPKD[2,13]

In the neonate, on ultrasonography the kidneys are greatly enlarged and retain their reniform shape with accentuated fetal lobulation. The myriad of diffusely spread microcysts are too small to demonstrate anechoic (cystic) areas, but provide innumerable reflective surfaces. This obscures normal corticomedullary differentiation and calyces so that a diffuse highly 'echogenic' (bright) appearance is generated. Liver involvement may or may not be demon-

strable. The IVP picture is almost pathognomonic. There is a delayed nephrogram; it may not develop for up to 24 h. The dye is then retained within the medullary and cortical microcysts producing a mottled nephrogram which may persist for 7–10 days. Dye is excreted so slowly from these cysts that the pelvicalyceal system is often not visualized at all and is always very poorly seen. Opacification of dilated cortical ducts produces radially arranged streaks of contrast medium in the outer portions of the kidney and in dilated medullary collecting ducts produce linear, brush-like medullary opacification, tubular ductal ectasia (Figure 25.5). There is debate as to whether or not IVP is required as well as ultrasound. The ultrasound merely demonstrates diffuse microcysts. The combination of this with IVP appearances is probably more specific to RPKD. We have seen one child with bilateral massively enlarged kidneys with typical bright echo pattern who had no evidence of liver involvement and in whom the IVP showed prompt excretion into a normal pelvicalyceal system. She remains with enlarged kidneys but normal function at the age of 5 years.

Though highly suggestive of RPKD the ultrasound and IVP changes are not absolutely pathognomonic. The most difficult differential diagnosis is the rare neonatal presentation of DPKD. This is virtually indistinguishable from RPKD (see below).[2,15] These appearances have been reported very rarely in normal newborns.[18] Familial hypoplastic glomerulocystic kidney disease gives an identical ultrasound picture.[13] In this condition the liver is normal and the renal function remains normal or stable into adulthood. Inheritance is autosomal dominant. The radiology must, therefore, be interpreted in the light of all the information available, including genetic, clinical and biochemical features and other organ involvement.

Appearances in older children are very variable, reflecting the evolving pathological process. With regression of the cysts the kidneys become smaller, and the typical appearances are lost. A mottled nephrogram is unusual beyond the age of 2 years. Thereafter the appearances will depend on the degree of renal impairment and the extent of persisting cysts. Occasional macrocysts up to 2 cm can develop in older patients which can be visualized on ultrasound and IVP, but they are never as large or as widespread as occurs in DPKD (or tuberous sclerosis). Tubular ductal ectasia remains and is a virtually diagnostic sign.[13] The diffusely bright echo pattern regresses, but medullary echogenicity is maintained with often small foci of very brightly increased echogenicity (simulating nephrocalcinosis) because of focal tubular cysts. The liver is enlarged with evidence of periportal fibrosis and decreased visualization of the peripheral portal venous vasculature. Macrocysts may occasionally be seen in the liver and pancreas. Splenomegaly is usually noted.

Clinical variants

RPKD has generally been referred to as infantile polycystic kidney disease because of its clinical presentation. Perinatal, neonatal, infantile and juvenile variants have been described. Blyth and Ockenden suggested that these were four more or less discrete groups and might represent four different mutant genes.[17] Subsequent reports have been almost equally divided between those reporting concordant expression in siblings within any one family, suggesting different genes and discordant presentation compatible with varying expression of the same gene.[2,15] This problem will probably only resolve when the gene(s) is identified. The use of RPKD to cover all these variants is much to be preferred and on available information it is not possible to predict how severely a subsequent child might be affected.

Autosomal dominant polycystic kidney disease

This is a common problem (for adult physicians), with estimated incidence between 1:200 and 1:1000,[13] and accounting for 8% of adult patients who require end-stage renal failure management in Europe.[19] It is transmitted as an autosomal dominant with almost complete penetrance by the eighth and ninth decade of life. The gene has been localized to chromosome 16, closely linked to the α-haemoglobin gene. This allows for presymptomatic even antenatal diagnosis in informative families (see Chapter 23). It has also led to the demonstration of genetic heterogeneity.[20,21]

Clinical features[2,13,22]

Many patients will have symptomless abdominal masses. The clinical problems which may develop include hypertension, abdominal pain, haematuria, proteinuria and chronic renal failure. With increasing use of ultrasound examination, cysts are being detected at an earlier age in children. Probably 10% of affected individuals demonstrate cysts by the age of 10 years.[2,22] By the age of 19 years, 95% of affected individuals will have cysts demonstrable on ultrasound. Symptoms rarely develop in childhood but have been reported.[22] Five per cent of affected individuals have symptoms by the age of 20 years. By the age of 35 years, 17% of patients have symptoms and 6% have developed uraemia. The liver is also involved in at least 30% of patients and occasionally portal hypertension is the major clinical problem.

Typically, symptomatic DPKD is an adult problem. The exception is the very rare severe neonatal presentation. More than 40 cases have now been reported.[2,15] There is no adequate explanation for this occasional severe neonatal presentation. The clinical presentation, clinical course and findings on imaging are virtually indistinguishable from early onset RPKD (see below).

Pathology

Macroscopically the kidneys may be asymmetrical in size, with an irregular distribution of small cysts throughout cortex and medulla. Histologically these are both glomerular and tubular cysts with intervening areas of normal renal parenchyma. Microdissection studies show that these cysts can be derived from any part of the nephron. The liver is involved in 30% of patients with DPKD. There may be occasional large cysts, but the usual histological appearances are those of groups of dilated bile ducts widely scattered throughout normal liver parenchyma. The lesion is much more irregularly distributed compared with the changes seen in RPKD and liver biopsy may be a useful diagnostic tool in distinguishing between the two forms of the disease. Cysts in other organs, such as the pancreas, spleen and lung, occur occasionally. The well-known association of berry aneurysms and cerebral arteriovenous malformations in adults is rare in childhood.

Imaging in DPKD[2,13]

Ultrasonography is a sensitive way of detecting the cysts, which are varying sized macrocysts spread throughout cortex and medulla of both kidneys. This typical appearance is virtually always present by the age of 19 years. Before then, cysts are initially absent and develop progressively. On IVP the cysts do not opacify but their presence is indicated by the stretching of the calyces.[3] Large filling defects can be demonstrated on a static renal scan. Rarely if ever is IVP or radioisotope scanning required, particularly in families known to have the DPKD gene. Although diagnostic in an affected family, the appearances are not absolutely pathognomonic and in sporadic cases other diagnoses should be considered. The appearance of similar cysts in tuberous sclerosis is a particular confusion, but the large macrocysts in this condition are present at a much younger age in children than the macrocysts of DPKD[2,10,13]

In the rare neonatal form the imaging appearances are identical to those of RPKD.

Differentiation between RPKD and DPKD

The typical presentations of RPKD and DPKD are so different that a clear distinction is usually easy. Difficulty in differentiation is considerably more complicated and may be impossible in the sporadic case with no family history, particularly in the newborn and to a lesser extent in the older child and adolescent.

The clinical and imaging features of RPKD and the extremely rare cases of DPKD presenting in the neonate are usually indistinguishable.[2,15] Localization of the gene to chromosome 16 is of no use in the single case with no other affected family members (see Chapter 23). An extended family history and clinical and ultrasound examination of parents and siblings is essential and might establish the diagnosis. It is surprisingly common for information about DPKD to be deliberately concealed in families and this should be borne in mind. If the parents are young, absence of cysts on ultrasonography does not exclude DPKD (see above).

Demonstration of 'biliary dysgenesis' by ultrasound of the liver is very suggestive of RPKD, but it cannot detect microscopic bile duct ectasia and the problem is further complicated by reports in DPKD of hepatic lesions resembling those in RPKD.[2] Liver biopsy is not advised, though typical liver involvement can be demonstrated. In the patient with a normal hepatic ultrasound, the liver biopsy may provide no information if the specimen is too small or superficial. Some authorities advocate a renal biopsy,[2] but this procedure has an increased risk in 'polycystic kidneys' and it is frequently difficult to identify the origin of the cysts. In our view, renal biopsy is even less helpful than liver biopsy. Thus it can be difficult and may be impossible to accurately differentiate between RPKD and DPKD in the neonate. From a clinical point of view this creates little problem, as both conditions have a very similar clinical course at this age. There are more problems from a genetic counselling viewpoint. Again these, though real, are not such a problem in practice. RPKD clearly has a 1:4 recurrence rate. Though DPKD has a 1:2 risk, recurrence of the severe neonatal presentation in the same family is uncommon. Thus all parents of neonates with 'polycystic kidney disease' should be warned of the risk of recurrence, and the risk of 1:4 of the *severe neonatal presentation* would seem reasonable.

RPKD and DPKD also overlap in late childhood and adolescence, though this is less of a problem. At this age in surviving patients with RPKD, the microcysts may have been replaced by macrocysts.[13] With increasing use of ultra-

Table 25.6   Differential diagnosis of cystic diseases in infancy (After Kaplan *et al.*[13])

Recessive polycystic kidney disease
Dominant polycystic kidney disease
Bilateral multicystic dysplastic kidneys
Cystic disease associated with tuberose sclerosis
Meckel–Gruber syndrome and variants
Zellweger cerebrohepatorenal syndrome
Jeune's asphyxiating thoracic dystrophy
Aneuploides (trisomes 9, 13 and 18)
Familial hypoplastic glomerulocystic disease

sound, 10–20% of affected children with DPKD can be demonstrated to have renal involvement by the age of 10 years.[22] Thus demonstration of macrocysts at this age does not distinguish between DPKD and RPKD. Full evaluation of the child and family as detailed above may again elucidate the situation. If this is unhelpful, the clinical situation is usually discriminating. In late childhood and early adolescence, even when cysts can be demonstrated in the kidney, the lesion is virtually always clinically silent in DPKD, whereas late presentations of RPKD at this age will almost always have evidence of renal functional decline and often signs of significant hepatic involvement.

Glomerulocystic disease

This is now recognized to be a heterogeneous condition.[23] Glomerular cysts are commonly seen in syndromic and non-syndromic forms of renal dysplasia, as an early manifestation of DPKD and perhaps as a sporadic case. Familial hypoplastic glomerular cystic kidney disease may be a more specific entity of some clinical importance.[13] They present more of a problem in differential diagnosis for the pathologist than the clinician.

Differential diagnosis of multiple renal cysts in infancy

The problem of differential diagnosis of multiple renal cysts[13] is predominantly one of the neonatal period and infancy. The 90% of cases of cystic dysplasia associated with urinary tract obstruction should present no diagnostic problem. Although there are innumerable multiple

malformation syndromes in which cystic renal disease can occur, only a small number are both frequent and cause severe renal involvement. Thus a manageable list of likely causes emerges which should allow for systematic evaluation (Table 25.6).

The problems of differentiation of RPKD and DPKD at this age have already been extensively discussed.

Bilateral multicystic dysplasia may have been suspected antenatally. Some features of the Potter's sequence will be evident. Patients usually have pulmonary hypoplasia and severe renal failure. This latter feature is uncommon (as opposed to severe oliguria) in RPKD in the newborn period. Absence of hepatic involvement would be another distinguishing feature.

Tuberous sclerosis is an important differential diagnosis.[10,13] In an infant with multiple macrorenal cysts, the diagnosis is almost certainly DPKD and tuberous sclerosis should be excluded. Other features of the syndrome are usually present if sought for or soon emerge.

Meckel's syndrome is characterized by post-axial polydactyly, micro-ophthalmos, encephalocele, cystic kidneys and hepatic fibrosis. It should be easy to recognize and may have been suspected antenatally if there was an encephalocele and/or a raised AFP. Partial expression may prove a much greater diagnostic problem.

Not only does Zellweger's syndrome exhibit characteristic features but there is now a specific biochemical test. The disease arises because of a generalized defect of peroxisomal biogenesis and in this context measurements of plasma very long chain fatty acids and the enzyme dehydroxy acetone phosphate acyltransferase are diagnostic. The clinical features in addition to cerebral, renal and hepatic involvement include skeletal abnormalities and severe hypotonia.

In Jeune's syndrome the narrow thorax, short ribs, stubby hands, cone-shaped epiphysis of the phalanges and trident-shaped iliac bones should allow for easy recognition. In some cases, however, rib cage anomalies may be relatively occult.

The chromosal syndromes should present no major diagnostic problem and additionally chromosomes should be requested in any neonate with unexplained cystic kidneys.

Familial hypoplastic glomerulocystic disease is difficult to distinguish from RPKD on ultrasound, but not only is there absence of liver

Table 25.7 Medullary cystic diseases

Medullary cycstic diseases
   Familial juvenile nephronophthisis and
   variants (AR)
   Medullary cystic diseases (AD)
   Medullary cystic lesions in inherited syndromes
   (usually AR):
      Bardet–Biedl syndrome
      Jeune's syndrome, etc.

Medullary sponge kidney

involvement but renal function which may be normal or impaired is preserved into adulthood. Inheritance is autosomal dominant.

Medullary cystic lesions

Here again there is confusion of terminology. Familial juvenile nephronophthisis (FJN), which is an autosomal recessive condition with onset in childhood, is sometimes referred to as medullary cystic disease. This latter specific term is better reserved for the adult condition medullary cystic disease in which the pathology is identical but there is onset in adulthood and it is dominantly inherited.[2,24] Unfortunately, medullary sponge kidney is also sometimes wrongly referred to as medullary cystic disease. A classification of medullary cystic lesions derived from Kissane[1] is given in Table 25.7

Familial juvenile nephronophthisis

FJN is considered to be an uncommon condition but as there are few specific clinical features, even with renal biopsy, the diagnosis is not always certain. It is likely that the condition is under-diagnosed. Some reports suggest that FJN may account for 20–40% of end-stage renal failure in children.[25]

Symptoms normally appear at 2–5 years, but may be delayed to 8–10 years. Polyuria and polydipsia are the most common presenting features and occur at an early stage when renal function is often relatively well preserved. Moderate proteinuria is often an early feature and this is usually of a tubular pattern with predominance of low molecular weight proteins such as β_2-microglobulin. Salt-wasting and hypokalae-

mia are usually present. Less commonly, other tubular problems such as acidification defect and amino aciduria may be present. Anaemia develops at an early stage in 30% of patients and growth retardation in 40–50%. There is gradual deterioration in glomerular function, with end-stage failure supervening by 10–15 years of age. An interesting and clinically useful association is the high frequency of red and blonde hair in these patients.

Pathology
The gross pathology and histological appearances vary with the stage of the disease. Renal biopsy in the early stages may show little or no change but in specimens received from patients in end-stage failure, the kidneys are markedly reduced in weight and size and show severe cortical atrophy. Seventy per cent demonstrate cysts at the corticomedullary junction and in the medulla. Microdissection studies show that the cysts are derived mainly from distal convoluted tubules and collecting ducts. Histologically, cysts are lined by a single layer of flattened epithelium and surrounded by abnormal basement membrane. By transmission electron microscopy there may be thickening, thinning or splintering of the basement membrane or a combination of these feature.[26] The cortex shows patchy glomerular sclerosis, severe tubular atrophy and interstitial fibrosis.

Imaging
Translucent cysts have been demonstrated on IVP using a high dose of contrast medium and tomography.[27] Renal arteriograms may also show lucent cysts and distortion of the renal arteries.[28] In the authors' experience neither of these features has usually been present and, as macroscopic cysts are not invariably present, this is perhaps not a surprising finding. In addition, contrast studies are often done at a stage at which renal function is severely impaired, further reducing the chances of demonstrating medullary cysts even if they are present. Usually, therefore, kidneys in FJN appear normal or small in size with smooth outlines and undistorted calyces. For the same reasons, normal ultrasound or CT scans do not exclude FJN. Ultrasound usually shows uniformly small kidneys but the microcysts in the medulla may produce a bright medullary echo pattern.

Associated malformations

Tapetoretinal degeneration is the most common association with FJN and is then described as renal-retinal dysplasia. This syndrome may have additional features with cerebral and cerebellar abnormalities. Hepatic fibrosis has been associated with FJN and there is a report of renal-retinal dysplasia and hepatic fibrosis occurring together in monovular twins. The authors have seen a child with tapetoretinal degeneration and hepatic fibrosis without clinically apparent renal disease. Some children have skeletal chondrodysplasia with or without ocular involvement. New variants of the disease[29] continue to appear in the literature.

Medullary cystic involvement in inherited syndromes

In some inherited syndromes with cystic kidney disease, the cysts are predominantly medullary so that the presentation of the renal lesion overlaps with FJN/MCD. The most important differential diagnosis is Bardet–Biedl syndrome (obesity, mental retardation, genital hypoplasia and polydactyly). Renal involvement has been reported with increasing frequency and is now considered to be a sixth cardinal feature of the syndrome.[30] One of the earliest manifestations of functional renal involvement is polyuria/polydipsia which may be so severe as to suggest nephrogenic diabetes insipidus. Varying degrees of renal glomerular failure have been reported which may or may not be progressive. The medullary cysts frequently communicate with the calyces (unlike FJN/MCD) and this is often demonstrated on contrast studies.

Different forms of predominantly medullary involvement with or without cyst formation are observed in other inherited syndromes, and this may be the predominant renal lesion in some cases of Jeune's syndrome.

Medullary sponge kidney

This is a developmental defect of distal collecting ducts in the medullary pyramids characterized by dilatation or ectasia and must be distinguished from the FJN/MCD complex.

It is rarely seen in childhood[2,31] and usually presents as an incidental finding on IVP or plain abdominal X-ray. Excretory urography reveals linear and saccular cystic areas of opacification within the renal pyramid. The cysts themselves are asymptomatic but symptoms may develop as a result of complications – calculus formation and pyelonephritis.

Most of the cases reported in the literature occurred sporadically, but there have been groups of children with a wide spectrum of congenital malformation in whom the typical radiological findings of medullary sponge kidney are found.

Simple renal cysts

Simple renal cysts are rare in children and especially in neonates. The majority of children are asymptomatic and present with an abdominal mass which is initially diagnosed as a renal malignancy or a duplication anomaly. A few patients present with enuresis, haematuria or rarely hypertension.[32,33]

IVP examination shows an avascular mass which may either bulge out from the kidney or be located more centrally, displacing the renal collecting system. Ultrasound of a simple renal cyst reveals an anechoic mass with a smooth posterior wall showing enhancement and is easily differentiated from the sonographic appearances of a tumour.

Treatment used to consist of marsupialization of the cyst or even of nephrectomy. Current practice appears to be cyst puncture to confirm the diagnosis, followed by yearly ultrasound evaluation. Surgery is reserved for those rare patients who may have associated obstructive urinary tract pathology.

Acquired renal cysts

Acquired renal cyst have been a well-recognized feature of native kidneys in adult patients with end-stage renal disease undergoing dialysis. In the larger series in the literature,[34] acquired cystic disease occurs in 35–47% of all patients on intermittent maintenance haemodialysis. Of these cysts, 10–20% show gross or microscopic 'adenomas', while 3–6% show 'adenocarcinomas'. There appears to be a direct correlation between the duration of dialysis and the subsequent appearance of cysts, epithelial hyperplasia and epithelial neoplasia. In a recent study in children undergoing long-term dialysis,[35] patients were evaluated by MRI and ultrasonography for evidence of acquired cystic disease. One-third of the patients had developed bilateral multiple cysts, one-third solitary cysts and one patient who had been on dialysis for 37 months developed multiple tubular adenomas in her native kidney. The study suggests that all children undergoing dialysis for more than 2 years should have regular evaluation by MRI or sonography for the detection of acquired cystic disease.

Antenatal diagnosis of cystic renal disease[2,13]

(This is discussed more fully in Chapter 23.)

In obstructive dysplasia the associated obstruction dominates the antenatal ultrasound findings. This is usually a serendipitous finding. The exception is the multicystic dysplastic kidney which is an important differential diagnosis of antenatal hydronephrosis. If unilateral, it may be difficult to distinguish from unilateral hydronephrosis. If bilateral, it presents as a differential diagnosis of severe oligohydramnios and the Potter's sequence.

Prenatal diagnosis of RPKD is possible but not reliable. The ultrasonographer must be aware that the enlarged bright echo pattern is the feature that should be sought not discrete cysts. Unfortunately this appearance develops after 22 weeks in 50% of affected fetuses. Differential diagnosis is as for the neonatal form of RPKD. No genetic markers are currently available. An increased amniotic fluid AFP, or trehalase, are non-specific adjuncts to diagnosis.

The severe neonatal form of DPKD may be detected by antenatal ultrasonography as with RPKD but given the extreme rarity of this presentation it clearly has no role in the systematic detection of DPKD. Molecular genetic techniques, however, allow for the accurate diagnosis in embryos only a few weeks old in informative families. The therapeutic and ethical problems produced by this are enormous, given the benign natural history of this condition in at least 85% of affected individuals for the first 35 years of life.

Routine antenatal ultrasound has resulted in the termination of many pregnancies at 16–18 weeks of gestation for 'polycystic kidneys'. The morphology of these fetal cystic kidneys may be extremely confusing. The presence of glomerular cysts is a useful distinguishing feature of DPKD. It should be clear, however, from the previous discussions that the overwhelming majority of these lesions are not 'polycystic kidneys' in the strict and accurate sense used in this chapter. This is an extension of the tendency to use this term to describe any multiple renal cysts. This should be avoided. Presumably most of these lesions occur for the various other reasons that give rise to renal cyst formation.

References

1. Kissane J.M. Renal cysts in pediatric patients. *Pediatr. Nephrol.* 1990, **4**, 69–77
2. Gagnadoux M.-F., Habib R., Levy M., Brunelle F. and Broyer M. Cystic renal diseases in children. *Adv. Nephrol.* 1989, **18**, 33–58
3. Greene L.F., Feinzaig W.M. and Dahlin D.C. Multiple dysplasia of the kidney with special reference to the contralateral kidney. *J. Urol.* 1971, **105**, 482
4. Vinocur L., Slovis T.L., Perlmutter A.D., Watts F.B. and Chang C.-H. Follow-up studies of multicustic dysplastic kidneys. *Radiology* 1988, **167**, 311–315
5. Hartman G.E. The dilemma of the multicystic dysplastic kidney. *Am. J. Dis. Child.* 1986, **140**, 925–929
6. Stuck K.J., Koff S.A. and Silver T.M. Ultrasonic features of multicystic dysplasic kidney: expanded diagnostic criteria. *Radiology* 1982, **143**, 217–221
7. Mentser M., Mahan J. and Koff S. Multicystic dysplastic kidney. *Pediatr. Nephrol.* 1994, **8**, 113–115
8. Mir S., Rapola J. and Koskimes O. Renal cysts in paediatric autopsy material. *Nephron* 1983, **33**, 189–195
9. Bernstein J. Renal hypoplasia and dysplasia. In: Edelmann C.M. (ed.) *Pediatric Kidney Disease*, 2nd edn. Boston, Little, Brown, 1992: 1121–1137
10. Bernstein J., Robbins T.O. and Kissane J.M. The renal lesions of tuberous sclerosis. *Sem. Diagn. Pathol.* 1986, **3**, 97–105
11. Al-Saadi R.A., Yoshimoto M., Bree R., Chang C.H., Sahney S., Shokeir M.H.K. and Bernstein J. A family study of renal dysplasia. *Am. J. Med. Genet.* 1984, **19**, 667–670
12. Kaplan B.S., Milner L.S., Jequier S., Kaplan P. and Chadarevian J.P. de. Autosomal dominant inheritance of small kidneys. *Am. J. Med. Genet.* 1989, **32**, 120–126
13. Kaplan B.S., Kaplan P., Rosenbert H.K., Lamoth E. and Rosenblatt D.S. Polycystic kidney diseases in childhood. *J. Paediatr.* 1989, **115**, 867–880
14. Kaarianen H., Jaaskelainen J., Koskimies D., Rapola J. and Norio R. Polycystic kidney disease in children: differential diagnosis between the dominantly and recessively inherited forms. *Prog. Clin. Biol. Res.* 1989, **305**, 55–59
15. Kaariainen H., Koskimies V. and Norio R. Dominant and recessive polycystic kidney disease in children: evalu-

ation of clinical features and laboratory data. *Pediatr. Nephrol.* 1988, **2**, 296–302

16. Kaplan B.S., Fay J., Shah V., Dillon, M.J. and Barratt T.M. Autosomal recessive polycystic kidney disease. *Pediatr. Nephrol.* 1989, **3**, 43–49

17. Blyth H. and Ockenden B.G. Polycystic disease of the kidneys and liver presenting in childhood. *J. Med. Genet.* 1971, **8**, 257–284

18. Stapleton F.B., Hulton S., Wilcox J. and Leopold G.R. Transient nephromegaly simulating polycystic disease of the kidneys. *Pediatrics* 1981, **67**, 534–539

19. Milutinovic J., Phillips L.A., Bryant J.I., Fialkow, P.J., Agoda L.Y., Denny J.D. and Rudd T.G. Autosomal dominant, polycystic disease: early diagnosis and data for genetic counselling. *Lancet* 1980, **i**, 1203–1206

20. Grantham J.J. Polycystic kidney disease – an old problem in a new context. *New Engl. J. Med.* 1988, **319**, 944–946

21. Reeders S.T., Germino G.G. and Gilespie G.A.J. Recent advances in the genetics of renal cystic disease. *Mol. Biol. Med.* 1989, **6**, 81–86

22. Sedman A., Bell P., Manco-Johnson M., Shrier R., Warady B.A., Heard E.D., Butler-Simon N. and Gabow P. Autosomal dominant polycystic kidney disease in childhood: longitudinal study. *Kidney Int.* 1987, **31**, 1000–1005

23. Bernstein J. and Landing B.H. Glomerulocystic kidney disease. *Prog. Clin. Biol. Res.* 1989, **305**, 27–43

24. Gardner K.D. and Bernstein J. Familial juvenile nephro–nophthisis: medullary cystic disease complex. In: Edelmann C.M. (ed.) *Pediatric Kidney Disease*, 2nd edn. Boston, Little. Brown. 1992: 1171–1188

25. Helin I. and Winberg J. Chronic renal failure in Swedish children. *Acta Pediatr. Scand.* 1980, **69**, 607–611

26. Cohen A.H. and Hoyer J.R. Nephronthisis. A primary tubular basement membrane defect. *Lab. Invest.* 1986, **55**, 564–572

27. Spicer R.D., Obb S.J., Saxton H.M. and Symonon J.S. Renal medullary cystic disease. *Br. Med. J.* 1969, **1**, 824–825

28. Mena L., Bookstein J.J., McDonald F.D. and Gikus, P.W. Angiographic findings in renal medullary cystic disease. *Radiology* 1973, **110**, 277

29. Gagnadoux M.F., Bacri J.L., Broyer M. and Habib R. Infantile chronic tubulo-interstitial nephritis with cortical microcysts: variant of nephronophthisis or new disease entity? *Paediatr. Nephrol.* 1989, **3**, 50–55

30. Frazick R.A., Leichter H.E. and Sheth K.J. Early diagnosis of Bardet–Biedl syndrome. *Pediatr. Nephrol.* 1990, **4**, 264–265

31. Patriquin H.B. and O'Regan S. Medullary sponge kidney in childhood. *Am.J.Radiol.* 1985, **145**, 315

32. Kramer S.A., Hoffman A.D., Aydin G. and Kelalis P.P. Simple renal cysts in children. *J.Urol.* 1982, **128**, 1259

33. Bartholomew T.H, Slovis T.L, Kroovand R.L. and Corbett D.P. The sonographic evaluation and management of simple renal cysts in children. *J.Urol.* 1980, **123**, 732

34. Welling L.W. and Grantham J.J. Cystic diseases of the kidney. In: Tisher C.C. and Brenner B.M. (eds) *Renal Pathology*, Vol. 2. Philadelphia, J.B Lippincott, 1989: 1250–1254

35. Leichter H.E., Dietrich R., Salusky I.B, Foley J., Cohen A.H., Kangarloo H. and Fine R.N. Acquired cystic kidney disease in children undergoing long-term dialysis. *Pediatr. Nephrol.* 1988, **2**, 8–11

26

The neuropathic bladder

A.R. Mundy

Introduction

It is essentially incorrect to talk about a 'neuro-pathic bladder' because in the vast majority of affected children the entire lower urinary tract is involved; indeed, in many, the urethral dysfunction is more important than the bladder dysfunction. It is more accurate, although rather more cumbersome, to describe the problem as neuropathic vesico-urethral dysfunction. Even then it is important to remember that there are often related rectal and genital dysfunctions in addition to the urinary tract problems.

There are many neurological causes of vesico-urethral dysfunction in children, such as sacral agenesis, dysraphism, transverse myelitis and trauma, but by far the most common is spina bifida. This chapter will therefore be directed principally towards the problems of spina bifida, but the principles of investigation and treatment can be equally applied to any other condition.

It is only in the past 20 years or so that substantial numbers of children with spina bifida have survived to show the urological problems to which they are prone. Initially the general policy of early back closure and the use of shunting devices for hydrocephalus produced a large group of children with multiple handicaps of which incontinence was but one and often a comparatively minor one. The more recent selective policy has meant that smaller numbers of children are surviving, but these have far fewer handicaps and the bladder problem is often the major if not the only problem.

Early on it was apparent that incontinence was not the only urological problem; a substantial number of children showed deterioration of renal function as well. Because of this and because of the problems of treating incontinence in a largely female population with a high incidence of physical and intellectual disabilities, there was a vogue for treating many of these children by urinary diversion.

It subsequently became apparent that urinary diversion was not a 'fit and forget' procedure. There was a high incidence of stomal problems but, more importantly, there was an alarming incidence of upper tract deterioration on long-term follow-up. The role of diversion began to be questioned.

Simultaneously, the application of sophisticated electromanometry to the lower urinary tract led to a more thorough investigation of bladder and urethral function and dysfunction and subsequently to improved methods of treatment for incontinence. The era for diversion therefore ended and selective treatment is now the aim, although there is now a new vogue which has replaced diversion in general esteem – intermittent catheterization.

Pathophysiology

We have four expectations of our lower urinary tracts:

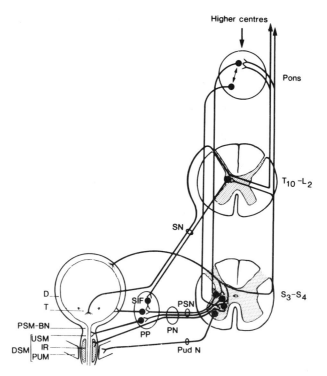

Figure 26.1 A concept of the structure and innervation of the bladder and sphincter-active urethra as described in the text. Key: D, detrusor; T, trigone; PSM, proximal sphincter mechanism; BN, bladder neck; DSM, distal sphincter mechanism; USM, urethral smooth muscle; IR, intrinsic rhabdosphincter; PUM, peri-urethral musculature; SN, sympathetic nerves; PSN, parasympathetic nerves; PN, pelvic nerves; PP, pelvic plexus; SIF, small intensely-fluorescent cell; Pud N, pudendal nerve (From Mundy,[1] by permission)

- that the bladder should fill to a good capacity
- that it should empty to completion
- that emptying should be under voluntary control
- that filling and emptying should not be detrimental to upper urinary tract function and thereby to renal function.

Any or all of these aspects may be deranged in neuropathy. As a result the affected child may present in one of two ways: with incontinence which is almost always present, or with impaired renal function which is less common but far more serious. The voiding dysfunction may be due to failure to fill adequately, failure to empty adequately or to a combined failure.

In health, the bladder fills to a good capacity partly because the viscoelastic elements of its wall allow filling, to a certain extent, without a corresponding rise in bladder pressure and partly because there is a neurological mechanism which controls the transmission of nerve impulses through the parasympathetic ganglia of the pelvic plexuses and therefore prevents the detrusor from contracting until voiding is voluntarily initiated. As a result, a normal capacity is accommodated with little or no rise in intravesical pressure.

This inhibitory neurological mechanism is poorly understood, but is thought to have two components – a 'gating' system such that preganglionic parasympathetic nerve impulses are not transmitted through the ganglia of the pelvic plexuses until they reach a critical frequency; and an inhibitory reflex which also inhibits ganglionic transmission at subthreshold levels of afferent activity, in this case via pelvic nerve afferents and efferents in the sympathetic nerves which seem to produce their effect by activating small intensely fluorescent cells (SIF cells) within the ganglia of the pelvic plexuses (Figure 26.1).

Throughout the filling phase urine is held in the bladder by the bladder neck sphincter mechanism (the proximal sphincter mechanism), which should remain closed at all times except when the detrusor contracts. Even if the bladder neck were to be rendered incompetent, by disease, by surgery, or simply by contraction of the detrusor, the urethral sphincter mechanism (the distal sphincter mechanism) should still be able to maintain continence. This sphincter mechanism has three components (Figure 26.1): the urethral smooth muscle which is innervated by the autonomic nerves of the pelvic plexus, the striated muscle within the urethral wall, known as the intrinsic rhabdosphincter which is innervated by somatic nerves which travel with the autonomic nerve supply, and the peri-urethral striated muscle, innervated by the pudendal nerve, which surrounds the urethra in the region of the intrinsic rhabdosphincter and which is part of the levator ani. In health, it is the intrinsic rhabdosphincter which maintains urethral closure under normal conditions (except of course during voiding) and this is supplemented under stress conditions by voluntary or reflex activation of the peri-urethral musculature.

When the bladder is full the child should be able to distinguish that sensation and go to an appropriate place to void or to defer voiding until the circumstances are more appropriate. Voiding is then initiated voluntarily by a simultaneous contraction of the detrusor and relaxation of the distal sphincter mechanism; indeed, urethral relaxation normally precedes detrusor contraction by a few seconds. It is this reciprocal and co-ordinated activity of the detrusor and the distal sphincter mechanism (particularly the intrinsic rhabdosphinter component) that is the hallmark of normal voiding and it is disturbance of this relationship which is the single most important factor in the vesico-urethral dysfunction of neuropathy.

Detrusor contraction is produced by impulses in the pelvic parasympathetic nerves which run from the (S2), S3 and S4 segments of the spinal cord to the ganglia of the pelvic plexuses and from there to the bladder. These impulses arise in the 'micturition centre' in the nucleus locus coeruleus in the rostral pons (Figure 26.1) which initiates detrusor contraction and coordinates it with sphincter relaxation. The supraspinal origin for bladder–sphincter co-ordination explains the frequency with which this co-ordina-tion is disturbed in patients with suprasacral cord lesions such as those found in many patients with spina bifida (see below).

In health, the pontine centre is only active (once bladder control has been acquired) when facilitated by the higher centres in the brain, as occurs when voiding is voluntarily initiated in response to an adequate afferent stimulus from the sensory nerves of the bladder and urethra. These sensory nerves are found in both the sympathetic and the parasympathetic components of the autonomic supply to the lower urinary tract.

Contraction of the detrusor causes opening of the bladder neck and voiding proceeds until the bladder is empty whereupon the detrusor relaxes, thereby causing closure of the bladder neck, and the distal sphincter mechanism resumes its occlusive role.

With this outline of normal function in mind (for a more detailed review see, for example, Reference 1), it will be apparent that failure to fill in disease may be due to:

1   A rise in intravesical pressure due to 'stiffness' of the bladder wall – called low compliance – due either to hypertrophy or fibrosis affecting the viscoelasticity of the bladder or to excessive neuromuscular activity.
2   Involuntary detrusor contractions – called detrusor hyper-reflexia – causing involuntary voiding. If sensation is deficient, this may be insensible; if sensation is preserved, the involuntary contraction will give rise to the symptom of urgency.
3   Incompetence of the bladder neck and distal sphincter mechanism – together called sphincter weakness incontinence – causing leakage of urine because of an inability either to resist involuntary detrusor contractions or, more commonly, to resist stress incontinence due to raised intra-abdominal pressure as on coughing, laughing, straining or changing position.

Similarly, failure to empty in children with congenital cord lesions may be due to:

1   Failure to generate a detrusor contraction of adequate amplitude or duration.
2   Failure of the distal sphincter mechanism (and particularly the intrinsic rhabdosphincter) to relax when the detrusor contracts. Commonly, the sphincter actually contracts tighter when the detrusor contracts – so-

Table 26.1   Incidence of urinary tract infection, vesico-ureteric reflux and outflow obstruction at different ages in children with neuropathic bladder dysfunction (From Mundy,[2] by permission)

	3 months	*1 year*	*5 years*
Infection	25%	50%	50%
Reflux	15%	25%	20%
Obstruction	10%	20%	50%

called detrusor–sphincter dyssynergia – so that little or no flow may be generated even with a very high voiding detrusor pressure. Sometimes the distal sphincter mechanism does not relax or contract but maintains a constant closure pressure against a non-contracting or poorly contracting bladder (here perhaps the urethral smooth muscle is an important factor). In this case the obstruction to voiding induced by straining or compression is called a static distal sphincter obstruction

These two types of obstruction can be very serious, particularly static distal sphincter obstruction as this is commonly associated with persistently elevated bladder pressures due to poor compliance (see below, 'Intermediate dysfunction').

3 Failure of the bladder neck to open when the detrusor contracts. This is very rare in neuropathic dysfunction and I have only seen it once, in a child with transverse myelitis. Far more commonly, failure of bladder neck opening is due to failure of the detrusor to contract.

In summary, the bladder may be of normal or low compliance; the detrusor may be acontractile or contractile (in which case it is usually hyper-reflexic); the bladder neck may be competent or incompetent; and the distal sphincter mechanism may be normal, incompetent or obstructive (in which case it might be either a detrusor–sphincter dyssynergia or a static distal sphincter obstruction). Furthermore, abnormalities in each of these four anatomical areas may coexist in any combination; and at the level of the distal sphincter mechanism, sphincter weakness incontinence and obstruction may both be present if the distal sphincter mechanism is of insufficient strength to hold urine in during the filling phase and also fails to relax during voiding.

These lower tract abnormalities and the neurological lesions that cause them often affect the upper urinary tract. About 25% of children develop vesico-ureteric reflux either because of denervation or outflow obstruction due to detrusor–sphincter dyssynergia or a combination of the two. Obstructive uropathy is usually due to detrusor–sphincter dyssynergia or static distal sphincter obstruction, but vesico-ureteric junction obstruction due to a thick-walled bladder and a large residual urine are other causes. The combination of detrusor–sphincter dyssynergia and reflux is particularly sinister – children with this combination inevitably develop impaired renal function if it is left untreated.

Finally, this is not a static situation (Table 26.1); the pattern of dysfunction tends to change with time.[2] Vesico-ureteric reflux tends to develop between 18 months and 3 years of age. Low compliance is variable in onset. Detrusor–sphincter dyssynergia is often not apparent until about 5 years of age and there is commonly a deterioration of vesico-urethral behaviour in the late teens. Overall the trend is for compliance, detrusor–sphincter dyssynergia and sphincter weakness incontinence to deteriorate.

For all these reasons – the complexity of the functional abnormality; the variable interrelationship between bladder, bladder neck and distal sphincter mechanism behaviour; and the changing pattern with time – an accurate diagnosis is impossible on the basis of symptoms alone. The lower urinary tract needs to be assessed objectively in each child, specifically to detect those at risk of impaired renal function, and this assessment needs to be repeated at intervals as the child grows to detect any change in the pattern of the dysfunction.

Assessment

There are three aspects to the assessment of a child with a neuropathic vesico-urethral dysfunction:

- the assessment of the child as a whole
- the assessment of the upper urinary tract
- the assessment of the lower urinary tract.

The child as a whole

Before planning investigation and management

it is important to assess the child as a whole. The management of the child will be influenced by the age, sex, type and extent of neurological lesion, intelligence, spinal deformity, obesity, mobility, motivation, manipulative skills and the degree of independence that the child has and is likely to have in the future. At one extreme there is the 'windswept' teenager with a severe spinal deformity, hydrocephalus and low IQ who is confined to a wheelchair, in whom a permanent indwelling catheter is likely to be the only realistic form of treatment for the urinary tract problem. Such a child will not require detailed investigation of the upper or lower urinary tract because the results are not likely to influence treatment. At the other extreme is the youngster with little or no problem except for the bowel and the bladder, but who may nevertheless be refused a place in a 'normal' school because of urinary incontinence. This is obviously a totally unacceptable situation and detailed investigation is therefore indicated so that specific treatment options may be sensibly and selectively applied.

The upper urinary tract

This is traditionally assessed by an intravenous urogram (IVU) and a blood urea. Unfortunately, although the IVU gives good anatomical delineation of the upper urinary tract, it gives little in the way of functional information, and repeated exposure to X-rays in the serial studies that the child is likely to require is undesirable. As a measure of renal function, the blood urea is also less than perfect. For these reasons it is useful to assess the child initially with an IVU, ultrasound and serum creatinine and then, because obstruction and reflux are the most likely upper tract problems that the child is likely to develop, to follow the child with serial ultrasound and serum creatinine measurements.

If the IVU shows the changes of obstructive or reflux nephropathy (or any other abnormality), then total renal function is assessed by measurement of the GFR using the ^{51}Cr-EDTA clearance method and differential function with a ^{99m}Tc-DMSA renal scan. If obstructive uropathy is suspected a ^{99m}Tc-DTPA renal scan will confirm and quantify the obstruction, and a comparison between scans performed before and after catheterization will differentiate outflow obstruction from vesico-ureteric junction obstruction when this is in doubt.

Assuming that any active cause of renal impairment has been excluded or treated, it is our practice to repeat the ultrasound and serum creatinine studies annually in most children. In those children with detrusor–sphincter dyssynergia who are at risk of developing obstructive uropathy, the studies are repeated 6-monthly; in those children with a GFR below the lower limit of normal, the ^{51}Cr-EDTA clearance is reassessed annually.

About 15% of children have upper tract complications at birth and, as shown in Table 26.1, this increases to about 50% by the age of 5, after which it stabilizes. Hence, early childhood is the critical period; those children who have passed the age of 5 uneventfully are unlikely to run into upper tract problems if they do not have a predisposing urodynamic abnormality at that age.

The IVU, and the DMSA or DTPA scans when used, is only repeated when a definitive episode such as outflow obstruction or some form of surgical intervention has taken place, or when indicated by an abnormal ultrasound or serum creatinine result.

The lower urinary tract

The lower urinary tract needs to be assessed for the presence or absence of vesico-ureteric reflux, urinary tract infection and filling–voiding dysfunction. These are traditionally assessed by a micturating cysto-urethrogram (MCUG) and by culture of a mid-stream urine specimen (MSU). Unfortunately, whereas these investigations will reliably detect reflux and urinary infection, they are little help in assessing the filling–voiding dysfunction. This is because the radiological configuration of the bladder (such as the so-called 'fir tree' bladder) is not a reliable indicator of bladder behaviour and because the static films of an MCUG are not applicable to the dynamic nature of the bladder problem. The most important factors in this respect are detrusor contractility, bladder compliance, sphincteric competence and outflow obstruction, and these can only be assessed reliably with synchronous radiological and intravesical pressure studies – in other words by video-urodynamics.

A video-urodynamic study is a filling and voiding cystometrogram with a synchronous video-MCUG. The two are simultaneously displayed on a television screen (and may be recorded on videotape for playback at a later date) and intravesical pressure changes may thereby be correlated exactly with the behaviour of the bladder neck and distal sphincter mechanism as assessed radiologically. For details about urodynamics in general,[3] in children in particular[4] and specifically in the neuropathic bladder in children,[5,6] the reader is referred elsewhere.

The timing of these investigations is related to their purpose. Assessment of the upper tract is intended to detect problems before they become clinically significant and should therefore be performed early and regularly. Assessment of the lower tract is less pressing: when incontinence requires treatment – usually just before school age – unless there is deterioration of renal function suggesting outflow obstruction. On the other hand, an early MCUG is likely to be required to look for reflux, and the addition of the intravesical pressure studies is no extra burden for the child if the facilities are available.

It is our practice to perform a urodynamic study when the child is first seen and to repeat it anually until the age of about 6 or 7 when the danger period for the upper tracts is past. We then restudy the child every 2 years thereafter until growth has ceased, unless there is a clinical indication to repeat the study in the interim.

To some extent the likely vesico-urethral behaviour can be predicted on the basis of three neurological signs, although direct correlation with the anatomical level of the lesion is poor. If the anocutaneous reflex is positive, then the detrusor is likely to be contractile, although the contrary does not hold so well; if anal tone is normal it is unlikely that there will be a severe degree of sphincter weakness incontinence, and if the child can voluntarily squeeze the examining finger, then there may be some voluntary control of continence; if perineal and perianal sensation is normal, then bladder and urethral sensation are likely to be normal. Indeed, if all three of these signs are positive, the child is likely to be among the 25% or so who will in time develop some semblance of normal control. This does not, however, mean that they will not be prone to upper tract problems – quite the reverse. Those with lesser degrees of incontinence are more likely to suffer outflow obstruction and therefore are more at risk than their incontinent counterparts.

Classification of the vesico-urethral dysfunction

Traditionally, neuropathic problems were classified according to the type of voiding pattern (e.g. the reflex or the autonomous bladder), the level of the neurological lesion (e.g. the upper motor neuron or lower motor neuron bladder) or hypothetical interpretations based on peripheral neurological signs (e.g. hypertonic or atonic bladder). The thinking underlying these classifications was concerned with effect on the *voiding* behaviour of the *bladder* of *complete* lesions of the *preganglionic parasympathetic* nervous system and took little or no account of incomplete lesions, of postganglionic parasympathetic or sympathetic nerve activity, of behaviour during the filling phase or of urethral and pelvic floor activity. To consider all of these factors with our present limited understanding of the relevant pathophysiology would produce a system of classification that was hideously complex and therefore useless. For this reason the current approach is based on the urodynamic findings[6] and the overall ability to hold and void urine.[7] In this system the lower urinary tract is regarded as contractile, acontractile or intermediate and in each group may exhibit storage failure, voiding failure, combined failure or, by contrast, balanced function.

Contractile dysfunction

In general, these patients have normal bladder compliance and normal bladder neck competence with no sphincter weakness during the filling stage and with involuntary high-pressure voiding due to a hyper-reflexic detrusor contraction trying to empty against an obstructive distal sphincter mechanism as a result of detrusor–sphincter dyssynergia (Figure 26.2).

Those children with incomplete lesions may have some sensation of bladder fullness or urgency and some ability to resist urine leakage by voluntary contraction of the pelvic floor. If detrusor–sphincter dyssynergia is not severe, these children will have balanced function.

Storage failure in the remainder is usually due to detrusor hyper-reflexia and voiding failure to detrusor–sphincter dyssynergia.

Acontractile dysfunction

These children usually have normal bladder

DETRUSOR PRESSURE

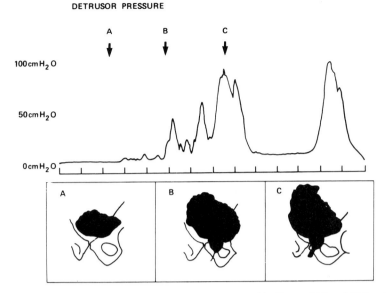

Figure 26.2 Contractile dysfunction – video-urodynamic features. (In this and in Figures 26.3 and 26.4, only the detrusor pressure trace is shown, although in an actual urodynamic trace, total bladder pressure, abdominal pressure, flow rate and filling volume would also be shown. The detrusor pressure is the most important parameter and is electronically derived from total bladder pressure minus abdominal pressure which are measured by catheters in the bladder and rectum, respectively). Detrusor pressure trace shows high amplitude swings in detrusor pressure (detrusor hyper-reflexia). Synchronous video MCUG shows initial bladder neck competence and trabeculation (A); opening of the bladder neck with a detrusor contraction (B); but failure of opening of the distal sphincter mechanism (C) due to detrusor–sphincter dyssynergia

compliance and little or no evidence of detrusor contractility at any stage. Incontinence occurs due to sphincter weakness (both the bladder neck and distal sphincter mechanism), but paradoxically during voiding induced by straining or abdominal compression there is often a relative obstruction due to static distal sphincter obstruction (Figure 26.3).

Storage failure is due to sphincter weakness incontinence and voiding failure to static distal sphincter obstruction or to ineffective straining or compression. Balanced function is found in those children with sufficient static distal sphincter obstruction to resist leakage during filling, but not sufficient to prevent adequate emptying by straining/compression.

Intermediate dysfunction

This is the commonest group with the worst bladder behaviour. These children tend to have poor bladder compliance and sphincter weakness incontinence during filling, causing a low bladder capacity, with ineffective low-pressure detrusor contractions causing voiding (Figure 26.4). The end result is usually a series of small voids off the top of a residual urine made worse by a variable degree of outflow obstruction at the distal sphincter mechanism – in this case static distal sphincter obstruction.

Storage failure is usually due to a combination of poor compliance, sphincter weakness incontinence and detrusor hyper-reflexia. Voiding failure is due to static distal sphincter obstruction. Combined failure is common and balanced function is rare.

Assessing bladder dysfunction when video-urodynamic studies are not available

Video-urodynamic studies are widely available and should be available to every unit which treats children with spina bifida and related problems on any scale. There are, however, some hospitals where these studies are not available and, even when they are, there are some paediatricians who are reluctant to use them in the very young. Although no child should ever undergo any form of surgical treatment without a full video-urodynamic assessment, it is quite

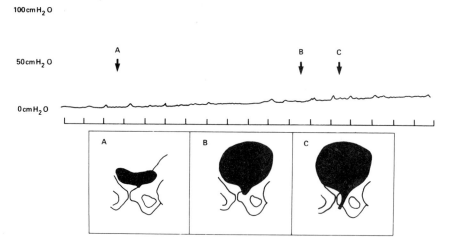

Figure 26.3 Acontractile dysfunction. Detrusor pressure trace shows no evidence of detrusor contractility. Synchronous video MCUG shows bladder neck incompetence with early 'beaking' of the bladder neck (A), which becomes more marked with filling (B). On coughing (or attempted voiding by straining), sphincter weakness incontinence occurs (C), but the urethra in the region of the distal sphincter mechanism fails to open adequately because of static distal sphincter obstruction

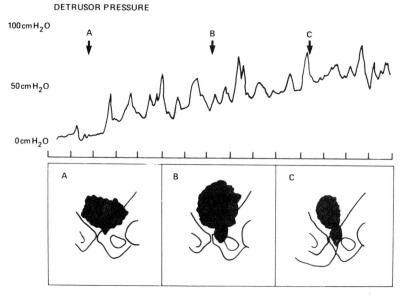

Figure 26.4 Intermediate dysfunction. Detrusor pressure trace shows a steady rise in baseline pressure (low compliance) and constant detrusor activity of varying amplitude. However, as distinct from Figure 26.2, this activity is poorly sustained and is therefore ineffective – it is sufficient to restrict filling but insufficient to produce voiding. Synchronous video MCUG shows bladder neck incompetence (A) which gets progressively worse (B) with detrusor–sphincter dyssynergia during detrusor contractions (C)

reasonable to start conservative treatment on empirical grounds assuming that ultrasound scanning of the kidneys (or any other investigation) shows no evidence of impaired renal function.

The correlation, albeit loose, between sacral reflex activity on physical examination and lower urinary tract function has already been mentioned. When combined with an ultrasound assessment of residual urine volume, and the statistical observation that 65% of children fall into the 'intermediate' group, 25% into the 'contractile' group and only 10% into the 'acontractile' group, these findings can allow a reasonably good guess as to what type of problem the affected child has and how to proceed.

Thus a child with a partial cord lesion, positive sacral reflexes and no residual urine probably has a 'contractile bladder'; a child with an extensive thoracolumbar lesion and a significant residual urine probably has an 'intermediate' bladder and should do well with clean intermittent self-catheterization; and a child with absent anal reflexes and a permanently empty bladder may well have an 'acontractile' bladder.

Management

The guiding principles of management are:

- that preservation of renal function takes priority
- that the vesico-urethral dysfunction should be treated according to the nature of the objectively demonstrated abnormalities
- that both of these principles should be interpreted and realistically applied in the light of the child's general neurological condition, as indicated above
- that infection should be controlled: the principles are the same as for urine infection in general and are specifically discussed in Chapter 14.

A plan of management is outlined in Figure 26.5 and shows the phases of management for each individual child. Phase 1 involves the identification and treatment of those with, or at risk of developing, impaired renal function (Figure 26.6). Impaired renal function is almost always due to outflow obstruction – either detrusor–sphincter dyssynergia in children with a 'contractile' bladder, or static distal sphincter obstruction in children with an 'intermediate' type, in which case the problem of obstruction is compounded by the persistently elevated intravesical pressures associated with poor bladder compliance.

In both types of dysfunction there is a higher than usual incidence of vesico-ureteric reflux which is generally attributed to the 'blow-out' effect of persistent obstruction. When present in association with obstruction, reflux accelerates the renal damage caused by obstruction. Urinary tract infection alone probably does not cause severe renal damage but will accelerate damage induced by either obstruction or reflux or both. Likewise, reflux in the absence of obstruction is not usually harmful and impaired renal function is therefore directly or indirectly attributable, in most children, to outflow obstruction. The preservation of renal function is therefore mainly the management of obstruction; this will be discussed below.

Phase 2 of management requires a decision as to whether or not incontinence is a problem that needs to be treated at the present time; thus the management of 'incontinence' in a 2- or 3-year-old child may be deferred until the child reaches an age at which the incontinence acquires a social or educational significance. When this applies, phase 3 involves the assessment of whether the child's general condition allows a selective approach to treatment. When this is unrealistic because of gross neurological, intellectual or skeletal problems, the incontinence is best dealt with by an indwelling catheter or, in boys, by sphincter ablation and the use of an external appliance or, in either sex, by a urinary diversion.

It is perhaps worth emphasizing that neither indwelling catheterization nor urinary diversion are always the simple solutions they appear to be. Both may be fraught with problems, particularly leakage around a catheter and stomal problems with a diversion.

Phase 4 assumes that the incontinence requires treatment and that a selective approach is possible (Figure 26.7). At this stage a urodynamic study is necessary to identify the urodynamic problems. The most important parameter in the first instance is bladder capacity and the main limiting factor in this respect is sphincter weakness incontinence as most other problems can usually be managed, at least to a degree, without recourse to surgical interference. Gross sphincter weakness, however, can only be treated surgically and usually the only effective method is by implantation of an artificial sphincter.

Having established that there is an adequate bladder capacity, phase 5 must ensure that this capacity is used to the full by ensuring adequate emptying. This may be achieved in one of four ways. In a very few children (and only those in the contractile group), a hyper-reflexic voiding contraction may be induced by various stimuli,

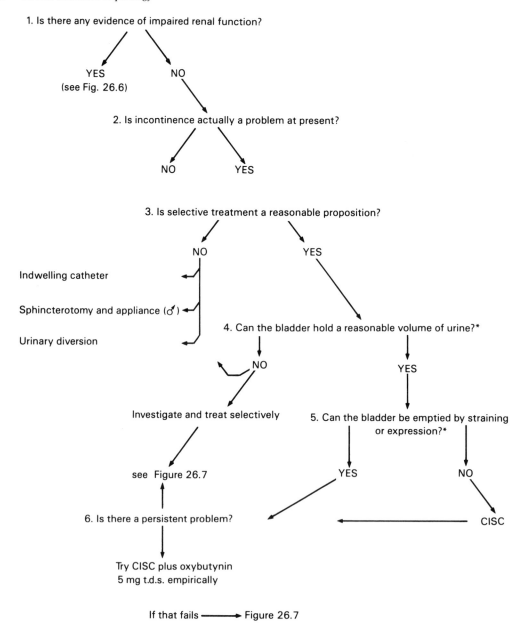

Figure 26.5 Scheme of management for the child with neuropathic vesico-urethral dysfunction – see also Figures 26.6 and 26.7 (CISC, clean intermittent self-catheterization). *Patients with partial cord lesions who have contractile bladders and preservation of sensation (see text), with frequency, urgency and urge incontinence, enter the scheme at these two points.

but even when a contraction can be induced in this way, voluntary control does not usually result. In the acontractile and intermediate groups, either abdominal compression or straining may be used. Straining requires normal abdominal muscles and the understanding

which is often lacking in the younger child; the disadvantage of compression is that it may be easy for someone else, particularly if the neurological level is above T12, but it is not usually easy for the patient unless outflow resistance is low, in which case bladder emptying is

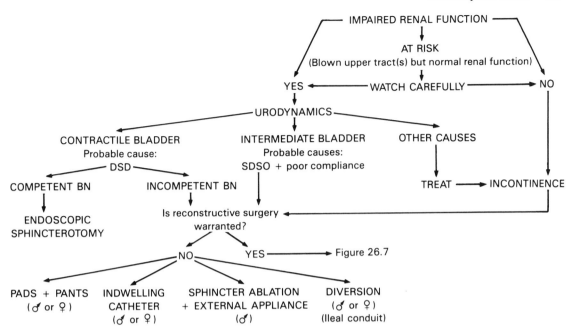

Figure 26.6 Management of impaired renal function – see also Figures 26.5 and 26.7 (DSD, detrusor–sphincter dyssynergia; BN, bladder neck; SDSO, static distal sphincter obstruction)

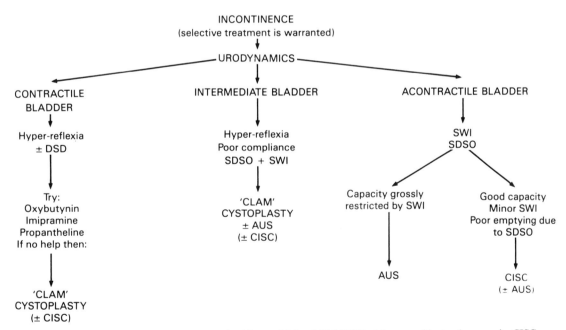

Figure 26.7 Management of incontinence – see also Figures 26.5 and 26.6 (DSD, detrusor–sphincter dyssynergia; CISC, clean intermittent self-catheterization; SDSO, static distal sphincter obstruction; SWI, sphincter weakness incontinence; AUS, artificial urinary sphincter)

not usually a problem compared with the sphincter weakness incontinence associated with such a low outflow resistance.

Finally, clean intermittent self-catheterization (CISC) may be used. This is currently in vogue and it is therefore important to recognize its limitations. To be regarded as effective it must be capable of securing 3 h (or thereabouts) of continence between emptyings by day, with minimal reliance on pads or nappies to absorb leakage, and should be a technique used by the child herself/himself to ensure independence. It is unfortunately all too common to see children on CISC who are catheterized 2-hourly and are still using 12 pads or so a day to keep socially dry. CISC is only really a way of draining off residual urine and cannot be expected to improve incontinence due to detrusor hyper-reflexia or sphincter weakness or to enlarge the poorly compliant bladder. Thus CISC is not applicable to many children because they lack the motivation and manipulative skills necessary, and not effective in many, usually because of either detrusor hyper-reflexia or sphincter weakness incontinence (which is the commonest limiting factor). Having said that, CISC must be regarded as one of the major advances in the management of the neuropathic bladder in recent years and for many children is the only way they are likely to achieve voluntary emptying.

It is important to stress that CISC is a clean technique and not a sterile technique, something that often goes unrecognized outside the hospital environment, and that the aim of it is to make life easier rather than more complicated. A home liaison nurse or similar individual is invaluable in helping to resolve difficulties or misunderstandings at home or school. The aim is catheterization with the minimum of fuss about 4 or 5 times a day. Night-time catheterization is not usually required and may be counter-productive. Small children have to be catheterized by their carers, but most children over the age of 6 can catheterize themselves and should be encouraged to do so to become independent. Physical handicap *per se* is not a bar.[8] A simple Nelaton-type catheter about 12 Fr in calibre or appropriate to the child's age, passed without preamble, washed after use, kept between times in a convenient container such as a freezer bag, and changed weekly, is suitable for most children.

At this stage, all of our original criteria for lower urinary tract function (to fill, to empty, to have 'voluntary' control and to be free of risk of renal impairment) have been satisfied to a degree. Phase 6 involves the correction of individual urodynamic abnormalities which may be limiting the response of the child to the

manoeuvres that have been employed so far. When treating these voiding dysfunctions, it is important to remember that a 'cure' is rarely possible. The best that is usually achieved is an improvement of incontinence from a socially unacceptable to a socially acceptable degree. The specific treatment modalities to achieve these aims are directed at the objectively demonstrated urodynamic abnormalities and, as these are often multiple, combinations of treatment modalities are often necessary.

In the child who is voiding by straining or expression, the reason for a limited response so far may be obstruction, either due to detrusor–sphincter dyssynergia or to a static distal sphincter obstruction, in which case the problem is a failure to empty properly, or it may be detrusor hyper-reflexia, sphincter weakness incontinence or poor compliance which all cause a failure to fill to an adequate capacity.

In the child using CISC, only the latter three problems apply. In such a child, outflow obstruction does not cause problems as long as the catheterization provides complete emptying; indeed, a degree of obstruction is an advantage because it reduces or abolishes the risk of sphincter weakness incontinence between catheterizations.

These individual problems will now be considered in turn.

Sphincter weakness incontinence

This is the most important reason for failure to achieve dryness without recourse to an appliance. Minor degrees of sphincter weakness incontinence may be helped by ephedrine 2.5 mg kg^{-1} day^{-1} in 3 divided doses, or phenylpropanolamine 2.5 mg kg^{-1} two or three times daily. For reasons given above, degrees of sphincter weakness incontinence and outflow obstruction due to static distal sphincter obstruction frequently coexist in children with 'intermediate'-type bladders, giving some a large residual urine. Improvement in bladder emptying (see below) will therefore sometimes help sphincter weakness incontinence when ephedrine alone fails.

Similarly, when sphincter weakness and obstruction coexist with poor compliance and elevated intravesical pressures in the 'intermediate' group, a reduction in intravesical pressure by drugs or surgery (cystoplasty – see below)

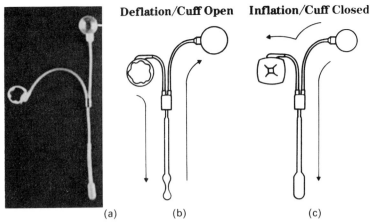

Figure 26.8 The Brantley Scott artificial urinary sphincter (AUS). This consists of a circumferential cuff that is placed around the bladder neck or bulbar urethra, a pressure balloon that lies extraperitoneally in the pelvis and a pump which lies subcutaneously in either the scrotum or a labium majus, all of which are fluid filled and connected by the control assembly which lies in the inguinal canal (a). The pressure inside the system is controlled by the pressure balloon and this is predetermined. In this way the pressure is kept inside a range of say 60–70 cmH$_2$O by choosing to implant a pressure balloon with this specific pressure range. This pressure is transmitted to the cuff which thereby occludes the bladder neck (or bulbar urethra) constantly unless the pump is squeezed. When the pump is squeezed 2–3 times, fluid is rapidly transmitted from the cuff (b) through the control assembly to the balloon and then slowly back from the balloon to the cuff through a series of delay-resistors in the control assembly until the occlusive pressure of the cuff is fully restored (c) – this allows about 3–4 min for the patient to void.

There is another model – the AS800 – in which the control assembly and the pump are incorporated into a single component, the control pump. The principle and the rest of the device are the same

usually improves continence, although simultaneously increasing the residual urine volume and therefore the need for CISC. If sphincter weakness persists in such patients, a bladder neck suspension procedure, like those used in adult women with stress incontinence, will often help.

For more severe degrees of sphincter weakness incontinence (when there is rarely a significant obstructive element), the only reliable method of treatment is implantation of an artificial urinary sphincter (Figure 26.8). This is now of proven benefit in selected cases,[9] although only available at present in certain specialist centres.

Outflow obstruction

This will almost always be due to either detrusor–sphincter dyssynergia in the contractile group or static distal sphincter obstruction in the acontractile or intermediate groups. Minor degrees of obstruction may respond to phenoxybenzamine 0.5 mg kg^{-1} day^{-1}, but not regularly or predictably, and the only effective way of treating the problem is by endoscopic sphincterotomy in boys or urethrotomy (which

does the same thing) in girls. This will almost certainly improve bladder emptying, but unfortunately it does not usually improve continence; indeed if the bladder neck is incompetent it will make incontinence worse. It is therefore only of use in those few children with 'contractile'-type bladders and marked detrusor–sphincter dyssynergia who have a competent bladder neck and in whom the associated detrusor hyper-reflexia can be controlled.

For this reason, much the best solution for most children is to use the obstruction to the child's advantage and to institute CISC to bypass the obstruction although, again, detrusor hyper-reflexia may limit the degree of continence achieved in this way.

Detrusor hyper-reflexia

This is usually treated with the anticholinergic drug propantheline 1 mg kg^{-1} day^{-1} in 3 divided doses. This is effective to some degree in about 50% of patients and the response rate can be further improved in many children by the addition of imipramine 1.5–3 mg kg^{-1} day^{-1} in 3 divided doses. The mode of action of imipramine is not fully understood, but there are

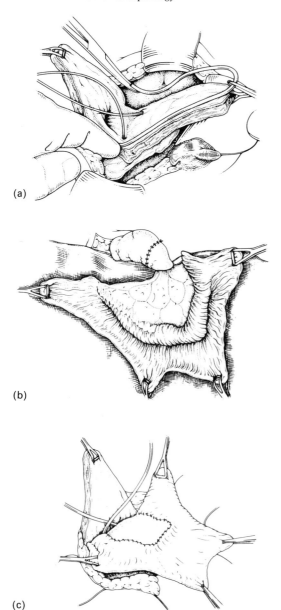

(a)

(b)

(c)

Figure 26.9 'Clam' ileocystoplasty: (a) the bladder is almost completely bisected in the coronal plane; (b) a segment of ileum is isolated and opened to form a patch; (c) the ileal patch is sewn in place to close the bladder (From Mundy,[11] by permission)

at least three separate effects on the lower urinary tract which make it a useful agent.

A more recent introduction is oxybutinin which, although widely used now, is still only obtainable in the UK on a named-patient basis. This is without doubt the most important phar-macological advance in the treatment of the hyper-reflexic and the unstable bladder in recent years and is a significant improvement on pro-pantheline, mainly because of its longer dura-tion of action. It is prescribed in children of 5 years of age and upwards at a dose of 0.2 mg/kg two to four times daily. It has anticholinergic effects and a papaverine-like action on detrusor smooth muscle, the relative contribution of each varying from patient to patient.

If oxybutynin fails to help, detrusor hyper-reflexia is readily corrected surgically by 'clam' ileocystoplasty, which is a form of augmenta-tion cystoplasty. Along with CISC, oxybutynin and artificial sphincters, this is one of the major developments in the treatment of the neuro-pathic bladder in recent years. The technique is illustrated in Figure 26.9. The crucial point is to bisect the bladder almost completely and then to interpose a section of ileum of the appropriate length, opened to form a patch, to close the bladder but to keep the two contractile halves apart and thereby prevent them contract-ing effectively. As with all treatments which suppress detrusor activity or otherwise reduce intravesical pressure, these goals are achieved at the expense of increased voiding inefficiency and an increased requirement for CISC as a result.

Poor compliance

This is a much more difficult problem to treat and usually occurs in association with a degree of superimposed detrusor hyper-reflexia in the 'intermediate' – type bladder. Drugs rarely help, but oxybutinin is worth trying. If this fails to help and particularly when persistently elevated intravesical pressure combined with static distal sphincter obstruction has led to the develop-ment of obstructive uropathy, 'clam' plasty ile-ocystois indicated, as for detrusor hyper-reflexia.

Other treatment modalities

Neurosurgical ablative procedures (such as sacral rhizotomy) for detrusor hyper-reflexia, bladder neck reconstruction, electronic stimula-tion for bladder emptying or sphincter stimula-tion, drugs such as carbachol, bethanechol or distigmine to improve bladder contractility, drugs such as dantrolene to reduce detrusor–sphincter dyssynergia and pudendal neurectomy are, as a general rule, useless. Techniques of electronic stimulation are helpful in some cases of neuropathic bladder dysfunction, principally following spinal cord injury,[10] but anatomical factors restrict their usefulness in most children with congenital cord lesions.

Bladder neck incision or Y–V plasty should never be used unless an obstruction has been objectively demonstrated to exist at that point in the presence of an adequate detrusor contraction. This is extremely rare. The widespread empirical use of these techniques in the past has meant that subsequent sphincterotomy to eliminate the actual obstruction (detrusor–sphincter dyssynergia) has inevitably caused total incontinence when this might easily have been avoided.

When these measures are inappropriate

The commonest reasons why one or more of these treatments is inappropriate are low intelligence or poor mobility – the greater the degree of incapacity, the greater the demand on continence. Whereas 2-hourly voiding is acceptable in a mobile child, it is unacceptable in a child confined to a wheelchair with multiple handicaps, because of the time needed to transfer to a toilet and back again. In such a situation, a permanent indwelling catheter for girls or a penile urinal for boys (after a sphincterotomy if any obstruction is present) is much the most realistic approach.

References

1. Mundy A.R. Clinical physiology of the bladder, urethra and pelvic floor. In: Mundy A.R., Stephenson T.P. and Wein A.J. (eds) *Urodynamics: Principles, Practice and Application.* Edinburgh, Churchill Livingstone, 1984

2. Mundy A.R. The prognosis of the neuropathic bladder in childhood. In: Brodehl J. (ed.) *Proceedings of the 6th International Symposium of Paediatric Nephrology.* Berlin, Springer Verlag, 1984

3. Mundy A.R., Stephenson T.P. and Wein A.J. (eds) *Urodynamics: Principles, Practice and Application.* Edinburgh, Churchill Livingstone, 1984

4. Koff S.A. and Mundy A.R. Urodynamics in children. In: Mundy A.R., Stephenson T.P. and Wein A.J. (eds) *Urodynamics: Principles, Practice and Application.* Edinburgh, Churchill Livingstone, 1984

5. Mundy A.R., Borzyskowski M and Saxton H.M. Urodynamic evaluation of neuropathic vesicourethral dysfunction in children. *Br. J. Urol.* 1982, **54**, 645–649

6. Rickwood A.M.K. The neuropathic bladder in children. In: Mundy A.R., Stephenson T.P. and Wein A.J. (eds) *Urodynamics: Principles, Practice and Application.* Edinburgh, Churchill Livingstone, 1984

7. Raezar D.M., Benson G.S., Wein A.J. and Duckett J.W. The functional approach to the management of the paediatric neuropathic bladder: a clinical study. *J. Urol.* 1977, **117**, 649–653

8. Robinson R.O., Cockram M. and Strode M. Severe handicap in spina bifida: no bar to intermittent self catheterisation. *Arch. Dis. Child.* 1985, **60**, 760–762

9. Mundy A.R. Artificial urinary sphincters. *Arch. Dis. Child.* 1986, **61**, 1–3

10. Brindley G.S. Electrical stimulation in vesicourethral dysfunction. In: Mundy A.R., Stephenson T.P. and Wein A.J. (eds) *Urodynamics: Principles, Practice and Application.* Edinburgh, Churchill Livingstone, 1984

11. Mundy A.R. Augmentation and substitution cystoplasty. In: Frank J.D. and Johnston J.H. (eds) *Operative Paediatric Urology.* Edinburgh, Churchill Livingstone, 1990: 77–94

General reading

Borzyskowski M. and Mundy A.R. (eds) *Neuropathic Bladder in Childhood. Clinics in Developmental Medicine No. 111.* London, MacKeith Press, 1990

27

Common non-obstructive urological problems

A.P. Dickson

Almost all common urological problems in children result from a malformation of the urinary tract. The development of the urinary tract is exceedingly complex and is therefore liable, in a similar way to the cardiovascular system, to developmental misadventure. Most of the serious anomalies which occur cause either obstruction or dilatation to develop in the urinary tract at some point (see Chapters 28 and 30). There are, however, a very large number of other abnormalities occurring in the urinary tract. Most of these are rather uncommon, but this chapter intends to cover the most common.

In these days of maternal antenatal ultrasonography, lesions which cause dilatation of the urinary tract are commonly suggested even before the child is born. Only some of the conditions which are to be discussed here fall into this group. Most are likely to appear in the postnatal period or early childhood or indeed not at all. One can do little to help the outcome of a cryptic lesion, but the early appropriate management of overt anomalies is a challenge to the paediatric surgeon, and essential for the good health and psychological welfare of the child also.

Cystic disease, dysplasia and agenesis of the kidney

(Cystic diseases of the kidney are discussed fully in Chapter 25.)

Renal agenesis

Renal agenesis describes a total absence of one or both kidneys. The condition is different from renal aplasia. Renal agenesis is the complete absence of any renal tissue; renal aplasia suggests a rudimentary kidney without normal structure and with dysplasia throughout.

Agenesis may occur as a result of an isolated failure of ureteral bud development or alternatively it may follow interference of the pronephric–mesonephric–metanephric systems and then be associated with partial or total absence of the genital duct system and of the gonads and adrenals. In keeping with this, in girls, a unicornuate or bicornuate uterus is common and aplasia of the vagina also occurs. In boys, anomalies affecting the external genitalia are seen. The condition may be unilateral or bilateral and the prevalence is about 1 : 5000[1] live births. In renal agenesis, the ureter on the affected side is usually absent or atretic.

Obviously bilateral renal agenesis is not compatible with a normal fetus. The child has a typical Potter's facies at birth[2] and is either stillborn or dies in the first few days of life from pulmonary insufficiency or renal failure. In the unilateral condition the other kidney is usually normal and may be hypertrophied. The condition is usually found incidentally on routine investigations.

Renal fusions and ectopia

Renal fusions and ectopia result following disturbance in renal embryogenesis. These include horseshoe kidney,[3] crossed renal ectopia[4] and pelvic kidney.[5]

Renal fusion

Renal fusion may be complete, the kidney presenting as a disc-shaped mass, or fusion can occur at the renal poles.

Polar fusion

Upper to lower pole fusion occurs in crossed ectopia where the crossed kidney lies below and medial to the normally sited one (see below). Fusion of the lower poles occurs with horseshoe kidney and presents characteristic pyelographic appearances. Both kidneys are situated at a lower level in the abdomen than usual, with the lower poles lying closer to the spine than normal. The lower pole calyces show an antero-medial rotation. The isthmus, formed by the fused lower poles, may sometimes be visible on the nephrogram phase of an intravenous urogram, but is best seen on DMSA radioisotope scanning. Horseshoe kidneys are more common in males, and show an association with various syndromes, including Turner's syndrome. This lesion commonly gives no problems but some-times can be associated with urinary infection, vesico-ureteric reflux and pelvi-ureteric obstruc-tion. The horseshoe kidney is rarely, if ever, obstructed by its isthmus, and it is rarely neces-sary to divide it.

Complete fusion

The fusion of both kidneys to form a single renal mass is most commonly found in a pelvic situation. The blood supply is abnormal and may be multiple, derived from the aorta and iliac arteries. Short subsidiary vessels may enter the renal mass posteriorly, while the major supply lies on the anterior surface. The renal pelves are anteriorly placed and are often intra-renal. The fused mass presents as a disc-like mass in the midline overlying the sacrum. The most important differential diagnosis is an ab-dominal tumour. The lesion itself may well be trouble free. Pelvi-ureteric obstruction, how-ever, is not uncommon on one or both sides. Furthermore, the short ureters may follow ir-regular courses to the bladder and are prone to

vesico-ureteric reflux and dilatation. As a result, urinary tract infection occurs.

Ectopia

Ectopic kidneys may occur anywhere from the pelvis to the thorax. They may be of abnormal shape and size with a vascular supply that may be multiple with accessory vessels entering the posterior surface. The contralateral kidney may be entirely normal or be totally absent.

The most common situation for a simple ectopic kidney is in the pelvis (Figure 27.1) where the ureter is short and the renal pelvis usually intrarenal. It may be of little clinical significance but this is not always so. Often the kidney is smaller than usual but it can be ap-proaching normal size, and present as a pelvic mass, requiring differentiation from a neo-plasm. Pelvic kidneys are often associated with other and multiple congenital abnormalities. Problems affecting the kidney itself include pelvi-ureteric obstruction and vesico-ureteric reflux with accompanying infection. Surgical reconstruction is therefore sometimes required and is often extremely problematical because of the difficult anatomy. Results of surgery are therefore often disappointing.

Crossed ectopia

This lesion is also associated with other distant congenital abnormalities. The occurrence of both kidneys on the same side of the abdomen is almost always associated with fusion of the two organs. The crossed organ lies below and medial to the normal one and usually shows an abnormal rotation (Figure 27.2). The ureter from the ectopic kidney crosses the midline and passes to the appropriate side of the bladder.

Both kidneys may be entirely normal, but in many there are hydronephrosis and infection and even stones secondary to lower tract abnor-mality such as pelvi-ureteric obstruction, reflux, posterior urethral valves and ectopic ureters. Many patients will therefore come to surgery.

Duplications of the upper urinary tract

Duplication is one of the most frequent urinary tract anomalies.[6] It arises as the end result of the development of an accessory ureteric bud which arises from the Wolffian duct and commu-

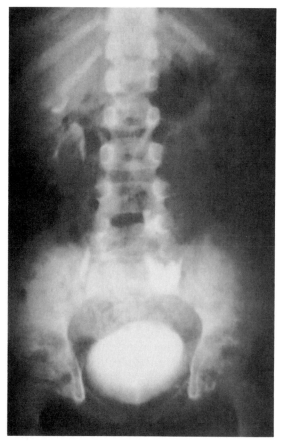

Figure 27.1 Normal right kidney with pelvic left kidney showing abnormal size, shape and rotation

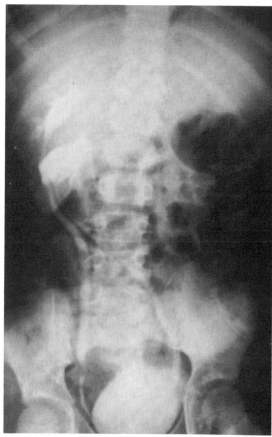

Figure 27.2 Left crossed renal ectopia showing polar fusion and abnormal rotation. The ureter from the ectopic kidney crosses the midline to drain into the appropriate side of the bladder

nicates with the metanephrogenic ridge cranial to the normal ureter. The condition carries a familial incidence and occurs predominantly in females. Although, in the majority of cases, both ureters and renal moieties function normally, the incidence of complications is high.

Varying degrees of duplication occur so that only the pelvis and upper ureter are involved, or the duplication may be complete with both ureters opening into the bladder (Figure 27.3). When the duplication is incomplete, the ureteric bifurcation is commonly over the sacroiliac joint, but may occur at any point along the ureters. Sometimes disorders of peristalsis occur at this site, so that urine passes from one limb into the other rather than down towards the bladder, and mild hydronephrosis may develop. Athough the vast majority of incomplete duplications require little specific therapy, the occur-

rence of recurrent urinary infection and/or pain may be indications for surgery. A low bifurcation is usually excised and both ureters are reimplanted into the bladder. Where the junction is at a higher level, it is preferable to convert the system into a bifid pelvis, by excising the upper pole ureter and anastomosing the upper to the lower pole pelvis.

When the duplication is complete, both ureters enter the bladder with the ureter from the upper renal moiety opening lowermost and more medially on the trigone. Reflux is the most common complication, affecting the lower pole ureter much more commonly than the upper. Sometimes the upper pole ureter is stenosed at its vesico-ureteric junction. Developmental dysplastic changes in the renal parenchyma often accompany primary reflux and obstruction in this situation. Minor degrees of reflux

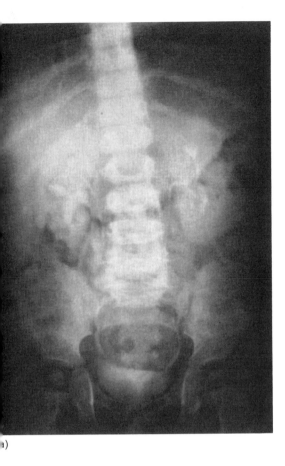

(a)

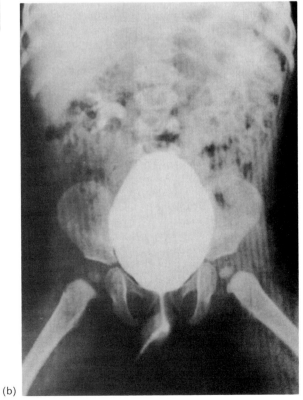

(b)

Figure 27.3 (a) Right duplex kidney and ureters with normal function of both moieties; (b) ureteric reflux into the lower moiety of duplex kidney demonstrated at cystography, showing a 'drooping flower' appearance

can be treated conservatively but ureteric dilatation, persistent infection and pyelonephritic scarring in the presence of reflux are indications for surgery. Obstruction is always an indication for surgery. If the renal moieties are well preserved a reconstructive procedure such as reimplantation of both ureters or uretero-ureterostomy should be performed. Heminephro-ureterectomy is indicated, however, for the severely scarred renal moiety.

Ectopic ureter associated with duplex kidney

If the ureteric bud arises from the Wolffian duct far from the normal site, then the ureteric orifice is not taken up into the bladder. It may then come to lie in the bladder neck area, in the posterior urethra, in the Wolffian derivatives in the male or the Muellerian duct derivatives in the female. More commonly, ectopic ureteric buds are accessory and the ectopic ureter is found in association with a duplex kidney.[7] The accessory ureter drains the upper pole of the duplex kidney. Its orifice may lie low on the trigone and may then be associated with normal anatomy and function. If it opens further away and is definitely ectopic in position, then the ureter is usually dilated and the renal moiety which it drains can be dysplastic.

Some ectopic orifices allow reflux, some are stenosed and obstructed, and others are associated with a ureterocele (because it is associated with an ectopic ureteric orifice the ureterocele is known as an ectopic ureterocele). All of these are liable to lead to dilatation of the ureter and renal pelvis and may therefore be suggested by antenatal scans and confirmed by postnatal investigations. If not, clinical presenting features include urinary tract infection and urinary incontinence. Sometimes, an ectopic ureterocele may present with acute pyuria, urinary retention from bladder neck obstruction, contralateral ureteric obstruction or prolapse of the ureter down the urethra to the vulva.

The diagnosis and assessment of duplications, ectopic ureters and ectopic ureteroceles demands the use of all available modes of urinary tract imaging. Ultrasound allows the initial identification of collecting system dilatation and ureteroceles, intravenous urography displays characteristic diagnostic signs of a dilated poorly functioning upper pole ('drooping flower') and ectopic ureterocele ('cobra's head'), and micturating cystography is essential because vesico-ureteric reflux is so common. Radioisotope scanning is extremely useful in assessing the function of the respective moieties of a duplex kidney, thereby giving guidance regarding the choice of operative intervention. (See also Chapter 28, particularly Figure 28.1.)

In most situations where the ectopic ureter of a duplex system is associated with either reflux, obstruction or ureterocele, the required treatment will be upper polar heminephro-ureterectomy because of the accompanying dysplasia of the upper pole. Very often this proves definitive therapy, even in the case of ectopic ureterocele, and no further intervention is required. Sometimes, when some reasonable function is preserved in the upper pole, it may be possible to reconstruct the situation using a ureteropyelostomy as previously described, a uretero-ureterostomy or a reimplantion of the ureters into the bladder.

Bladder diverticulum

A diverticulum of the bladder is a herniation of a pocket of mucosa through a defect in the muscular wall. Diverticula may be congenital or acquired. If acquired, they are secondary to infravesical or bladder neck obstruction (e.g. posterior urethral valves or neuropathic bladder), and their management is essentially that of the primary condition.

The congenital diverticulum is usually a solitary lesion with its neck high on the posterolateral wall of the bladder. The lesion usually occurs in males and is due to a developmental defect in the detrusor musculature. The sac wall consists of mucosa covered by compressed paravesical tissue, but a few muscle fibres are sometimes seen. Para-ureteric diverticula also occur, particularly in association with vesico-ureteric reflux of obstruction. In reflux they are said to mitigate against successful conservative therapy.

A large and narrow-necked diverticulum leads to a large amount of residual urine and predisposes to infection.[8] Other complications include stone formation and adenocarcinoma in later life. The diagnosis is made on cystoscopy or cystography, and the full extent of the lesion is determined at fluoroscopy on micturition. Definitive treatment is total excision of the diverticulum with repair of the muscular defect usually through the intravesical route.

Para-ureteric diverticula are dealt with during the definitive surgery for reflux or obstruction.

Bladder extrophy and epispadias

Bladder extrophy has an incidence of between 1 : 10 000 and 1 : 50 000 live births[9] and is twice as common in males. A familial incidence is rare. The condition is due to a failure of invasion of the cloacal membrane by mesoderm, so that the ectoderm and the endoderm are in abnormal contact in the developing lower abdominal wall. The unstable membrane subsequently disintegrates, so that the pelvic viscera are laid open on the abdominal surface.

At birth the bladder bulges outwards because of the raised intra-abdominal pressure. Exposure and infection rapidly lead to a thick fibrotic muscle layer and a polypoid friable mucosa which may later undergo squamous metaplasia. In boys, the penis is always epispadiac with a wide-splayed glans which carries a wide dorsal groove. The urethra is virtually absent, represented only by a strip of mucosa on the dorsum of the severely upturned penis (dorsal chordee). The scrotum is wide and shallow and the testes may be undescended. Girls also show epispadias with a hemiclitoris on each side, and the labia widely separated anteriorly. The pubic bones, in both sexes, are widely separated and the anus is displaced anteriorly.

Historically, the results of extrophy repair have been very poor. Total primary repairs have broken down, as have repeated salvage procedures. The end result was often a disturbed child with a very scarred abdomen, constantly leaking urine from a fistulated short upturned unpleasant penis. In addition, the kidneys became damaged secondary to high pressure, reflux and infection arising within a small non-compliant bladder. It is now felt that a normally functioning continent bladder is an unrealistic hope and aims of treatment should be to achieve a safe low-pressure bladder which can be drained by clean intermittent catheterization through a constructed urethra or a continent (Mitrofanoff) abdominal wall stoma.

A successful approach is therefore to close the bladder only, in the neonatal period, allowing the baby to pass urine easily through the epispadias at the bladder neck. This facilitates primary healing of the bladder wall. Later the severe epispadias can be repaired, and at the

same time the bladder can be augmented (cystoplasty) with bowel if its capacity is small or the intravesical pressure is high. Extremely useful additions to the epispadias repair, developed in London, include:[10] (a) the placing of vascularized omentum around the repaired proximal urethra, which aids primary healing and facilitates catheterization later; and (b) cavernocavernostomy, which is a direct anastomosis between the derotated corpora cavernosum within the shaft of the reconstructed penis, a manoeuvre which both corrects the severe dorsal chordee and lengthens the phallus significantly.

Epispadias without extrophy

The epispadias component may occur in isolation from extrophy. In this situation, the deformity may be confined to the penis and just affect the glans and/or shaft or may extend all the way through the proximal urethra and sphincters to the bladder neck. In the more distal deformities, repair involves creation of a urethra, usually from foreskin, release of the chordee, and perhaps later, some form of penile lengthening. Results are usually good in terms of function, and acceptable in terms of appearance.

In the severe forms of isolated epispadias, the approach is essentially the same as outlined above for the epispadias part of bladder extrophy. It is only in recent years that reports have appeared in the literature detailing successful repair of proximal epispadias deformity.

Hypospadias

Hypospadias is a common anomaly in boys, with an incidence of about 1 : 130 to 1 : 200 live births. It involves a combination of abnormalities, including a ventral situation of the external urethral meatus which can open anywhere on the ventral surface of the penis from the glans to the perineum, a hooded foreskin, and sometimes chordee which is ventral curvature of the erect penis, particularly distal to the meatus. In the most severe form, when the meatus lies perineally, care should be taken to exclude female pseudohermaphroditism, e.g. congenital adrenal hyperplasia.

In hypospadias, the urethral abnormality is due to failure of fusion of the urethral folds on the ventral aspect of the penis, and the chordee is due to bands of fibrous tissue (replacing the absent urethra and corpus spongiosum) anterior to the urethral orifice, lying centrally and expanding laterally and distally towards the glans over the ventral surface of the corpora cavernosum.

Hypospadias causes several problems:

- The abnormality is clearly visible and is therefore usually unacceptable.
- The urinary stream is usually diverted posteriorly because of the ventral situation of the orifice and often also because of a bar of tissue commonly situated on the distal edge of the hypospadiac meatus. This diversion of stream also affects the seminal fluid and may lead to difficulty with ejaculation, impregnation and resulting fertility.
- The presence of chordee during erection may severely affect sexual intercourse later in life.
- The primary abnormality and the resulting attention and surgery to the external genitalia can lead to long-standing psychological problems.

The management plan commences with early detection of the condition and parental counselling and reassurance. Sometimes meatal stenosis is present in the newborn and early relief may be required by meatotomy. Definitive management is clearly surgical and is planned for the second year of life, hopefully completed before the child will have established any long-term memory, thereby minimizing psychological sequelae. The surgical approach depends on (a) the position of the meatus, (b) the quality of the distal urethra, (c) the presence or absence of chordee, and (d) the quality and size of the foreskin.

There have been many operations described for hypospadias repair. Most situations, however, can be managed by one of two well-tried procedures. The Mathieu operation,[11] described early this century, lenthens the urethra using a meatal-based skin flap, raised from the proximal ventral surface of the penis. The flap is reflected distally and sutured to the distal ventral skin and glans. The glans is reconstructed around the neo-urethra to give an excellent cosmetic result. The abnormal foreskin is excised to give the appearance of a normal circumcised penis. This procedure is ideal for the common distal hypospadias without chordee and with a good penile urethra.

The transverse preputial island flap (Duckett) operation[12] is used if the meatus is sited more proximally than the distal third of the penile shaft, if there is chordee or if the distal urethra is of poor quality. This operation includes the denuding of skin off the penile shaft facilitating (a) the excision of chordee tissue, (h) the release of the distal urethra and, if necessary, (c) the excision of the distal urethra.

The neo-urethra is created from the inner aspect of the foreskin. The tubularized flap is swung round onto the ventral aspect with its blood supply maintained and anastomosed to the hypospadiac meatus proximally. Because this new tube is not attached to skin it can be tunnelled through the glandular tissue, thereby giving an excellent cosmetic result.

Both these procedures give good results in experienced hands and well-selected patients. The results of the Mathieu operation are optimal, complications occurring in less than 5%. The island flap repair may give an incidence of up to 30% local complications, including breakdown, fistula and stricture. Results of secondary surgery for hypospadias and its complications are unfortunately not as good, and all possible efforts should be made to ensure a successful primary operation.

Circumcision

Broadly speaking, there are three reasons for circumcision: religious circumcision, social circumcision and circumcision for medical indications.

Religious and cultural circumcision will go on as long as time. The ritual, even in Western countries, is still usually performed by non-medical personnel, and in the main there seems to be little in the way of severe complications which subsequently present to hospitals. Nevertheless, serious acute problems can occur, including haemorrhage, glandular injury, denuding of penile skin and urethral trauma. In the long term, meatal stenosis commonly follows neonatal circumcision. These problems may be more frequent than are commonly supposed.

Social circumcision is practised widely in America, but much less in the UK, Canada and Australasia. The pendulum of medical opinion has probably swung against routine circumcision currently, and it is performed less now than previously. The American Academy of

Paediatrics now supports this view and provides a brochure advising about the care of the uncircumcised boy.

Reasons suggested for routine circumcision include:

- Urinary tract infections: a higher incidence of urinary tract infection has been shown to occur in non-circumcised boys in several large American studies.[13]
- Prevention of common foreskin problems in childhood: local infection, phimosis and paraphimosis.
- Prevention of foreskin problems in adulthood: local problems requiring adult circumcision, increased risk of penile cancer, and the possible association of the foreskin with cervical cancer.

Circumcision, however, has complications and there is inadequate medical knowledge to support its routine practice for any of the above reasons. Proper care and hygiene of the foreskin prevent almost all the above local problems and it is important that parents are aware of this. Medical indications for circumcision vary from one surgeon to another. There is a view which suggests that almost all problems can be managed locally and the foreskin will eventually become normally retractile in the fullness of time without surgical intervention.

Balanitis xerotica obliterans, a primary non-infective aggressive fibrosis of the foreskin, is however always an indication for circumcision, as it is irreversible and causes discomfort, meatal stenosis and other local problems.

Any of the following conditions may also become indications for circumcision depending on their severity, and possibly the ability of the parents to care for the foreskin adequately.

Phimosis is a tight foreskin which cannot therefore be retracted. Most phimoses do, however, resolve in time provided that there is not fibrosis present and other local complications do not develop.

Paraphimosis is a most unpleasant and painful acute condition, caused by retracting a phimotic foreskin over the glans, so that the phimosis acts as a partial tourniquet around the base of the glans. This causes glandular oedema and swelling, making reduction of the foreskin extremely painful and very difficult. Sometimes, an emergency dorsal slit operation is performed to allow reduction. Subsequently, a circumcision should be performed to prevent recurrence, and should also be considered for cosmetic reasons if the foreskin has had to undergo dorsal slit.

Local infection (balanitis and posthitis) occurs usually, but not always, in association with phimosis and retention of trapped underlying smegma. Management of the acute infection is with systemic antibiotics and this is extremely effective. The infection is liable to recur, however, if normal local hygiene of the foreskin cannot be, or is not, maintained. In such a situation, circumcision is indicated. Local infection may also cause meatitis and meatal stenosis and in this situation also, circumcision is advisable. A single episode of balanitis should not usually be an indication for circumcision since, although a single episode is relatively common, further episodes are much less so.[14]

Undescended testis

The testis develops on the posterior abdominal wall close to the mesonephric ridge. Between the seventh and ninth month of intra-uterine life, it passes from an intra-abdominal position through the inguinal canal to lie in the scrotum. The incidence of undescended testes at birth in a full-term normal male infant is 2.8%. There is a higher incidence in premature infants. Further testicular descent occurs during the first year of life so that at age 1 year, only about 1% remain outside of the scrotum.[15]

Not all testes that are not palpable in the scrotum are undescended. The normal 'retractile testis' frequently lies in the superficial pouch in the groin. It can be clearly differentiated from the true undescended or ectopic testis because it may be manipulated with ease into the lower scrotum without tension.

The true undescended testis is thought to be held up in its path of descent and is then classified under the heading of 'incomplete descent'. It may lie intra-abdominally, in the inguinal canal or at the external inguinal ring. On the other hand, the testis may have come to lie in an 'ectopic' position, and should be searched for at the base of the penis (pubic), over the femoral vessels (femoral) in the groin crease, or laterally in the superficial layers of the abdominal wall. Very occasionally it may lie in the perineum where it will remain undiscovered unless great care is taken during physical examination.

The undescended testis may be associated with several complications. The processus vaginalis fails to ablate and may present as a hernia for which urgent treatment is required. The unusual position of the testis renders it unstable, and predisposes the testis to torsion. The higher environmental temperature of the undescended testis leads to impaired spermatogenesis in later life. Psychological problems may occur in late childhood or adolescence. Undescended testes carry a risk of malignant degeneration. The increased risk relates to the position of the testis, the intra-abdominal situation being the maximum risk. Sixty per cent of tumours are seminomas, but other types of tumour do occur including teratomas. Malignant change occurs maximally around the age of 40 years.

The management of the undescended testis is essentially surgical, although stimulation with chorionic gonadotrophin or luteinizing hormone-releasing hormone by nasal spray is sometimes effective. All children should be examined at birth and again at 1 year of age. Orchidopexy is best performed before the second birthday in order to maximize future fertility and minimize the risk of future malignant change. The surgery required at this age is technically demanding, and should only be contemplated by one with considerable experience in order to minimize the possibility of cord structure damage. Impalpable testes should not be presumed absent. The incidence of true anorchism is 3% for unilateral and 0.6% for bilateral cryptorchids. A definite attempt should be made by laparoscopy to locate the impalpable testis. High inguinal testes can usually be placed in the scrotum after full mobilization of the cord. The intra-abdominal organ will require either testicular transfer to the scrotum, based on microvascular testicular revascularization, or a staged orchidopexy following previous *in situ* division of the testicular vessels.

The acute scrotum

The acute scrotum is one of the commonest causes of emergency surgical admission of boys to hospital. The most frequent problems are torsion of a testicular appendage, acute idiopathic scrotal oedema, torsion of the testis and acute epididymo-orchitis, in that order. It should be noted that torsion of an appendage is much more common than torsion of the testis

itself.[16] (Other causes which may have to be considered include local trauma, incarcerated inguinal hernia and certain viral infections.)

Although there is an increasing tendency to manage the acute scrotum conservatively, most surgeons agree that all acute scrotums should be explored with the exception of acute idiopathic scrotal oedema, which is a scrotal rather than testicular condition and can easily be diagnosed as such. This condition is probably an allergic condition resulting from some unknown stimulus. Certain insects have been incriminated, but generally there is no history of insect bites and the predisposing cause is unclear. The important feature, as already stated, is that it is usually very clearly a problem of acutely tender oedematous swelling affecting the scrotal wall (but not the underlying testis) and extending into the groin and perineum. The condition is self-limiting within 48 h, although the use of antihistamine drugs may relieve the pain and swelling more rapidly. The possibility of generalized oedema, such as occurs in nephrotic syndrome, should be borne in mind.

Torsion of the testis is most frequent in the perinatal period and around puberty. Most commonly the testis twists on the cord inside the tunica vaginalis (intravaginal). However, perinatal torsion is usually due to a twist outside the tunica. Perinatal cases are often symptomless, the torsion having occurred prenatally. Clinically the testis is hard and the scrotum has a bluish colour. Torsion may occur bilaterally. Since the diagnosis is almost always made late, the opportunities for saving the testis are rare. Treatment is generally confined to orchidectomy and fixation of the contralateral testis.

In older children, the onset of symptoms is often gradual with abdominal pain and eventually discomfort in the groin and testicle. The testis is swollen and tender and is drawn up to the top of the scrotum. The testis becomes congested and, if unrelieved, will undergo infarction. For this reason it is wise urgently to explore all acute scrotums for fear of missing an early twisted testis which could be saved. It is often very difficult to differentiate between the different conditions clinically. Since the underlying anatomical abnormality which allows torsion of the testis to occur is usually bilateral, the contralateral testis should always be fixed to the scrotum.

Torsion of a testicular appendage (most commonly the hydatid of Morgagni) may present with either just modest local inflammation or a much more florid, red swollen hemiscrotum. Often the small black nodule is apparent on close inspection through the scrotal skin at the upper pole of the testis. Even if the diagnosis is clear and one can exclude torsion of the testis, it is still wise to operate and remove the appendage, as conservative watching tends to be associated with persistent local discomfort.

Acute epididymo-orchitis is extremely rare in children and is always secondary to either an abnormality of the lower urinary tract (e.g. posterior urethral valves, urethral stricture) or recent iatrogenic instrumentation of the bladder or urethra (e.g. cystoscopy or urethral dilatation). This condition should always be fully investigated because specific treatment of the underlying condition is usually required.

Anomalies of the female external genitalia

Labial adhesions

Fusion of the labia minora across the midline, obscuring the vaginal orifice, most often occurs congenitally and is noticed by the parents some time after birth. Occasionally it may not be noted until other symptoms such as dysuria, mild enuresis or diversion of the urinary stream occur. Occasionally, similar labial adhesions may develop after local vulval or vaginal infection. The best and most simple treatment is locally applied dienoestrol cream which usually separates the labia within 2 weeks. The adhesions can also be physically separated, but this is usually painful and causes distress to the children and their mothers. Furthermore, recurrent adhesions are more likely.

Hydrocolpos

Hydrocolpos is usually encountered at birth when the vagina is obstructed by an imperforate hymen or a vaginal septum situated at a higher level. Septal vaginal obstruction has a familial incidence, the anomaly being inherited as an autosomal recessive disorder. The vagina and, less frequently, the uterus and fallopian tubes are distended with a mucinous secretion from the fetal and vaginal glands. At birth the child is found to have a tense lower abdominal mass due to vaginal tension. Vulval examination often reveals a bulging membrane. This must be distinguished from a para-urethral cyst or a prolapsed ectopic ureterocele. Simple vaginal occlusion at the vaginal orifice is easily treated by incision and drainage. Higher septal vaginal obstruction requires vaginoscopy for diagnosis. Such complex forms require specialized management to avoid injury to surrounding structures.

Urogenital sinus anomalies

In this condition the urethra and vagina share a common terminal channel with a single opening at the vulva. Urogenital sinus stenosis is not uncommon and is associated with massive hydrocolpos and urinary tract obstruction. This anatomical situation is common to a number of diverse conditions. These include virilization of the female fetus, as in congenital adrenal hyperplasia, vulval obstruction with pseudopenis from fusion of the labial folds, female hypospadias with the urethral opening on the anterior vaginal wall, vaginal atresia with a wide urethra where the atretic vagina opens into the posterior wall of an incompetent urethra, and urovaginal confluence with absent bladder neck and urinary incontinence. Biochemical, radiological and endoscopic investigations allow differentiation of the various anomalies. Treatment is complex and should only be undertaken in specialized units.[17]

Genito-urinary malformations in imperforate anus

Almost all babies born with imperforate anus have associated genito-urinary anomalies. More than 90% of babies with so-called intermediate or high lesions (i.e. those without a cutaneous fistula) have a fistula between the rectum and the urinary tract in the male, or a rectovaginal fistula in the female. Almost 50% of babies with imperforate anus have other genito-urinary abnormalities quite apart from the rectogenito-urinary fistula itself.[18] The incidence and severity of other genito-urinary anomalies is directly related to the level of the fistula between the blind-ending rectum and the genito-urinary tract. High-level fistulae to the bladder neck in males and into the cloaca in females have a 90% incidence of associated anomalies, while lower-level fistulae into the perineum show only a 14% incidence. In addition, the presence of a

Table 27.1   Most common urinary anomalies associated with imperforate anus

Anomaly	%
Renal agenesis	18.0
Vesico-ureteric reflux	14.4
Neurogenic bladder	6.5
Renal dysplasia	4.5
Renal ectopia	4.1
Mega-ureter	4.1
Hydronephrosis	3.7
Ectopic ureter	3.7
Ureterovesical junction obstruction	2.5
Duplication	3.2
Ureteropelvic junction obstruction	2.5
Malrotation	2.0

lumbosacral anomaly greatly increases the risk of having a genito-urinary abnormality. Table 27.1 shows the most common major urinary lesions, renal agenesis and vesico-ureteric reflux being by far the most common. Some other non-listed lesions occur less commonly, as well as a wide range of minor anomalies including cryptorchidism, ureteral duplication and hypospadias.

The importance of proper urological assessment of children with imperforate anus cannot be over-emphasized. Commonly, abnormalities are missed early in life and the child presents much later with avoidable irreversible renal damage. All children should undergo ultrasound scanning of the urinary tract even before performing a colostomy or an early local perineal procedure. This simple procedure often gives useful information. Sometimes, however, the information is vital such as in children with a high fistula, including females with a single perineal orifice compatible with a persistent cloaca as well as all males with a poorly-formed sacrum and a flat perineum. It is important in these high malformations to be aware of the condition of the genito-urinary tract before the colostomy is fashioned, because sometimes these infants require some form of urinary diversion and this can be performed at the same time as the colostomy.

The children then require further urological assessment after the primary surgery. This includes mandatory micturating cystography in all cases, and intravenous urography and renography as required.

By defining the patients at significant urologi-

cal risk, it should be possible to minimize some of the serious avoidable complications by careful assessment and surveillance. Long-term follow-up is imperative because of the risks of late-presenting problems such as neuropathic bladder.

References

1. Emanuel B., Nachiman R. and Arouson N. Congenital solitary kidney: review of 74 cases. *J. Urol.* 1974, **111**, 394
2. Potter E.L. Facial characteristics of infants with bilateral renal agenesis. *Am. J. Obstet. Gynecol.* 1956, **51**, 885
3. Pitts W.R. Jr. and Muecke E.C. Horseshoe kidneys: a 40 year experience. *J. Urol.* 1975, **113**, 743
4. Hendren W.H., Donahoe P.K. and Pfister R.C. Crossed renal ectopia in children. *Urology* 1976, **7**, 135
5. Dretler S.P., Olsson C. and Pfister R.C. The anatomic, radiologic and clinical characteristics of the pelvic kidney: an analysis of 86 cases. *J. Urol.* 1971, **105**, 623
6. Barrett D.M., Malek R.S. and Kelalis P.P. Problems and solutions in surgical treatment of 100 consecutive ureteral duplications in childhood. *J. Urol.* 1975, **114**, 126
7. Stevens F.D. *Congenital Malformations of the Rectum, Anus and Genito-urinary Tracts*. Edinburgh, E. and S. Livingstone, 1963: 191
8. Johnston J.H. Vesical diverticula without obstruction in childhood. *J. Urol.* 1960, **84**, 535
9. Lattimer J.K. Extrophy closure: a follow-up on 70 cases. *J. Urol.* 1966, **95**, 356
10. Ransley P.G., Duffy P.G. and Wollin M. Bladder extrophy closure and epispadias repair. In: *Rob and Smith's Operative Surgery – Paediatric Surgery*, 4th edn. London, Butterworths, 1988: 620
11. Mathieu P. Traitment en un temps de l'hypospadias balanique et juxtabalanique, *J. Chir.* 1932, **39**, 481
12. Duckett J.W. Jr. Transverse preputial island flap technique for repair of severe hypospadias. *Urol. Clin. North Am.* 1980, **7**, 423
13. Wiswell T.E. and Roscelli J.D. Corroborative evidence for the decreased incidence of urinary tract infections in circumcised male infants. *Pediatric*, 1986, **18**, 96
14. Escala J.M. and Rickwood A. Balanitis. *Br. J. Urol.* 1990, **63**, 196
15. Scorer C.G. The descent of the testis. *Arch. Dis. Child.* 1964, **39**, 605
16. McCombe A.W. and Scobie J. Torsion of scrotal contents. *Br. J. Urol.* 1988, **61**, 148
17. Hendren W.H. Surgical management of urogenital sinus abnormalities. *J. Pediatr. Surg.* 1977, **12**, 339
18. Rich M.A., Brock W.A. and Pena A. Spectrum of genitourinary malformations in patients with imperforate anus. *Pediatr. Surg. Int.* 1988, **3**, 110

28

The dilated urinary system

D.C.S. Gough

Introduction and pathophysiology

Acute complete urinary tract obstruction causes effects which are rapid in onset with dramatic clinical presentation. Stimulation of stretch receptors in the wall of the urethra, bladder and ureter causes pain as the rise in pressure in the collecting system leads to acute hydronephrosis or hydro-ureter.

With acute unilateral upper tract obstruction, the kidney becomes enlarged, tender and hydronephrotic, with rapid development of interstitial oedema.

There is a decrease in renal blood flow, possibly caused by the rise in interstitial pressure, which makes imaging of the kidney difficult in this acute phase, and is responsible for the dense nephrogram and late pyelogram seen radiologically in this situation. Ultrasound seldom shows gross hydronephrosis with acute complete obstruction, unless there has been long-standing previous hydronephrotic change. The acute tenderness and pain make palpation of the kidney difficult, but the perinephric oedema causes a mass to develop in the flank.

Glomerular filtration is maintained initially by pyelovenous and pyelotubular back-flow of urine with evidence of enhanced reabsorption of sodium and water from the proximal tubule.[1]

Despite this reabsorption of urine, the kidney becomes tense, inflamed,[2] and the rise in interstitial pressure and decrease in renal blood flow leads to progressive nephron loss. Half the functioning nephrons will be dead within 6 days and all within 6 weeks if the obstruction is total and unrelieved.[3] This type of clinical presentation is a urological emergency as such rapid deterioration in function occurs.

Acute or chronic obstruction may be precipitated by trauma, with blood clot occluding the lumen, or the complication of infection in a partly obstructed system may lead to complete occlusion of the ureter, and pyonephrosis, which further adds to the urgency of the clinical problem.

Chronic obstruction, in which much slower functional deterioration occurs, may lead to presentation with the secondary effects of infection, features of renal insufficiency or stone formation. The pathological process which causes this type of obstruction is not understood, and almost universally affects either the pelvi-ureteric junction or the vesico-ureteric junction.

Urologists have difficulty in defining chronic incomplete obstruction and its natural history. There is therefore real disagreement about the diagnosis and the treatment of patients who have apparent upper tract obstruction of a chronic nature.

There would, however, be universal agreement on one point and that is that hydronephrosis is an inevitable consequence of chronic obstruction, and that hydronephrosis may well persist after the obstruction has been relieved.

It used to be thought that idiopathic hydronephrosis 'pelvi-ureteric junction obstruction' and idiopathic hydronephrosis/hydro-ureter 'vesico-ureteric junction obstruction' were chronically progressive conditions in which functional deterioration always occurred. It is now realized that hydronephrosis may well persist for years without any evidence of change in renal concentrating ability, or glomerular filtration rate, and therefore the place of surgery in these conditions has recently come under more close scrutiny (see below).

Clinical causes of acute urinary obstruction

Urinary retention

This is a situation common in adults but rare in paediatric practice. Because of its rarity and the lack of specific symptoms in small children, it can often pass unnoticed, especially where there is some urine overflow. Most of the conditions which cause acute obstruction are in fact quite rare, but in general paediatric practice the three commonest causes of acute retention in children are:

- gross constipation with pelvic impaction of faeces
- local genital problems such as balanitis, vulvovaginitis and ulceration of the meatus
- pelvic abscess following acute appendicitis.

Most patients with acute urinary retention therefore do not require extensive urological investigation which is only needed if a diagnosis cannot be made from the history, clinical and rectal examination. More specific urological problems can cause acute retention and, for convenience, are divided into those presenting in the newborn and then older child.

1 *In the newborn period*
     Posterior urethral valves (male)
     Hydrocolpos or prolapsing ureterocele (female)
     Pelvic tumours
     Spinal tumour with compression of the cord
     Traumatic delivery with spasticity
     Neuropathic bladder

Most newborn infants will pass urine within 24 h of birth, sometimes creamy coloured, and usually in small amounts. The symptoms of retention are sometimes missed until illness and irritability lead to a thorough clinical examination or serum is sent for biochemical investigation. In some patients with posterior urethral valves, the bladder is in fact small and not easily palpable, and it is only when the serum biochemistry returns, revealing hyponatraemia and uraemia, that attention is drawn to the urinary tract.

2 *In the older child*
     Male: Posterior urethral valves
                  Unrecognized or unadmitted trauma
                  Rhabdomyosarcoma bladder/prostate
                  Prolapsing ureterocele
                  Meatal polyp
     Female: Prolapsing ureterocele (Figure 28.1)
                  Trauma
                  Pelvic tumours, 'usually rhabdomyosarcoma'

Stone formation is not usually the cause of acute symptoms or retention of urine in Western cultures, yet bladder stone would be one of the commonest problems causing voiding difficulties in childhood in global terms.

Management

Once the diagnosis of acute urinary retention has been made, symptomatic relief and improvement in renal function can be obtained by passage of a urinary catheter. Adequate drainage can be obtained in the female with an 8 or 10 Fr. gauge Foley balloon catheter. The male urethra, however, especially in the newborn period, may be much smaller than this, and the passage of a fine 5 Fr. gauge feeding tube may be all that is possible. Silastic catheters should always be used to reduce urethral damage and lessen the risk of traumatic stricture. There can be difficulty maintaining drainage by this method in the male, and in general rapid treatment of the primary cause should be undertaken following resuscitation and improvement in the patient's fluid and electrolyte balance. Drainage of hydrocolpos or excision of a pelvic tumour leads to improvement in the baby's ability to micturate and catheter drainage can be discontinued within a few days of surgery. Prolapsing ureterocele from a duplex system can cause diagnostic difficulty, but with appropriate techniques of visualization, such as ultrasound and cystography, should become obvious as a potential cause of obstruction, and cystoscopy will confirm the diagnosis. Heminephro-ureterectomy will cure this condition, as when the secret-

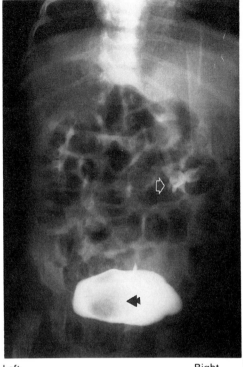

(a)   Left   Right

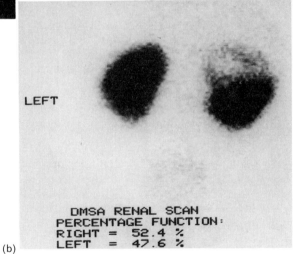

(b)

Figure 28.1 Duplication of urinary tract with ureterocele. IVU shows 'drooping flower' appearance (arrowed) (a) and filling defect in bladder – ureterocele. The poorly functioning upper pole supplying this moiety is not visualized on the pyelogram but is shown on the DMSA scan (b)

ing part of the kidney is removed, the uretero-cele empties, collapses and relieves the ball-valve effect on the bladder outflow.

The treatment of rhabdomyosarcoma of the urinary tract is beyond the scope of this chapter, but in essence modern management consists of biopsy to confirm the diagnosis, followed by

chemotherapy and radiotherapy to the lesion, rather than extensive surgical extirpation as an initial form of treatment.

Bladder drainage may be necessary for some weeks and suprapubic percutaneous drainage may be more comfortable for the patient during this time.

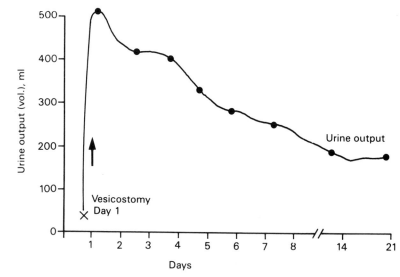

Figure 28.2 Daily urinary volumes in newborn with urethral valves following relief of obstruction. Diuresis persists for 5 days

Posterior urethral valves

Within the first year of life, the commonest cause of acute obstruction is congenital posterior urethral valves. This condition occurs only in the male, and there are two anatomical varieties:

- valve leaflets rather like venous valves coming off below the verumontanum in the posterior urethra (common)
- a circular diaphragm in the urethra below the verumontanum but above the urethral bulb (rare).

Urethral valves are a congenital malformation and may cause profound effects on the upper tracts and bladder during antenatal development with hydronephrosis, reflux and impaired renal function. Children present with an antenatal or postnatal diagnosis from the ultrasound department, or with clinical evidence of failure to thrive or renal failure in the first few weeks or months of life. Patients presenting in renal failure with obstruction usually have a palpable bladder and abdominal ultrasound which shows hydronephrosis. Hyponatraemia and metabolic acidosis are frequent findings in association with high creatinine and urea. Drainage of the urinary tract is important under these circumstances and a fine feeding tube is passed into the bladder and fixed to the penis

with adhesive tape. Antibiotics are begun immediately, as infection complicating this situation can be fatal. All such patients should be transferred to the care of paediatric nephrologists and urologists. Following relief of acute obstruction, there is a diuretic phase which lasts between 5 and 7 days, and obligatory salt and water loss occur needing careful monitoring during this period (Figure 28.2). Daily weight, serum biochemistry and estimation of urinary sodium loss are important factors in the careful management of these children.

The treatment of the urethral valves themselves will be dictated somewhat by the patient's basic condition and most acutely ill children will be treated with temporary urinary diversion through a urethral or suprapubic catheter.

Resection of the urethral valves is usually delayed until the patient's condition has improved. Surgical treatment in the newborn period may be cutaneous vesicostomy, endoscopic ablation through a cystoscope, or the use of a diathermy hook. Treatment is dictated by the size of the patient's urethra, and secondary urethral injury and stricture from instrumentation which is sometimes associated with direct endoscopic attack on the valves in the newborn period can be prevented by diversion, delaying valve resection until 6 months of age when these complications are then minimized. The combination of better surgical and medical treatment has led to an improvement in the results and the overall mortality is now 7.4% in the UK.[4] Careful continued follow-up of these children is mandatory and it may be anticipated that a number who survive with impaired renal function may well develop end-stage renal failure later, with early proteinuria being a bad prognostic sign. Subsequent renal failure will occur in approximately 7% of patients during childhood.[5]

Acute unilateral obstruction

The child presents with pain and frequently a mass lesion palpable in the abdomen. The admission may have been precipitated by trauma or infection, but the situation is clinically an acute one, and the obstruction complete or nearly so.

Calculi are not a major cause, but a plain X-ray can help with early recognition that this might be the case. The two basic lesions causing this problem are idiopathic obstruction in the pelvi-ureteric junction or the vesico-ureteric junction. The reason some patients present acutely with these lesions is not always obvious, but unrecognized mild trauma or infection may be responsible for precipitating an acute change in a chronically obstructed system. Sudden stress or fluid load is known to precipitate acute pelvi-ureteric junction obstruction in adults, and although rare, this form of intermittent obstruction can occur even in very small children. Ultrasound examination should be able to distinguish between obstruction at the upper or lower end of the ureter.

Initial conservative treatment with analgesics to relieve the pain, and complete bed rest, should allow spontaneous resolution of the acute obstruction in the majority of patients within 48 h.

Where infection in an obstructed system is suspected, or where the symptoms persist beyond 48 h, then drainage of the kidney is vital, allowing cultures to be accomplished and relieving the acute rise in pressure, and encouraging rapid return of function.

The way that drainage is accomplished depends on local circumstances, but in major centres it should be possible to do this percutaneously under ultrasound control or with radiographic screening. In some circumstances, formal surgical nephrostomy will still be necessary.

One significant diagnostic trap for the unwary is Wilms' tumour. This lesion can present with an acute pain from haemorrhage or small rupture of the kidney, and on clinical examination a mass lesion is discovered which is tender. Intravenous urography in this situation can sometimes show a mild to moderate hydronephrosis, and in the first MRC Wilms' tumour trial 3% of the lesions were initially thought to be hydronephrotic, and approached with this diagnosis, and incorrect surgery performed. What is important in this situation is to correlate the size of the mass lesion, which is often very gross, with the relatively small pyelographic size of the kidney. Further investigation with ultrasound should now prevent unnecessary exploratory surgery. In acute unilateral obstruction, once the patient's symptoms have been relieved, and the pressure in the system released, the urine should be cultured, and antegrade pyelography down the draining catheter will confirm the level of obstruction (Figure 28.3). Most patients do not require emergency drainage procedures as the symptoms resolve within 48 h, and renography and pyelography then confirm the anatomical site of obstruction and early surgery is planned. This clinical situation is nearly always obstruction at the pelvi-ureteric junction, and only occasionally at the vesico-ureteric junction. Surgical treatment can now be planned and proceed with relative safety once it has been established that the urine is sterile, and the function of the kidney guaranteed by drainage. Where treatment has been expeditious, and the lesion dealt with before infection supervenes, excellent functional recovery can be expected.

Chronic obstruction

Far more subtle and less easily understood are those patients who present with non-specific abdominal symptoms, urinary infection, or serendipitous ultrasound report of hydronephrosis. Before proceeding further, it must be realized that hydronephrosis is not a diagnosis, but a pathological definition, and there are four basic causes of this phenomenon:

- obstruction (Figure 28.3)
- vesico-ureteric reflux (Figure 28.4)
- dysplasia of the urinary system (Figure 28.5)
- high urinary flow.

Each of these conditions will require specific

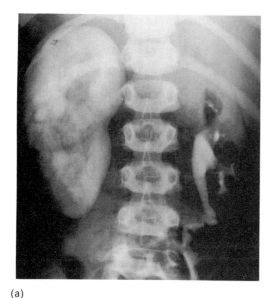

(a)

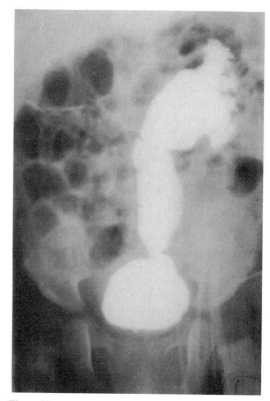

Figure 28.4 Grade 5 vesico-ureteric reflux causing hydronephrosis

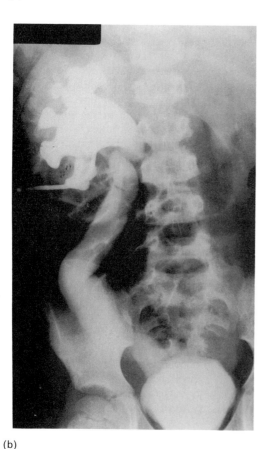

(b)

Figure 28.3 Acute upper tract obstruction. Delayed nephrogram (a) and subsequent nephrostogram (b) after drainage showing VUJ obstruction

diagnosis and exclusion with appropriate radiological investigation. There is still a tendency to equate hydronephrosis with obstruction, but this tendency must be resisted at all costs. A flow diagram which illustrates a method progressing to diagnosis of patients with hydronephrosis is shown in Figure 28.6.

The diagnosis of obstruction in these chronic hydronephrotic states is difficult and controversial, but rests essentially on appreciation of diuresis renography and contrast radiology. In some instances the use of antegrade pressure perfusion tests is added to the diagnostic armamentarium, especially where function is poor and dilatation great. Until the introduction of pressure perfusion tests for obstruction in 1973 by Whittaker,[6] or radioisotopes in the diuresis renogram by O'Reilly and colleagues in 1978,[7] there was no satisfactory technique, other than intravenous urography, for determining who might benefit from surgery. It was Whittaker who first showed clearly that dilatation does not necessarily mean obstruction.

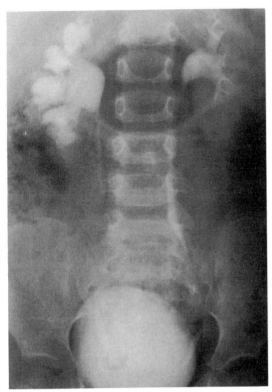

Figure 28.5 Hydronephrosis – non-obstructive. Calyces are blunted, but normal pelvis and ureter: megacalicosis

Despite its theoretical merit, the Whittaker test has not found great popularity because of its invasive nature, requiring needling of the collecting system for performance of the study. Contrast material is perfused into the renal pelvis at a steady rate and the pressure required to perfuse the urinary tract is measured. A bladder catheter is inserted to ensure free drainage. It is believed that the urinary system can normally accommodate 10–15 ml/min, without the pressure rising above 22 cmH$_2$O. Should the pressure rise above this level, then obstruction is thought to exist. General anaesthesia is required for all children, and the procedure takes at least 1 h.

Diuresis renography, however, has become the mainstay of diagnosis because of its relative clinical simplicity, and sedation rather than general anaesthetic is the usual form of preparation.

In children, careful technique is required in order to produce high-quality curves from the gamma camera; the patient must be still for at least 15 min if the isotope used is MAG3 or ^{123}I-hippuran, and for 30 min if DTPA is used. Unfortunately there is no standardization of this investigation, and therefore there would be differences of opinion about what the time activ-

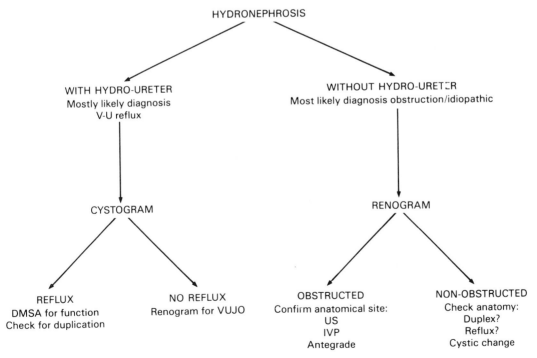

Figure 28.6 Flow diagram for investigating children with hydronephrosis

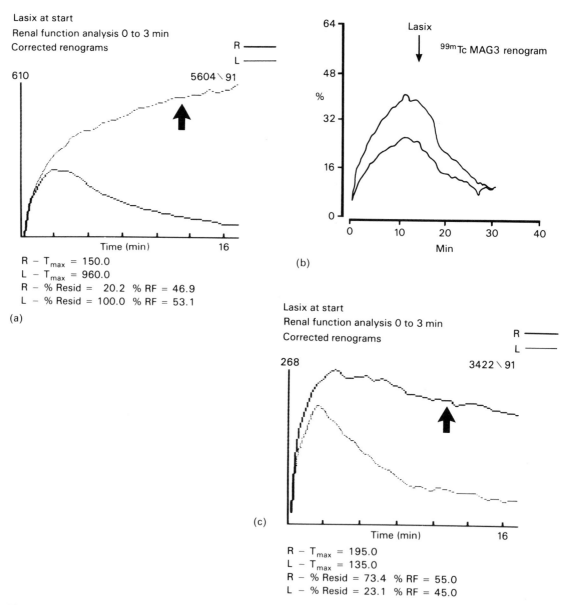

Lasix at start
Renal function analysis 0 to 3 min
Corrected renograms

R ———
L ———

610   5604 \ 91

R – T_{max} = 150.0
L – T_{max} = 960.0
R – % Resid = 20.2 % RF = 46.9
L – % Resid = 100.0 % RF = 53.1

(a)

(b)

Lasix at start
Renal function analysis 0 to 3 min
Corrected renograms

R ———
L ———

268   3422 \ 91

(c)

R – T_{max} = 195.0
L – T_{max} = 135.0
R – % Resid = 73.4 % RF = 55.0
L – % Resid = 23.1 % RF = 45.0

Figure 28.7 (a) Type 2 obstructive curve on renography, normal type 1 curve also seen; (b) type 3a curve, non-obstructive falling after Lasix, plus normal curve; (c) type 3b curve, slow fall with Lasix diuresis, plus normal curve

ity curves over the kidney actually mean. The normal curve (Figure 28.7), as designated type 1 by O'Reilly, is clearly seen in normal individuals, and type 2 is deemed obstructive. This type of curve is often seen in obviously symptomatic obstructions, and improves rapidly following relief of obstruction.

Equivocal washout from the kidney is seen in type 3a and type 3b curves, which are not

thought to be obstructive in nature, and our own work in children tends to confirm this fact. Equivocal results can be minimized by ensuring maximal diuresis during the performance of the renogram, by giving furosemide (Lasix) at the start of the test. Recent work suggests that giving Lasix 15 min before the start of the test[8] may minimize the number of equivocal curves seen in individual patients. It should also be remembered that poorly functioning hydronephrotic kidneys may not respond to Lasix and continue to show slow washout of isotope from the upper tracts.

If obstruction is suspected in the distal ureter or at bladder neck level, then considerable washout of the isotope from the upper tracts can occur into the lower collecting system during the study, and give apparently normal excretion curves over the kidney. This makes diagnosis of obstruction at these lower levels quite difficult.

A number of authors have compared the diagnostic accuracy of the Whittaker test and the diuresis renogram, and the general results of these comparisons suggest that they agree in about two-thirds of cases. Where they disagree there is quite understandably a lack of information about which investigation might be right or wrong, and a genuine dilemma continues to exist in some patients. Where the level of renal function is very poor in an individual kidney which is hydronephrotic, and particularly where the obstruction is thought to be distal in the urinary tract, most urologists would prefer the Whittaker test under these circumstances, in deciding whether surgical therapy was indicated.

It has always been encouraging to urologists that removing an anatomical obstruction usually causes the diuresis renogram or the Whittaker test to return towards normal, and that this is especially true where the level of obstruction is at the pelvi-ureteric junction.

Despite almost incessant investigation, the common sites of obstruction such as the pelviureteric and the vesico-ureteric junction remain areas full of mystery, and all attempts to create animal models of progressive chronic obstruction that is apparently seen in humans seem doomed to failure, limiting research potential. Acute complete obstruction is a readily identifiable condition whose clinical and pathological effects are well known and reproducible in the experimental animal. Yet at the other end of the spectrum, the silent asymptomatic incomplete obstruction sometimes takes decades to cause its deleterious effects.

Evidence that the natural history of these conditions is not always progressive has recently come to light, and in many instances spontaneous improvement can occur, particularly in patients diagnosed antenatally. Careful audit of surgical results has further identified areas where complication rates of treatment are higher than we would wish, and perhaps surgical treatment is not always indicated.

Difficulties in diagnosis can be emphasized by studying the two most common clinical situations, that of idiopathic hydronephrosis, pelviureteric junction (PU) 'obstruction' and idiopathic mega-ureter or vesico-ureteric junction 'obstruction'.

Pelvi-ureteric junction obstruction

Where the patient presents with pain and intermittent hydronephrosis, there is no doubt that surgery will relieve the symptoms, and improve the radiological appearance and often the functional contribution of the kidney on renography (Figure 28.8). The intravenous urogram may still look abnormal after surgical treatment because of chronic change, but the absence of symptoms postoperatively confirms the value of surgical treatment. When the patient presents without apparent symptoms, it would be helpful to know the natural history of the condition and the long-term results of treatment. Roberts reviewed some 200 patients with this particular anatomical abnormality, in order to discern the natural history.[9] Of the 30 cases in which the diagnosis was made at post mortem, half the patients had severe parenchymal damage, with calculi being found in 4 kidneys. The cause of death was renal in 10% of these patients. It was clear that the majority of cases eventually gave rise to symptoms of pain, haematuria or dysuria, although infection was unusual. Of 26 patients treated expectantly, only 6 had no progression of the disease, and in 10 patients severe renal damage occurred within 1–3 years. One can therefore deduce that in this particular anatomical site, obstruction produces progressive changes in the kidney which eventually will lead to symptoms, parenchymal damage and the complications of obstruction in the majority of patients.

What is unpredictable is the speed with which all this will occur, but once glomerular damage has occurred, relief of obstruction is most unlikely to cause any measurable improvement in glomerular function. Can surgery influence the natural history? Long-term studies of the effects of pyeloplasty have been performed in adults, which show that in general the natural course of deterioration is halted, and symptoms relieved.[10] The clinician is therefore on relatively solid ground when a diagnosis of idiopathic hydronephrosis is made, and there is no doubt that pyeloplasty is the treatment of choice, and can be

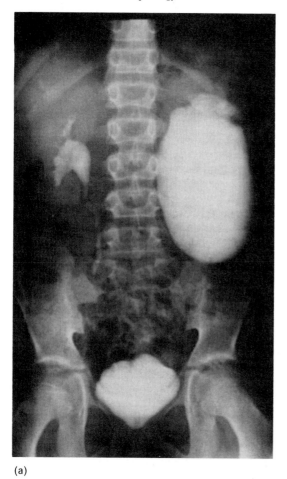

(a)

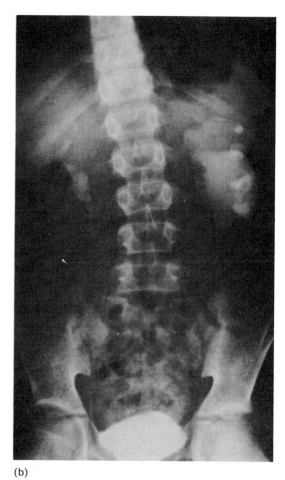

(b)

Figure 28.8 (a) Symptomatic pelvi-ureteric junction obstruction – preoperative IVU; (b) post pyeloplasty – symptom free

expected to improve the patient's symptoms and the prognosis for the kidney. In most series, about 10% of patients have a nephrectomy rather than a reconstruction, as functional impairment of the kidney has reached such a level as to render the kidney practically useless. Where the DMSA scan shows that the kidney has 10% or less of the total renal function, then nephrectomy would usually be indicated, although depressed function on MAG3 or ^{123}I-hippuran renography may well improve after surgical treatment.

The surgical complication of reconstruction of the pelvi-ureteric junction is low. In our own series of 110 cases, only 1 patient required reoperation. Following pyeloplasty, a dynamic scan 6 months after treatment should usually show a dramatic improvement in the drainage pattern of the kidney, and if it does not, would signal the need for further studies, such as an antegrade pyelogram or Whittaker test.

Where no clear evidence of obstruction exists on renography or pressure perfusion tests, and vesico-ureteric reflux has been excluded on cystography, and the patient is asymptomatic, it would be foolish to recommend surgical treatment. Such patients are labelled as having idiopathic non-obstructive hydronephrosis, and managed conservatively with ultrasound follow-up.

If the diagnosis of apparent pelvi-ureteric junction obstruction has been made antenatally, further evidence of hydronephrosis should be obtained postnatally, and imaging of the kidney undertaken to confirm the anatomical site of the apparent obstruction. When intravenous urography is used to confirm the ultrasound report, 10% have normal upper tracts.

Most authors looking after such patients find that idiopathic hydronephrosis frequently resolves after birth without surgical intervention and in our own experience more than half do not require any form of surgical intervention.

This topic is covered in greater detail in Chapter 30.

Vesico-ureteric junction obstruction

This is a much rarer lesion in childhood practice, and therefore obstruction at the vesico-ureteric junction causing hydronephrosis and hydro-ureter often presenting with infection has not been the subject of such detailed investigation. It has been realized for many years that the apparent obstructed mega-ureter is a relatively benign condition in adults, yet children in whom this problem was identified seldom escaped surgery because they usually presented with urinary tract infection, and often pyonephrosis. The lesion was usually managed surgically by excision of the stenotic end of the ureter, reimplantation of the widened ureter in the bladder with some form of anti-reflux procedure. Where a very large bulky ureter was encountered, it has been difficult to reimplant the ureter in the bladder without leaving the patient subject to vesico-ureteric reflux, and there have been significant complication rates in dealing with mega-ureters. Some surgeons rely on implanting a large ureter in a long submucosal tunnel, but others recommend folding of the ureter before reimplanting and Hendren popularized the surgical excision and tapering of ureters. Each method has its advocates and complications, and persistent vesico-ureteric reflux occurs in at best 5% of each group, and the hydronephrosis deteriorates in approximately 10% of those who have tapering of the ureter surgically performed.

The results of surgery are generally good for this lesion,[11] but as might be anticipated, the large chronically obstructed kidney with parenchymal damage and gross dilatation of the ureter is going to be the case which functions poorly in the long term and may well be the subject of continued infection.

Recent experience with apparent vesico-ureteric junction obstruction diagnosed antenatally has led many surgeons to change their view about vesico-ureteric junction obstruction. Most patients diagnosed antenatally show resolution rather than deterioration in their hydronephrosis/hydro-ureter, and the functional contribution by the kidney does not seem to deteriorate.[12] It is not yet clear whether symptomatic patients could also be managed conservatively, but currently the author has experience of 3 patients presenting with infective complications of vesico-ureteric junction obstruction who are undergoing conservative treatment over periods of between 6 months and 18 months, without any evidence of functional deterioration or further infection while on chemoprophylaxis.

Patients who present with painful episodes of obstruction with hydronephrosis/hydro-ureter without evidence of reflux should, however, continue to receive surgical treatment, as their symptoms will be relieved. As with obstruction at any point in the urinary system, some form of assessment of the relative function of each renal unit should be made before surgery is undertaken. If the affected kidney is functioning poorly at a level of less than 10% of its partner on a DMSA scan, then the value of extensive reconstructive surgery has to be questioned. Many people would advise nephrectomy or nephro-ureterectomy when function has deteriorated to this level, because it is seldom possible to improve the overall renal function in chronic obstruction.

Chronic urethral obstruction

Obstruction to the bladder outflow can occur with prolapsing ureterocele or with meatal polyp. A rare form of urethral diverticulum can cause voiding difficulties in the male, or urethral stricture secondary to catheterization or trauma may be to blame. Phimosis does not cause chronic obstruction.

Bilateral hydronephrosis/hydro-ureter and enlargement of the bladder can be seen in patients with an occult neuropathic bladder where no evidence of spinal abnormality or tumour exists; patients present with a palpable bladder and symptoms usually related to incontinence or infection. Reflux may well be associated with bladder outflow obstruction in children, and therefore the possibility of occult neuropathy should be entertained in all patients presenting with these symptoms.

Prune-belly syndrome

It is important again to stress that not all patients with dilated urinary systems have obstruction, and the prune-belly syndrome

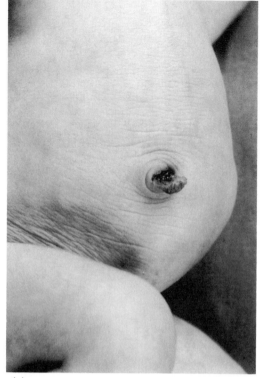

(a)

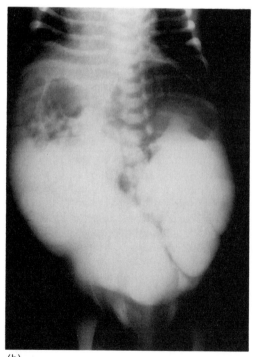

(b)

Figure 28.9 (a) Prune-belly syndrome; (b) prune-belly syndrome, showing megacystis mega-ureter

(Figure 28.9) is a prime example of this particular statement.

Otherwise known as the triad syndrome, the patient has undescended testicles, abdominal wall muscle deficiency and muscle deficiency in the urinary system with dilatation. It may be associated with urethral atresia, the baby dying *in utero*, or presenting with a patent urachus bypassing the urethra at birth. Many patients, however, have apparently few, if any, symptoms related to quite awful-looking urinary tracts. Provided that instrumentation is not performed, they escape most infective complications and have stable urinary tracts over many years. The condition can occur in the female, and in the male without undescended testis, being part of a complex in which a forme fruste of the prune-belly syndrome is therefore suspected.

The aetiology of the prune-belly syndrome and its allied conditions is essentially unknown; they are thought to occur when temporary urethral obstruction occurs early in antenatal development. Obstruction in some cases then relieves, leaving the patient with a chronically dilated, and poorly functioning, urinary system. The value of surgical treatment in 'tailoring' the urinary tract to a more normal appearance is questionable, and the current concept of persisting urethral obstruction requiring urethrotomy is still controversial.

The challenge that the clinician then faces in these patients is the challenge faced in every situation with hydronephrosis:

- the careful assessment of the urinary system, and the exclusion of an organic obstruction which may require bypass or surgical relief
- the maintenance of sterility within the urinary system by ensuring adequate drainage and the abolition where necessary of residual urine following micturition
- the realization that surgery has its limitations, and its complications, and the mere fact that a urinary tract is dilated and/or refluxing does not necessarily mean the surgeon should intervene.

References

1. Suzuki S., Saito Y., Nishiyama A., Fukuzaki A. and Orikasa S. Effect of ureteral obstruction on proximal tubular functions of rat kidney. *J. Urol.* 1988, **139**, 158–161
2. Schreiner G.F., Harris K.P.G., Pukerson M.L. and

Klahr S. Immunological aspects of acute ureteral obstruction: immune cell infiltrate in kidney. *Kidney Int.* 1988, **34**, 487–498

3. Gillenwater J.Y. Clinical aspects of urinary tract obstruction. *Sem. Nephrol.* 1982, **2**, 46–54

4. Atwell J.D. Posterior urethral valves in the British Isles. A multicentre BAPS review. *J. Pediatr. Surg.* 1983, **18**, 237–243

5. Dixon-Walker R. and Padron M. The management of posterior urethral valves by initial vesicostomy and delayed valve ablation. *J. Urol.* 1990, **144**, 1212–1214

6. Whittaker R.H. Methods of assessing obstruction in dilated ureters. *Br. J. Urol.* 1973, **45**, 15–22

7. O'Reilly P.H., Testa H.J., Lawson R.S., Farrar D.J. and Charlton-Edwards E. Diuresis renography – equivocal urinary tract obstruction. *Br. J. Urol.* 1978, **50**, 76–80

8. Upsdell S.M., Testa H.J. and Lawson R.S. The F-15 diuresis renogram in suspected obstruction of the upper urinary tract. *Br. J. Urol.* 1991 (in press)

9. Roberts J.B.M. and Slade N. The natural history of primary pelvic hydronephrosis *Br. J. Surg.* 1964, **51**, 759–762

10. Notley R.G. and Beaugie J.M. The long term follow up of Anderson Hynes pyeloplasty for hydronephrosis. *Br. J. Urol.* 1973, **45**, 464–467

11. Cox R., Strachan J.R. and Woodhouse C.R.J. Twenty year follow up of primary mega-ureter. *Eur. Urol.* 1990, **17**, 43–46

12. Keating M.A., Escala J., Snyder H. McC., Heyman S. and Duckett J.W. Changing concepts in the management of obstructive megaureter. *J. Urol.* 1989, **144**, 636–640

29

The antenatal diagnosis of renal abnormalities

W.E. Grupe

Introduction

The first successful *in utero* diagnosis of polycystic kidneys using ultrasound was reported slightly over 20 years ago. Five years later, the first report of ultrasonographic detection of obstructive nephropathy in a fetus appeared. Subsequent advances in technical capability have produced a rapid improvement in the ability to study fetal anatomy. For many, prenatal ultrasonographic examination has become a routine procedure, even when no specific indication is evident. With this, the discovery of unexpected malformations has quickly expanded. The prevalence of abnormalities approximates 1–2 per 1000 ultrasound procedures, of which 20–33% are anomalies of the genito-urinary tract.[1,2] In some series, this is second only to malformations of the central nervous system.[3]

An improved capability for intra-uterine diagnosis is of unquestioned value. Congenital anomalies of the genito-urinary tract can be detected as early as 12–15 weeks' gestation.[4-7] Almost 90% of the fetal kidneys can be identified by 17–20 weeks' gestation, and 95% by the 22nd week.[8] The rate of renal growth has been sufficiently well measured beyond the 20th week that renal size by ultrasonography can be used as a guide to gestational age.[9] Anomalies that require immediate postnatal treatment are detected which would have remained unrecognized in the otherwise asymptomatic child by routine nursery examinations.[10] A time, mode and place of delivery that will maximize postnatal care can be selected.[1,11,12] The possibility to evaluate renal function *in utero* is offered.[13] Even the potential for intra-uterine correction emerges.[14] An opportunity for the parents to receive counsel and to adjust to the situation is presented.[6,15] The benefit receiving the broadest clinical support is the opportunity to organize the postnatal management prospectively, to be initiated promptly.[10-12]

As with all new and expanding capabilities, however, the potential problems require examination.[6,15] Although the errors in ultrasound diagnosis are currently few, the consequences can be considerable. Not all retroperitoneal masses, for example, are renal. In the presence of renal agenesis, the adrenal is misshapen and can appear deceptively like a kidney.[16] The enlargement of the stomach produced by duodenal atresia can be easily confused with ureteropelvic junction abnormality.[8] In like fashion, a large dilated renal pelvis has been interpreted as duodenal atresia.[17] Some malformations discovered after birth can escape intra-uterine detection.[18,19] Other lesions are pleomorphic by ultrasonography.[20] The distinction between multicystic kidneys and ureteropelvic junction obstruction is not as sharp in the fetus as it is postnatally.[8,18,21] The dilated calyces of ureteropelvic stenosis can mimic renal cysts.[22] Physiological dilatation can be confused on ultrasonography with obstruction.[5,8,20,22-24]

Potential for error

A potential for error exists, even in experienced hands. In a 1982 report, 8 of 13 patients (61%) with proven obstructive disease at birth had an incorrect diagnosis made at the time of prenatal ultrasound examination.[25] Several studies in 1984 had error rates of 23–41%.[3,18] Some had no obstruction found at postnatal examination. In others, a bilateral renal lesion was thought to be unilateral.[18] In a 1986 report, the reason for the urinary tract dilatation was not recorded for 33 of 73 fetuses,[14] while a 1987 report had 31% erroneously diagnosed.[21]

There is every reason to believe that accuracy will improve with experience. Nevertheless, even when the accuracy of prenatal diagnosis is excellent, problems can arise. Reports from centres with considerable experience and diagnostic accuracy above 89% detail such problems.[10,19,24] In one report, 13% of the pregnancies were terminated for the wrong reason, even when 96% of the diagnoses were accurately made.[24] In a similar study, 18 fetuses were defined as having urinary abnormalities with an accuracy of 89%.[19] However, two additional children had unrecognized abnormalities of the bowel in addition to their renal lesions and in another with a prenatal diagnosis of unilateral disease, the contralateral kidney was absent at birth.[19] Seven infants died of renal or pulmonary failure (39%); for these seven, an early diagnosis was of no help.[19]

A third study of 46 pregnancies, in which 24 of 25 antenatal diagnoses were confirmed postnatally, noted that the prenatal knowledge of renal disease was of value to the infant in only 20%.[10] Twelve neonates had physical signs at birth which rendered the prenatal diagnosis unnecessary or non-beneficial.[10] The renal disease was sufficiently mild in 15% to make the diagnosis of doubtful value, while useful information about unilateral disease was obtained in 35%.[10] All three groups of investigators ultimately agreed that the main potential advantage of accurate intra-uterine diagnosis was not selection for early delivery or intra-uterine intervention, but the opportunity for earlier postnatal treatment.[1,10,19,24]

It is difficult to differentiate physiological dilatation from high-pressure obstruction.[5,8,17,18,21,24] Most agree that marked dilatation of the pelvicalyceal system with dilatation of the infundibulum and calyces is distinctly abnormal.[20,22,23] Transient modest obstruction, however, is a normal component of the canalization of the urinary tract. Thus, a delay in canalization or a delay in the rupture of the cloacal membrane can produce transient dilatation.[8] Similarly, urachal closure at 32 weeks produces the first high-resistance outflow for the collecting system, producing a temporary dilatation.[8] Conversely, a delay in the closure of the urachus or some other site of urinary egress could produce a factitious period of decompression for a system with more distal obstruction;[8] by ultrasound, such a tract would appear normal at first, then become worse as pregnancy progresses. With all these hydrodynamic variables, it is not surprising that transient dilatation has been reported in as high as 10–20% of fetuses in the third trimester.[5,8,17,18,24] Although not physiologically significant to the fetus, such findings are ultrasonographically confusing for the medical care team. To date, the only accurate way to define transient non-obstructive dilatation of the genito-urinary tract is through serial examinations of the fetus.

Urinary tract dilatation, even when it is reflective of obstructive uropathy, does not completely define the anatomical or functional status of the developing kidneys. Other means to acquire this information have been devised. Attempts to determine the presence and severity of renal dysplasia by ultrasonographic techniques have been only partially successful, however. Increased renal echogenicity, renal cortical cysts, severe hydronephrosis and definite calyceal changes are strongly suggestive of significant renal dysplasia.[26] Even with experienced personnel, however, an appreciable number of fetuses with physiologically significant dysplasia will be missed. For example, the detection of hydronephrosis has been meaningless in 25% of fetuses, whereas in 60% of those with subsequently proven severe dysplasia none or only minimal calyceal blunting was noted *in utero*.[26] Increased echogenicity of the renal cortex has been found in 20% of normal fetuses, whereas 25% of those with dysplasia were not detected on this basis.[26,35] Cortical cysts, when present, are highly specific; however, more than half of the dysplastic kidneys do not display cysts and in one-quarter of the fetuses with renal dysplasia, neither sonographically visible cysts nor increased echogenicity are present.[26] Thus, ultrasound will define the diagnosis accurately in only a minority of fetuses. More disturbingly, the technique cannot be used to positively exclude the presence of renal dysplasia in any fetus.

The *in utero* appearance of multicystic dysplastic kidneys can change dramatically throughout pregnancy, as well. In one study of 9 neonates, repeated ultrasound examinations disclosed a progressive regression of 'multicystic kidneys' that, by delivery, appeared as unilateral renal agenesis, including the absence of a detectable ureter and renal artery in three.[39]

The assessment of renal function by ultrasonographic techniques is also not completely reliable. Non-invasive tests cannot accurately define intra-uterine renal function or predict the potential for renal recovery. The volume of amniotic fluid remains the most useful and reliable reflection of renal function, since the formation of amniotic fluid depends on the ability to form urine. The amount of amniotic fluid is predictive only at extremes, however. Although severe oligohydramnios was associated with poor renal function and poor fetal outcome in a representative study, one-third of the pregnancies with only a mild reduction in amniotic fluid volume resulted in an infant with severe renal dysfunction, whereas one-third moderately severe oligohydramnios had a positive outcome.[13] Normal amniotic fluid volume early in pregnancy is no assurance of normal renal function;[5] a precipitous drop in amniotic fluid volume during the third trimester is more predictive of a poor prognosis.[23]

Attempts to use the rate of fetal urine formation as a predictor of renal function are only modestly successful.[27,28] The urine volume is calculated from changes in bladder size following a spontaneous void. In a normal fetus, the flow rate increases from 0.6 ml/h to 27 ml/h during the last trimester.[27] Two methods have been proposed to enhance the value of these measurements as a rough measure of renal function. The first involves giving furosemide to the mother, which normally should increase fetal urine output by 80–150%.[28] A second method is to aspirate the bladder, then directly measure the rate at which it refills.[27] Both of these methods fail on at least three counts. First, at any age, the volume of urine does not reflect the glomerular filtration rate. It is well recognized, in fact, that polyuria, not oliguria, is the usual response to renal damage. Secondly, massive reflux, which is often present with obstruc-

tion, makes an accurate measure of urine flow impossible; the bladder can fill quite well from the urine drained from the upper tract. Thirdly, the state of maternal hydration alone can affect the rate of fetal urine production.[29] Finally, failure to see the fetal bladder by ultrasound, even after furosemide, does not necessarily indicate absent renal function.[30]

One well-presented case clearly outlines how complex the problems can be.[5] At 28 weeks' gestation, dilatation of the posterior urethra, megacystis, and minimal right hydronephrosis were diagnosed by ultrasound. The amount of amniotic fluid was normal, and the bladder promptly filled at a normal rate following aspiration. A repeat ultrasonogram at 20 weeks showed the hydronephrosis to be bilateral. Again there was a normal amniotic fluid volume and the bladder refilled once more at a normal rate. At 26 weeks, oligohydramnios was noted for the first time. By 30 weeks, however, the ultrasonographic examination had improved, the bladder was normal in size, and the hydronephrosis had resolved. At 36 weeks, the infant was vaginally delivered, but died at 16 hours of age with profound pulmonary insufficiency. A urethral valve with severe bilateral dysplasia was found at autopsy. In this particular case, the disappearance of urinary tract dilatation was the ominous sign of deteriorating function rather than an indication of the resolution of transient physiological hydronephrosis.

The direct analysis of fetal urine has been used to define the extent of intra-uterine renal functional loss.[13] Those who subsequently had a poor renal outcome had urinary sodium concentrations greater than 100 mmol/litre, urinary chloride concentration greater than 90 mmol/litre, urinary osmolarity greater than 210 mosmol/kg and urine flow rates less than 2 ml/min.[13] Ten per cent of the fetuses in the study were misclassified, however.[13] Even when the urine data were combined with the amniotic fluid volume and the ultrasonographic appearance of the fetal kidneys, prognostic criteria remained correct in 90% of the fetuses evaluated. Fetal glomerular filtration rate, urinary potassium concentration and urinary creatinine concentration were not predictive of outcome.[13] Although urinary sodium, chloride, osmolarity and flow rate can define those at high risk, there is currently no evidence that the ultimate outcome can be altered by any intervention. In fact, in the study presented, 3 of 6 fetuses with predicted good outcome were lost *in utero* secondary to procedure-related chorio-amnionitis.[13]

The definition of renal size *in utero* is another important diagnostic detail. For example, both dysplastic kidneys and polycystic kidneys are hyperechoic; size, therefore, is a major point for differentiation, with infantile polycystic kidneys larger than normal for gestational age and dysplastic kidneys smaller. As early as 1980, Grannum and colleagues followed a group of normal pregnancies from 12 weeks until delivery at term.[7] The circumference of the kidney (KC) was compared with the abdominal circumference (AC). Throughout observation, with repeated examinations, the KC/AC ratio remained constant between 0.27 and 0.30. A later study examined cross-sectional areas, rather than circumference, noticing a similar constancy of the KA/AA ratio from 20 weeks to term.[31] Although growth-retarded fetuses have smaller than normal kidneys for gestational age, the KA/AA ratios remained generally within the normal range.[31]

As might be anticipated, the ability to detect urinary tract malformations *in utero* was almost immediately followed by efforts toward intra-uterine intervention. The first attempt, reported in 1981, was considered quite successful.[27] Subsequent reports have failed to define a consistent role for the intra-uterine relief of obstruction, however. Only three procedures have been used to any degree: (a) percutaneous needle aspiration of the bladder; (b) placement of a permanent shunt between the fetal bladder and the amniotic space; and (c) intra-uterine surgery to decompress the urinary tract.[5,8,18,27]

The reasons for attempting intra-uterine intervention include the prevention of dysplasia, the preservation of renal function and the prevention of pulmonary hypoplasia. Unfortunately, there is little evidence in humans that the intra-uterine drainage of urine by any means has any direct influence on any of these concerns. In several series, the number of infants with severe oligohydramnios who have been delivered with adequate renal function is very small, even after intra-uterine drainage, so that the benefit to the child of any intra-uterine manipulation is far from obvious.[5,6,8,18,27] In one representative report, intra-uterine bladder drainage in 8 fetuses had rather poor results.[32] Three infants died soon after delivery with Potter's syndrome; 2 more were lost *in utero* after attempts at

drainage, and 2 others were terminated at the ages of 13 and 17 weeks. The only infant to survive with adequate renal function was diagnosed postnatally with bilateral ureteropelvic junction obstruction; because the site of obstruction is so high in the tract, it is doubtful that bladder drainage would have been helpful in the first place. A subsequent report from the same group involved 12 additional fetuses.[13] In 4 pregnancies, poor renal function was predicted from *in utero* measurement; 2 of these pregnancies were terminated electively, 1 infant was stillborn and the fourth succumbed to respiratory failure at 15 hours of age. In 2 other pregnancies, good renal function was predicted, but the subsequent appearance of associated fetal anomalies led to elective abortion. Three pregnancies were lost secondary to procedure-related fetal infection. In the 3 remaining pregnancies, good renal function was predicted by *in utero* measurements. One fetus did well without any further intra-uterine intervention, the second did well despite multiple problems with indwelling catheter shunts, and the third fetus did well subsequent to the creation of a supra-pubic vesicotomy.

A contemporary review that did not attempt intra-uterine drainage can be used for comparison.[1] Thirty urinary tract anomalies, of which 23 were unilateral, were discovered in 9453 pregnancies. One-quarter of the anomalies were detected prior to 20 weeks' gestation. Six died in the immediate postnatal period from multiple associated anomalies; only 1 of these 6 had bilateral hydronephrosis. Four other infants had bilateral hydronephrosis; 3 were successfully treated in the neonatal period, whereas 1 required no surgery.[1] Other investigators have also raised concern that intra-uterine intervention offers no advantage to the fetus, particularly in terms of the number of survivors and the post-natal level of renal function.[10–12]

A report from the International Fetal Surgery Registry reviewed the placement of 73 catheter shunts for fetal obstructive uropathy between 17 and 36 weeks' gestational age.[14] The shunt was successfully placed on the first attempt in only 8%, while the others took 2 to 7 attempts. Twenty per cent of the fetuses failed to reach term; 11 fetuses were electively aborted and 3 others were lost as a direct result of the intra-uterine procedure. Twenty-seven infants died within hours of delivery from pulmonary hypoplasia and respiratory insufficiency, with no evidence that the vesico-amniotic shunt altered the course of pulmonary development for those infants. Thirty fetuses survived the intra-uterine procedure. Survival was not related to the fetal age at diagnosis, treatment, the volume of amniotic fluid, or the duration of shunt function. Data on the renal function of the survivors were not presented. Thus, this survey readily documents the feasibility and risks of intra-uterine intervention, but cannot be used to define the benefits.[14] It may be that the only realistic intra-uterine intervention currently available is termination of the pregnancy; such drastic intervention, of course, assumes that the original diagnosis is correct.

If the goal of intra-uterine intervention is to prevent renal dysplasia and preserve renal function, there is virtually no evidence in humans that dysplasia can be ameliorated at any stage of gestation.[4,8,18] That dysplasia is commonly associated with obstructive uropathy cannot be used as evidence that the two conditions are causally related or that relief of obstruction will reverse the abnormal development of the kidney.[33] Experiments in fetal lambs have shown that the reactive and regressive components of renal dysplasia can be produced through a mid-trimester urinary tract obstruction.[34,35] As in humans, the severity of the renal parenchymal damage varies with the timing, severity and duration of the obstruction.[34] Further, relief of the obstruction before birth alters the extent of progressive damage.[35] Although these data suggest that at least a portion of the parenchymal injury is related to obstruction, they do not address that portion of the process related to nephronic dysgenesis.[33] If, for example, dysplasia evolves from a primary abnormality in the origin of the ureteric duct, as other evidence suggests, then the relief of obstruction could not be expected to change the pattern of nephron induction.[36] The presence of irreversible dysplasia at 15 weeks' gestation in one case report suggests that, at least for some, even successful intervention would not alter the course of abnormal embryogenesis.[4]

A third reason for intervention is the prevention of pulmonary hypoplasia. When the amount of amniotic fluid is experimentally reduced in the rat or lamb, pulmonary hypoplasia develops.[37] Such data suggest that oligohydramnios from urinary tract obstruction could also be responsible for pulmonary hypoplasia in the human.[38] If the release of obstruction lessened the degree of pulmonary dysfunction, then intra-uterine drainage would have clear value. Unfortunately the human experience is not that positive; the degree of oligohydramnios does not always relate to the risk of subsequent pulmonary disease. For example, as one case report illustrates, the successful relief of intra-uterine obstruction at 32 weeks of age resulted in an infant born with the 'prune-belly' syndrome and adequate renal function, who at 4 months of age was still using a home respirator for pulmonary disease.[5]

The risks of intervention are not minor and include haemorrhage, chorioamnionitis, intestinal perforation, sepsis, abortion, premature labour, and fetal and maternal death. Vesico-amniotic catheter shunts are not technically easy to place and usually require multiple attempts.[13,14] The catheters commonly fail to remain patent and occasionally migrate to unwanted sites.[13,18,23] These problems must be considered seriously in any programme of intra-uterine intervention. At the moment, none of the therapeutic manipulations currently undertaken *in utero* can be considered to have clear benefit.[9-12,14,18,23] Nevertheless, the technical availability of fetal intervention tends to encourage an unrealistic attitude towards its role and importance.

Even with more accurate diagnosis and improved intra-uterine intervention techniques, the ultimate outcome for the fetus may depend on conditions beyond the urinary tract.[13] There is a frequent association of congenital renal disease, diagnosed ultrasonographically, with other major structural anomalies.[38] Although unilateral multicystic dysplasia is generally thought to have an almost invariably good prognosis postnatally, one study found that 37% of those detected *in utero* had a severe life-threatening associated anomaly that eclipsed the significance of the renal disease.[21] In another study that included all renal diagnoses, those detected with bilateral renal disease had a 33% mortality, with coexisting major non-renal anomalies present in 56%.[10] Ford and colleagues also noted that almost one-third of the fetuses died with unsalvageable anomalies.[11]

Effect of diagnosis on parents

One aspect not frequently discussed is the effect that intra-uterine diagnosis has on the parent.[6,15,19] By the very nature of the ultrasonographic or intra-uterine studies, it is virtually impossible to conceal that a diagnostic problem exists. Even though most problems are detected late in the third trimester, there are increasing instances where diagnoses are made much earlier.[1,4,14] Thus, parents can have more than 5 months to wonder and to worry. Feelings of inadequacy, guilt, fear and anger, or a refusal to bond to the infant or to anticipate delivery, would be expected behaviour. It is exceedingly difficult to reassure parents when the diagnosis may still be in question. A parent's quest for precise answers therefore must often be met by a facade of uncertainty and equivocation. It is almost impossible to provide adequate counsel when the diagnosis has a reasonable chance of being either incorrect or incomplete. An incorrect diagnosis can produce inappropriate antenatal advice. The consequences of an inaccurate antenatal diagnosis can be devastating; to advise termination for the wrong reasons could even qualify as a disaster.[24]

Because the problems with intra-uterine diagnoses are still poorly resolved, guidelines for management that protect the fetus and parents as much as possible are needed. Several protocols have been offered.[8,13,18,27] First, a single examination is never enough to either include or exclude fetal abnormalities.[32,39] Secondly, early delivery is rarely necessary. One must avoid the natural urge toward active intervention, and resist those same pressures from the family. Prematurity generally worsens the prognosis of postnatal surgery. With our current knowledge, it is probably more beneficial to the infant to plan and arrange for appropriate postnatal management.

Thirdly, fetal surgery, so far, is limited to drainage of the bladder only.[13] Upper tract lesions, such as ureteropelvic junction anomalies, do not benefit.[12] Unilateral disease rarely needs intra-uterine intervention.[8,18] If there is bilateral dilatation with adequate amniotic fluid, intervention is probably not required until after delivery.[13,26] If obstruction is bilateral with severe oligohydramnios, and ultrasonographic evidence of dysplasia is present, current evidence suggests that interventions are futile.[5,8,10,13,14,23,26,32] More difficult are the small number of fetuses in whom bilateral obstruction is present with equivocal amounts of amniotic fluid. Although some authors feel this group might benefit most from intra-uterine bladder drainage, particularly if fetal urine

analysis predicts good renal function, there is still no definitive evidence that intra-uterine manipulation alters the course for these children.[10–14,23] In no circumstance is there clear evidence in the human that early drainage avoids dysplasia, improves renal function, avoids a pulmonary complication, or offers any advantage over appropriate postnatal surgery following a full-term delivery. Finally, studies must be repeated post delivery no matter how convincing the prenatal evidence is.[12] What existed *in utero* may no longer exist. Repeat evaluation on the first day of life, however, may not be optimal and might only add to the confusion.[29]

Intra-uterine diagnosis identifies the child at risk who is in need of further and more reliable evaluation.[11,12] Well over half of these children would have otherwise remained undetected.[10] A system must be available to support the parents extensively.[6,15,19] Early knowledge of an anomaly, even with counselling, is not an assurance that the parents will adjust to the situation calmly, gradually or successfully. Communication between all providers of care becomes essential if an appropriate postnatal plan is to be formulated. This includes co-ordination between the obstetrician, the ultrasonographer, the paediatrician, the neonatologist, the nephrologist and the urologist.

References

1. Grisoni E.R., Gauderer M.W.L., Wolfson R.N. and Izant R.J. Antenatal ultrasonography: the experience in a high risk perinatal center. *J. Pediatr. Surg.* 1986, **21**, 58–61

2. Scott J.E.S. and Renwick M. Antenatal diagnosis of congenital abnormalities of the urinary tract. *Br. J. Urol.* 1988, **62**, 295–300

3. Vandenberghe K., De Wolf F., Fryns J.P. *et al.* Antenatal ultrasound diagnosis of fetal malformations: possibilities, limitations, and dilemmas. *Eur. J. Obstet. Gynecol. Reprod. Biol.* 1984, **18**, 279–297

4. Bellinger M.F., Comstock C.H., Grosso D. *et al.* Fetal posterior urethral valves and renal dysplasia at 15 weeks gestational age. *J. Urol.* 1983, **129**, 1238–1239

5. Diamond D.A., Sanders R. and Jeffs R.D. Fetal hydronephrosis: considerations regarding urologic intervention. *J. Urol.* 1984, **131**, 1155–1159

6. Editorial: When ultrasound shows fetal abnormality. *Lancet* 1985, **1**, 618–619

7. Grannum P., Bracken M., Silverman R. and Hobbins J.C. Assessment of fetal kidney size in normal gestation by comparison of ratio of kidney circumference to

abdominal circumference. *Am. J. Obstet. Gynecol.* 1980, **136**, 249–254

8. Kramer S.A. Current status of fetal intervention for congenital hydronephrosis. *J. Urol.* 1983, **130**, 641–646

9. Jeanty P., Dramaiz-Wilmet M., Elkhazen N. *et al.* Measurement of fetal kidney growth on ultrasound. *Radiology* 1982, **144**, 159–162

10. Thomas D.F., Irving H.C. and Arthur R.J. Prenatal diagnosis: how useful is it? *Br. J. Urol.* 1985, **57**, 784–787

11. Ford W.D., Ahmed S., Verco P.W. and Jureidini K.F. Fetal urinary tract abnormalities detected on maternal ultrasound. *Aust. Paediatr. J.* 1984, **20**, 67–72

12. Koyle M.A. and Ehrlich R.M. Management of ureteropelvic junction obstruction in neonate. *Urology* 1988, **31**, 496–498

13. Glick P.L., Harrison M.R., Golbus M.S. *et al.* Management of the fetus with congenital hydronephrosis. II: Prognostic criteria and selection for treatment. *J. Pediatr. Surg.* 1985, **20**, 376–387

14. Report of the International Fetal Surgery Registry. Catheter shunts for fetal hydronephrosis and hydrocephalus. *N. Engl. J. Med.* 1986, **315**, 336–340

15. Mervyn-Griffiths D. and Gough M.H. Dilemmas after ultrasonic diagnosis of fetal abnormality. *Lancet* 1985, **1**, 623–624

16. Dubbins P.A., Kurtz A.B., Wapner R.J. *et al.* Renal agenesis: spectrum in *in utero* findings. *J. Clin. Ultrasound* 1981, **9**, 189–193

17. Sanders R. and Graham D. Twelve cases of hydronephrosis *in utero* diagnosed by ultrasonography. *J. Ultrasound Med.* 1982, **1**, 341–348

18. Broyer M., Guest G., Lestage F. *et al.* Prenatal diagnosis of urinary tract malformations. *Adv. Nephrol.* 1985, **14**, 21–38

19. Hutson J.M., McNay M.B., MacKenzie J.R. *et al.* Antenatal diagnosis of surgical disorders by ultrasonography. *Lancet* 1985, **1**, 621–623

20. Glazer G.M., Filly R.A. and Callen P.W. The varied sonographic appearance of the urinary tract in the fetus and newborn. *Radiology* 1982, **144**, 563–568

21. Rizzo N., Gabrielli S., Pilu G. *et al.* Prenatal diagnosis and obstetrical management of multicystic dysplastic kidney disease. *Prenat. Diagn.* 1987, **7**, 109–118

22. Blane C.E., Koff S.A., Bowerman R.A. *et al.* Nonobstructive fetal hydronephrosis: sonographic recognition and therapeutic implications. *Radiology* **147**, 1983, 95–99

23. Fleischer A.C., Kirchner S.G. and Thieme G.A. Prenatal detection of fetal anomalies with sonography. *Pediatr. Clin. North Am.* 1985, **32**, 1523–1536

24. Gauderer M.W.L., Jassani M.N. and Izant R.J. Ultrasonographic antenatal diagnosis: will it change the spectrum of neonatal surgery? *J. Pediatr. Surg.* 1984, **19**, 404–407

25. Mahan J., Gonzales R., Godec C.J. *et al.* Intrauterine obstructive uropathy: is early detection and intervention beneficial? Read at Annual Meeting of the North Western Pediatric Society, Chanhassen, Minnesota

26. Mahoney B.S., Filly R.A., Callen P.W. *et al.* Sonographic evaluation of renal dysplasia. *Radiology* 1984, **152**, 143–146

27. Harrison M.R., Filly R.A., Parer J.T. *et al.* Management of the fetus with a urinary tract malformation. *J. Am. Med. Ass.* 1981, **246**, 635–639

28. Wladimiroff J.W. and Campbell S. Fetal-urine production rates in normal and complicated pregnancy. *Lancet* 1974, **1**, 151–154

29. Laing V.D., Burke V.C., Wing V.W. *et al.* Postpartum evaluation of fetal hydronephrosis: optimal timing for follow-up sonography. *Radiology* 1984 **152**, 423–424

30. Raghavendra B.N., Young B.K., Greco M.A. *et al.* Use of furosemide in pregnancies complicated by oligohydramnios. *Radiology* 1987, **165**, 455–458

31. Sato A., Yamaguchi Y., Liou S.M. *et al.* Growth of the fetal kidney assessed by real time ultrasound. *Gynecol. Obstet. Invest.* 1985, **20**, 1–5

32. Golbus M.S., Harrison M.R. and Filly R.A. Prenatal diagnosis and treatment of fetal hydronephrosis. *Sem. Perinatol.* 1983, **7** 102–108

33. Bernstein J. The morphogenesis of renal parenchymal maldevelopment (renal dysplasia). *Pediatr. Clin. North Am.* 1971, **18**, 395–407

34. Glick P.L., Harrison M.R., Adzick N.S. *et al.* Correction of congenital hydronephrosis *in utero*: III. Early mid-trimester ureteral obstruction produces renal dysplasia. *J. Pediatr. Surg.* 1983, **18**, 681–687

35. Glick P.L., Harrison M.R., Adzick N.S. *et al.* Correction of congenital hydronephrosis *in utero*: IV. *In utero* decompression prevents renal dysplasia. *J. Pediatr. Surg.* 1984, **19**, 649–657

36. Henneberry M.O. and Stephens F.D. Renal hypoplasia and dysplasia in infants with posterior urethral valves. *J. Urol.* 1980, **123**, 912–915

37. Symchych P.S. and Winchester P. Potter's syndrome. Animal model: Amniotic fluid deficiency and fetal lung growth in the rat. *Am. J. Pathol.* 1984, **90**, 779–782

38. Quinlan R.W., Cruz A.C. and Huddleston J.F. Sonographic detection of fetal urinary-tract anomalies. *Obstet. Gynecol.* 1986, **67**, 558–565

39. Pedicelli G., Jequier S., Bowen A.D. and Boisvert J. Multicystic dysplastic kidneys: spontaneous regression demonstrated with US. *Radiology* 1986, **161**, 23–26

30

Antenatal hydronephrosis: postnatal management

D. C. S. Gough

You saw me before I was born and scheduled each day of my life before I began to breathe . . . (Psalm 139, v. 16, *The Living Bible*)

Introduction

Although considerable anxiety will have developed during the pregnancy in the minds of the parents and their medical attendants, it is fairly predictable what will happen immediately after the baby is born. Infants will enter the world without a visible abnormality, feed normally, pass urine within the first 24 h and will have no detectable renal enlargement. These children pose no particular management problem in the newborn period, and can be investigated at leisure, and 80% of all children with antenatal hydronephrosis fall into this category. The need for referral will depend on local radiological expertise, and its ability to produce images of diagnostic quality in the small baby.

The second group of children will apparently be well at birth, but then show signs of a palpable bladder, suggesting outflow obstruction to the urinary tract. Ultrasound will confirm the enlarged bladder with unilateral or bilateral hydronephrosis/hydro-ureter. These children will require urgent medical intervention to preserve their upper tract function and prevent infection and should be transferred to a specialist unit for investigation forthwith. About 5% of patients fall into this category.

Those children with a solitary palpable kidney make up about 10% of all patients, and the need for referral will depend upon the underlying diagnosis, but where outflow obstruction to the bladder is not suspected, referral can take place within the first few weeks of life.

A much rarer event is the delivery of an obviously ill child, who may well show signs of respiratory distress, exhibiting features of Potter's syndrome. This will usually have been anticipated antenatally because of oligohydramnios and may well have been the subject of interventional antenatal procedures for sampling fetal urine or draining the urinary tract into the amniotic cavity. They may well require emergency resuscitation procedures and artificial ventilation, and will best be delivered in a centre able to cope with their immediate problems. The prognosis for such patients is very poor.

Our own experience is that severe renal impairment is an extremely rare event, only occurring in 3% of our series, and therefore the paediatrician's first responsibility to the family is one of reassurance in an endeavour to counter the anxiety that will have been building up during the latter part of the pregnancy. The normal appearance of a well child, coupled with the natural excitement of child birth, goes a long way to help the paediatrician in these circumstances.

When we looked at serum creatinine at the age of 1 month as a measure of renal impairment, we found that 89% of all children had no evidence of renal impairment when presenting with antenatal hydronephrosis, and a further

8% had only modest elevations of creatinine at this time. Serum creatinine should be measured in all children at some time in the first month, depending on the clinical circumstances.

Coming to a diagnosis

It is important for the paediatrician to realize that hydronephrosis is not a diagnosis in itself, but merely an expression of the fact that the urinary tract may be obstructed, dysplastic, the subject of vesico-ureteric reflux, or a combination of these conditions. Ultrasound examination of the urinary tract gives approximately 10% false positive investigations; when the urinary tract is imaged by other means, no abnormality is identified.

The following are some general principles which will help the clinician in deciding what to do:

- In the absence of respiratory distress, palpable bladder or other obvious clinical abnormality, the investigation is non-urgent.
- Early repeat ultrasound may be normal. The volume of urine produced each hour falls dramatically from prenatal levels in the first week of life, and there may be under-filling of a dilated system which makes ultrasound diagnosis difficult. Repeat all normal investigations at 1 month of age. Vesico-ureteric reflux is a condition where the hydronephrosis may be variable.
- The most significant complication of hydronephrosis is infection. Most practitioners would advise chemoprophylaxis with trimethoprim 2 mg kg^{-1} day^{-1}, at least until the diagnosis is established.
- Renal function matures quickly after birth and both isotope images and contrast studies will produce clearer diagnostic information if delayed beyond 1 month of age.

Approaches to investigation

A number of algorithms have been produced over the past few years which are deemed to guide the paediatrician and the radiologist in investigating children with this anomaly, designed to minimize radiation exposure and limit the collection of information to that which

will determine management decisions (Figure 30.1).

Individual centres will have varying expertise at their disposal for the radiological imaging of the urinary tract of the newborn, and decisions will have to be taken as to whether referral for a diagnosis will be appropriate. With the current level of controversy over management and the difficulty of coming to a precise diagnosis, sharing the responsibility for diagnosis and initial treatment with the regional centre would seem appropriate.

Radiological imaging

Micturating cystography should be within the remit of most radiological departments, and should be performed with antibiotic cover in all patients where the hydronephrosis is confirmed to exclude infravesical obstruction and vesico-ureteric reflux. Indirect methods for assessing reflux at this age are not recommended. Care must be taken in interpreting reflux cystography, so that abnormalities such as duplication or diverticulum are not missed. Where the dilatation is shown to be due to vesico-ureteric reflux, then upper tract assessment is best made using dimercaptosuccinic acid-labelled technetium scans (DMSA).

If there is no evidence of outflow obstruction to the bladder or reflux, then the upper tract needs to be assessed with some form of functional imaging, which is most likely to be a radioisotope such as technetium-labelled MAG3. This not only gives functional information if the first 3 min of the uptake of isotope are analysed during the renogram by suitable computer program, but also evidence of poor drainage, often associated with dilatation of the upper urinary tract.

Clinicians still argue about the accuracy of diagnostic information from radiosotope scans of the kidney, and whether they will or will not predict the presence of urinary tract obstruction. A certain amount of prognostic information, however, will be forthcoming from an isotope renogram when related to the anatomical site of apparent obstruction on the urinary tract.

Very strong opinions are held with regard to the value of intravenous urography in this clinical setting. Our own experience has been quite extensive, and we have always used urography

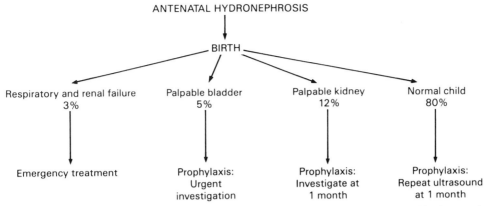

Figure 30.1 Postnatal management of children with antenatal hydronephrosis – used in conjunction with ultrasound at birth and clinical judgement. Significant hydronephrosis is taken to be anteroposterior diameter of renal pelvis > 10 mm at term. Anteroposterior diameter of 75 mm at term is equivocal hydronephrosis

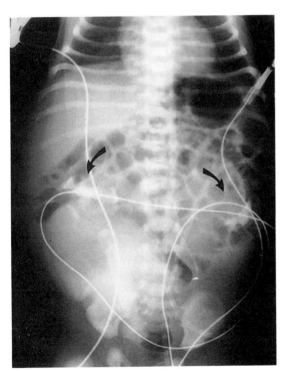

Figure 30.2 Bilateral duplication of the urinary tract with ureterocele, evident as filling defects in the bladder and depression of lower pole calyces

hydrocalicosis has been obtained by ultrasound.

Modern ultrasound equipment, however, can be superior to urography where function is poor, and this is particularly helpful in patients with duplication and ureterocele where the side of the duplication related to the ureterocele in the bladder can be accurately determined by ultrasound examination.

The clinician must be aware that reflux obstruction and dysplasia can all occur in the same patient. An example is given in Figure 30.2 of a patient who has bilateral duplication with ureteroceles which are causing outflow obstruction to the bladder and the whole process is complicated by vesico-ureteric reflux into the lower pole of the duplex system.

Diagnostic possibilities

There is no substitute for the awareness of potential diagnoses and careful radiological assessment of each patient before coming to a diagnosis which leads to treatment. Our own figures show that where ultrasound is used alone in the pre- and postnatal period, then only one diagnosis in three is actually correct,[1] and supported by further radiological imaging. Based on our own experience with 350 patients referred for further investigation of antenatal hydronephrosis, we can identify some common clinical patterns and diagnoses, as outlined in Table 30.1

Again it should be stressed that more that one diagnosis may exist in each patient, but by

for precise anatomical diagnosis, and have been surprised by the number of mega-ureters, both refluxing and obstructing, that have been missed on ultrasound, and the number of normal upper tract studies on urography when quite confident prediction of hydronephrosis/

Table 30.1   Final diagnosis in 335 children with hydronephrosis after the neonatal period

Primary diagnosis	No.
Idiopathic hydronephrosis	85
PUJ obstruction	73
Multicystic dysplastic kidney	48
VUJ obstruction	34
Vesico-ureteric reflux	21
Posterior urethral valves	16
Ectopic ureterocele	11
Others	47
Total	335

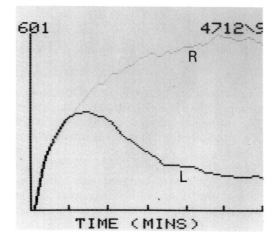

Figure 30.3 Diuresis renogram. Both kidneys take up isotope equally, displaying equal function. The right kidney shows obstructed and the left normal drainage curves

far the most common problem is unilateral upper tract hydronephrosis in the patient suspected as having a pelvi-ureteric junction obstruction.

Pelvi-ureteric junction – obstruction or not?

Nearly half of our cases have this diagnosis on ultrasound and very few have clinical signs of renal enlargement. All have normal measurable renal function and will require further investigation to elucidate the problem and make a diagnosis. Nearly 90% are male.

The diuresis renogram has been the most useful method of visualizing the kidney. The isotope study is best performed in a specialized unit, as the baby needs to be strapped into a

cradle and remain quite still during the 15 or 20 min that the study takes to perform. Frusemide is given to induce diuresis, either at the commencement of the investigation or at a fixed time during the study. Any movement of the patient under the camera will cause serious problems with interpretation of the function and drainage pattern of the kidney, and irregular patterns in the computer-generated excretion curve and blurring of the gamma camera image would make the investigation invalid.

Renograms give information about

- Rapidity of uptake – computer analysis of the area under the renogram curve at 3 min gives a figure for individual renal function.
- Rapidity of drainage – the computer-generated drainage curve may be: (a) normal (Figure 30.3), (b) clearly obstructed (Figure 30.3), and (c) slow to drain and therefore equivocal (Figure 30.4).
- Anatomical information from the gamma camera images can often confirm the anatomical site of apparent obstruction, showing for instance pooling in the renal pelvis alone, suggesting poor drainage from the pelvi-ureteric junction, or at the lower end of the ureter, suggesting obstruction at the vesico-ureteric junction.

Considerable controversy currently exists about which is the most valuable aspect of the diuresis renogram in guiding the clinician as to what to do in patients with unilateral upper tract hydronephrosis.

One view states that it is the functional element of the renogram which is the most important, and that if the individual kidney function is more than 40%, then even if obstruction is present, it has not damaged the kidney at this stage, and the patient can be followed conservatively on the basis of serial renograms until the patient either (a) recovers, or (b) shows functional deterioration, when surgical treatment is then instituted.[2]

Published results from this type of approach led to between 30% and 40% of patients ultimately receiving surgical treatment in the form of a pyeloplasty.

A different view has been that the most valuable part of the renogram is in fact the drainage curve. Whatever the level of renal function, provided that the drainage curve does not show clear obstruction, the patient can be followed

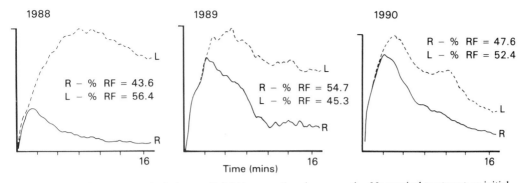

Figure 30.4 Progressive improvement in drainage of left kidney on diuresis renography. No surgical treatment, as initial drainage curve not clearly obstructed

conservatively and improvement will always ensue. Treatment based on this assessment of the initial renogram leads to approximately 40% of patients receiving a pyeloplasty for clear evidence of obstruction on the renogram associated with hydronephrosis and hydrocalicosis on urography.[3] Figure 30.4 shows progressive improvement in the drainage of a hydronephrotic kidney.

It is of considerable interest that both attitudes towards the renogram lead to about 40% of patients receiving a pyeloplasty, and there is no consensus to date as to what is the correct approach.

What is clear is that fewer and fewer patients are having urgent surgical intervention within the first few months of life, and this is not leading to any permanent handicap or renal damage, where careful clinical observation is maintained.

There is no doubt that a number of patients have received unnecessary surgical treatment during the evolution of our understanding of antenatal hydronephrosis, and that as time progresses we should become more adept at identifying those patients who will benefit from pyeloplasty and those who are going to improve spontaneously.

Vesico-ureteric reflux

When postnatal investigations reveal that the patient has vesico-ureteric reflux, the clinician must ensure that the reflux is not secondary to some other remediable cause, and should carefully scrutinize the radiology.

Full views of the male urethra need to be taken and voiding films without the catheter *in situ* to be certain that posterior urethral valves or urethral diverticulum is not causing outflow obstruction to the bladder.

So-called occult neuropathic bladder – not associated with spinal dysraphism – can present in the newborn period with upper tract dilatation and vesico-ureteric reflux. The condition is rare and bladder pressure studies for precise diagnosis are not reliable in this age group. It should be suspected where there is obvious retention of urine without evidence of urethral obstruction, or where the bladder ruptures during delivery, or where large diverticula are present around the bladder base or the urachus is patent.

Other structural malformations associated with vesico-ureteric reflux are usually related to duplication of the urinary tract. The 'drooping flower' appearance (see Chapter 28, particularly Figure 28.1) should alert the clinician to the presence of duplication. A ureterocele in the bladder is usually easily diagnosed both on cystography and ultrasound, and may itself cause outflow obstruction by prolapsing into the urethra during the child's attempts at micturition.

If the child is not already on antibiotics, they should be started immediately, as vesico-ureteric reflux predisposes to early infection and may well cause serious upper tract changes. The author believes that the most appropriate upper tract assessment of patients with reflux which is deemed to be primary in nature, or secondary to structural malformation such as duplication, should be a DMSA scan. It has been dispiriting to discover the extent of reflux nephropathy at birth in this group of patients. We found that one-quarter had evidence of renal damage associated with the reflux at birth,[4] which supports the theory proposed by Mackie and Stevens that congenital reflux is often associated with renal dysplasia secondary to developmental abnormalities of the ureteric bud.[5]

The concept that congenital reflux can subsequently present with infection was supported by Smith *et al.*,[6] and our own study showed that when patients presented with urinary tract infection associated with reflux in the first year of life they had a greater incidence of reflux nephropathy, more than two-thirds showing evidence of renal parenchymal damage on DMSA scan, associated with the refluxing kidney.[4]

Based on this evidence it would seem sensible to place all such patients on chemoprophylaxis, hopefully preventing infection, but alerting the parents to the need of prompt investigation and treatment of all febrile episodes in the first few years of life.

The natural history of vesico-ureteric reflux presenting at this age and in this fashion has not yet been established, but our own figures suggest that even high-grade reflux can undergo spontaneous cure within the first few years of life, and it is to be hoped that the current successful medical management will prevent the upper tract changes seen in those patients presenting with pyelonephritis. Studies from Leeds and London suggest at least one-third of all infants with congenital VUR will cure spontaneously by 3 years.

All febrile episodes in these patients should be carefully investigated and upper tract changes documented with DMSA scan. Renal growth is assessed on an annual basis with ultrasound, and repeat cystogram at 3 years of age used to identify those who spontaneously improve. Early surgical treatment is not advised, as the results of reimplantation surgery in the first 6 months of life are poor, with large numbers of patients showing persisting reflux or developing obstruction after surgery. We have not chosen to perform injection treatment for reflux in this age group either, preferring to identify the natural history of the condition before practising intervention. There is, however, a body of opinion who would suggest that endoscopic injection for reflux in this group had a significant part to play in their management. Time will tell.

Most patients with congenital reflux are male, and where there is evidence of breakthrough infection, circumcision can help reduce the incidence of urinary sepsis. It has been previously noted that urinary tract infections are almost unknown in circumcised male infants.

Hydronephrosis/hydro-ureter – vesico-ureteric junction obstruction

The diagnosis of this condition rests on the exclusion of vesico-ureteric reflux and bladder outflow obstruction as the cause of the dilatation of the renal pelvis and ureter. Renography identifies the relative function of the affected kidney and its drainage pattern, which then compared with subsequent imaging helps determine the sort of management that is best for the individual. Urography has been used in our department to define the radiological anatomy.

Most patients with apparent obstruction at the level of the vesico-ureteric junction will show spontaneous improvement over the first few years of life, with not only resolution of the hydronephrosis, but improvement of the drainage curve.[7] Complications during conservative management are rare, and all related to infection. Chemoprophylaxis is routinely advised, but is not always 100% effective in preventing these complications. We have seen acute infective complications in three patients, two of whom responded to conventional conservative medical management with intravenous antibiotics, but one who had bilateral vesico-ureteric junction obstruction becoming anuric, requiring a period of percutaneous drainage of the upper urinary tract.

Our experiences, however, have not deterred us from the routine medical management of vesico-ureteric junction obstruction, in the firm belief that the majority of patients will have spontaneous cure of their problem, without medical complications.

Where spontaneous improvement is going to occur, it happens within the first 3-years of life, and in our own patients where dilatation persists or worsens beyond this period, or where the drainage curve or function deteriorates, we advise surgical intervention. Intermittent pain in the loin associated with this condition is uncommon, and in small children it is difficult to be certain that the pain is renal in origin, but where present, would indicate surgical treatment.

Careful anatomical and functional evaluation of all patients with hydronephrosis/hydro-ureter should be mandatory, as this may indicate the presence of an underlying duplication in the urinary tract. If present, the obstructed segment is always the upper pole, which may be connected to a ureterocele, obvious on ultrasound, or an ectopic ureter draining into the urethra or perineum. These obstructed segments are frequently either non-functionning or very poorly functioning, and should be the subject of surgical excision. Lower pole vesico-ureteric reflux may be present in such patients, and confuse the clinical picture. Antegrade pyelography may help to determine the precise anatomy.

Multicystic dysplastic kidney

This abnormality, easily diagnosed on ultrasound and confirmed by total absence of function on DMSA scan, is far more common than previously suspected.

Historically, cystic dysplasia was associated with significant abnormalities in the contralateral kidney, but currently most patients seem to have normal renal function (see Table 25.2) and can be anticipated as having a normal life span. This creates a dilemma, which has been fully discussed in Chapter 25.

Many authors have pointed out that the complications of cystic dysplasia are few and far between, and recommended that all such patients should be treated conservatively, and that routine nephrectomy of the cystic element is unnecessary.[8]

We must remain aware, however, that the condition is not totally benign, and in choosing such a course of action, need to explain the reasons for continuing supervision. With cases of carcinoma occurring in cystic dysplastic kidneys beyond the sixth decade of life, it would be foolish to recommend that patients can or should be discharged from follow-up while this approach prevails.

Our own experience with cystic elements that have disappeared on ultrasound for 2 consecutive years has been that reniform tissue is still present and histologically identifiable in the renal fossa, and we are a little uneasy about the conservative approach.

Where there are other abnormalities of renal function or when long-term follow-up is anticipated, we have no hesitation in recommending this course of observation to the parents, but will remove a multicystic dysplastic kidney when the contralateral urinary tract is normal and then discharge the patient from further follow-up.

Duplication of the urinary tract

Partial duplication of the urinary tract (see also Chapters 28 and 29) is a common developmental variant, but where hydronephrosis or hydro-ureter is associated with duplication, it will usually be complete, with two separate ureteric orifices.

The earlier the budding of the ureteric bud, the more abnormal the kidney that it induces. There are certain rules governing the development of duplication and its effects on the urinary tract:

- the upper pole orifice always opens more distally in the urinary tract
- the more distal the opening, the more dysplastic the upper pole kidney
- if obstruction is present in an upper pole duplication, it is always at the lower end of the ureter
- reflux is associated with duplication, but only into the lower pole of the kidney
- if obstruction is present in the lower pole of a duplex system, it is always at the pelvi-ureteric junction.

Treatment will depend on the level of function in the affected segment of the duplex system, but where ureterocele or ectopia are found, it is usual to perform upper pole heminephro-ureterectomy.

Where reflux or obstruction is present in the lower pole, then some form of functional assessment of this part of the kidney should be undertaken before any surgical or medical treatment is offered, as function may be extremely poor. Surgical removal of the dysplastic obstructed or refluxing segment may be more appropriate than reconstruction.

Reflux in association with duplication has a lower chance of spontaneous cure, and where it persists beyond the age of 3, or fails to respond to medical treatment, thought should be given to endoscopic or open methods of surgical correction.

References

1. Clarke N.W., Gough D.C.S. and Cohen S.J. Neonatal urological ultrasound: diagnostic inaccuracies and pitfalls. *Arch. Dis. Child.* 1989, **64**, 578–580
2. Ransley P.G., Dhillon H.K., Gordon I. and Duffy P.G. The post natal management of hydronephrosis diagnosed by prenatal ultrasound. *J. Urol.* 1990, **144**, 584–587
3. O'Flynn K., Gupta S., Gough D.C.S. *et al.* Prediction of recovery in antenatally diagnosed hydronephrosis *Br J. Urol.* 1993, **71**, 478–480.
4. Sheridan M., Jewkes F. and Gough D.C.S. Reflux nephropathy in the first year of life – the role of infection. *Pediatr. Surg. Int.* 1991, **6**, 214–216

5. Mackie G.G. and Stevens F.D. Duplex kidneys, a correlation of renal dysplasia with position of ureteral orifice. *J. Urol.* 1975, **114**, 274–280
6. Smith D., Egginton J.A. and Brookfield D.S.K. Detection of abnormality of foetal urinary tract as a predictor of renal tract disease. *Br. Med. J.* 1987, **294**, 27–28
7. Keating M.A., Escala J., Snyder H. III *et al.* Changing concepts in management of primary obstructive megaureter. *J. Urol.* 1989, **142**, 636–640
8. Gordon A.C., Thomas D.F.M., Arthur R.J. *et al.* Multicystic dysplastic kidney: is nephrectomy still appropriate? *J. Urol.* 1988, **140**, 1231–1234

31

Renal disease in neonates

R.L. Chevalier

To maintain homeostasis during transition from fetal to extra-uterine life, renal structure and function must change rapidly in the neonate. As care improves for very low birthweight infants as well as term neonates, the influence of gestational age on renal function becomes an important consideration. In this chapter, normal renal development will first be reviewed, followed by consideration of specific renal disorders in the newborn.

Renal embryogenesis

Renal development in the human takes place with the sequential appearance of three distinct excretory organs: the pronephros, mesonephros and metanephros. The first two organs appear during the third to fifth weeks of gestation, and the mesonephros produces urine through the eleventh week. Disordered embryogenesis during this period may result in renal agenesis because the mesonephric duct must contact the metanephric blastema to induce formation of the metanephros, or definitive kidney.[1] A branch of the mesonephric duct becomes the ureteric bud during the fourth week, and after growing into the metanephric blastema, branches repeatedly to form the pelvis, calyces and papillary ducts by the twelfth week. Branching continues until the 34th week, at which time nephrogenesis is complete. As a consequence of this process, the most mature nephrons are juxtamedullary, while superficial nephrons are immature. The change in nephron number during human fetal development is shown in Table 31.1.

Each nephron is initially formed by induction of cells of the metanephric blastema by the tip of the ureteric bud. After formation of a cavity, the cells become the renal vesicle which assumes an S shape. Over a period of 5 weeks the vesicle eventually develops into the renal tubule, extending from Bowman's capsule to the distal tubule. The tubule continues to grow in length into adulthood, and may demonstrate additional hypertrophy if renal mass is reduced. The glomerulus is formed by growth of a small vessel into the cleft in the S-shaped renal vesicle. From this vessel, glomerular capillaries develop with primitive mesenchyme becoming the mesangium. Interaction of mesenchymal tissue with epithelial cells forming Bowman's capsule results in production of the glomerular basement membrane which becomes progressively more permeable during maturation. The surface area available for filtration also increases during fetal and postnatal growth.

While abnormalities of renal development in

Table 31.1 Human renal development (Data from Potter[1])

Gestational age (weeks)	Body weight (g)	No. of nephrons
8		200
20	508	350 501
24	1065	608 260
28	1490	766 663
40	3380	822 300

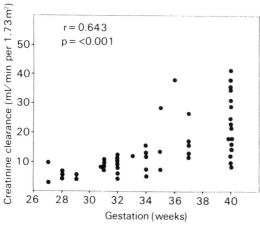

Figure 31.1 Correlation between creatinine clearance and gestational age (From Siegel and Oh,[2] by permission)

the first trimester may result in hypoplasia (decreased number of nephrons), obstruction of the collecting system at any point from the ureteropelvic junction to the urethra can cause cystic dilatation of nephrons and de-differentiation, resulting in deposition of cartilage or primitive mesenchyme typical of dysplastic kidneys.[1] An extreme example of this is multicystic dysplasia, in which the affected kidney is non-functional. Obstruction of some of the tubules may result in polycystic kidney disease, but the relative role of tubular obstruction and toxic or metabolic injury to the tubular epithelium in pathogenesis of cystic disorders remains controversial. An improved understanding of both morphological and metabolic aspects of renal development is necessary before pathological processes will be elucidated.

Fetal renal function

The fetus is unique in that excretory function is accomplished by continuous highly efficient 'haemodialysis' by the placenta, which receives approximately 50% of the infant's cardiac output. In contrast, the fetal kidneys receive less than 5% of cardiac output as a result of high renal vascular resistance relative to the placenta. Renal blood flow in the fetus is maintained at a low rate by low mean arterial blood pressure, by high renin secretion rates, and by increased sensitivity to catecholamines. Glomerular filtration rate increases with gesta-

tional age, but remains very low (less than 15 ml/min per 1.73 m²) until the 34th week (Figure 31.1).[2] This is presumably due to incomplete nephrogenesis as well as to reduced renal blood flow, glomerular capillary pressure and ultrafiltration coefficient (the product of glomerular permeability and surface area for filtration).

It is not surprising that tubular as well as glomerular function is reduced in the fetus. Presumed to be similar to the human, tubular sodium reabsorption increases during gestation in the fetal sheep, and changes in response to osmotic stimuli or vascular volume. Potassium excretion increases during gestation, and correlates with a rise in fetal plasma aldosterone concentration. Glomerulotubular balance for glucose has been demonstrated in the fetal lamb kidney by mid-gestation and is preserved through parturition. While fetal serum phosphate concentration is elevated in the face of low renal phosphate clearance, numerous studies have shown that phosphate excretion may be increased by acute volume expansion or parathyroid hormone secretion. Similarly, although the threshold for tubular bicarbonate reabsorption is normally reduced (to approximately 18 mmol/litre) in the fetal sheep, renal carbonic anhydrase is present and the bicarbonate threshold varies with intravascular volume as it does postnatally. In addition, the fetal kidney is capable of generating an acid urine pH in response to acid infusion. As with all tubular functions, however, excretion of acid is primarily by placental clearance (80%), with less than 5% appearing in amniotic fluid.

Urine production by the human fetus has been determined by ultrasonography, and was found to rise from 12 ml/h at 32 weeks' gestation to 28 ml/h at 40 weeks. The net flux of water *in utero* is from mother to fetus to amniotic fluid, and back to the fetus by swallowing. Approximately 3500 ml/h are exchanged at term. The role of fetal kidneys in fluid exchange during normal pregnancy is therefore relatively unimportant, but when the dynamic balance is disrupted by oligohydramnios due to renal agenesis or malformation, pulmonary development may be impaired. In the fetal sheep, an intrarenal gradient for sodium and urea is present by mid-gestation, and tubular responsiveness to vasopressin may be demonstrated in the third trimester. Although fetal urine is normally hypotonic to plasma, vasopressin has been identified in the human fetal pituitary by 10 weeks' gesta-

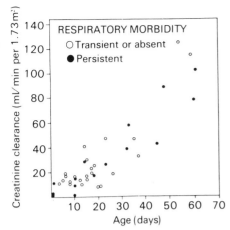

Figure 31.2 Correlation between creatinine clearance and postnatal age of low birth weight infants (birth weight 1000–1928 g) (From Ross *et al.*,[3] by permission)

tion, and fetal vasopressin secretion increases perinatally. By maintaining vascular tone, this hormone may have other important functions in the fetus subjected to hypoxia or hypovolaemia.

Fetal surgery

This is discussed in Chapter 29.

Perinatal and postnatal renal function

Glomerular filtration rate

As reviewed above, most known renal homeostatic mechanisms are operative in the fetus, although fluid and electrolyte regulation is accomplished almost entirely by the placenta. At the time of birth, the functional demand is placed entirely on the kidney, whose performance will be largely dependent on gestational age. In the term infant, glomerular filtration rate increases 50–100% during the first week of life, after which the rate of increase diminishes, reaching adult levels (corrected for body surface area) by the second year. For infants born before 34 weeks of gestational age, glomerular filtration rate rises slowly, if at all, until reaching a post-conceptional age of 34 weeks, after which a rapid increase is also observed. While glomerular filtration rate of term infants at birth is approximately 25 ml/min per 1.73 m², that of 31-week gestational age infants is 10–20 ml/min per 1.73 m² and remains low for the first 2–3 weeks of life (Figure 31.2).[3] As described above, this relates to the timing of completion of nephrogenesis at 34 weeks.

Sodium homeostasis

The relationship of tubular function to gestational age is more complex and remains incompletely understood. After an initial diuresis, the neonate is in a state of positive sodium balance which is a component of normal growth. Following an acute sodium load, the rate of sodium excretion is significantly lower than in the older child or adult, and this may relate to enhanced distal tubular sodium reabsorption under the influence of circulating aldosterone rather than to reduced filtration rate. While term infants are capable of sodium conservation during sodium deprivation, the infant with gestational age less than 35 weeks may develop negative sodium balance with resultant hyponatraemia. This apparent glomerulotubular imbalance may be due to proximal or distal tubular immaturity. As glomerulotubular balance for glucose (reabsorbed proximally) is present in infants as early as 24 weeks' gestation, diminished distal tubular responsiveness to aldosterone is probably more important. The higher rates of natriuresis in small premature infants has led to the recommendation that such infants receive higher sodium intake (i.e. greater than the customary 3 mmol kg⁻¹ day⁻¹) during the first week of life. However, normal gestation is associated with a significant redistribution of body fluid compartments, with relative decrease in extracellular fluid and increase of intracellular fluid space. This change necessitates a reduction in body sodium content from 120 mmol/kg at 8 weeks' to 80 mmol/kg at 40 weeks' gestation. It is therefore not surprising that the extra-uterine trend is similar, and must be taken into account in caring for the infant deprived of a placenta prematurely. The natriuresis occurring during the first few days of life in the preterm infant is associated with initially high levels of plasma atrial natriuretic peptide, which decrease as right atrial size is reduced and body weight falls.[4] It is likely that increased plasma concentration of atrial natriuretic peptide plays a role in postnatal natriuresis, and constitutes a link between cardiopulmonary and renal homeostasis.

Water homeostasis

Reduction in body water content also constitutes a normal aspect of gestation, and correlates with increasing fetal urine production during the third trimester. For the premature infant to assume at birth a body composition similar to that of the term neonate, greater water and sodium losses would be expected. During the first several hours of life, urine volume of the 28-week infant averages 4 ml $kg^{-1} h^{-1}$, while that of the term infant is 1 ml $kg^{-1} h^{-1}$. Diluting capacity of infants with gestational age greater than 30 weeks actually exceeds that of adults, such that urine osmolality can be lowered to 30–50 mmol/kg. Despite this capability, the results of recent studies suggest that excessive rates of fluid administration to premature infants (greater than 150 ml $kg^{-1} day^{-1}$) are associated with expanded extracellular volume and increased incidence of patent ductus arteriosus, bronchopulmonary dysplasia and necrotizing enterocolitis. Thus, interference with normal homeostatic mechanisms by iatrogenic fluid overload may carry significant morbidity.

Unlike diluting capacity, the maximal urinary concentrating capacity of the neonate is initially little higher than plasma osmolality, and ranges from 425 to 670 mosmol/kg in premature and term infants 4–6 weeks of age. Even when a 13–15% loss in body weight is permitted by the fifth day of life in infants with birth weight 750–1500 g, urine-specific gravity remains isotonic to plasma.[5] This may be explained in large part by relatively short loops of Henle and diminished tubular response to circulating vasopressin.

Calcium and phosphorus homeostasis

While fetal serum calcium and phosphorus concentrations are higher than those of the mother, birth results in an abrupt decrease in calcium and more gradual increase in phosphorus concentration.[6] Despite elevated blood phosphorus levels and reduced filtered load of phosphorus secondary to low filtration rate, tubular phosphate reabsorption is enhanced. Tubular reabsorption of phosphorus at birth is approximately 85% in infants of 28 weeks' gestation, and increases to 98% at term. This trend is related to the gradual increase in tubular sodium reabsorption with increasing gestational age. With the commencement of feedings, tubular reabsorption of phosphorus decreases, preventing a further rise in blood concentration. While tubular response to parathyroid hormone in the premature infant is diminished compared to the adult, serum concentration of this hormone does not rise significantly despite a rapid decline in serum calcium concentration in the first postnatal day. There is no general agreement regarding the role of parathyroid hormone in calcium and phosphorus homeostasis in the neonate, and the interplay with vitamin D metabolites is even less clear.[6]

Acid-base homeostasis

Following birth, control of acid-base balance of the neonate shifts from the placenta to the infant's kidneys and lungs. While normal arterial pH of premature and term infants is similar to that of adults, plasma bicarbonate concentration increases from 18 mmol/litre at birth to 20 mmol/litre by 3 weeks, and to 26–28 mmol/litre in adulthood. The observed reduced threshold for bicarbonate reabsorption in the premature infant is probably due to a larger extracellular volume and diminished proximal tubular sodium reabsorption. A phenomenon frequently reported in the past, 'late metabolic acidosis' of the premature, refers to the association of plasma bicarbonate (or total CO_2) less than 18 mmol/litre with impaired weight gain and high protein intake. In a study of 114 low birth weight infants, Schwartz and colleagues[7] found that plasma total CO_2 as low as 14.5 mmol/litre may be normal in the first 3 weeks of life. Furthermore, they detected no difference in growth rate between infants whose total CO_2 was maintained above 21 mmol/litre by administration of bicarbonate and those given a similar amount of isotonic saline. It is therefore likely that many infants previously thought to have significant metabolic acidosis may have simply represented the lower range of normal for this population. Net acid excretion by the kidney is also lower in premature than term infants, and ammonium secretion increases with increasing gestational age. Titratable acid excretion by premature infants 3 or more weeks of age is not different from that of term infants, probably as a result of increased phosphate availability for acid buffering.

In summary, the neonate is capable of rapid adaptation to the extra-uterine environment

Table 31.2 Signs associated with urinary tract disease in the neonate

General
Lethargy
Pallor
Vomiting
Poor feeding
Seizures
Oliguria
Elevation in serum creatinine
Hypertension
Oedema and ascites

Malformations
Head:
  Potter's facies
  Auricular anomalies
Chest:
  Pulmonary hypoplasia
  Pneumothorax
  Supernumerary nipples
Trunk and abdomen:
  Palpable abdominal mass
  Absent abdominal muscles
  Single umbilical artery
  Myelomeningocele
  Imperforate anus
  Cryptorchidism
  Scoliosis
Extremities:
  Radial anomalies
  Single palmar crease

Urinary abnormalities
Haematuria
Proteinuria
Pyuria
Bacteriuria

Table 31.3 Time of first void in 500 infants (Data from Clark[8])

| Age (h) | Cumulative percentage in each group | | |
	Term	Preterm	Post-term
0–8	51	84	38
9–16	91	99	84
17–24	100	100	100

such that homeostasis is normally maintained. The previously described 'functional immaturity' of the newborn kidney was the result of inappropriate comparison of renal function with that of the adult, who has quite different body composition and homeostatic requirements. However, when the neonate is subjected to stress, disease or injudicious fluid and electrolyte therapy, renal adaptation may be inadequate.

Renal disorders in the neonate

Identification of the neonate with renal disease

General signs suggestive of renal disease in the neonate are non-specific, and include lethargy, pallor, vomiting, poor feeding and convulsions (Table 31.2). These signs are also compatible with urinary tract infection, septicaemia, congenital heart disease, and a host of other neonatal disorders. Fever and jaundice are also suggestive of urinary tract infection.

Urine output

As shown in Table 31.2, oliguria is a most helpful sign of renal impairment in the newborn, and the first clue to renal status is the time of first void. Clark[8] found that each of 500 normal infants voided within the first 24 h regardless of gestational age (Table 31.3). The majority of term and preterm infants voided within the first 8 h of life, while post-term babies generally voided during the next 8 h. Therefore, any infant remaining anuric beyond the first day should be investigated for renal insufficiency. Because the neonatal bladder protrudes into the abdominal space, percussion and palpation of the abdomen may reveal a distended bladder secondary to urethral obstruction such as posterior urethral valves. Sterile urethral catheterization with a small feeding tube allows assessment of urine production, urinalysis and measurement of urinary indices (see below).

Based on the average dietary solute load and renal concentrating capacity of the neonate, the minimum urine output of the neonate remaining in solute balance is approximately $1 \, ml \, kg^{-1} \, h^{-1}$, and any infant producing less urine beyond the second day of life may be oliguric. However, critically ill newborns are often administered a lower osmotic load (particularly in the first days of life), such that a more stringent criterion for oliguria, $0.5 \, ml \, kg^{-1} \, h^{-1}$, may be more appropriate in these patients. In addition, non-oliguric renal failure has become more widely appreciated in recent years,[9] and a measure of glomerular filtration should also be sought.

Elevation in serum creatinine

Renal dysfunction in hospitalized infants is frequently first identified by an elevation in serum creatinine obtained in the general evaluation of the patient. Because of difficulties in obtaining accurately timed urine collections, lack of a steady state in transition from intra-uterine to postnatal life, and lack of reliability in measuring serum creatinine at the low concentrations present in infants, determination of glomerular filtration rate in newborns is problematic. Despite these concerns, the most commonly available index of glomerular filtration remains the

Table 31.4 Normal serum creatinine concentration (Data from Trompeter *et al.*[10])

Age	Concn in term babies (μmol/litre)		Concn in preterm babies (μmol/litre)	
	Mean	*Range*	*Mean*	*Range*
Cord blood	87	64–115		
2 days	76	56–106	83	62–120
7 days	56	39–79	76	49–91
10–15 days	62	43–74	86	60–130

serum creatinine concentration. After the first 2 days of life, a serum creatinine concentration greater than 88 μmol/litre in the preterm infant (132 μmol/litre in the preterm infant) suggests filtration failure. These values are obtained from the commonly used autoanalyser technique, and are somewhat lower when the more precise kinetic method is employed. Normal values for serum creatinine concentration during the first 2 months of life are listed in Table 31.4.[10] Perhaps more importantly, the serum creatinine concentration should not rise significantly after birth, and a daily increase of 44–88 μmol/litre indicates falling filtration rate regardless of urine output. For purposes of following glomerular filtration rate during growth of the infant, creatinine clearance (ml/min per 1.73 m²) may be estimated from the formula:

$$C_{Cr} = k \times L/P_{Cr}$$

where k = an empiric constant (30 in preterm and 40 in term infants), L = body length in cm, and P_{Cr} = plasma creatinine concentration in μmol/litre.[11] Although serum urea nitrogen has also been used as a measure of glomerular filtration rate in the newborn, its dependence on dietary protein intake and effective circulating volume make it unreliable.

Hypertension

Hypertension is another sign of renal dysfunction in the neonate. Infants having an indwelling umbilical artery catheter may be predisposed to renal embolization and development of renin-dependent hypertension.[12] The current practice of positioning the catheter tip below the level of the renal arteries should result in decreased incidence of this entity. Additional causes of hypertension include polycystic kidney disease, obstructive nephropathy, renal or adrenal neoplasm, and acute or chronic renal failure. However, non-renal causes of hypertension should also be kept in mind, including aortic coarctation, congenital adrenal hyperplasia, subdural haemorrhage and corticosteroid administration. Normal systolic blood pressure in term infants is less than 90 mmHg during the first week of life, and less than 110 mmHg in the second month. In preterm infants, systolic pressure greater than 70 mmHg in the first week and 90 mmHg in the second month of life should be considered elevated.

Oedema and ascites

The differential diagnosis of oedema in the neonate includes all of the causes of hydrops foetalis, such as Rh isoimmunization and fetal supraventricular tachycardia. Thus, evaluation should include a careful haematological and cardiological examination. The most important renal causes of congenital oedema are lower urinary tract obstruction and congenital nephrotic syndrome. Severe obstructive nephropathy may result in rupture of a renal calyx, and urinary ascites. This is not infrequently found in infants with posterior urethral valves, in whom the urinary leak may actually serve as a protective mechanism by reducing intrapelvic pressure and preserving functioning renal mass. The diagnosis can be made by abdominal ultrasonography and nuclide scan using ^{99m}Tc-diethyltriamine penta-acetic acid (DTPA), or cystourethrography, if vesico-ureteral reflux is present. Congenital nephrotic syndrome may be suspected *in utero* if the maternal serum alpha fetoprotein is elevated, or if oedema is detected by prenatal ultrasonography. These infants will have heavy proteinuria, and urinary losses of thyroxine may result in abnormal thyroid function tests during neonatal screening. Since virtually all infants with congenital nephrotic syndrome develop hypothyroidism, it is imperative that thyroid function be monitored closely in infancy even if the initial values are normal. Appropriate thyroid replacement should be instituted early to prevent the development of overt hypothyroid signs and symptoms.

Malformations

Renal malformations are frequently associated with anomalies of other organs. The typical facial features of renal agenesis (Potter's syndrome) include large flat ears, infraorbital skin folds sweeping laterally from the inner canthus, and a flat nasal profile.[1] These findings, as well as pulmonary hypoplasia and bowing of the feet, are thought to result from oligohydramnios due to fetal oliguria or anuria. Although originally described in association with bilateral renal agenesis, any severe bilateral renal malformation resulting in oliguria (including hypoplasia, dysplasia or cystic kidney disease) can result in these non-renal features. The most life-threatening of the effects is pulmonary hypoplasia, which may make the patient dependent on respiratory support. In addition to pulmonary hypoplasia, pneumothorax may be a sign of underlying renal maldevelopment, including hypoplasia, dysplasia, hydronephrosis, or bilateral cystic kidney disease. There appears to be a close association between malformations of the pinna and renal anomalies such as double collecting system, hydronephrosis and cystic kidney.[13] In cases of unilateral renal involvement, the ipsilateral ear is more often involved.[13] Infants with significant malformation of one or both ears should therefore undergo screening renal ultrasonography.

A palpable abdominal mass in the newborn most likely represents renal enlargement due to obstructive nephropathy, cystic renal disease, renal vein thrombosis or tumour. The finding of 'prune-belly' (redundant, wrinkled abdominal skin) indicates hypoplastic abdominal musculature, which is frequently associated with undescended testes and dilatation of the urinary collecting system (also known as the 'triad' or Eagle–Barrett syndrome). However, the abdominal defect may also result from severe intra-uterine hydronephrosis and distension of the abdominal wall. Moreover, cryptorchidism may be associated with renal anomalies even in the absence of abdominal wall defects.[14]

The combination of vertebral defects, imperforate anus, tracheoesophageal fistula and radial dysplasia constitutes the VATER association. Since renal and cardiac defects are also present in nearly 75% of reported cases, a thorough evaluation of the urinary tract is essential is all affected infants. Myelomeningocele is associated with varying degrees of bladder dyssynergia, and if untreated leads to hydro-ureteronephrosis and/or vesico-ureteral reflux, and to progressive renal insufficiency. These patients should have lifetime monitoring of their renal status, and may require urinary tract diversion or intermittent bladder catheterization to optimize renal function.

Whereas the association of renal anomalies with Potter's facies, prune-belly and imperforate anus is well established, the significance of supernumerary nipples, scoliosis or single umbilical artery in the neonate is less clear. There does, however, appear to be sufficient evidence to justify at least a screening renal sonogram in all infants with these physical findings.

A number of dysmorphic features may also suggest a chromosomal defect, many of which are associated with renal malformations.[15] Down's syndrome, commonly associated with a single palmar crease, is associated with hydro-ureteronephrosis, while Turner's syndrome is associated with horseshoe kidney or duplicated collecting system.[15]

Haematuria (Table 31.5)

Although microscopic haematuria is not uncommon in the critically ill preterm infant (usually associated with sepsis or hypoxia), gross haematuria is distinctly rare. As shown in Table 31.5, renal vascular insults and congenital renal anomalies account for haematuria in most instances. Renal venous thrombosis typically results in a palpable abdominal mass due to extension of thrombi in one or both kidneys, and presents with brick-red urine. There is usually an acute drop in the haematocrit and platelet count. Renal arterial embolization may result from umbilical artery catheterization, and should be suspected in the infant with haematuria and hypertension. Extensive occlusion of either the arterial or venous renal circulation of the neonate can lead to renal cortical necrosis. This is usually patchy, and the extent of recovery depends on the severity of the insult and the promptness of restoration of circulation.

Table 31.5   Renal causes of haematuria in the newborn (After Brem[31])

Renal vascular disorders secondary to sepsis, asphyxia, hypertension
Ischaemic acute renal failure
Renal venous thrombosis
Renal cortical necrosis
Renal arterial embolization

Renal anomalies
Partial urinary tract obstruction
Cystic renal diseases

Tumours
Wilms' tumour
Mesoblastic nephroma (hamartoma)
Nephroblastomatosis

Drugs
Antibiotics
Anticoagulants
Diuretics
Anticonvulsants

Inflammatory
Glomerulonephritis
Urinary tract infection

Table 31.6   Causes of proteinuria in the newborn (After Brem[31])

Physiological (first week)
Renal vascular disorders
Congenital nephrotic syndrome
Inflammatory renal disease (infection)
Drugs

Obstructive nephropathy due to ureteropelvic junction obstruction, posterior urethral valves or other congenital lesions, may also present with haematuria, particularly if there is marked hydronephrosis and a difficult vaginal delivery. Autosomal recessive (infantile) polycystic kidney disease should be suspected in the infant with bilateral renomegaly, hypertension and haematuria. Although uncommon, autosomal dominant (so-called 'adult') polycystic kidney disease may also present in the neonate, and should be considered if there is a positive family history for cystic renal disease. Multicystic dysplasia is usually unilateral, and does not generally cause haematuria. Whereas Wilms' tumour is rare in the neonate, mesoblastic nephroma or nephroblastomatosis are occasionally seen, and carry a more favourable prognosis than renal neoplasms in older infants and children.

Drugs which may result in haematuria in the neonate include aminoglycosides, penicillins, heparin, anticonvulsants, aminophylline and diuretics. Furosemide, particularly when combined with corticosteroid administration for treatment of pulmonary disorders, may result in hypercalciuria and secondary gross haematuria. In contrast to the older infant and child, in whom the urinary calcium to creatinine concentration ratio is below 0.69 mmol/mmol, the ratio may be as high as 2 in the normal term infant, and 4 in the preterm infant.[16]

Unlike in the older infant or child, glomerulonephritis is a very rare cause of haematuria in infants in developed countries. Neonatal infections that may cause inflammation of the renal parenchyma include syphilis, toxoplasmosis and cytomegalovirus. Idiopathic chronic glomerulonephritis (such as IgA nephropathy, membranous nephropathy or membranoproliferative glomerulonephritis) is even less likely than the post-infectious types.

Proteinuria (Table 31.6)

Urine protein excretion is greatest during the first day of age (approximately 0.5 g/litre) and rapidly falls to normal adult concentrations by the second week of life. As described above, proteinuria may also be associated with vascular disorders or with inflammatory renal disease. The congenital nephrotic syndrome is described in detail in Chapter 19.

Pyuria and bacteriuria

Normally, uncentrifuged urine collected from neonates contains less than 5 leucocytes per mm³. Increased numbers of urinary leucocytes generally suggests the presence of a urinary tract infection, although inflammatory renal diseases, drug reactions or hypercalciuria should also be considered.

The prevalence of bacteriuria in neonates is less than 1% in term and preterm infants, and screening for bacteriuria is probably not warranted in otherwise healthy infants. It should be noted that the bacterial contamination rate for urine collected by the plastic bag method in neonates is 6%. In febrile infants, however, the prevalence of bacteriuria is 7.5%,[17] and urine culture in these neonates should be obtained by suprapubic aspiration or bladder catheterization.

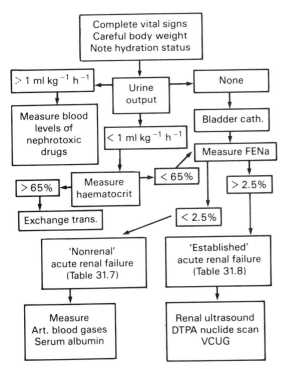

Figure 31.3 Evaluation of the neonate with elevated serum creatinine due to suspected acute renal failure (see text for details)

Table 31.7 **Non-renal causes of oliguria in the newborn**

Fractional sodium excretion < 2.5%
Hypotension
    Early cord clamping
    Hypothermia
    Sepsis
    Increased insensible water loss
Congestive heart failure
Hypoproteinaemia

Fractional sodium secretion variable
Hyperviscosity
Hypoxia
Respiratory distress syndrome

Evaluation of the neonate with renal disease

After identification of the infant with renal disease by history, physical examination or serum creatinine measurement, appropriate diagnosis should be sought.

Acute renal failure (Figure 31.3)

Because renal insufficiency in the newborn often accompanies circulatory disorders associated with birth or prematurity (Table 31.7), it is necessary to separate renal parenchymal disease from non-renal causes. Reduced renal perfusion due to hypovolaemia and hypotension may result from perinatal blood loss, an asphyxiated myocardium, sepsis, or increased insensible water loss due to exposure to a radiant warmer. Decreased cardiac output from any cause, including congenital cardiac anomalies and arrhythmias, may also impair renal perfusion. Severe hypoproteinemia resulting from congenital nephrotic syndrome may cause diminished glomerular filtration secondary to lowered colloid oncotic pressure and decreased effective circulating volume. In each of these conditions, tubular sodium reabsorption is enhanced. Because a random urine sample may be used, determination of fractional sodium excretion (FE_{Na}) is practical in the neonate (see Chapter 21).

Unlike in the older child or adult, neonatal sodium reabsorptive capacity is limited in the first week of life, and a higher value for FE_{Na} may represent normal maximal sodium conservation. The results of several studies indicate that values lower than 2.5–3.0% in the oliguric neonate (gestational age 28–44 weeks) suggest circulatory insufficiency rather than intrinsic renal disease.[18]

For the infant with low FE_{Na} and suspected hypovolaemia without oedema or evidence of congestive heart failure, urine output may be restored by infusion over 1 h of 20 ml/kg of plasma. In the very low birthweight infant, vascular volume must be expanded cautiously to avoid complications such as intraventricular haemorrhage. If oliguria persists, a single intravenous dose of frusemide, 2 mg/kg, may result in diuresis. Due to the risks of hyperosmolarity in the neonate, mannitol infusion is not recommended.

There are several additional disorders which may cause renal insufficiency as a result of circulatory disturbances, but FE_{Na} may be higher. Polycythaemia (defined as venous haematocrit exceeding 65%) occurs in 2–5% of neonates, and causes hyperviscosity, reduced cardiac output, decreased renal plasma flow and glomerular filtration rate. Reduction in haematocrit by dilutional exchange transfusion is followed by increase in glomerular filtration and urine output. While it is generally agreed that hypoxia results in vasoconstriction and decreased urine flow rate, glomerular filtration rate may not fall acutely. Because sodium reabsorption is reduced during hypoxia, FE_{Na} would be expected to rise. Due to the complex physiological perturbations caused by idiopathic respiratory distress syndrome, renal involvement is unclear at present. Decreased

---

Table 31.8   Renal causes of filtration failure in the newborn

Prolonged ischaemia
Hypotension
Congenital heart disease
Hypoxia

Vascular disorders
Renal venous thrombosis
Renal cortical necrosis
Renal artery embolization

Renal anomalies
Renal agenesis (Potter's syndrome)
Renal dysplasia (including multicystic kidney)
Renal hypoplasia
Polycystic kidney disease

Obstructive nephropathy
Ureteropelvic junction obstruction
Posterior urethral valves
Ureterovesical obstruction
Vesico-ureteral reflux
Megacystic syndrome
Renal tumours

---

glomerular filtration rate in this syndrome[19] may be dependent more on the infant's state of hydration than on pulmonary function. More important than filtration rate, mobilization of fluid from the pulmonary interstitium and resultant diuresis appears to herald recovery. The mechanisms responsible for these fluid shifts are not established, but may involve decreasing production of vasodilator prostaglandins or increased secretion of atrial natriuretic peptide.[20] Although sodium excretion is enhanced by respiratory distress syndrome, continuous positive airway pressure administered to improve oxygenation inhibits sodium excretion. As a result, calculated FE_{Na} is not a useful index of renal perfusion in these infants (see Table 21.11).

Once established, renal parenchymal disease generally results in diminished tubular sodium reabsorption as well as glomerular filtration rate, and FE_{Na} exceeds 2.5% despite oliguria. If prolonged, any of the conditions listed in Table 31.7 could result in acute renal failure not reversible by volume expansion, exchange

transfusion or cardiopulmonary therapy. Table 31.8 shows additional causes of neonatal acute renal failure. Possibly as a result of increased renal vascular resistance, the newborn appears to be at risk of renal vascular thrombosis. Renal venous thrombosis should be considered in the infant with oliguria, gross haematuria, palpably enlarged kidneys, and a precipitous fall in haematocrit and platelet count. Predisposing factors include asphyxia, dehydration, cyanotic congenital heart disease, and administration of radiographic contrast material for angiography in critically ill infants.

Renal ultrasonography reveals unilateral or bilateral renal enlargement and possibly increased echotexture without evidence of hydronephrosis. Radionuclide scintiscan may show decreased function, and possibly no detectable uptake of isotope.[9] However, lack of visualization by scintigraphy does not preclude recovery in this condition. Treatment is generally supportive, including peritoneal dialysis if necessary to correct congestive heart failure, electrolyte imbalance, or intractable acidosis in cases of bilateral involvement. The use of heparin and surgery remains controversial, but is probably indicated in bilateral cases and those with inferior vena caval involvement in whom it should be continued until platelet count and clotting studies normalize. Following an initial intravenous dose of 100 u/kg, the hourly infusion rate should be 25 u kg^{-1} h^{-1}.

Renal cortical necrosis is a serious complication of severe renal ischaemia, usually in the context of sepsis and disseminated intravascular coagulation. Infants recovering from cortical necrosis may have intrarenal calcification detectable on abdominal radiographs. In contrast, the severity of renal arterial embolization depends on the extent of involvement, and may present with hypertension out of proportion to renal insufficiency. As described above, renal embolization is usually a complication of umbilical artery catheterization, and hypertension is renin-mediated. Care of these patients is also supportive, and includes treatment of hypertension. In general, management of hypertension follows the principles set out in Chapter 15. Although angiotensin converting enzyme inhibitors are theoretically ideal for the management of severe renin-dependent hypertension, several reports indicate that neonates may be unusually sensitive to their effects, and may develop renal insufficiency or neurologic sequelae unless the

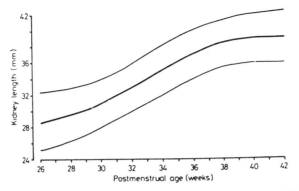

Figure 31.4 Correlation between sonographic renal length and post-menstrual age (mean ± 2 SD) (From de Vries and Levene,[23] by permission)

dose is markedly reduced.[21] A starting dose of captopril of 0.01 mg/kg has been recommended.

Congenital renal anomalies (including obstructive nephropathy) are responsible for over half of the cases of renal failure in infancy. These entities are discussed in detail in Chapters 7 and 27–30, and their diagnosis in the newborn depends largely on radiological studies.[22] Renal ultrasonography should be performed first in any infant with a palpable abdominal mass or suspected renal anomaly. The procedure is non-invasive, not dependent on renal function, and permits assessment of renal size, position, presence of cysts, and hydronephrosis. Normal renal length for infants of varying gestational age measured sonographically within the first 3 days of life is shown in Figure 31.4.[23] It should be noted that the limit of resolution of transducers is 5 mm, and smaller cysts, such as are present in neonates with polycystic kidney disease, cannot currently be detected by this technique. To determine function of each kidney, sonography should be followed by renal scintigraphy using ^{99m}Tc-DTPA to determine differential kidney function. ^{131}I-ortho-iodohippurate (hippuran) should be avoided because of the higher dose of radiation involved. Scintigraphy is superior to intravenous pyelography (IVP) in the neonate because radiation exposure is reduced, the infant is not subjected to the osmotic and toxic hazards of radiocontrast infusion, and kidneys are usually poorly visualized by IVP until at least 2 weeks of age. In addition to its value in determining the relative contribution of each kidney to total renal function, scintigraphy also provides an index of prognosis in neonatal acute renal failure.[9] Infants demon-

strating uptake of nuclide during the initial period of renal insufficiency are likely to make an excellent recovery, while those without detectable uptake are likely to have irreversible renal damage. Caution must be exercised, however, as occasional patients (particularly those with bilateral renal vein thrombosis) may fail to reveal renal uptake of nuclide and yet recover significant function. Because low rates of renal perfusion may be undetected by scintigraphy, confirmation of suspected Potter's syndrome should include aortography. Renal biopsy should also be considered in any infant with renal failure persisting for longer than several weeks in whom the diagnosis or prognosis remains uncertain.

Multicystic dysplasia is a frequent cause of abdominal mass in the neonate (see Chapter 25). Ureteropelvic junction obstruction, the most common cause of obstructive nephropathy in the newborn,[24] is often bilateral, causing renal failure in infancy. Posterior urethral valves are frequently found in males with hydronephrosis and result in dilated ureters and thickened bladder wall which may be detected sonographically. Although vesico-ureteral reflux and megacystis syndrome are not characterized by identifiable anatomical obstruction, the effect on renal parenchyma and radiographic appearance may be similar. Voiding cysto-urethrography is an important adjunct to evaluation of neonatal renal anomalies and should be performed whenever vesico-ureteral reflux is suspected. Renal tumours such as hamartoma or Wilms' tumour are rare in the neonate, but are an additional cause of urinary tract obstruction. In patients with complex anomalies or neoplasms involving the kidney, more precise anatomical definition may by accomplished using computerized axial tomography. Optimal management of infants with obstructive nephropathy involves participation of the paediatric urologist in planning appropriate urinary diversion or primary surgical correction.

Urinary tract infection

As stated above, urinary tract infection may be manifested in the newborn by poor weight gain, fever, lethargy, vomiting, diarrhoea and jaundice. Haematuria and proteinuria are infrequently associated with neonatal urinary tract infection, and leucocyturia is not a consistent finding. Using suprapubic bladder aspiration, the prevalence of asymptomatic infection has been shown to be less than 1% in term infants,[25] and symptomatic infection occurs in approximately 2% of high-risk neonates.[26] The slight preponderance of infection in male preterm and post-term infants remains unexplained. The route of infection in the neonate is also poorly understood, and is presumed to be haematogenous, although bacteriuria is rare in infants with documented septicaemia. The role of circumcision in predisposing infants to urinary tract infection remains controversial, but several studies suggest an increased incidence of urinary tract infection in uncircumcised infants.[27] Urinary tract infection without bacteraemia is more common in infants over 72 hours of age. Any infant with urinary tract infection should be given a 10–14-day course of appropriate intravenous antibiotics.

There is significant disagreement regarding the prevalence of urinary tract abnormalities in neonates with documented urinary tract infection, with figures ranging from less than 10% to nearly 50%. In view of the susceptibility of the developing kidney to damage from obstruction or infection, it would seem prudent to perform renal ultrasonography to rule out gross anomalies, and cysto-urethrography to rule out vesico-ureteral reflux. Intravenous pyelography may be performed in selected infants after 2 weeks of age.

Inflammatory renal disease

Glomerular and interstitial inflammatory renal disease is far less common in the neonate than the older infant or child. There are scattered

reports of acute pyelonephritis in newborns who present with signs of sepsis or urinary tract infection. Most affected infants have pyuria and azotaemia in addition to bacteriuria and septicaemia. Necropsy has revealed leucocytic interstitial infiltration, glomerular sclerosis and paucity of cortical scarring. It is likely, however, that scars would have developed had these infants survived. It is in fact possible that most renal cortical scars detected in later childhood are the result of intrarenal reflux of infected urine in early infancy. Evaluation of infants with suspected pyelonephritis should include culture of urine obtained by suprapubic puncture as well as of blood and spinal fluid. Renal ultrasonography should be performed to rule out major urinary tract malformation, and voiding cysto-urethrography is required to rule out vesico-ureteral reflux. If reflux is demonstrated, urine cultures should be carefully monitored for recurrence of bacteriuria and intravenous pyelography may be performed after several months. Blood pressure should also be carefully monitored as these infants are at risk for development of hypertension.

Glomerulonephritis in the neonate is generally due to congenital infection. Syphilis may result in congenital nephrotic syndrome, and serological tests for syphilis should be performed in any infant with unexplained haematuria or proteinuria, even in the absence of other signs of disease. Hypertension, azotaemia and hypocomplementaemia may also be present in congenital syphilitic nephropathy, unlike the secondary type occurring in older patients. Immune complex nephrosis may also result from congenital toxoplasmosis, and appropriate serological studies should be obtained in the proteinuric infant with clinical signs of infection. Renal biopsy reveals proliferative nephritis and tubulo-interstitial changes which may respond to corticosteroid treatment. Viruria with typical intracellular inclusion bodies is not uncommon in infants with cytomegalovirus disease, but overt glomerulonephritis is rare with congenital infection.

In all renal inflammatory diseases of the newborn, evaluation should include complete bacterial cultures, serological titres of antibodies to infections common in the neonate, urine cytology and viral culture, and measurement of serum complement components. Renal biopsy may be necessary to diagnose the renal lesion.

Table 31.9 Parameters to follow in the neonate with renal insufficiency

Serial body weight
Serial serum creatinine
Daily urine output
Cardiopulmonary status
Fluid, sodium, potassium protein intake
Serum electrolytes, calcium, phosphorus
Blood levels of nephrotoxic drugs

Table 31.10 Insensible water loss in the neonate ($ml\,kg^{-1}\,h^{-1}$) (Data from El-Dahr and Chevalier[28])

Weight of infant (kg)	Incubator	Radiant warmer
0.6–1.0	1.5–3.5	2.4–5.2
1.0–1.5	1.5–2.3	1.5–2.7
1.5–2.0	0.7–1.0	0.5–1.5
3.0	0.5	1.0

Treatment of the neonate with renal disease

Management of the newborn with renal impairment requires a complete understanding of neonatal renal physiology and close collaboration with the attending neonatologist, urologist or paediatric surgeon.

Acute renal failure

Established acute renal failure unresponsive to volume expansion or cardiopulmonary care may result in complications similar to those present in the older infant or child (Chapter 21). Initial objectives of management include treatment of proven or suspected infection with broad-spectrum antibiotics, maintenance of adequate tissue perfusion, oxygenation, blood pressure, acid-base and electrolyte balance. Some of the most important parameters to follow are listed in Table 31.9.

It cannot be overemphasized that every effort must be made to monitor body weight accurately at least every 12 h, as cumulative changes of several grams may be significant in the critically ill neonate. Fluid replacement for insensible losses may be estimated initially at 0.5–1 $ml\,kg^{-1}\,h^{-1}$ for a term infant, but must be reassessed daily (Table 31.10).[28] Humidification of air administered by mechanical ventilation will decrease water requirements, while exposure to a radiant warmer will increase evaporative losses. Due to the greater surface/volume ratio, preterm infants have greater insensible losses (at least 1.5 $ml\,kg^{-1}\,h^{-1}$ for a 1000 g infant) (Table 31.10).[28] All insensible losses should be replaced with 10–15% dextrose in water without added electrolytes. Fluids infused as a result of flushing vascular catheters may constitute a significant fraction of daily requirements and should be taken into account. Additional losses in urine, gastrointestinal and surgical drainage should be replaced with fluids of similar composition or altered to correct electrolyte imbalance. With appropriate fluid administration, body weight should decrease 0.5–1% daily for several days until the patient is no longer catabolic. Unless the patient is initially volume contracted, progressive increase in weight indicates overhydration.

Arterial pH should be maintained above 7.2 by adequate ventilation and sodium bicarbonate infusion. In the neonate with intractable acidosis, repeated administration of hypertonic sodium bicarbonate will result in hypernatraemia and possible hypertension, congestive heart failure, patency of the ductus arteriosus, and intracranial haemorrhage. Peritoneal dialysis allows correction of acidosis without volume expansion in such patients.

In the setting of acute renal failure, hyponatraemia generally indicates overhydration, but adrenal insufficiency with severe hyponatraemia, hyperkalaemia and vascular collapse should also be kept in mind, particularly in the child with ambiguous genitalia. If the infant is clearly volume expanded based on increased weight, blood pressure or presence of oedema, fluid intake should be further restricted to allow correction by insensible losses. If dehydration is present, 20 ml/kg volume expansion should result in improvement. It should be noted that FE_{Na} is high ($>2.5\%$) in infants with adrenal insufficiency regardless of renal function or state of hydration. If serum sodium is less than 120 mmol/litre or the infant is convulsing, 3% sodium chloride solution should be infused to raise serum sodium above 125 mmol/litre. A dose of sodium (in mmol) equal to three times the infant's weight (kg) should raise the serum sodium by 5 mmol/litre.

In the neonate, serum potassium concentrations up to 7 mmol/litre are generally tolerated. For higher potassium concentrations or electrocardiographic evidence of hyperkalaemia, emergency treatment is instituted as for the older child (see Chapter 21). Exchange transfusion with low potassium washed red blood cells reconstituted with fresh frozen plasma has recently been shown to effectively reverse hyperkalaemia in the neonate and may avert necessity for dialysis.

In the infant deprived of oral feedings, renal insufficiency may result in hypocalcaemia which may lead to tetany during rapid correction of acidosis. Infusion of calcium gluconate to maintain normal ionized serum calcium concentration should prevent this complication. To minimize phosphate and potassium intake, infants able to tolerate feedings should be given formulae with a high calcium/phosphorus ratio and low potassium content. Calcium carbonate, administered orally in divided doses, may be added to maintain serum inorganic phosphate between 1.6 and 2.3 mmol/litre. Aluminium-containing compounds are contra-indicated in the neonate due to the risks of aluminium toxicity to the developing nervous system and bone mineralization. For infants with prolonged renal failure unable to receive oral feedings, adequate nutrition (100 kcal kg^{-1} day^{-1}) should be provided by parenteral alimentation consisting of dextrose, lipid and amino acids.

Severe hypertension should be treated along the principles set out in Chapter 15. Intravenous hydrallazine (0.2 mg/kg), labetalol and probably nitroprusside have probably superceded intravenous diazoxide (3 mg/kg repeated in 20–30 min if necessary). Because of inhibition of myocardial contractility, use of labetol and β-adrenergic blockers must be carefully considered in the infant with cardiac disease.

If life-threatening electrolyte imbalance or hypertension is unresponsive to these measures and the infant remains oliguric, peritoneal dialysis should be instituted (see Chapter 21). Because temporary rigid peritoneal catheters in the neonate are subject to leakage, poor outflow and bacterial invasion, they are generally unsatisfactory. Instead, an appropriate-sized single-cuff Tenckhoff silastic catheter should be surgically placed, allowing prolonged dialysis if necessary. Although techniques of peritoneal dialysis cannot be delineated here, it should be noted that critically ill neonates are often unable to metabolize the acetate or lactate in commercial dialysate, and the dialysis solution may need to be specially prepared using sodium bicarbonate as a source of alkali. Continuous arteriovenous

haemofiltration is a newly developed technique for the treatment of fluid and electrolyte imbalance in critically ill oliguric infants. This involves cannulation of a major artery and vein, and circulation of the blood through a cartridge containing a semipermeable membrane allowing rapid ultrafiltration to relieve pulmonary oedema or congestive heart failure. The technique is described in detail in Chapter 21.

As tubular and glomerular function recover, urine output increases, resulting in electrolyte loss. It is important to recognize this 'polyuric' phase of acute renal failure, and to monitor the urine content of sodium and potassium and phosphate for proper replacement. Dietary restrictions should be eased and medications should be adjusted to the changing glomerular filtration rate.

Chronic renal failure

Infants with presumed acute renal failure not recovering within 4–6 weeks, as well as those with severe congenital renal anomalies, may have irreversible renal failure. It may be necessary to perform renal biopsy in selected cases in attempts to establish diagnosis and prognosis at this point. Until recently, neonates with severe renal insufficiency were not offered long-term support. As a result of advances in peritoneal dialysis, including continuous ambulatory and continuous cycling peritoneal dialysis, several centres have reported growth in infants to a weight of 7–10 kg over a period of months. Infants with chronic renal failure have a number of special needs, including a frequent requirement for nasogastric feeding to enhance caloric intake and to permit sodium supplementation to replace that lost in the dialysate. Although some infants receive calcium carbonate or calcium citrate to bind dietary phosphorus, many actually require phosphate supplementation to allow normal skeletal growth.

Transplantation of a parent donor kidney is feasible in infants weighing 7–10 kg, and the success rate is far more encouraging than for cadaveric transplants at this age. This is a rapidly advancing field, and short-term results at a number of centres are quite promising. However, the long-term outcome of these children is less certain, as the neurological sequelae of chronic renal insufficiency during infancy may become more apparent in the future.

Renal pharmacology in the neonate

Due to the reduced glomerular filtration rate in the neonate, dosage of drugs excreted by the kidneys must be adjusted appropriately. As prematurity and renal disease result in additional reduction in glomerular filtration, monitoring blood concentrations of nephrotoxic drugs becomes necessary.

Aminoglycoside antibiotics are commonly prescribed in the high-risk infant, and the recommended dose for gentamicin in the term infant with normal renal function is 2.5 mg/kg per dose every 12 h during the first week and every 8 h during the second week of life. For the infant with gestational age less than 35 weeks, the interval should be prolonged to 18 h, and even to 36 h if renal insufficiency is present. The desired one-hour post-dose peak serum concentration is 4–8 μg/ml, and pre-dose (trough) concentration is 0.5–2 μg/ml. Peak and trough concentrations should be measured on the second day of treatment and on alternate days thereafter. Experimental evidence suggests that aminoglycosides may be proportionately less nephrotoxic in the newborn than in the adult, but by the time an increase in serum creatinine is detected, significant tubular damage has occurred. Monitoring blood levels is therefore the most prudent approach to management in the infant.[29]

Another drug frequently administered to the critically ill neonate is frusemide, whose half-life in the first 3 weeks of life (20 h) is considerably longer than in adults. Daily doses exceeding 2 mg/kg may place the patient at risk for development of ototoxicity.[30] Furthermore, long-term use of frusemide, particularly when combined with glucocorticoids for treatment of bronchopulmonary dysplasia, may lead to hypercalciuria, urolithiasis, and skeletal demineralization. Urine calcium/creatinine ratio should be measured periodically in these infants to detect hypercalciuria (see above).

Administration of indomethacin to induce closure of patent ductus arteriosus causes transient decrease in urine flow, creatinine clearance and sodium excretion. However, successful closure of the ductus results in reversal of these trends, presumably as a result of restoration of effective circulating volume.

Numerous additional drugs used in the neonatal period have significant effects on renal function and in turn are affected by impaired renal function. The undesired as well as therapeutic effects of medications must be considered in the evaluation and management of any infant with renal disease.

References

1. Potter E.L. *Normal and Abnormal Developmenet of the Kidney*. Chicago, Year Book, 1972
2. Siegel S.R. and Oh W. Renal function as a marker of human fetal maturation. *Acta Paediatr. Scan.* 1976, **65**, 481–485
3. Ross B., Cowett R.M. and Oh W. Renal functions of low birth weight infants during the first two months of life. *Pediatr. Res.* 1977, **11**, 1162–1164
4. Bierd T.M., Kattwinkel J., Chevalier R.L., Rheuban K.S., Smith D.J., Teague W.G. *et al.* The interrelationship of atrial natriuretic peptide, atrial volume, and renal function in premature infants. *J. Pediatr.* 1990, **116**, 753–759
5. Lorenz J.M., Kleinman L.I., Kotagal U.R. and Reller M.D. Water balance in very low-birthweight infants: relationship to water and sodium intake and effect on outcome. *J. Pediatr.* 1982, **101**, 423–432
6. Greer R.R. and Chesney R.W. Disorders of calcium metabolism in the neonate. *Sem. Nephrol.* 1983, **3**, 100–115
7. Schwartz G.J., Haycock G.B., Chir B., Edelmann C.M. and Spitzer, A. Late metabolic acidosis: a reassessment of the definition. *J. Pediatr.* 1979, **95**, 102–107
8. Clark D.A. Times of first void and first stool in 500 newborns. *Pediatrics* 1977, **60**, 457–459
9. Chevalier R.L., Campbell F. and Brenbridge A.N. Prognosis in neonatal acute renal failure. *Pediatrics* 1984, **74**, 265–272
10. Trompeter R.A., Al-Dahhan J., Haycock G.B., Chik G. and Chantler C. Normal values for plasma creatine concentration related to maturity in normal term and preterm infants. *Int. J. Pediatr. Nephrol.* 1983, **4**, 145–148
11. Schwartz G.J., Brion L.P. and Spitzer A. The use of plasma creatinine concentration for estimating glomerular filtration rate in infants, children, and adolescents. *Pediatr. Clin. North Am.* 1987, **34**, 571–590
12. Buchi K.F. and Siegler R.L. Hypertension in the first month of life. *J. Hypertension* 1986, **4**, 525–528
13. Hilson D. Malformation of ears as sign of malformation of genitourinary tract. *Br. Med. J.* 1957, **2**, 785–789
14. Fallon B., Welton M. and Hawtrey C. Congenital anomalies associated with cryptorchidism. *J. Urol.* 1982, **127**, 91–93
15. Egli F. and Stalder G. Malformations of kidney and urinary tract in common chromosomal aberrations. *Humangenetik* 1973, **18**, 1–15
16. Karlen J., Aperia A. and Zetterstrom R. Renal excretion of calcium and phosphate in preterm and term infants. *J. Pediatr.* 1985, **106**, 814–819

17. Crain E.F. and Gershel J.C. Urinary tract infections in febrile infants younger than 8 weeks of age. *Pediatrics* 1990, **86**, 363–367

18. Mathew O.P., Jones A.S., James E., Bland H. and Groshong T. Neonatal renal failure: usefulness of diagnostic indices. *Pediatrics* 1980, **65**, 57–60

19. Guignard J.P., Torrado A., Mazouni S.M. and Gautier E. Renal function in respiratory distress syndrome. *J. Pediatr.* 1976, **88**, 845–850

20. Kojima T., Hirara Y., Fukuda Y., Iwase S. and Kobayashi Y. Plasma atrial natriuretic peptide and spontaneous diuresis in sick neonates. *Arch. Dis. Child.* 1987, **62**, 667–670

21. O'Dea R.F., Mirkin B.L., Alward C.T. and Sinaiko A.R., Treatment of neonatal hypertension with captopril. *J. Pediatr.* 1988, **113**, 403–406

22. Chevalier R.L., Campbell F. and Brenbridge A.N.A.G. Nephrosonography and renal scintigraphy in evaluation of the newborn with renomegaly. *Urology* 1984, **24**, 96–103

23. de Vries L. and Levene M.I. Measurement of renal size in preterm and term infants by real-time ultrasound. *Arch. Dis. Child.* 1982, **56**, 145–147

24. Chevalier R.L. and El Dahr S. In: *Urologic Surgery in Neonates and Young Infants* King L.R. (ed.). Saunders, Philadelphia, 1988

25. Edelmann C.M., Ogwo J.E., Fine B.P. and Martinez A.B. The prevalence of bacteriuria in full-term and premature new born infants. *J. Pediatr.* 1982, **58**, 145–147

26. Maherzi M., Guignard J.P. and Torrado A. Urinary tract infection in high-risk newborn infants. *Pediatrics* 1978, **62**, 521–523

27. Wiswell T.E. and Roscelli J.D. Corroborative evidence for the decreased incidence of urinary tract infections in circumcised male infants. *Pediatrics* 1986, **78**, 96–99

28. El-Dahr S.S. and Chevalier R.L. Special needs of the newborn infant in fluid therapy. *Pediatr. Clin. North Am.* 1990, **37**, 323–336

29. Craft J.C. Monitoring antibiotic therapy in the newborn infant. *Clin. Perinatol.* 1981, **8**, 263–272

30. Mirochnick M.H., Miceli J.J., Kramer P.A., Chapron D.J. and Raye J.R. Furosemide pharmacokinetics in very low birth weight infants. *J. Pediatr.* 1988, **112**, 653–657

31. Brem A.S. Neonatal hematuria and proteinuria. *Clin. Perinatol.* 1981, **8**, 321–332

32

Hypercalciuria, stones and nephrocalcinosis

T.L. Chambers, G. Moss

Urinary stones (calculi) are composed of a crystalline aggregate incorporated into a mucoid matrix accounting for up to 10% of the stone's weight and mainly composed of protein and carbohydrate. Crystal aggregation may occur within the renal tubule, but stone formation occurs in the calyces, renal pelvis and bladder.

Nephrocalcinosis is the deposition of calcium salts within the renal parenchyma: it is associated (but not invariably) with urinary stone disease (urolithiasis).

Renal stones[1,2]

Incidence and geography

There are several patterns of urolithiasis[3-6] throughout the world. In the less developed countries, bladder stone disease is extremely common,[7] with urate stones predominating in the Middle East, North Africa and India. A similar pattern of disease was seen in Britain in earlier centuries. Dietary factors are important in this group, and in some instances have been very carefully identified – such as in the calcium oxalate stone formers in Thailand[8] who consume large amounts of rice, which is metabolized to oxalate, and leafy oxalate-rich vegetables. In the UK, the incidence of stone is less common, affecting about 1.5 children per million population per annum (compared with an incidence in adult males of 2 per thousand). Upper tract magnesium ammonium phosphate stones are more common and usually associated with urinary tract infection by *Bacillus proteus*, whereas pure metabolic stones (oxalosis, cystine) are rarer. In the USA, the infective/metabolic ratio is reversed.[9] The following discussion will apply to children in Britain unless stated otherwise.

Pathogenesis

Interest has centred on the relative contributions of the crystals or matrix to the initiation of stone formation. The matrix component has been largely discounted but, because of its importance in the genesis of infection stones, this view may need re-examining.[10,11] Precipitation of compounds from solution has been more widely investigated: the stimulus is easily identified when it occurs in an abnormal urinary tract with stasis or one that is catheterized. Idiopathic stone formation has been a greater challenge: Table 32.1 shows the common stone types with contributory factors.

Hydration plays a part: solute will obviously crystallize out if there is insufficient solvent. A liberal fluid intake is basic therapy for recurrent stone formers. In hard water areas the calcium intake will also be greater: the significance of this is debatable.

Solute concentration is particularly important in metabolic urolithiasis. When the solubility threshold of a compound in urine is exceeded it will crystallize. Reduction of solute concentration is a major principle of therapy.

Urine pH influences stone formation. Alkaline urine favours calcium phosphate and mag-

Table 32.1   Characteristics of urinary stones (From Rose,[11] by permission)

Type	Appearance	Causes	Radio-opaque*
Magnesium ammonium phosphate	Very soft white toothpaste or gravel fragments	Infection with urea-splitting organisms, especially with urinary stasis	0
Calcium phosphate	Large smooth pale friable	Renal tubular acidosis Idiopathic hypercalciuria Vitamin D toxicity Immobilization Hyperparathyroidism Sarcoidosis	+
Calcium oxalate	Jagged brown crystalline	Oxalosis (1 or 2) Idiopathic 'Dietary' bladder stone	+
Cystine	Pale-yellow crystalline Maple sugar	Cystinuria	+
Uric acid	Hard yellow	Inborn metabolic errors (Lesch–Nyhan syndrome) Dietary Induction of remission in haematological malignancies	0
Xanthine	Smooth soft Brown/yellow	Xanthinuria	0
Dihydroxyadenine	Friable Grey-blue	Adenine phosphoribosyl transferase deficiency	0

*This depends on the amount of calcium in the stone and an individual patient may have more than one type of stone each with different radiolucencies.

nesium ammonium phosphate precipitation, whereas uric acid and cystine are more likely to precipitate in acid urine. Calcium oxalate solubility does not vary significantly with urine pH.

Inhibitors are present in normal urine preventing the growth of crystal aggregate. A balance exists in urine between the degree of saturation by the stone-forming salts and the protective capacity of the pyrophosphate and mucopolysaccharide inhibitors. Recurrent idiopathic stone formers have a different solute/inhibitor relationship than normal individuals. Urinary pyrophosphate concentration may be increased by oral phosphate or thiazide diuretics. Magnesium salts and citrate both increase the solubility of calcium ions and their excretion has been found to be lower in stone formers:[12] both are used therapeutically.

Diet

Calcium absorption is reduced when the fibre content of the diet is high and this approach has been used to reduce urinary calcium concentration. Otherwise the total calcium and vitamin D intake influence the urinary calcium concentration: oxalate (in tea, strawberries) consumption affects urinary oxalate excretion and animal protein intake may increase the urinary uric acid concentration and lower the urinary fibrolytic activity.[13]

Other influences

Diurnal variations in urinary calcium excretion are related to intake and, although quantitatively small, may profoundly affect saturation. Fluid intake is likely to be low at night, favouring crystallization. Seasonal variations in calcium and oxalate excretion may also be important.

Clinical aspects

Symptoms of renal stones in children vary: they may be asymptomatic or cause non-specific recurrent abdominal pain, microscopic or macroscopic haematuria, classical renal colic, urinary infection or even renal failure. Otherwise the child may pass the stone or gravel, or have symptoms related to micturition such as dysuria and strangury. Nevertheless, it must be remembered that in the majority of children in Britain who complain of these symptoms (renal colic apart), there will be some other cause.

The diagnosis is either made from inspection of the passed stone or by imaging techniques. Current imaging of the urinary tract involves ultrasound examination combined with a plain abdominal X-ray. Stones and renal tract dilatation or other malformation should be revealed by this simple method. An intravenous urogram (IVU) may show an opaque stone on the plain film or else urographic features of obstruction with a radiolucent defect caused by the stone. Adolescents may demonstrate conditions seen in adults such as medullary sponge kidney (see Chapter 25) or papillary necrosis. The urine may contain red cells, white cells, protein or bacteria; none is specific for renal stones. Calcium oxalate crystals often form in normal urine that has been standing for a few hours and are of no significance. A general history should be obtained, with emphasis on the family history and consanguinity, as many metabolic causes of urolithiasis are inherited, and the diet. Physical examination should include the routine, including blood pressure, and the recherché (gouty tophi). Renal function should be assessed by plasma creatinine estimation.

The general management of renal stones is to relieve and treat obstruction and infection – whether primary or secondary to stone formation. The ultrasound in renal colic may show major ureteric dilatation, but this will rapidly resolve with passage of the stone and a measured approach is indicated: if the IVU shows a non-functioning kidney, rapid relief of obstruction is required. The main consideration is preservation of renal parenchyma. Stones in the renal pelvis causing obstruction should be removed by pyelolithotomy as should infection stones and, occasionally, nephrectomy is required in pyonephrosis with major renal tissue destruction. Newer techniques for management of renal stones include destruction by ultrasonic lithotripsy[14] or removal via a dilated nephrostomy tract; both have been used in children and have advantages in that open operations are not required. It is too early to judge their longer term benefits or risks. Ureteric stones may be removed by a Dormia basket, but ureterolithotomy will be needed in the young child. Similarly, stone-crushing techniques will

occasionally be appropriate for bladder stones in the young and a suprapubic cystolithotomy is employed. Some 8% of children will have a recurrence (in the absence of metabolic disease), a much lower incidence than in adults, and some of these will be small stones missed at operation. If stone clearance is absolute and infection prevented, stone recurrence is very rare. Correction of obstruction and infection is common management in all childhood stone formers.[16] In children with metabolic stones attempts should be made to dissolve them by medical therapy, and surgery should be reserved for obstruction, particularly where infection supervenes.

Specific investigations in urolithiasis

In addition to the general investigations listed above, the diagnosis of urinary stone in children should be followed by ascertainment of the underlying cause – at least in the Western world. The rigorousness of this investigation will vary; in a child with *Proteus* infections and magnesium ammonium phosphate stones, there may be little point in searching for inborn metabolic errors, although some would argue that this should be done in all cases. One investigational protocol is detailed in Table 32.2 and it should be noted that it differs from the investigation of adults in that hyperparathyroidism is rare in children and is usually not searched for so diligently. The importance of analysis of the stone if this is available cannot be stressed too greatly.

Calcium-containing stones[17]

Calcium oxalate or phosphate is the main constituent of one-third of all stones and 80–90% of non-infection associated calculi.

Although often idiopathic, risk factors for the production of calcium stones include those affecting supersaturation (hypercalciuria, hyperoxaluria, hyperuricosuria and decreased urine volume) and those altering ionic strength such as hypocitraturia and urine pH.

Hypercalciuria

The upper limit of normal for urinary calcium excretion is $0.1\ \text{mmol}\ \text{kg}^{-1}\ \text{day}^{-1}$ as measured in a 24 h urine collection.[18] The urinary cal-

Table 32.2   Specific investigation of renal stone disease (From Rose,[15] by permission)

Sample	Analysis	Reference range	Primary disease
Stone (preferably quantitatively)	Calcium oxalate	–	Idiopathic, oxalosis
	Calcium phosphate	–	Hypercalciuria, foreign body
	Magnesium ammonium phosphate	–	Infection
	Uric acid	–	Gout, acid urine, leukaemia, Lesch–Nyhan syndrome
	Cystine	–	Cystinuria
	Xanthine	–	Xanthinuria
	Dihydroxyadenine*	–	Adenine phosphoribosyl transferase deficiency
Blood (plasma)	Creatinine	30–100 μmol/litre‡	Infection, renal failure
	Calcium (fasting)	2.13–2.62 mmol/litre	Hyperparathyroidism
	Bicarbonate	20–26 mmol/litre	Renal tubular acidosis
	Urate	60–462‡ μmol/litre	Uric acid stones
Urine	pH < 5.3		*Excludes* distal renal tubular acidosis
	Culture		Infective
	Calcium (24 h)	< 0.1 mmol/kg	Hypercalciuria from any cause
	Oxalate (24 h)	0.18–0.33 mmol/1.73 m²	Oxalosis (but may be marginally raised in idiopathic stone formers)
	Cystine† (24 h)	0.04–0.42 mmol/1.73 m²	Cystinuria
	Uric acid (24 h)	< 5 mmol/1.73 m²	Uric acid stones

*Probably not available routinely.
†Or a nitroprusside test on random urine.
‡Varies with age.

cium: creatinine (Ca: Cr) ratio in a single urine sample is a useful index of calcium excretion for general screening and monitoring purposes with obvious practical advantages. The Ca:Cr ratio measured in the second morning urine sample after an overnight fast most accurately reflects daily calcium excretion: the 97th percentile level for British children eating an unrestricted diet found in a recent study was 0.69 mmol/mmol.[19] Measurement of the fasting Ca:Cr ratio will not identify those with the absorptive pattern of idiopathic hypercalciuria and if this is suspected, a 24 h urine collection or oral calcium loading test[20] is required.

Normocalcaemic hypercalciuria

Idiopathic hypercalciuria (IH). Defined as normocalcaemic hypercalciuria occurring in the absence of any identifiable factors increasing urinary calcium excretion, is the commonest metabolic anomaly found in those with calcium stones. There is a familial incidence consistent with autosomal dominant inheritance.[21] In addition to urolithiasis, other urinary tract symptoms and signs occur (see below) but many individuals are asymptomatic.

The pathogenesis is debated. The oral cal-

cium loading test[20,22] differentiates two subtypes:

- Absorptive hypercalciuria, characterized by normal fasting calcium excretion with hypercalciuric response to standardized oral calcium load (Ca:Cr ratio greater than 0.76 mmol/mmol).
- Renal hypercalciuria, characterized by fasting hypercalciuria; there is usually a further increase in calcium excretion after a calcium load. This is the commoner type in childhood.

Care should be taken when interpreting the results of this test as available data is derived mainly from North American children.

The pattern obtained may be indeterminate and different underlying pathogenic mechanisms for the increased intestinal absorption and decreased tubular reabsorption of calcium, respectively, cannot necessarily be assumed. Assessment of the calcium-vitamin D-parathyroid hormone axis has revealed overlapping features in the subtypes leading to the hypothesis that they represent different aspects of one underlying disorder, perhaps altered vitamin D metabolism. Alternatively, recent work has raised the possibility of a primary defect of calcium transport across cell membranes.[23]

Distal renal tubular acidosis (dRTA). Hypercalciuria results from the increased bone resorption and decreased tubular reabsorption of calcium associated with systemic acidosis. Other factors promoting stone formation are hypocitraturia, which may be due to both systemic acidosis and an associated tubular defect, and high urinary pH which *per se* decreases calcium phosphate solubility.

Frusemide. Frusemide increases urinary calcium excretion and its long-term use in pre-term infants with chronic lung disease is associated with hypercalciuria, calcium urolithiasis and nephrocalcinosis. Withdrawal of frusemide or the addition of chlorothiazide does not always resolve the calcium deposits and in some there has been concern about long-term renal sequelae.[24] It is suggested that prolonged frusemide therapy should be used only where alternative treatment is ineffective (e.g. thiazide diuretics, which decrease urinary calcium excretion).

Hypercalcaemic hypercalciuria

Increased bone resorption. Increased calcium excretion during prolonged immobilization most commonly occurs in older children who have had extensive burns, fractures or orthopaedic surgery. Long-term or high-dose corticosteroid therapy is associated with calcium urolithiasis. Osteolytic metastases secondary to malignancy may produce hypercalcaemia, but calculi have not been reported. Although uncommon in childhood, primary hyperparathyroidism promotes calcium stone formation. More rarely, hypercalciuria secondary to increased bone resorption occurs in hypo- and hyperthyroidism, hypoadrenalism and Cushing's disease, but calculi have been described only in the latter.

Increased intestinal absorption of calcium. This may be secondary to excessive vitamin D administration, high circulating levels of $1,25(OH)_2D$ found in those with the infantile hypercalcaemia of Williams' syndrome (see below) where studies have suggested an abnormal regulation of vitamin D metabolism; extrarenal production of $1,25(OH)_2D$ in sarcoidosis or immoderate ingestion of calcium salts together with absorbable alkalis (milk-alkali syndrome). All these conditions are rare and are associated with hypercalciuria: urolithiasis is seen only occasionally, but ultrasound examination of the kidney may demonstrate microscopic deposits of calcium.

Williams' syndrome[25] consists of typical facial features: maldevelopment of the facial skeleton, with depression of the nasal bridge, prominent maxillae and receding mandible, resulting in elfin facies. There is failure to thrive and sometimes hypertension and congenital valvular heart disease. Hypercalcaemia and hypercalciuria are common but not invariable. Treatment is by lowering the calcium and vitamin D intake, but nutritional rickets must be avoided. The cause is unknown; familial cases are described but it is usually sporadic. Intellectual development is often poor and there is little evidence that it can be enhanced by dietary manipulation of calcium metabolism.

Other hypercalciuric states

Prolonged use of non-absorbable antacids such as magnesium or aluminium hydroxides may produce severe phosphorus depletion with hypercalciuria secondary to increased $1,25(OH)_2D$ production. Hypercalciuria may complicate long-term parenteral nutrition; risk factors such as the amount of calcium and vitamin D given, hypophosphataemia, relative immobilization, use of corticosteroids and the nature of the underlying disease may be present but in some the mechanism is uncertain.

Hyperoxaluria

Data concerning oxalate excretion in idiopathic calcium urolithiasis in childhood is not available, but adult studies suggest that mild hyperoxaluria, urinary oxalate above the 95th percentile not due to primary or enteric hyperoxaluria, is a considerably more important factor than the level of calcium excretion in the genesis of 'idiopathic' calcium oxalate stones because of a proportionately greater effect on calcium oxalate supersaturation.[26]

Hyperuricosuria

An association between hyperuricosuria, most commonly due to a purine-rich diet, and calcium stone formation is reported in adults with putative mechanisms of epitaxial growth of calcium oxalate on uric acid seeds or binding of inhibitors by uric acid. However, evidence suggests that hyperuricosuria is not a major risk factor in childhood urolithiasis.

Hypocitraturia

Urinary citrate, by chelating calcium, inhibits growth of calcium oxalate and calcium phosphate crystals. Hypocitraturia has been documented in dRTA, gastrointestinal malabsorption secondary to inflammatory bowel disease or jejuno-ileal bypass and as a complication of thiazide therapy. Idiopathic hypocitraturic calcium oxalate urolithiasis has not been described in childhood; this may be partly due to the inverse relationship between urinary citrate excretion and age.

Urinary volume and pH

Low urine output is a major risk factor in all types of urolithiasis. Recent results suggest that this is of particular importance in idiopathic calcium calculi. The solubility of calcium oxalate is not significantly altered by changes which occur in urine pH in the physiological range. The solubility of calcium phosphate increases with decrease in urine pH and therefore these stones are more common in infected and alkaline urine, renal tubular acidosis and where excessive bicarbonate therapy for cystinuria or uric acid calculi has been given.

Management of calcium stones

Acute

Pain, especially that resulting from passage of a stone, may be particularly severe requiring potent analgesics. An adequate urine output must be maintained, but the measures required will depend on renal function and degree of any obstruction. Prompt treatment must be given for suspected urinary tract infection after collection of samples for culture. Although rare, urgent correction of associated severe hypercalcaemia (plasm calcium > 3.8 mmol/litre) may be necessary. Liberal intravenous fluids and electrolyte, isotonic saline, are required; frusemide will promote calcium excretion, but should accompany rehydration. Corticosteroids are useful in certain malignancies, sarcoid, vitamin D intoxication and Williams' syndrome. Short-

term reduction in plasma calcium will occur with calcitonin 25–150 u intravenously; mithramycin 15 μg/kg, is used in hypercalcaemia complicating malignancies, but some authors recommend rehydration, frusemide and prompt chemotherapy. In renal failure complicated by hypercalcaemia, dialysis against a low calcium dialysate will be required.

Long term

A high fluid intake, distributed throughout the 24 h period, should be encouraged in all forms of urolithiasis. Apart from milk products and tea, any fluids may be used. Calcium intake will be increased by drinking a large volume of tap water, especially in areas with hard water; the effect on urinary calcium excretion is likely to be insignificant, with the benefit of diluting urinary constituents outweighing any potential disadvantage. Relief of persistent obstruction and treatment of infection are essential.

Hypercalciuria
Initial management of idiopathic hypercalciuria is directed by the result of the oral calcium loading test. In absorptive IH a high-fibre diet and avoidance of an excessive intake of calcium are advocated. The decreased calcium-oxalate binding in the gut increases oxalate absorption thereby encouraging calcium stone formation; concomitant reduction of dietary oxalate is therefore advised. Additional measures have included sodium cellulose phosphate, orthophosphates and occasionally thiazide diuretics, but their merits should be weighed against the severity of the symptoms.

Induction of a negative calcium balance by aggressive application of these measures will increase bone resorption and calciuria and have a deleterious effect on growth. In absorptive IH, the hypocalciuric effect of chlorothiazide is not associated with decreased intestinal absorption, plasma calcium remains normal and the retained calcium presumably accretes in bone; while this may have advantages in growing children, the long-term effect is unknown.

Chlorothiazide is usually sucessful in treating renal IH. Tubular reabsorption of calcium is increased by a direct effect on the distal nephron and an indirect effect on the proximal tubule by causing relative ECF volume depletion.

Other potential advantages are increased excretion of magnesium and zinc which inhibit calcific crystallization and decreased concentration of urinary calcium phosphate and brushite. A low calcium diet does not alleviate the hypercalciuria of renal IH.

Calcium excretion may be increased by a high sodium intake; some individuals exhibit sodium-dependent hypercalciuria. Measurement of sodium excretion and prescription of a no-added-salt diet is sometimes recommended.

Correction of acidosis with oral sodium bicarbonate rectifies the biochemical and pathophysiological disturbances of dRTA; additional potassium supplements may be required. Potassium citrate alone has also been shown to correct the metabolic abnormalities.

Urolithiasis resulting from immobilization should be generally preventable by ensuring adequate hydration, encouraging frequent changes in position, avoiding instrumentation of the urinary tract and promptly treating any urinary tract infection. Appropriate treatment of the specified endocrine diseases corrects the associated hypercalciuria.

Where hypercalciuria is secondary to increased intestinal absorption, dietary calcium should be limited, vitamin D supplements discontinued and adequate hydration ensured. Corticosteroids are often beneficial.

Hyperoxaluria
The presence of hyperoxaluria will prompt assessment of possible underlying causes. If mild and idiopathic, oxalate-rich food (rhubarb, spinach, chocolate and tea) should be restricted. Vitamin C is a substrate for oxalate synthesis; any supplements should be stopped where possible.

Hyperuricosuria
A high animal protein intake will increase uric acid excretion in addition to reducing urinary citrate; therefore such dietary excesses should be avoided. Strict restriction or specific drug therapy are indicated only for those with hyperuricosuria.

Hypocitraturia
Treatment of the underlying disease combined with potassium citrate as necessary will rectify the hypocitraturia. Universal citrate supplementation is not warranted.

Non-calculi disorders associated with idiopathic hypercalciuria

In contrast to adults, several non-calculi disorders are described in association with IH in childhood.

Haematuria

Otherwise unexplained haematuria occurring prior to detectable urolithiasis is the major non-calculus manifestation of IH.[27] Intermittent, painless, gross haematuria is most commonly seen but it may be microscopic. The exact pathogenesis is uncertain: a glomerular origin is unlikely and it is suggested to result from epithelial damage secondary to microcrystallization. Haematuria occurs in both subtypes of IH; no metabolic differences between those presenting with calculi or haematuria have been found.

Moderation of calcium and sodium intake may be useful. Thiazides are effective in resolving the haematuria and hypercalciuria but their prolonged use is controversial. A short-term diagnostic trial of 3–6 months to confirm the association between IH and the haematuria is suggested with restriction of long-term treatment to those who have persistent or frequent episodes of gross haematuria after stopping therapy or where calculi develop.

Other disorders

Dysuria alone or together with other symptoms such as frequency, back pain, abdominal pain, nocturnal enuresis and daytime incontinence is associated with IH.[28] Elimination of commoner causes and resolution of the symptoms on correction of the hypercalciuria are required for the diagnosis. Increasing fluid intake with dietary modification may suffice; in some, thiazides are required, sometimes with potassium citrate.

Far less commonly, recurrent urinary tract infection, isolated pyuria and mild proteinuria have been reported in connection with IH, although the causal link is not well established.

Hyperoxaluria

Excessive oxalate may be excreted in the urine because (a) there is excessive absorption (enteric hyperoxaluria)[29,30] or (b) excessive endogenous production of oxalate (oxalosis). Oxalate produced by these means may accumulate in the blood and tissues if renal clearance is not efficient or else the normal metabolic load of oxalate may accumulate with severe renal failure. Poisoning with the oxalate precursors ethylene glycol (antifreeze) and methoxyfluorane will cause an oxalate nephropathy.

Enteric hyperoxaluria

Here the normal dietary intake of oxalate is absorbed excessively – usually where there has been extensive small bowel resection or with intestinal malabsorptive states. The management is by reducing the oxalate content of the diet and liberal fluid intake.

Oxalosis

This is the term given to two recessively inherited inborn errors of metabolism causing excessive endogenous oxalate synthesis. The commoner type I (hepatic peroxisomal alanine: glyoxylate aminotransferase deficiency) results in excessive glycolate and oxalate excretion, whereas type II (D-glyceric acid dehydrogenase deficiency) causes excessive L-glyceric acid and oxalate excretion but normal glycolate. The metabolic enzyme defect can be demonstrated in the leucocytes of the peripheral blood in type II but not type I oxalosis, which is diagnosed biochemically in a liver biopsy specimen. Calcium oxalate is extremely insoluble and crystals readily precipitate in areas of high calcium ion concentration such as the kidney, metaphysis, myocardium and arteries.

Three patterns of clinical disease have been recognized: (a) a malignant infantile form with nephrocalcinosis resulting in early terminal renal failure[31] – it is possible that this is caused by an as yet unclassified form of oxalosis; (b) juvenile type with recurrent stones, renal infections and oxalate deposition – myocardial oxalosis may cause fatal conduction defects and arrythmias; (c) a more benign adult form with less oxalate excretion and longer survival. This classification is somewhat empirical and severity may be variable; infection, obstruction or renal failure may confuse the picture. The diagnosis is made from the finding of stones or nephrocalcinosis, demonstration of a high oxalate excretion and excess of either glycolate or glycerate depending on the type. The main diagnostic difficulty is when there is established

renal failure before diagnosis or typing, when the urinary excretion of oxalate and metabolites will be difficult to interpret because of the low GFR; furthermore, widespread oxalate deposition may occur in renal failure from other cause. The distinction is important because of the genetic implications and it is here that liver biopsy diagnosis of type I is most helpful.

Treatment is challenging. Provided that the dietary oxalate intake is not excessive, there is little point in reducing it as most of the oxalate is synthesized endogenously. The usual aspects of stone management apply – mainly a high fluid intake. Pyridoxine therapy in pharmacological doses varying from 250 mg to 1 g reduces urinary oxalate excretion in type I, and magnesium and phosphate should be given to inhibit calcium oxalate crystal formation in the urine. Patients have been treated by renal dialysis and transplantation; oxalate tends to recur in the grafted kidney but this may perhaps be ameliorated with aggressive pyridoxine/phosphate therapy.[32] A particularly disabling bone disease has also been described. The most recent approach to type I oxalosis is to perform orthotopic liver transplantation (with or without renal transplantation depending on the degree of renal insufficiency), thus correcting the primary liver defect.

Other causes of matabolic stones

Cystinuria

This recessively inherited renal tubular lesion is associated with urolithiasis and is described in Chapter 24.

Uric acid stones

These are most frequently seen when there is massive cell destruction in the induction chemotherapy of leukaemias and lymphomas. Otherwise it is associated with familial gout, Lesch–Nyhan syndrome, and has been reported complicating a ketogenic diet for intractable convulsions and type I glycogen storage disease. Treatment and prevention is by giving regular alkali[33] to keep the urine pH above 6.5 and by administering allopurinol to block uric acid synthesis. Stones can be dissolved using the fluid, alkali and allopurinol combination.

Table 32.3 Causes of nephrocalcinosis in children

Medullary nephrocalcinosis
Distal renal tubular acidosis*
Idiopathic hypercalciuria*
Oxalosis
Vitamin D toxicity†
Hypothyroidism*
Prolonged immobilization† ⎫
Sarcoidosis† ⎬ Adult pattern diseases and very rare in children in the UK
Hyperparathyroidism (1°)† ⎭
Medullary sponge kidney

Cortical nephrocalcinosis
Following renal cortical necrosis

*Conditions causing hypercalciuria.
†Conditions causing hypercalcaemia and hypercalciuria.

Xanthinuria

The primary form is excessively rare and results from xanthine oxidase deficiency with accumulation of xanthine, insoluble in acid urine. Radiolucent stones may develop with a very low plasma urine acid level. Treatment is by fluids, dietary purine restriction and alkali.

Secondary xanthinuria occurs during allopurinol therapy and if excretion is excessive xanthine stones may be produced.

Dihydroxyadenine stones

A recessively inherited deficiency in adenine phosphoribosyl transferase results in excessive urinary excretion of 2,8-dihydroxyadenine.[34] Its solubility does not vary much across the pH range, so alkalinization is not helpful (and some would say harmful). Allopurinol is extremely effective in blocking 2,8-dihydroxyadenine formation and thus stopping stone formation. Surgery may be needed to remove persistent stones.

Nephrocalcinosis

This should be regarded as a syndrome rather than a specific diagnosis; it is a feature of the many renal and non-renal diseases shown in Table 32.3. The mechanism of calcium deposition is poorly understood; studies in children receiving vitamin D have shown that calcium deposits may be present without radiological nephrocalcinosis.[35] A relationship has been found between prostaglandins and calciuria; experimental nephrocalcinosis has been prevented by use of prostaglandin synthetase inhibitors.[36] Management of nephrocalcinosis is that of the primary cause; in distal renal tubular acidosis, the urinary calcium excretion should be reduced by the therapy described in Chapter 24. Control of calcium oxalate deposition in oxalosis is attempted by pyridoxine, phosphate and magnesium. Vitamin D toxicity is now rarely seen and the likeliest cause today is from excessive doses of calciferol and its synthetic metabolites in the management of the various types of vitamin-D-resistant rickets (hypophosphataemia, cystinosis, chronic renal failure) described in Chapters 5, 22 and 24.

References

1. Wickham J.E.A. and Buck A.C. *Renal Tract Stone: Metabolic Basis and Clinical Practice.* Edinburgh, Churchill Livingstone, 1990
2. Resnick M.I. and Pak C.Y.C. *Urolithiasis: A Medical and Surgical Reference.* Philadelphia, Saunders, 1990
3. Ghazali S. Childhood urolithiasis in the United Kingdom and Eire. *Br. J. Urol.* 1975, **47**, 739–743
4. Sinno K., Boyce W.H. and Reswick M.I. Childhood urolithiasis. *J. Urol.* 1979, **121**, 662–664
5. Reiner R.J., Kroovand R.L. and Perlmutter A.D. Unusual aspects of urinary calculi in children. *J. Urol.* 1979, **121**, 480–481
6. Scott R. Epidemiology of stone disease. *Br. J. Urol.* 1985, **57**, 491–497
7. Ashworth M. Endemic bladder stones. *Br. Med. J.* 1990, **301**, 826–827
8. Prasongwatana V., Sriboonlue P. and Suntarapa S. Urinary stone composition in north-east Thailand. *Br. J. Urol.* 1983, **55**, 353–355
9. Broadus A.E. and Thier S.O. Metabolic basis of renal-stone disease. *N. Engl. J. Med.* 1979, **300**, 839–845
10. Nishio S., Yukichi A., Watatsuki A., Hidenobu I., Ochi K., Takeuchi M. *et al.* Matrix glycosaminoglycan in urinary stones. *J. Urol.* 1985, **134**, 503–505
11. Rose G.A. Biochemical aspects of urinary stones. *Proc. R. Soc. Med.* 1977, **70**, 517–520
12. Martinez M.E., Salinas M., Miguel J.L., Herrero E., Gomez P., Garcia J., Sanchez-Siulia L. and Montero A. Magnesium excretion in idiopathic hypercalciuria. *Nephron* 1985, **44**, 446–450
13. Margetts B.M., Barker D.J.P., Kavanagh J.P. and Blacklock N.J. Do stone formers have lower urinary fibrinolytic activity than controls? *Br. J. Urol.* 1990, **66**, 581–584
14. Abara E., Merguerian P.A., McLorie G.A. *et al.* Lithostar extracorporeal shock wave lithotripsy in children. *J. Urol.* 1990, **144**, 489–491
15. Rose G.A. Screening techniques for investigating the cause of urinary calculi. In: Chisholm G.D. and Williams D.I. (eds) *Scientific Foundations of Urology*, 2nd edn. New York, Heinemann, 1982: 329–331

16. Laiyer J. and Boichis H. Urolithiasis in children: current medical management. *Pediatr. Nephrol.* 1989, **3**, 317–331

17. Goldwasser B., Weinerth J.L. and Carson C.C. Calcium stone disease: an overview. *J. Urol* 1986, **135**, 1–9

18. Ghazali S. and Barratt T.M. Urinary excretion of calcium and magnesium in children. *Arch. Dis. Child.* 1974, **49**: 97–101

19. Shaw N.J., Wheeldon J. and Brocklehurst J.T. Indices of intact serum parathyroid hormone and renal excretion of calcium, phosphate and magnesium. *Arch. Dis. Child.* 1990, **65**, 1208–12

20. Stapleton F.B., Noe N., Jerkins G. *et al.* Urinary excretion of calcium following an oral calcium loading test in healthy children. *Pediatrics* 1982, **69**, 594–597

21. Coe F.L., Parkes J.H. and Moore E.S. Familial idiopathic hypercalciuria. *N. Engl. J. Med.* 1979, **300**, 337–340

22. Hymes L.C. Idiopathic hypercalciuria of childhood: response to oral calcium loading in children with and without urolithiasis. *J. Urol.* 1985, **133**, 436–438

23. Bianchi G., Vezzoli G., Cusi D. *et al.* Abnormal red-cell calcium pump in patients with idiopathic hypercalciuria. *N. Engl. J. Med.* 1988, **319**, 897–901

24. Ezzedean F., Adelman R.D. and Ahlfors, C. Renal calcification in preterm infants: pathophysiology and long term sequelae. *J. Pediatr.* 1988, **113**, 532–539

25. Harrison H.E. and Harrison H.C. Idiopathic hypercalcaemia (Williams' syndrome). In: Harrison H. E. and Maurison H.C. (eds.) *Disorders of Calcium and Phosphate Metabolism in Childhood and Adolescence.* Philadelphia, Saunders, 1979: 109–115

26. Robertson W.G. and Peacock M. The cause of idiopathic calcium stone disease: hypercalciuria or hyperoxaluria? *Nephron* 1980, **26**, 105–110

27. A report of the South West Pediatric Nephrology Study Group prepared by F. Bruder Stapleton. Idiopathic hypercalciuria: association with isolated haematuria and risk for urolithiasis in children. *Kidney Int.* 1990, **37**, 807–811

28. Heiliczer J.D., Canonigo B.B., Bishof N.A. *et al.* Non calculi urinary tract disorders secondary to idiopathic hypercalciuria in children. *Ped. Clin. North Am.* 1987, **34**, 711–718

29. Coe F.L. Uric acid and calcium oxalate nephrolithiasis. *Kidney Int.* 1983, **24**, 392–403

30. Watts R.E. and Mansell, M.A. Oxalate, livers and kidneys. *Br. Med. J.* 1990, **301**, 772–773

31. Morris M.C. Chambers T.L., Evans P.W.G., Malleson P.N., Pincott J.R. and Rose G.A. Oxalosis in infancy. *Arch. Dis. Child.* 1982, **64**, 782–788

32. Rose G.A., Arthur L.J.H., Chambers T.L., Kasides S.P. and Scott I.V. Successful treatment of primary hyperoxaluria in the neonate. *Lancet* 1982, **i**, 1298–1299

33. Sakhaee K., Nicar M., Hill K. and Pak C.Y.C. Contrasting effects of potassium citrate and sodium citrate therapies on urinary chemistries and crystallization of stone-forming salts. *Kidney Int.* 1983, **24**, 348–352

34. Witten F.R., Morgan J.W., Foster J.G. and Glenn J.F. 2,8-Dihydroxyadenine urolithiasis: review of the literature and report of a case in the United States. *J. Urol.* 1983, **130**, 938–942

35. Moncrieff M.W. and Chance G.W. Nephrotoxic effect of vitamin D therapy in vitamin D refractory rickets. *Arch. Dis. Child.* 1969, **44**, 571–579

36. Buck A.C., Davies R.L.L., Leaker B. and Moffat D.B. Inhibition of experimental nephrocalcinosis with a prostaglandin synthetase inhibitor. *Br. J. Urol.* 1983, **55**, 603–608

Index